PROCEED WITH CARE

V O L 1 U M E

PROCEED WITH CARE

FINAL REPORT
OF THE
ROYAL COMMISSION ON
NEW REPRODUCTIVE TECHNOLOGIES

VOLUME 1

This Report is available in both official languages as a set or as individual volumes.

Available in Canada through your local bookseller
or by mail from
Canada Communications Group — Publishing
Ottawa, Canada K1A 0S9

CANADIAN CATALOGUING IN PUBLICATION DATA

Canada. Royal Commission on New Reproductive Technologies

Proceed with Care: Final Report of the Royal Commission on New Reproductive
Technologies

Issued also in French under title: Un virage à prendre en douceur.
Complete work consists of 2 v.
ISBN 0-660-15359-9 (set)
ISBN 0-660-15365-3 (v.1); 0-660-15366-1 (v.2)
Cat. no. Z1-1989/3E (set);
Z1-1989/3-1E (v.1); Z1-1989/3-2E (v.2)

1. Human reproductive technologies — Canada. 2. Infertility — Treatment —
Canada. 3. Human reproductive technologies — Canada — Moral and ethical
aspects. 4. Infertility — Treatment — Canada — Moral and ethical
aspects. 5. Embryology, Human — Canada. I. Title. II. Title: Final report of the
Royal Commission on New Reproductive Technologies.

RG133.5C2 1993   618.1'78   C94-980002-3

The Royal Commission on New Reproductive Technologies and the publishers wish to
acknowledge with gratitude the following:

- Translation Services, Government Services Canada, for their contribution to the
  translation of this report and related studies. Special thanks are due to the Privy
  Council Translation Service, the Scientific Translation Service and the Montreal Health
  and Criminology Translation Service. We also gratefully acknowledge the contribution
  of the Parliamentary Documents Translation Service to the revision and preparation of
  the French version of this report.
- Canada Communications Group, Printing Services
- Biomedical Communications at the University of British Columbia

> Consistent with the Commission's commitment to full
> equality between men and women, care has been
> taken throughout this text to use gender-neutral
> language wherever possible.

Royal Commission on
New Reproductive Technologies

Commission royale sur les
nouvelles techniques de reproduction

TO HIS EXCELLENCY
THE GOVERNOR GENERAL IN COUNCIL

MAY IT PLEASE YOUR EXCELLENCY

By Order in Council dated October 25, 1989, we were requested to
inquire into and report upon current and potential medical and scientific
developments related to new reproductive technologies, considering in
particular their social, ethical, health, research, legal and economic
implications and the public interest, recommending what policies and
safeguards should be applied.

We have been honoured to have the responsibility of working to
fulfil this mandate, and beg to submit our Final Report in each official
language.

Respectfully submitted,

Patricia Baird
Patricia Baird, Chairperson

Grace M. Jantzen
Grace Jantzen

Bartha Maria Knoppers
Bartha Maria Knoppers

Susan E.M. McCutcheon
Susan E.M. McCutcheon

Suzanne Rozell Scorsone
Suzanne Rozell Scorsone

November 15, 1993
Ottawa, Canada

Biographical Notes on Commissioners

Dr. Patricia A. Baird is a paediatrician, professor in medical genetics at the University of British Columbia, and a member of the Population Health Program of the Canadian Institute for Advanced Research.

Grace M. Jantzen is currently a Reader in Philosophy of Religion, Department of Theology and Religious Studies, King's College, University of London, England.

Bartha Maria Knoppers is an Associate Professor, Faculty of Law, at the University of Montreal, and a Senior Researcher with the Centre de Recherche en Droit public de l'Université de Montréal.

Susan E.M. McCutcheon began her career as a teacher, and was active in the business community. She currently takes part in several community organizations, and holds several corporate directorships.

Suzanne Rozell Scorsone is spokesperson for the Archdiocese of Toronto on family and women's issues, and is the Director, Office of Catholic Family Life. Dr. Scorsone is an anthropologist.

Contents

Volume 1

Part One: New Reproductive Technologies and Canadian Society

Part Two: New Reproductive Technologies: Examination of Conditions, Technologies, and Practices

6 Developing a Comprehensive Picture of Technologies and Practices   129

⟨19⟩ Infertility Treatments: Assisted Insemination   425

21 Handling of Eggs and Embryos   581

22 Embryo Research   607

Volume 2

23 Preconception Arrangements   661

◇24◇ Commercial Interests and New Reproductive Technologies **695**

◇25◇ Prenatal Diagnosis and Genetic Technologies: Introduction and Social Context **729**

30 Judicial Intervention in Pregnancy and Birth   949

31 Uses of Fetal Tissue   967

Part Three: Overview of Recommendations

Part Four: Annex, Glossary, and Appendices

◇ Annex: Suzanne Rozell Scorsone

◇ Glossary

◇ **Appendices**

Tables

Figures

Preface from the Chairperson

♦

When Commissioners were given the task of recommending how new reproductive technologies should be handled in this country, we recognized that it was a complex and demanding task and that there were no easy answers. It is difficult because there is tension between the potential benefits the technologies can bring — which are to enable people to have a family and healthy children, goals important to most of us — and the potential harms to health and well-being they can also bring to individuals, groups, and social institutions.

We are facing unprecedented choices about procreation. Our response to those choices — as individuals and as a society — will say much about what we value and what our priorities are. It is therefore important that policies be based on very wide input and consultations. In this report, with our understanding deepened by the many views and perspectives we have heard and the evidence we have reviewed, the other Commissioners and I have made it clear what we believe our choices, as a caring society, should be.

We reached three overall conclusions about the delivery of new reproductive technologies. First, there is an urgent need for well-defined boundaries around the use of new reproductive technologies, so that unethical use of knowledge is not permitted. Second, within those boundaries, accountable regulation is needed to protect the interests of those involved, as well as those of society as a whole. Third, given the ongoing and, indeed, increasing pace of knowledge and development, a flexible and continuing response to evolving technologies that involves wide input from Canadians is an essential component of their responsible delivery.

We set three broad goals for our work: to provide direction for public policy by making sound, practical, and principled recommendations; to leave a legacy of increased knowledge for Canadians and others about new reproductive technologies; and to enhance public awareness and understanding of the issues surrounding new reproductive technologies, so that ongoing public participation in determining the future of the technologies and their place in Canadian society would be facilitated.

The first goal has been achieved in the two volumes of this report. Our recommendations provide a detailed blueprint for how Canadians can deal with new reproductive technologies in this country, so that any use made of the technologies is in the service of our values. Throughout the report, we have made clear the evidence and the explicit framework we used to arrive at our policy recommendations — so as to make the reasoning behind our conclusions and recommendations evident.

The second goal has been fulfilled in the publication of the 15 volumes of research studies that accompany this report. The Commission developed and gathered an enormous and comprehensive body of information and analysis on which to base its recommendations, much of it available for the first time in Canada or indeed anywhere. The most qualified researchers in Canada participated in our research program — over 300 scholars and academics across the country representing more than 70 disciplines, including the social sciences, humanities, medicine, genetics, life sciences, law, ethics, philosophy, and theology.

Our third goal was to bring the issues before the public so as to encourage ongoing participation by Canadians in determining the future of the technologies and their place in our society. Although inquiries in other countries have addressed these issues and made recommendations, our Commission was the first that was able to consult widely and directly with citizens and benefit from substantial public input and participation. Many thousands of people attended public hearings or panel discussions, saw those discussions broadcast on cable television across the country, made written submissions, called our toll-free telephone lines for information or to express their opinions, talked to us about their own experiences with new reproductive technologies, or participated in research colloquia, workshops, and other consultations — in all, more than 40 000 Canadians participated. We sent out a newsletter, *Update*, and the research studies published in advance of this report were collected by academics, students, women's groups, and other groups working in this area and are available in libraries across the country. All these activities were important in helping us reach our conclusions, but they will also better equip Canadians to participate in and have input into how we will deal in an ongoing way with the issues as they evolve in Canada.

In a changing field of knowledge such as new reproductive technologies, new developments will require continuing attention by society regarding their implications and what needs to be done. Implementation of our recommendations will put in place the framework for this needed ongoing discussion, dialogue, limitation, and monitoring of the technologies.

Along with the other Commissioners, I wish to thank the very many Canadians who were involved in all facets of the Commission's work. Their contribution has been invaluable.

I would also like to acknowledge the efforts of a wide range of groups, for example the Canadian Coalition for New Reproductive Technologies, to have this Commission created, and the federal government for heeding their calls. We hope that the government will listen equally carefully to the calls for change that we make in this report and act promptly to implement our recommendations.

Appreciation and thanks are due to the researchers and to the external reviewers, who have given tremendous amounts of time, expertise, and thought to the Commission. I would also like to say how grateful I am to the Commission staff for their dedication, hard work, and commitment over the life of the Commission — they have gone many extra miles.

I would like to formally thank my four colleagues — my fellow Commissioners — for the spirit of collaboration, exploration, and cooperation with which they approached our work. We have all learned much and all felt a great responsibility to address the issues in as caring and wise a way as we can.

The issues this report has dealt with are important to us all. We hope governments and Canadians will use the detailed blueprint we have provided to make changes to the present unsatisfactory and harmful situation. Canada as a society can obtain benefits of technology for its members, but it also needs to protect them against harms from misuse.

We believe that, if we care about each other's well-being, the path we should take to deal with new reproductive technologies is clear. It is now up to governments and the people of Canada to decide whether they will take it. We believe it is critical that they do.

Patricia Baird

Patricia Baird

Chairperson
Royal Commission on New Reproductive Technologies

A Note on the Report

It is important that as many Canadians as possible, not just experts and academics, become aware of and understand the issues, so that they may participate in how we deal with new reproductive technologies in this country. In support of that goal, the Commission intends this report to be accessible to the general reader. The issues we are examining are complex and a certain amount of technical detail is unavoidable, but most of these details are provided in information boxes, which are set apart from the main body of the text.

In addition, quotations from the many groups and individuals who participated in the Commission's work are interspersed throughout the text; these reflect the extensive input the Commission received and the wide range of views we heard.

Executive Summary

♦

The mandate of the Royal Commission was to examine how new reproductive technologies should be handled in Canada. Having children and healthy families are important goals to most Canadians, but some people cannot reach those goals without help. If there are technologies that can be used to help, a caring society should provide these. But there are misuses and harms, as well as benefits, that may come from use of the technologies — harms to both individuals and society.

We undertook our task by consulting very widely. As well as public hearings and submitted briefs, we had toll-free telephone lines, public surveys, and other avenues for Canadians to have input. In all, more than 40 000 people were involved in our work. We carried out a canvassing and examination of the issues that was extensive in both width and depth, with research projects and analyses in many disciplines, among them the social sciences, ethics, law, and medicine. More than 300 researchers at institutions across the country conducted projects for us.

We came to our conclusions in light of this widely based input and evidence, with three considerations in mind: a set of explicit ethical principles, the values of Canadians, and a conviction that offering any medical procedure as a service must be based on evidence that it works.

In spite of the existence of standards and guidelines recommended by various professional associations, we found that a varied patchwork of practices exists. Some practices are dangerous, such as donor insemination using sperm from donors who have not been tested for HIV. Some are harmful to the interests of the children born through the use of various technologies, such as the lack of records kept on their origins. Some are not respectful of women's choices, such as the finding that a woman's chance of being referred for prenatal testing varied more than fourfold across the country, despite the fact that women's attitudes toward testing varied relatively little. We found insufficient emphasis on the prevention of infertility. We found some discriminatory practices in access to services, some clinics preparing to carry out procedures to allow surrogacy, and some commercial clinics existing to treat sperm to allow sex selection. Procedures are being offered as treatments without good evidence that they are effective, when they should be offered only in research trials. There are technologies on the horizon, such as embryo splitting and use of eggs from female fetuses for implantation. Our ethical analyses showed that some technologies and some uses of technology that are now possible or will be possible in the near future would contravene Canadian values.

It is clear that the situation with regard to the use of new reproductive technologies needs to be addressed; the issues will not go away — in fact, the field is growing, and potential uses are expanding. As this report went to press, the media were reporting the cloning of a human zygote. This vividly underscores the need to have in place a structure to deal with this evolving field in a way that takes into account the values and input of Canadians.

We conclude that government, as the guardian of the public interest, must act to put boundaries around the use of new reproductive technologies, and must put in place a system to manage them within those boundaries, not just for now, but, equally important, in an ongoing way. We therefore have two recommendations. First, we recommend legislation to prohibit, with criminal sanctions, several aspects of new reproductive technologies, such as using embryos in research related to cloning, animal/human hybrids, the fertilization of eggs from female fetuses for implantation, the sale of eggs, sperm, zygotes, or fetal tissues, and advertising for, paying for, or acting as an intermediary for preconception (surrogacy) arrangements.

Second, we recommend that the federal government establish a regulatory and licensing body — a National Reproductive Technologies Commission (NRTC) — with licensing required for the provision of new reproductive technologies to people. Only the federal government can set up such a system, and it is important that the government fulfil its responsibility to protect citizens and society by doing so.

Several requirements are common to all the technologies: the need for reliable information to guide policy and practice; the need for standards and guidelines for the organization and provision of services; the need for effective means to ensure compliance; and the need for accountability. The approach we propose builds on the best standards and practices of the medical specialties involved, which are already in use in some Canadian clinics. These standards should be expanded and should be embodied in a licensing system.

We recommend the NRTC be composed of 12 members, representing a broad range of experiences and perspectives. Consultation activities should be undertaken to further enhance public input and involvement.

Women should make up a substantial proportion — normally at least half — of the Commission's membership.

To ensure wide public input into the working of the system and to deal with setting policy as new issues evolve, we recommend that membership in the proposed NRTC should include persons with a broad range of experiences and perspectives, including the perspectives of those with disabilities, those who are infertile, and those who are members of racial minorities. A range of expertise should be represented, including reproductive medicine, ethics, law, and social sciences.

We recommend the NRTC have five areas of regulatory responsibility, in which the provision of services would be subject to compulsory licensing through five sub-committees established for that purpose. These areas are:

- sperm collection, storage, and distribution, and the provision of assisted insemination services;
- assisted conception services, including egg retrieval and use;
- prenatal diagnosis;
- research involving human zygotes (embryo research); and
- the provision of human fetal tissue for research or other specified purposes.

Licence hearings should be public, and a licence would be conditional on compliance with certain standards and stipulations of license. The major functions in these five areas of regulatory authority would be to:

- license, set standards, and monitor practice;
- collect, evaluate, store, and disseminate information;
- consult, help coordinate, and facilitate intergovernmental cooperation in the field; and
- monitor future technologies and practices and set policies for them.

In addition, we recommend the establishment of a sixth sub-committee, with primary responsibility in the field of infertility prevention. Its responsibilities would include the compilation and evaluation of data pertaining to the causes of infertility, the promotion of cooperative research efforts in Canada and internationally, and regulatory, public education, or other options for preventing or reducing the incidence of infertility.

With full implementation of these recommendations, a consistent country-wide system for the regulation of reproductive technologies and the provision of related services would emerge, with the following attributes:

- Assisted insemination, *in vitro* fertilization, and related infertility treatments would be provided only by licensed facilities, with national standards of service (related to matters such as counselling, informed disclosure and consent, standardized calculation of success rates, and consistent record keeping) as conditions for obtaining and keeping a licence to provide these services.

- A national sperm collection and distribution system would be in place to ensure the availability of safe sperm, quarantined until donors are tested for infectious diseases, for use in assisted insemination in a medical setting or in self-insemination. The system would include comprehensive confidential record keeping on donors and recipients, with non-identifying information on the donor available to the recipient and child, and personal identification kept secure and available only in court-ordered cases.

- Prenatal diagnostic services would be provided only by licensed facilities, with national standards established and monitored through the licensing system. Prenatal ultrasound and testing of pregnant women's blood for congenital anomalies or genetic disease in the fetus would be provided only through provincially licensed or mandated programs. The structure would assure Canadians that genetic knowledge is applied in human reproduction in an accountable way and within acceptable limits — for example, not used for purposes of sex selection.

- A mechanism would be in place to facilitate multicentre trials and other research needed to assess the safety and effectiveness of reproductive technologies. It would promote interprovincial co-operation to mount the large-scale research projects needed to provide information on which to base health care service provision and resource allocation decisions.

- Once their risks and effectiveness had been assessed, infertility treatment and prenatal diagnostic services would be provided solely through provincial health care systems. Other treatments or procedures would be provided only in the context of research, with fully informed participation by volunteer research subjects and with rigorous protections for them. To preclude the development of commercial services, licensing conditions would include a stipulation that services not be offered on a for-profit basis.

- Annual reporting to the National Commission by licensed facilities would provide data that would allow evaluation of any long-term effects of treatments on the health of women or on their children.

- Any provision of fetal tissue for research would be licensed, so that it is used only in an accountable and ethical way according to guidelines, with permission for tissue use obtained separately from and subsequent to the decision to terminate a pregnancy.

- Any embryo research would be conducted only in licensed facilities, so that such research is carried out in an accountable and ethical way and in accordance with guidelines, including limitations on the purposes for which research can be undertaken, and permitted only during the 14 days immediately following fertilization.

- A focal point for national action would be in place to support and encourage infertility prevention initiatives, to foster consultation and co-ordination of efforts among the many sectors involved, and to promote public education and research in Canada and internationally on the risk factors for and prevention of infertility.

- Canada would have a visible and continuing forum to monitor developments, promote public discussion, and develop public policy advice on the use of assisted reproductive technologies, prenatal diagnostic technologies, embryo research, research involving the use of fetal tissue, and other rapidly evolving or emerging technologies.

Getting There from Here

Commissioners are strongly of the view that the establishment of a National Reproductive Technologies Commission of the type we recommend must be an immediate federal priority. We believe that a National Commission presents the only feasible response to the clearly demonstrated need and justified public demand for coherent, effective, and appropriate national regulation of new reproductive technologies. The field is developing too rapidly, the consequences of inaction are too great, and the potential for harm to individuals and to society is too serious to allow Canada's response to be delayed, fragmented, or tentative.

A central goal of our recommendations is to enable individual Canadians to make personal decisions about their involvement with the technologies, confident in the knowledge that mechanisms are in place to assess their safety and effectiveness and to consider their ethical, legal, and social implications. Individuals have a responsibility to inform themselves as fully as possible before making such decisions, but government, on behalf of citizens, has a responsibility to ensure that inappropriate and unethical use of technology is prohibited and that the procedures and supports necessary for informed decision making are in place.

The regulatory framework we propose is essential to provide this assurance, but by itself it is not sufficient. Strong leadership and co-operation will be required among governments and professionals involved in the development and delivery of reproductive technologies, as well as among many other sectors of society. No group or institution can act effectively in isolation — partnership and cooperation among federal and provincial/territorial governments, professional organizations, patient groups, and other interested groups are critical.

Establishing such a system will take some time — although we should note that other countries have succeeded in putting their systems in place within a relatively short period after their own inquiries. Nevertheless, some time will be required to appoint members of the Commission, establish and appoint its sub-committees, and carry out detailed implementation of the licensing system. Time will be needed to hold an initial round of licensing hearings, design secure record-keeping systems, and identify specific data collection methods and reporting forms.

The need for comprehensive action at the national level does not preclude the need for provincial and professional responses. Nor do provinces or the professions need to wait for a federal response before taking action themselves.

Provinces can take immediate steps to control the provision and proliferation of reproductive technologies in the health care system through the evidence-based approach we recommend. Practitioners now offering services can respond to the concerns Canadians raised before the Royal Commission and to the issues we have identified in the report. Professional associations can ensure that all their members are aware of the existing guidelines for practice and can promote more complete adherence to these standards among their members. Technology users and groups representing them can use the report of the Royal Commission to press for government and professional action. In the meantime, individual Canadians contemplating the use of reproductive technologies can use the information we have provided, ask questions, and request information from providers about the effectiveness, consequences, and potential risks of the technology use they are considering. Indeed, an informed public is the most effective bulwark against misuse or abuse of technology.

But all of these are only stop-gap measures. Government should act as the guardian of the public interest to set limits and to regulate the use of new reproductive technologies. No other body is sufficiently broadly based or has the mandate to do this. It is important that we put in place now the structures and an open, broad process to enable Canadians to deal with these growing dilemmas, dilemmas that affect individual lives and what kind of a society we are. How we use reproductive technology is not at root a medical matter, but a social matter that reaches into law, prevention, education, commerce, science, and research policy. Matters so important to women and children, in terms not only of their health but of their legal status and how they are viewed, cannot differ from province to province. The field is growing rapidly and Canadians want the government to act. There is clearly precedent — radio and television broadcasting is regulated and monitored through a licensing agency for the Canadian public interest. The area of reproductive technology use is at least as important to us as individuals and as a society.

Conclusion

Commissioners have set out a blueprint for how Canada, with its unique institutions and social make-up, can deal with new reproductive technologies, regulate their use, and ensure that future developments or use are in the public interest. Our blueprint requires action and leadership from the federal government, but also involves the participation and commitment of provincial governments, the professions, and many sectors of society. The approach we propose is feasible and practical, and we have laid out a detailed plan for how it can be accomplished.

The reasons for such action are compelling: the potential for harm to individuals and the need to protect the vulnerable interests of individuals and society. Adopting our recommendations will enable this protection, but will also allow scientific knowledge to be used to better the lives of many Canadians. Implementing the blueprint will demonstrate that we care about each other's well-being and recognize collective values with respect to the importance people attach to having children. At the same time, it will ensure that only ethical and accountable use of technology is made, and demonstrate that Canadians have wisdom, humanity, and compassion in the way they choose to use technology.

The Commission has done its work and indicated the path it believes should be taken. The next steps belong to the government and people of Canada.

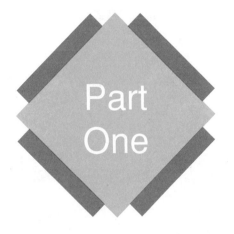

Part
One

New Reproductive Technologies
and Canadian Society

A Comprehensive Response to Issues of National Importance

As Canadians living in the last decade of the twentieth century, we face unprecedented choices about procreation, placed before us by what has been described as a revolution in reproduction. Our responses to these choices will say much about Canada as a society — what we value, what our priorities are, what kind of society we want to live in.

New reproductive technologies now make it possible to unlink fertilization from sexual intercourse and pregnancy, allow embryos to exist for a time outside a woman's body, and permit characteristics of a fetus to be known early in pregnancy. New reproductive technologies therefore open up major ethical dilemmas for individuals and for society as a whole, because, like most technologies, they have the potential for both benefit and harm. They offer new options and potential benefits for the people who can use the technologies to form a family, but scientific and medical interventions in procreation also challenge us as a society to be able to recognize their significance and control their development. Would they further entrench existing inequalities or create new ones? How could they potentially alter definitions of parent, family, and generation? What is their potential effect on the way women are viewed in society?

The Appointment of a Royal Commission

Although the debate about new reproductive technologies dated from a decade or more earlier, by the end of the 1980s the time had clearly come for more extensive public information and discussion on new reproductive technologies and their implications for Canadian society. Calls for public discussion and recommendations for policy development came from many sources, including women's groups, religious groups, legal and medical professional groups, federal-provincial/territorial working groups, academic organizations, and organizations of people with disabilities, as well as in forums such as international conferences on new reproductive technologies. Some of these organizations formed a coalition to advocate for the appointment of a royal commission; others supported the idea as a constructive way to deal with these complex issues.

In response to these developments, the Government of Canada appointed the Royal Commission on New Reproductive Technologies in October 1989 with a mandate to

> ... inquire into and report on current and potential medical and scientific developments related to new reproductive technologies, considering in particular their social, ethical, health, research, legal and economic implications and the public interest ...

The choice before Canadians is to decide to what degree our society will be driven by the pace of technological change, how to ensure that the further development of these technologies is conditioned by our priorities and values, and how those priorities and values will be identified and agreed upon. Technology is not beyond society's control. It can be shaped by policies adopted to guide our collective lives together and by personal choices in our private lives. This is the point from which the Commission began to explore its mandate, and it is the perspective that informs our recommendations. How we choose to use, or not to use, these technological capacities will shape society for our children and for their children. We need to evaluate the technologies and make decisions from the broadest possible perspective, using clear and explicit values and principles to guide our choices.

The Commission's Mandate

The establishment of the Commission therefore set in motion a comprehensive inquiry, based on a mandate that required the Commission to examine current and potential scientific and medical developments related to reproductive technologies, but also to go beyond them to consider

- the impact of the technologies on society as a whole;
- their impact on identified groups in society, specifically women, children, and families; and
- the ethical, legal, social, economic, and health implications of these technologies.

Although the past two decades have seen numerous examinations of certain aspects of new reproductive technologies in Canada and elsewhere, by and large these examinations did not include consideration of the causes and prevention of infertility, the use of prenatal diagnosis (PND), research

---

The Commission's Mandate .

The **Royal Commission on New Reproductive Technologies** will be established "under Part I of the *Inquiries Act*" and will "inquire into and report on current and potential medical and scientific developments related to new reproductive technologies, considering in particular their social, ethical, health, research, legal and economic implications and the public interest, recommending what policies and safeguards should be applied."

The Commission will examine, "in particular,

(a)   implications of new reproductive technologies for women's reproductive health and well-being;
(b)   the causes, treatment and prevention of male and female infertility;
(c)   reversals of sterilization procedures, artificial insemination, *in vitro* fertilization, embryo transfers, prenatal screening and diagnostic techniques, genetic manipulation and therapeutic interventions to correct genetic anomalies, sex selection techniques, embryo experimentation and fetal tissue transplants;
(d)   social and legal arrangements, such as surrogate childbearing, judicial interventions during gestation and birth, and 'ownership' of ova, sperm, embryos and fetal tissue;
(e)   the status and rights of people using or contributing to reproductive services, such as access to procedures, 'rights' to parenthood, informed consent, status of gamete donors and confidentiality, and the impact of these services on all concerned parties, particularly the children; and
(f)   the economic ramifications of these technologies, such as the commercial marketing of ova, sperm and embryos, the application of patent law, and the funding of research and procedures including infertility treatment."

—— *Order in Council No. P.C. 1989-2150*

---

involving human zygotes (or embryos*), or research involving the use of fetal tissue. Nor did they examine the broader context and implications of using the technologies — their social, health, and economic context, or

---

* There is a problem with terminology, as the term "embryo" is used in different ways. In the language of biologists, before implantation the fertilized egg is termed a "zygote" rather than an "embryo." The term "embryo" refers to the developing entity after implantation in the uterus until about eight weeks after fertilization. At the beginning of the ninth week after fertilization, it is referred to as a "fetus," the term used until time of birth. The terms embryo donation, embryo transfer, and embryo research are therefore inaccurate, since these all occur with zygotes, not embryos. Nevertheless, because the terms are still commonly used in the public debate, we continue to refer to embryo research, embryo donation, and embryo transfer. For accuracy, however, we also refer to the developing entity during the first 14 days as a zygote, so that it is clear that we mean the stage of development before implantation and not later.

their impact on the individuals and groups that make up society, particularly on women's health and well-being.

Central to the Commission's deliberations was how new reproductive technologies may affect women's reproductive health and well-being; their individual autonomy and scope for reproductive decisions; and their status, rights, and interests as members of society. Similarly, the Commission was concerned about the impact of the technologies on men, children, and families, and with ensuring that the technologies do not give rise to discrimination or exploitation related to socioeconomic, racial, or ethnic minority status.

Finally, given Canada's unique social make-up, the country's geography, our distinctive political and legal institutions, and our health and social systems, we had to evaluate new reproductive technologies and their implications from a Canadian perspective and to develop recommendations in light of our understanding of Canadians' collective values and attitudes.

The Commission's mandate was therefore broad and complex; we were asked to look at not only present technologies and procedures but also potential future developments, which meant also examining the implications of the technologies for future generations of Canadians.

The appointment of a royal commission was an opportunity to collect much-needed information, to foster the public awareness and debate that are necessary to create an informed social consensus, and, above all, to provide a principled framework for Canadian public policy on the use or restriction of these technologies. The Commission was thus placed squarely in the gap between technological development and policy development, with the task of helping to close it.

The Technologies

The term "new reproductive technologies," as used in the Commission's mandate, covers a broad range of conditions, technologies, procedures, and practices. By itself, the term is somewhat misleading, for it fails to convey the full scope of the Commission's mandate. Not all of the practices the Commission was asked to examine are new, not all involve technology, and not all are concerned with reproduction as it is usually understood.

Some of the practices the Commission was asked to examine are long-established. Assisted insemination (AI) in human beings, for example, has been practised in North America since at least 1884. Other practices, such as gene therapy, genetic alteration, and the use of fetal tissue for transplantation, are new but do not concern assisted human reproduction — which is the conventional understanding of what new reproductive technologies involve.

Some aspects of the Commission's mandate, such as infertility prevention, may require little technology; others, including prenatal diagnosis and therapy, involve highly complex technologies. Practices such as preconception agreements (surrogacy) may involve assisted reproduction; their main implications arise, however, not from the technology used but from the ethical, legal, and social issues surrounding them. In short, the questions embraced by the Commission's mandate cannot be considered in isolation from one another, for they are interdependent at several levels, and decisions about one often have repercussions for another — hence the need for a comprehensive, multidisciplinary approach to our task and a comprehensive public policy response.

Structure of the Report

Our report is divided into three major parts. Part One describes the context for our inquiry and the major considerations that guided our deliberations — the ethical and scientific framework for our review and assessment of new reproductive technologies, as well as the societal values and attitudes toward reproduction and the technologies. Part One concludes with an overview of our proposals for a legislative and regulatory framework for Canada's comprehensive response to these issues. Implementing it will require concerted, collaborative efforts on the part of the federal government, provincial and territorial governments, the health care system, and other key partners.

Part Two is devoted to our examination and assessment concerning the four principal areas of our mandate: the prevalence, risk factors, and prevention of infertility; assisted human conception and alternatives to it; prenatal diagnosis and genetics; and research involving human zygotes, embryos, and the use of fetal tissue. Our detailed findings on these topics are set out in the 15 research volumes accompanying publication of this report. Here we present the conclusions emerging from our research and analysis and the policy recommendations flowing from them.

Part Three provides a summary of our recommendations, organized by area of responsibility for implementation. This summary illustrates the importance of concerted and collaborative efforts among numerous key participants in achieving the success of the approach to new reproductive technologies that we propose.

To organize its research, the Commission grouped the conditions, technologies, and practices referred to in its mandate under four broad topics: the prevalence, risk factors, and prevention of infertility; methods of assisted human reproduction; prenatal diagnosis techniques and genetics; and research involving human zygotes and embryos and involving fetal tissue. These four areas of inquiry are described briefly in the following pages and provide the structure around which Part Two of our report is organized. Throughout the report, and unless otherwise indicated, we use the term "new reproductive technologies" to refer to this full range of conditions, technologies, and practices, not solely to interventions intended to assist conception.

Prevalence, Risk Factors, and Prevention of Infertility

Developing policy with respect to the use of reproductive technologies requires a clear understanding of infertility and its causes. Is infertility the inability to conceive within a particular time limit, to carry a pregnancy to term, or to produce a living child? What causes infertility in women and men? How common is it? Is infertility on the increase among people in Canada? Can it be prevented? If so, how and in what proportion of cases?

The answers to these kinds of questions will help to determine society's response to infertility. Understanding the causes and considering how to prevent infertility in women and men are therefore crucial in establishing a context for the other, more technologically oriented issues in the Commission's mandate.

Some of the questions we examined do not involve technology; for example, adoption is often thought of as an alternative to the use of reproductive technologies for people who are infertile. Others, such as preconception agreements, may involve assisted insemination or *in vitro* fertilization (IVF) but need not do so. These questions are discussed in Chapters 16 (adoption) and 23 (preconception arrangements).

Assisted Human Conception

This area of our inquiry examined procedures intended to help individuals or couples to conceive a child. Our examination included the practices and procedures usually included in the conventional definition of new reproductive technologies: the use of fertility drugs, assisted insemination using partner or donor sperm, *in vitro* fertilization, sterilization reversal, and newer developments such as gamete intra-fallopian transfer (referred to as GIFT).

Some of these procedures and practices require associated technologies. Assisted human conception using IVF and GIFT, for example, may involve other procedures, including the use of fertility drugs, frozen sperm, and, sometimes, frozen zygotes. Thus, the Commission also examined subjects such as the short- and long-term effects of fertility drug use, as well as the techniques and practices of facilities collecting sperm for donation, and freezing, storing, and handling human zygotes.

Prenatal Diagnosis and Genetics

Prenatal diagnosis (which encompasses a range of procedures for detecting medically relevant characteristics of the embryo or fetus) includes techniques such as ultrasound scanning and amniocentesis. Newer developments are less familiar: chorionic villus sampling (CVS), preimplantation diagnosis, maternal serum alpha-fetoprotein (MSAFP) screening, prenatal predictive testing for diseases that occur later in life, and gene therapy are examples of the newer technologies the Commission examined.

Of particular significance with some of the newer developments is that they make information about the embryo available earlier, thereby allowing knowledge of its status — and thus, potentially, various interventions — at earlier stages of development.

Research Involving Human Zygotes, Embryos, and Fetal Tissue

Fetal tissue use includes research aimed at understanding human development and functioning, as well as research to determine whether fetal tissue or its derivatives can be used to treat human diseases. An example of the latter is research to determine whether transplants of tissue from this source will help people with neurological diseases such as Parkinson disease. Embryo research involves efforts to understand fertilization, implantation, and very early human development so that this knowledge can be used subsequently in medical treatment.

Research involving human zygotes and the use of fetal tissue is carried out in relatively few places in Canada; society therefore has an opportunity to consider the issues they raise as the technologies develop. The rapid pace of development in both fields, in Canada and elsewhere, makes their consideration a priority. (See Chapters 22 and 31.)

Broader Questions

The Commission was directed to examine the technologies in their medical, ethical, social, scientific, and research dimensions, as well as their economic and legal aspects. As well as examining these aspects we commissioned research on questions related to the origins, development, alternatives to, and implications of the technologies, so that we could develop a comprehensive and integrated picture. This process is described more fully in Chapter 6. In addition, the Commission was asked to consider several questions related to the field of human reproduction though not related specifically to new reproductive technologies:

- judicial intervention in gestation and birth;

- the legal status of reproductive material such as gametes (sperm and eggs), zygotes, and embryos; and

- the economic and legal implications of commercial marketing of human eggs, sperm, and embryos, the application of intellectual property law, and methods of funding both research into and provision of these technologies.

Organization of the Commission's Work

To fulfil our mandate and ensure a sound basis for our findings and recommendations, we sought to develop effective and innovative ways to

- consult with Canadians from all sectors of society and listen to their views and experiences on the issues surrounding new reproductive technologies;

- assemble solid information about and critical analyses of the technologies and their implications; and

- develop an integrated approach to our work, so that what we heard from Canadians would inform specific research and evaluation projects, while research findings in turn would suggest specific questions to be addressed through the consultation process.

The Commission organized its work around two major streams of activities: consultations and communications, and research and evaluation. Through these activities we were able to appreciate the scope and complexity of the issues covered by our mandate, consider the far-reaching implications of the technologies, take into account the values and attitudes that Canadians bring to the debate, as well as the evolving social fabric of the country, and recommend a comprehensive approach to the technologies that recognizes and accommodates the dynamic nature of society, technology, and the interaction between them.

The Commission set three broad goals for its work:

1.   *To provide direction for public policy by making sound, practical, principled recommendations to help Canadians and our social institutions deal with the technologies now and to put in place mechanisms to ensure a continuing capacity to deal with them.*

In dealing with a subject with so many individual and social implications, we saw our task as being to offer recommendations that are principled, practical, and achievable, so that decision makers could formulate and implement sound policies in the interest of Canadian society now and in the future. We also wanted to provide the information and analysis that led to those recommendations.   To do this required documentation and analysis of the nature, effectiveness, and health effects of the new reproductive technologies currently in use, focussing on their social, ethical, health, research, legal, and economic implications. We were particularly concerned with the ethical bases for social and individual decisions — bases not unique to reproductive technologies. In offering practical and workable proposals to governments and other institutions, organizations, and professions regarding regulation of new reproductive technologies, we hope that these proposals can serve as a prototype for other emerging health care technologies.

2.   *To leave a legacy of increased knowledge in the field of Canadian and international experience with new reproductive technologies.*

Intelligent decisions require knowledge. The individual and societal choices surrounding new reproductive technologies must be founded on information and analysis about the capabilities, limitations, and implications of these technologies. This involves not only medical and scientific information, but also analysis of the values and the social, political, and economic forces shaping the development of new reproductive technologies and, conversely, how new reproductive technologies may shape Canadians' attitudes and values.

To expand our knowledge base, we commissioned research and analysis examining the origins, current practices in Canada, and future implications of all the technologies falling within our mandate. To consolidate existing information, the Commission conducted an inventory of the current state of research, collating and centralizing information for use by all those with an interest in the field. Fifteen volumes of research findings accompany this report. Together with the submissions, they constitute an enormous body of research findings and testimony, our assessment of which provided the basis for our conclusions and recommendations.

3.   *To enhance public awareness and understanding of the issues surrounding new reproductive technologies and to encourage public participation in determining the future of these diverse technologies and their place in Canadian society.*

In order to facilitate Canadians' participation in decision making at both the individual and collective level, we sought to expand the discourse around new reproductive technologies and to provide important information on the issues. To this end, our report is intended for the general reader, with only as much technical detail as is required to understand the implications of the technologies. We have also provided a chapter on the biology of human reproduction, definitions of terms used in each chapter, and a glossary at the end of the report. Readers with various degrees of expertise and familiarity with the technologies and the issues surrounding them who wish further detail may consult the 15 volumes of research studies.

The work of a royal commission is limited in certain ways inherent in its functions. A commission is not a permanent entity, so it cannot take on and manage research over the long term, deliver programs, or provide services. Nor can it ensure that its recommendations will be implemented — this is properly the function of elected governments and the democratic process. A royal commission's role is to clarify facts and issues, to analyze them from an ethical and social perspective, and to make principled recommendations chosen from among clearly described alternatives. The over-riding goal of the Royal Commission on New Reproductive Technologies was to do this for the consideration of the Government, Parliament, and the people of Canada.

Overall Results of Our Inquiry

After wide consultation with Canadians, ethical and social analysis of the implications, and careful examination of the scientific evidence relating to the current use of new reproductive technologies during the course of our mandate, the Commission has concluded that Canada must respond decisively and comprehensively to control development and use of these technologies; clear boundaries must be set and the technologies managed within these boundaries. As the Commission's detailed review of technologies and practices in Part Two of our report demonstrates, this response is necessitated by the technologies' profound ethical, social, health-related, and legal implications, both now and in the future.

The issues are not merely hypothetical; new reproductive technologies are already the subject of individual and systemic decisions about reproductive health, family formation, medical treatment, research, and health care resource allocation. Moreover, the field is evolving rapidly in Canada and elsewhere. As a society, we cannot turn back the clock. Nor can we live with the status quo, allowing the technologies to develop without clear societal direction grounded in collective values and priorities.

> Canada must move forward into the new reality with a clear, coordinated approach that permits us to resolve and manage the critical issues involved. To allow Canada's response to be delayed or fragmented by the existing web of jurisdictional and administrative arrangements would, in the view of Commissioners, be a mistake of enormous proportions.

Canada must move forward into the new reality with a clear, coordinated approach that permits us to resolve and manage the critical issues involved. To allow Canada's response to be delayed or fragmented by the existing web of jurisdictional and administrative arrangements would, in the view of Commissioners, be a mistake of enormous proportions. Failure to intervene constructively and decisively would amount to an abdication of social responsibility and a failure of political will.

The Commission sees a need to set clear limits based on what society considers to be acceptable activities in the field of reproductive research and treatment; to establish a system for managing the technologies within these limits; and to provide a mechanism for continuing review and evaluation as ethical and scientific issues in this field emerge and evolve. These are the principal goals of our recommendations.

Our detailed recommendations throughout Part Two are proposed in light of a long process of deliberation and consultation. In the remainder of this chapter we describe the broader overall framework into which these detailed and technology-specific recommendations fit.   With such a framework in place, our recommendations point the way to ensuring that future developments in this crucial, complex, and rapidly developing field are in the best interests of individual Canadians and of Canadian society generally.

The Call for National Action

Throughout our public hearings, in the many submissions and briefs we received, and in the surveys we conducted across the country, we found consistent and widespread demand for national leadership and action in relation to new reproductive technologies. This demand was expressed by women and men with widely varying backgrounds, experiences, and circumstances, in all age groups, and in all provinces. Since the issues and interests involved are of far-reaching importance for Canadian society as a whole, this response is not surprising. It reflected a prevailing belief that unconstrained development of new reproductive technologies is not in the public interest, and that the research and application of these technologies require clear boundaries and effective and appropriate management within those boundaries.

> The federal government must establish structures that will ensure the sound, fair and equitable development of NRTs [new reproductive technologies], by guaranteeing that standards are set through a process that is as representative as possible, and making certain that these standards are enforced. [Translation]
>
> *Brief to the Commission from Le comité "Vieillir au féminin" de l'Université du troisième âge de l'Université de Moncton, January 18, 1991.*

The need for a broad national framework within which to manage reproductive technologies was confirmed by the following results from our research, analysis, and consultations carried out over the course of the Commission's mandate:

- Some uses of reproductive technologies should be prohibited, as they violate ethical principles and contradict values widely held by Canadians. We were led to this conclusion by our ethical analysis, as well as our review of inquiries into and experience with reproductive technologies in other jurisdictions in Canada and abroad.

- Collective principles and values of Canadians include, at the societal level, non-commercialization of reproduction, fair and equitable access to services, and responsible use of public resources. At the individual level, they translate to the need to seek to prevent harm and to protect the health and safety of present and future technology users, and to ensure that they are fully informed of any risks and potential consequences of technology use.

- The status quo with respect to particular technologies is unacceptable from both an ethical and a medical perspective. Our review of evidence showed us that new and unproven medical procedures are being offered as treatment without the rigorous review and informed consent to which they should be subject; some practitioners are contravening guidelines established by their professional bodies; access to infertility treatment services is not equitable; and counselling and consent procedures for technology users are falling short of what is required.

- Our health care system cannot continue to respond to the demand for new medical technologies in the absence of clear evidence about their effectiveness. Such evidence constitutes a crucial component of the information necessary for individual decisions regarding treatment and collective decisions about resource allocation (including personnel, equipment, and facilities) needed to provide that treatment.

- More and better information on which to base informed choice and personal decision making with respect to reproductive health must become available. Our extensive consultations with Canadians revealed a need for public participation and public accountability in decision making; and a need for ongoing review of policies and decisions in the field of reproductive health and technologies.

- Canada's response to reproductive technologies must reflect constitutional values with respect to promoting equality and accommodating diversity, in the overall context of establishing congruence and consistency with Canadians' values and priorities and Canada's changing social fabric.

- Finally, no existing legislation or regulatory regime is broad enough and no public or private organization is equipped or has demonstrated the capacity to deal with all these questions in the comprehensive, timely fashion we believe is necessary.

Wide-Reaching Social, Ethical, and Public Policy Implications

The widespread call for national leadership heard by the Commission reflects a belief that it is unrealistic to expect self-regulating professional bodies, or the provinces, individually or together, to provide the necessary level of regulation and control on issues that transcend not only provincial but national and intergenerational boundaries and that have implications for all Canadians, regardless of where they live. It is the view of Canadians, and Commissioners' view as well, that given rapidly expanding knowledge and rapid dissemination of technologies, immediate intervention and concerted leadership are required at the national level. This does not obviate the need for decisive action by provinces and professional bodies as well, but action at the national level must provide the leadership and impetus for a new approach to managing reproductive technologies.

Public calls for national leadership reflect Canadians' recognition that a field with such wide-reaching social, ethical, and public policy implications could never be dealt with adequately by a single government ministry or department, no matter how well intentioned — the ethical and public policy questions are simply too broad for such a response to be effective. In the view of most of those who appeared before us, the inadequacy of existing piecemeal approaches to regulating the technologies, together with their implications for the future of our society, place a particular onus on this generation of Canadians to take immediate steps to deal comprehensively and consistently with these issues of national importance. Indeed, the appointment of the Royal Commission on New Reproductive Technologies reflected this recognition that public policy development in this field required a broad, multidisciplinary approach.

Canadians recognize that national leadership will provide the particular kind of impetus that is necessary in new reproductive technologies to ensure that the ethic of care and values such as equality, non-commercialization of human beings, privacy, and informed choice are reflected in services, that adequate standards of care are achieved and maintained, and that goals such as public accountability and responsiveness in decision making are realized.

In addition to calls for national leadership, many of the concerns we heard about the impact of new reproductive technologies took the form of calls for a moratorium on their development and use until such time as society is ready to deal with their implications.

> Given rapidly expanding knowledge and rapid dissemination of technologies, immediate intervention and concerted leadership are required at the national level. This does not obviate the need for decisive action by provinces and professional bodies as well, but action at the national level must provide the leadership and impetus for a new approach to managing reproductive technologies.

> We recommend that the federal, provincial, and territorial governments seriously examine the possibility of establishing a national organism for implementing reforms.
>
> *Brief to the Commission from the Law Reform Commission of Canada, November 21, 1990.*

Is a Moratorium the Appropriate Response?

The shortage of information on risks and effectiveness prompted calls during our public hearings for a moratorium on the development and use of new reproductive technologies. In the public debate that continued throughout our mandate, most intervenors who raised this issue expressed concern about women's inadvertent or uninformed exposure to risk because of lack of information and insufficient control over practices and procedures. It was in this context that some witnesses proposed a moratorium on the use of new reproductive technologies.

There was no consensus on what form a moratorium should take. Some intervenors spoke of legislative measures to suspend particular medical practices or types of research concerning reproductive technology, with the goal of allowing our collective knowledge and careful consideration of the issues to catch up to the developments themselves. Others used the term moratorium to mean a permanent halt to all current and future activity in an area of research or medical practice. Still others talked of maintaining activities at current levels without further expansion until results have been established and assessed. Opinion also varied on what technologies or research areas should be subject to a moratorium. Few aspects of reproductive research, assisted reproduction, prenatal diagnosis, gene therapy and genetic alteration, or research involving the use of fetal tissue were exempt from proposals to suspend or cease activity.

Calls for a moratorium are understandable in a field where the ethical and social implications are so far-reaching and knowledge is evolving so quickly. The Commission recognizes that there are certain technologies or areas of research that should be prohibited outright.   Our recom-mendations later in the report reflect this recognition.   However, we consider the imposition of a general moratorium inappropriate for several reasons:

- Some technologies and some uses of technology are beneficial. To deprive fully informed people of services that have been shown to make a difference in outcomes — services that may represent their only hope of having a biologically related child or of avoiding the birth of a child with a genetic disease or severe disabilities — would be inappropriate.

- It would be hard to ensure that only the specific activities covered by a research moratorium were put on hold and that necessary reproductive, endocrinological, or immunological research was not halted. This is because the boundaries between various research areas are not always clear, and because knowledge acquired through one type of research may have far-reaching beneficial applications in other fields that become apparent only later.

- A moratorium on research in Canada would not stop such research from occurring elsewhere; research results in other countries could easily be transferred and applied in Canada, just as they are now. This could have two consequences: first, it would be difficult to assess what the benefits and risks of an "imported" technology would be if applied in the Canadian clinical context, because it would not have been tested under Canadian conditions and controls. Second, Canada could become guilty of "ethical dumping" — taking the moral high road by banning research but later benefiting from the results of research conducted elsewhere and imported into medical practice in Canada.

- Leading researchers and research-oriented practitioners might leave the country, threatening the existence of Canadian centres of excellence, in which research and practice that have benefited Canadians have been linked.

Clearly, it is important to examine the concept of moratoria — what they are, what they can do, and when they are appropriate. However, a general moratorium is neither desirable nor feasible. The Commission believes that the best response in the area of new reproductive technologies is twofold: first, determining whether some forms of treatment or research are so ethically questionable, medically risky, or socially harmful that they should be banned. In cases where analysis shows that a practice or particular type of research violates fundamental ethical principles, or there is clear information that the potential for harm from a given practice is much greater than any anticipated benefit, a complete prohibition is the appropriate response. The second part of the response is to put in place mechanisms to manage research and treatment found to be potentially acceptable if they are carried out in an ethical, controlled, and accountable way. The result of this twofold response would be the establishment of boundaries, with unacceptable forms of research or treatment being prohibited, and potentially beneficial research or treatment activities being regulated and shaped by a publicly accountable body. Our recommendations reflect this stance.

We believe that the overall framework and the specific measures we propose not only will be capable of addressing the kinds of public concerns that gave rise to calls for a moratorium but will do so with greater precision and effectiveness than would be available through a general moratorium. At present, however, Canada has no mechanism for implementing such measures in a comprehensive, coordinated, and continuing way. Filling this regulatory void is the object of our recommendations in the remainder of our report.

A Matter of National Concern

As we were reminded repeatedly by the many groups and individuals that appeared before the Commission, the issues raised by new reproductive technologies defy neat categorization as solely a health problem, solely a legal problem, or solely an ethical problem. The research, development, and use of new reproductive technologies involve national concerns that cut across social, ethical, legal, medical, economic, and other considerations and institutions. This characteristic of new reproductive technologies generates the need for a distinct regulatory and organizational response — one capable of responding to and dealing with the issues in a comprehensive way.

New reproductive technologies are, in many ways, unique in Canada's health care system, in that they are administered under the jurisdiction of the provinces and territories, but, because of their profound social, ethical, and legal implications, raise issues that require national attention. Few individuals or families in this country are not touched in some way by new reproductive technologies.

Considering the overarching nature, profound importance, and fundamental inter-relatedness of the issues involved, we consider that federal regulation of new reproductive technologies — under the national concern branch of the peace, order, and good government power, as well as under the criminal law, trade and commerce, spending, and other relevant federal constitutional powers — is clearly warranted.

Just as the technologies themselves are highly complex, requiring careful and intelligent management, so are the ethical and social questions surrounding their use. A host of difficult issues and questions needs to be dealt with and resolved. A recurrent concern voiced to the Commission in our consultations with Canadians was that there is no single authority overseeing developments in the area of new reproductive technologies.

The Commission believes that the issues associated with new reproductive technologies must be resolved on a national basis. As we have already suggested, and as will become increasingly evident in our review of technologies and practices in Part Two of this report, it is not an exaggeration to say that chaos characterizes the regulation of the technologies in Canada today. The research, development, and application of new reproductive technologies are occurring in the absence of an overall framework for monitoring or controlling these developments. To allow this situation to continue is not in the interests of Canadians, and is not, in the Commission's opinion, an acceptable option.

Comprehensive Policies and Regulation Are Required

As it stands, no comprehensive law is in place, and no entity, public or private, has overall responsibility in this area. Existing family, health, contract, commercial, and related legal regimes apply to new reproductive technologies largely by inference, if at all, and few or no court cases have been decided. Thus, society lacks guidance on issues such as the status, liabilities, and responsibilities of participants; access to treatment; informed consent; privacy and confidentiality; and the boundaries between acceptable and unacceptable practices, procedures, and treatments.

For instance, prevention of infertility is not a health policy priority in Canada at present, and there is no coherent or comprehensive public policy response to factors that may put fertility at risk — for example, reproductive hazards in the environment and the workplace. Medical coverage of infertility treatments and access to them vary across the country and from clinic to clinic, there is marked variation in standards and practices, and there is no comprehensive system of keeping records on these treatments and their outcomes. Canada now depends on a patchwork of laws to address the bewildering challenges of medically assisted procreation. Other than the Yukon, Newfoundland, and Quebec, no province or territory has made provision for the unique situations created by the use of donated gametes, so that the legal status of the parents and children involved remains unclear. Similarly, with the exception of a provision in the Quebec *Civil Code*, there are no laws anywhere in Canada specifically governing preconception arrangements. Despite the existence of guidelines on prenatal diagnosis, a woman's access to this testing depends largely on the values and beliefs of her physician, which vary substantially from region to region, and from specialty to specialty. Canada has no national policy regarding the use of fetal tissues, and, in its absence, Canadian researchers rely on undocumented and unregulated individual agreements with facilities providing abortions.

> Accreditation and quality assurance functions [for IVF programs] should clearly be operated at a federal level. Furthermore, a registry could only effectively operate as a national registry.
>
> *D. Mortimer, Ontario Medical Association, Public Hearings Transcripts, Ottawa, Ontario, September 18, 1990.*

Issues such as these are too important to our society, their fundamental social, moral, legal, and ethical implications too profound, to be left to be resolved by a fragmented and disjointed sector-by-sector or province-by-province approach. The protection of the public interest, the well-being and interests of women, the creation of children, and the formation of families are national issues that must be addressed at a national level. Though not directly involved in the delivery of new reproductive technology services, the federal government has a critical role to play — that of facilitating societal inquiry, education, and reflection on new reproductive technologies, and then following this through with responsible regulation that is national in scope.

We believe that it is important that the approach of the 1980s, when many uses of new reproductive technologies proliferated with little control, does not continue in the future. Through our consultation activities, and through this report, we have brought forward and consolidated a considerable amount of information that will assist in ensuring this situation is rectified.

Given what we learned through extensive consultation, data collection, and analysis over the life of our mandate, we share the widely held public view that new reproductive technologies raise issues of a magnitude and importance that not only warrant but *require* a national response. We reject the argument that new reproductive technologies as a general matter should continue to be subdivided into component parts and left to the provincial legislatures, or delegated to self-governing professional bodies, for regulation on a province-by-province or even an institution-by-institution basis. Considering the overarching nature, profound importance, and fundamental inter-relatedness of the issues involved, we consider that federal regulation of new reproductive technologies — under the national concern branch of the peace, order, and good government power, as well as under the criminal law, trade and commerce, spending, and other relevant federal constitutional powers — is clearly warranted.

We recognize that the constitution assigns wide legislative jurisdiction to the provinces in the field of health. However, there is a clear basis for seeking national action in this area. In particular, Parliament has authority, under the national concern branch of the federal peace, order, and good government power, to regulate matters

> In Canada today, the development of IVF and related technologies can most charitably be described as anarchic.
>
> Provincial/territorial and federal levels of government have exercised little control or regulation concerning NRT practice and research. The medical profession and governments have done little in the way of formulating standards for the testing and monitoring of NRTs, thereby facilitating the confusion between research and treatment that marks NRTs.
>
> ... a national body [should] be established to review and approve research proposals, set ethical standards, set national standards of informed consent for NRT research and therapy, standardize data collection on NRTs, and monitor service access and provision.
>
> *Brief to the Commission from the Canadian Advisory Council on the Status of Women, March 1991.*

> The government [should] show leadership in this area [of creating] and perhaps emphasizing the importance of a national registry.
>
> *N. Barwin, Planned Parenthood Federation of Canada, Public Hearings Transcripts, Ottawa, Ontario, September 19, 1990.*

going beyond local or provincial interest that are of inherent concern to Canada as a whole.

Peace, Order, and Good Government

The Supreme Court has decided that the peace, order, and good government power can be invoked in support of federal legislative action, provided the matter Parliament seeks to regulate is of genuine national concern and possesses a degree of singleness, distinctiveness, and indivisibility that renders federal regulation compatible with provincial control over matters within their legislative jurisdiction.

The Supreme Court has held that provinces' ability to deal with a matter effectively through cooperative action, and the effect on extraprovincial interests of a province's failure to regulate the intra-provincial aspects of the matter, are of particular relevance, since it is the inter-relatedness of the intra- and extraprovincial dimensions of the problem that creates the need for single or uniform legislative treatment. We are firmly of the belief that new reproductive technologies, as defined in our mandate, meet the criteria established by the Supreme Court, so that federal intervention under the peace, order, and good government power is constitutionally justified.

New reproductive technologies possess a conceptual and practical integrity and distinctiveness. Their fundamental object is human reproduction, with all its distinct historical, social, and ethical implications. Viewed as a biological function, reproduction is easily distinguishable from other matters of human health. It has particular social significance, has particular ethical, political, and economic dimensions, and creates particular legal relations and responsibilities. Thus, although health issues are certainly involved, numerous other individual and societal issues converge in reproductive technologies, necessitating a broad, inclusive approach to dealing with them.

Focussing on human reproduction, new reproductive technologies are clearly identifiable and distinct from other areas of medical science, technology, research, and health service. Assisted conception services, for example, and the research, technologies, and medical interventions they involve, are not designed to cure illness or disease in a traditional pathological sense, but rather to address the problem of involuntary childlessness — a condition whose significance and implications for the individuals involved, and for society as a whole, are of a predominantly social rather than medical character. Prenatal diagnosis services, research involving human zygotes and the use of fetal tissue, and prenatal genetics research also have distinct ethical and social significance owing to their unique relationship to human reproduction. More than any other aspect of health-related technology or service, the research and application of new reproductive technologies have significance beyond the individuals directly involved.

Public control over the development and use of new reproductive technologies is therefore necessary to safeguard a wide range of interests. Some relate directly to the health and well-being of the individuals involved. Others relate to the welfare of particular groups such as women, for whom repro- duction has always had particu- lar social, economic, and legal consequences. Still others relate to the well-being of Canadian society as a whole, including that of future generations, and have implications beyond Canadian borders.

All of these interests are inter-related. It is hardly sur- prising, therefore, that at the level of both policy and practice, the effectiveness of regulation of one dimension of new repro- ductive technologies will depend greatly on the effectiveness of regulation of other dimensions of the technologies. For example, as the discussion in Part Two of our report makes clear, a legislative policy requiring disclosure of information about the medical and social family history of children born through assisted conception involving donated gametes (eggs or sperm) would be rendered meaningless by a failure to ensure that proper records on the donors are compiled and maintained. Similarly, requiring full and informed consent to any assisted conception intervention would be ineffective without information being available about the health status of donors or the safety of drugs and procedures. It would be ineffective to prohibit the donation of gametes or zygotes for research without being able to control the ultimate research use of such entities. And, similarly, a legislative policy discouraging or prohibiting preconception (surrogacy) arrangements would be compromised by a failure to ensure that practices surrounding embryo transfers are regulated appropriately.

Failure to regulate some or all aspects of new reproductive technologies in one province or region would also adversely affect the interests that such regulation seeks to promote elsewhere. Indeed, as we have indicated, detrimental consequences such as variations in access and

> Decisions about who will get how much of what in health care are made mostly in an ad hoc fashion, with different motives operating for the different levels of decision makers. Although some mechanisms exist for influencing technological adoption and diffusion, such as regulation under special programs for the purchase of expensive technologies ... or fee-for-service schedules that signal what services can be provided and how much the payment will be, ... policy mechanisms at present are neither coordinated nor applied consistently to ensure predefined and publicly articulated health goals. Moreover, prospective assessment of the consequences of technology decisions has not been part of the decision-making process.
>
> *A. Kazanjian and K. Cardiff, "Framework for Technology Decisions: Literature Review," in Research Volumes of the Commission, 1993.*

practices and inadequate record keeping have occurred already. Moreover, policies and practices that tended to allow the commodification of children or commodification of women's reproductive functions in one province would have significant social consequences that could not be confined to any particular jurisdiction where commodification was deemed acceptable. Allowing or ignoring the practice of preconception arrangements in one province while it is prohibited elsewhere would have a harmful impact, not only on the gestational mothers and other women in the province in question, but on Canadian women generally. Such permissiveness in one jurisdiction — quite apart from the "reproductive tourism" it would encourage — would convey tacit acceptance, or even affirmative state sanction, of a practice that is likely to undermine the value, dignity, reproductive capacity, and bodily integrity of Canadian women. Again, because of the great mobility of Canadians, failure to impose adequate controls on the safety of assisted conception technologies in one province or region would inevitably have social, health, and economic consequences as those affected moved elsewhere.

Some would argue that interprovincial variations in levels of access to, and control over, new reproductive technologies are an unavoidable fact of life in Canada, and that regional variations are one of the prices we pay for a federal system designed, in part, to accommodate diversity — and indeed this is true for many areas of our collective lives. In our view, however, the exacerbation of existing interprovincial discrepancies in access, monitoring, and control as the pace of technological developments accelerates — together with the fact that citizens in provinces with insufficient regulation may suffer harm and the fact that the technologies have social implications that are not containable within the boundaries of a single province — make new reproductive technologies a matter of national concern.

Some countries have already put in place nationally based measures to deal with the issues raised by new reproductive technologies; this enabled the Commission to learn from experiences elsewhere. The real difficulties in implementing a national system to regulate new reproductive technologies should not be underestimated, but other countries facing similar difficulties have established bodies to oversee developments in this area and have had them functioning within a relatively short period of time.

For instance, the British government established the Human Embryology and Fertilisation Authority to regulate all aspects of new reproductive technologies throughout the United Kingdom, including licensing of all clinics providing infertility-related services or conducting embryo research. Australia, which has a federal system of government, as does Canada, has opted for a national body, the Australian Health Ethics Committee, to encourage and enhance public debate on the ethical aspects of the technologies. France has created the National Advisory Committee for Health and the Life Sciences, the world's first permanent ethics committee, as well as a national self-regulating body, La Fédération

Française des Centres d'Étude et de Conservation des Oeufs et du Sperme humains (CECOS), while Denmark has a National Ethics Council.

In summary, the significance of research, development, and use of new reproductive technologies for Canadian society as a whole; the national as well as international character of the issues involved; the inter-relatedness of their intra- and extraprovincial dimensions; and the potential effects of provincial failure to regulate the intraprovincial aspects of the subject, taken together, indicate the need for national uniformity in legislative treatment rather than provincial or regional diversity. To safeguard the individual and societal interests involved, we believe that regulation of new reproductive technologies must occur at the national level, although provincial and professional involvement will be essential to the success of this endeavour. Only then will it be possible to overcome an increasing fragmentation of regulatory control and the difficulty of monitoring as practices and technologies expand and multiply.

The Commission therefore proposes that federal legislation be passed making some uses of the technologies illegal, thus establishing boundaries around what Canada considers acceptable use. To manage technology development and ensure only appropriate use within these boundaries, we propose the establishment of a National Reproductive Technologies Commission (NRTC) to fulfil policy, regulatory, and licensing functions in relation to specific activities in this field. We have also made relevant recommendations to the provinces and to professional and other bodies, which are essential partners in making the approach we propose workable and effective. An overview of the proposed regulatory framework is set out in Chapter 5, and further details are provided in the chapters devoted to our review of the specific conditions, technologies, and practices that our mandate asked us to examine. In Part Three, we provide the reader with an overview of how our recommendations work together, organized along the lines of who would be responsible for their implementation.

In the next three chapters, we set out the ethical and scientific principles that guided our review of current uses of the technologies and that provided a framework for reaching our conclusions and recommendations. In Chapter 5 we describe the broad outlines of our recommendations for establishing boundaries around the technologies whose use we consider acceptable and for managing them within those boundaries in an ethical and accountable way.

Social Values and Attitudes Toward Technology and New Reproductive Technologies

◆

Technology sparks strong emotions and debate among Canadians. The debate about technology has been intensified, however, by rapid changes in society, in Canadians' values and attitudes in general, and in the context of increasing globalization. Broad changes in society and the changing status of technology as a driving force in society come together in providing the framework within which reproductive decisions are made, individually and collectively. Commissioners were committed to under-standing new reproductive technologies in this Canadian social context, including such factors as sexism, racism, poverty, and other sources of discrimination. We believe that Canadians' values and attitudes must inform any policy decisions in this area.

To gauge Canadians' general attitudes the Commission conducted a series of national surveys measuring Canadians' familiarity with and values in areas related to new reproductive technologies. In total, representative samples involving more than 15 000 Canadians took part in personal interviews, focus groups, phone interviews, and/or answered written questionnaires. As well, Canadians from across the country attended public hearings and private sessions, sent written submissions or letters of opinion, and gave us their thoughts on our toll-free telephone lines. In all, more than 40 000* individuals contributed to the work of the Commission. Their contributions added immeasurably to the depth and the breadth of our understanding of Canadians' perceptions of technology in general and new reproductive technologies in particular, providing an

---

* Our consultations, communications, and research are discussed in Chapter 6, "Developing a Comprehensive Picture of Technologies and Practices."

important guide to, and source of wisdom about, the limits of what is ethically acceptable.

From Canadians' input, from survey research, and from analytic research projects, the Commission gained a sense of the values and attitudes that will carry Canada into the twenty-first century and that must form a context for all public policy decisions. We discuss these trends in the first part of this chapter. An over-riding theme emerging from this discussion is the need to consider reproductive technologies from the perspectives of the various groups and individuals who make up Canadian society. Therefore, in the second part of the chapter, we examine the impact of new reproductive technologies on these various sectors and groups. The issues concerning new reproductive technologies are not uniform, nor is Canadian society: both are diverse. Here we provide an overview of these complex issues, and we examine the implications of this diversity in much greater detail in Part Two of our report.

Technology and Society

Society has become fascinated by and dependent on science and technology, yet most people would be hard pressed to explain how many technologies work, let alone the scientific principles that underlie them. Scientific and technological advances have expanded the knowledge gap between technology experts and technology consumers. As a result, although public attitudes of 40 years ago — captured in the phrase "better living through modern technology" — are still prevalent, there are also increasing concerns about scientists "playing God" and technologies "tampering with nature." There is a growing unease on the part of some that the "genie has been let out of the bottle," and technology will never be "contained" again.

People are also recognizing that technological developments can give rise to unexpected problems, some of them very difficult to solve. Environmental degradation resulting from use of agricultural and industrial technologies is one example of unanticipated technological fallout. This has led to greater awareness that the cost of achieving short-term goals is sometimes long-term damage to the physical environment and resource base. By analogy, the complexity and delicacy of the human reproductive system necessitate a strong element of caution when scientific or technological intervention is contemplated, because of the risk of unintended or unforeseeable consequences. For example, the Commission heard from many people with concerns about the potential of reproductive technologies to change the genetic make-up of individuals and to change social relationships. Some people expressed concerns that technology in general, and medical developments in particular, are moving too fast for society.

National Surveys of Canadians' Attitudes Conducted by the Commission

Reproductive Technologies — Qualitative Research: Summary of Observations (*Angus Reid Group*)

Between May 15 and May 27, 1990, researchers conducted telephone interviews with a representative cross section of 1 503 Canadians. Respondents were asked about their knowledge, opinions, and perceptions concerning new reproductive technologies and the ethical, social, and economic issues concerning them.

Social Values and Attitudes of Canadians Toward New Reproductive Technologies (*Decima Research*)

Between December 1991 and July 1992, researchers conducted phone interviews with a representative sample of 7 664 Canadians, 2 722 of whom also completed a written questionnaire, which asked about the importance of family and children in the lives of Canadians, perceptions of social pressure to have children, and feelings and attitudes toward new reproductive technologies. The survey was controlled for demographic factors such as age, ethnicity, and region. Researchers also investigated the specific attitudes of Aboriginal peoples and members of racial and cultural minority communities by conducting 10 focus groups with members of these communities.

Canada Health Monitor (*Price Waterhouse*)

The Canada Health Monitor is an ongoing, semi-annual telephone survey of the Canadian population. One of its main purposes is to track the attitudes and behaviour of Canadians in a number of health-related areas, and each Canada Health Monitor survey has a "special theme" to investigate a specific subject more deeply. During 1991, two surveys (Canada Health Monitor #6 and #7) were devoted to "Health Issues Affecting Women." The Commission helped design a number of survey questions to determine attitudes toward the use of new reproductive technologies, attitudes toward adoption, and attitudes and perceptions of issues related to health care and the Canadian health care system. Canada Health Monitor #6 surveyed a representative sample of 2 723 Canadians, 15 years of age and older, between August and November 1991, with additional interviews on February 27 and 28, 1992. Canada Health Monitor #7 surveyed a representative sample of 2 725 Canadians, 15 years of age and older, between December 1991 and February 1992.

Survey of Ethnocultural Communities (*Shyla Dutt*)

This survey of 100 key representatives from ethnospecific and ethnocultural women's communities sought out the views and unique concerns of those sectors of the population with regard to new reproductive technologies. The qualitative summary of results showed that attitudes expressed by organizations reflected patterns similar to those in the general public.

An ambivalence toward technology was also apparent in the Commission's survey of values and attitudes. Although attitudes toward technological developments in general were quite positive, the data suggest that respondents tend to be more wary of specific procedures arising from these developments. A clear majority — 70 percent — said they welcomed new scientific developments, and 60 percent said they do not fear the impact of scientific developments (versus 30 and 40 percent who expressed reservations or fear). However, the number of respondents expressing caution, fear, or scepticism, when added to the number who said they had insufficient information on which to base an answer, rose to about half of all respondents as the survey questions became more specific ("I worry that medical science is moving too fast for our society to maintain control over its use"; "I worry that the medical technologies used to assist people to have children are not safe enough").

Ambivalence was again evident in responses to this statement: "I believe that even though there are some processes of human life, such as birth, that we increasingly know more about, we are not meant to alter these processes." Forty-two percent of respondents agreed with the statement, while 37 percent disagreed; the remaining respondents were neutral. What is noteworthy is that respondents were more likely to agree strongly (22 percent) than to disagree strongly (14 percent).

A national survey of ethnocultural communities also revealed a certain hesitation toward technology. Here too there was a strong feeling that medical science is moving too quickly for society to be able to control it. In addition to these concerns, minority groups expressed fears that technology could be used to exploit their members or to divide their communities. In discussions with Aboriginal people, Commissioners heard concerns that traditions passed on for centuries could be threatened.

> There was strong agreement for the suggestion that "medical science is moving too fast for our society to have control over its use" ... Those who had placed a higher value on preventing infertility also felt uncomfortable about the speed of medical innovation.
>
> There was virtually unanimous support for the statement "our community is more concerned with access to basic health care and overcoming discrimination than with technology to assist in reproduction." Only one respondent disagreed.
>
> S. Dutt, "Survey of Ethnocultural Communities on New Reproductive Technologies," in Research Volumes of the Commission, 1993.

In summary, the Commission's surveys of values and attitudes found that most Canadians are supportive of using technology to help people have children, even while having some concerns about the problems associated with their present or potential use. Concerns revolved around the health risks of the technologies and a general sense that technology is moving too fast at too great a cost to society. As we learned during our public consultations, Canadians are also aware of the ethical dilemmas raised by the existence of the technologies. Although in some cases this range of concerns led to calls for a moratorium on new reproductive technologies, as discussed in Chapter 1, many respondents, despite their concerns, did not want to deny the potential benefits of the technologies to those who wish to use them. For example, 73 percent of those surveyed agreed with the statement that "if the technology to assist people to have children is available, people should have the right to use it." In addition, there is a small group of Canadians who find new reproductive technologies unacceptable in principle and who believe that the risks to society far outweigh the potential individual benefits from their use.

Unquestionably, the challenge for Canadian society is to gather information about how specific technologies affect individuals and social groups, so that the attendant medical and psychosocial risks and benefits can be identified. This is particularly important for technologies that affect human biological processes and have the potential to affect how our society evolves.

Globalization

Technological development results in the blurring of national boundaries. This globalization received relatively little attention in earlier inquiries into new reproductive technologies. As with many endeavours that depend on the growth and dissemination of knowledge, what happens in the field of new reproductive technologies in one country affects developments in other countries — no country can isolate itself from events elsewhere in the world. We need to know how the actions of other countries with respect to the technologies may influence developments in Canada and how Canadian actions can influence other countries. Several aspects of globalization raised important issues for the Commission.

For instance, research done in one area of the world results in medical procedures and knowledge being exported to other areas through international conferences, journals, and movement of personnel — the scientific and medical community is global in membership and scope. It would be an abdication of ethical responsibility, however, to condone unethical research carried out elsewhere in the world, while prohibiting it in one's own country, and then to permit the results to be used to benefit one's own population. This "ethical dumping" has been criticized for exposing people in less developed countries to risks for the benefit of those in the developed world.

Given increased globalization and its implications, international cooperation is needed in the area of reproductive technologies, in forms such as harmonization of national regulations and record-keeping systems. Canada has an opportunity and a responsibility to contribute to the debate on the ethical, legal, social, and economic issues and their relevance in an international context. We believe that the appointment of this Commission — involving a commitment of time and resources thus far unmatched by any other country and leading to development of an extensive program of public consultation and original research — was a significant step in this direction.

Equality

As attitudes toward technology and society are changing, so too are Canadians' notions of equality and tolerance. This is reflected not only in constitutional and legislative arenas, such as the introduction of the *Canadian Charter of Rights and Freedoms* and various human rights laws, but also in workplace and other policies designed to promote more equitable opportunities for participation in society.

> With respect to the orientation of research and services and restrictions on practices, what we are recommending is that an international committee be set up under the auspices of a worldwide organization, the WHO [World Health Organization] for instance, which would exercise control at the international level over the orientation of research and restrictions on practices. This issue, which is being discussed here in Canada, in France, in the United States, is one that should be debated throughout the world — we cannot allow it to be discussed by only the industrialized countries. [Translation]
>
> *C. Coderre, Fédération des femmes du Québec, Public Hearings Transcripts, Montreal, Quebec, November 21, 1990.*

To gain a greater understanding of Canadians' general outlook with regard to a sense of tolerance and equality, the Commission's national survey of values and attitudes included several items asking about the principle of equality, attitudes toward immigration and the extent to which Canadians welcome others to our society, tolerance levels for homosexual relationships, and general attitudes toward women and women's role in society.

Most Canadians surveyed believed that all people should be treated equally. In fact, 90 percent agreed with the statement that "every individual should be treated equally regardless of ethnic origin, colour, religion, sex, age, or mental or physical disability," with over two-thirds of respondents strongly agreeing with this statement.

The majority of Canadians felt that equality between the sexes in terms of opportunities has not yet arrived. In our survey, for example, 69 percent of those interviewed agreed with the statement that "the opportunities for women are not equal to the opportunities for men in our society," while 18 percent disagreed and 13 percent neither agreed nor disagreed. Seventy-six percent of respondents indicated that they believe that women gaining more power and influence in the workforce has a positive impact on society, while 6 percent said that the impact has been negative, and 16 percent saw the impact as neither positive nor negative.

Survey respondents not only agree with the concept of equality of all individuals, most also believe that, as a society, Canadians welcome new immigrants from around the world. Two-thirds of respondents strongly agreed (30 percent) or agreed (36 percent) with the statement, "Canada welcomes people from different races, religions and cultures into society."

Although most people surveyed said they believed in the concept of equality, responses to specific issues of tolerance and acceptance varied. For example, with regard to acceptance of homosexual relationships, 35 percent of respondents believe they are acceptable; 21 percent had no opinion one way or another; 16 percent said they are unacceptable; and 27 percent found them totally unacceptable.

Pluralism and Diversity

Recognition of the need for more equitable participation in national life is reflected in increased awareness about human rights. The cumulative effect of these changes is that a more diverse range of voices is beginning to be taken into account in Canadian affairs. As a society based on immigration, Canada has seen a dramatic broadening of its cultural make-up, particularly in the past 30 years. Succeeding waves of immigrants are transforming labour markets, schoolrooms, and neighbourhoods of Canada's cities, especially in the large urban centres. Along with this greater cultural diversity have come new perceptions and new attitudes toward family, kinship, and parenthood.

It is our firm belief that it is our duty to future generations that we take actions today that are directed towards ending existing inequalities in society. We see the role of this Commission to recommend just such actions, actions that protect the interests of the most exploited and oppressed sectors of our society today.

S. Thobani, Immigrant and Visible Minority Women of British Columbia, Public Hearings Transcripts, Vancouver, British Columbia, November 26, 1990.

The trend toward diversity tells us something about what twenty-first-century Canada will be like and has significant implications for society's response to new reproductive technologies. For example, ethical questions related to use of some of the technologies will not be resolved by referring to an unchanging common set of social beliefs, assumptions, and values. Nor can we assume that established ways of setting priorities, making decisions, developing policies, and delivering services will be adequate to the task of accommodating Canadians' diverse aspirations and goals. Yet this is precisely what more and more Canadians expect of their systems and institutions — that they should not only listen to a more diverse range of voices but also embrace and accommodate diversity through their structures, personnel, and decisions.   As Canada becomes more heterogeneous, it will become increasingly important to make core values transparent and to ensure that consensus on technologies takes into account the diverse nature of the country.

Empowerment

There is a general belief in Canada that decisions about technology in general, and new reproductive technologies in particular, should be made in the context of common values and opinions, and with full public participation. Our inquiry into new reproductive technologies was sensitive to this growing trend toward empowerment.

"Empowerment" literally means the investing of power and authority. For many Canadians, the word has come to mean enabling or equipping individuals or groups to have power, with the aim of creating and fostering relationships of equals in society. Several developments reflect this new attention to equality in social relationships. Both nationally and internationally, the past two decades have seen greater emphasis on personal and collective rights. Individuals and groups have become more vocal with respect to their desires and priorities. In turn, such institutions and systems as governments, health care, and education have been striving with varying degrees of success to become more responsive to people's diverse expectations. Empowerment goes beyond this, however; it also requires active participation by these systems' clients and users in decisions that affect them.

On an individual level, empowerment is evident in the development of social trends with particular relevance to the Commission's mandate. Many Canadians are attracted to alternative forms of health and social services, for example, because they are seen as more empowering of the individual than traditional approaches to medical treatment. There has also been significant growth in self-help and mutual support groups dealing with issues once considered the domain of medical and other professionals. In response, people working in medical settings are increasingly endorsing empowerment and are changing their approach to include more information and greater involvement of patients in their own care.

During our public hearings we heard over and over that Canadians want more information to support their decisions about new reproductive technologies. In focus groups, submissions, and private meetings we heard repeatedly about a changing approach to making decisions about medical care, an approach that underscores individuals' need to comprehend their situation, to reflect on it, to understand the risks and benefits of medical treatment, to have all options explained to them, and to be counselled and supported throughout the decision-making process.

The empowerment of individuals thus has implications for traditional doctor/patient relationships. Individuals are no longer as accepting or trustful of "experts," particularly in fields such as medicine where the consumer movement has influenced people's perception of how they can participate in their own care. We found that Canadians are demanding a relationship with practitioners in which they are fully informed of their options — options that may include non-medical, non-interventionist approaches. Users of programs and services want relationships based on

> The fact of the matter is that the disability community feels as though doctors are a real problem, not just in this particular context but in general.
>
> *S. Day, Canadian Disability Rights Council, Public Hearings Transcripts, Vancouver, British Columbia, November 28, 1990.*

partnership rather than the focus on expert opinion that previously characterized such relationships.

The move to empowerment has also given rise, however, to a common perception that access to specific medical treatments is a right, regardless of whether a treatment is appropriate or likely to work or what the costs might be. With respect to new reproductive technologies, individuals often demand access to treatments and technologies as a right, seemingly without regard to the social implications or financial consequences for the health care system. Changes in attitudes and ways of relating to societal institutions therefore present both opportunities and problems, with implications for how and through what structures new reproductive technologies are made available.

> The right to have children is not like the right to have an object or an animal. Children are persons and must be treated as persons. The right to have children is, therefore, better understood as the right to take advantage of opportunities that are open to everyone as a matter of course. When those opportunities are not present, then society has an obligation to assist those who lack the opportunities. When such a lack can be remedied by the development or application of reproductive technologies, then society has a *prima facie* obligation to develop and apply them. However, any societal action in this regard must always be with an eye to the fact that children are persons.
>
> *Brief to the Commission from the Canadian Medical Association, February 1991.*

Advocacy groups present another facet of empowerment. In the health care sector, consumer groups and individuals with a shared condition or situation have organized to press for change in policies, programs, or services, to increase public awareness of an issue or problem, or to demand more effective participation in decisions that affect them. The rise of advocacy groups also reflects more extensive social participation by previously marginalized groups. Policy and law makers are being asked to ensure that the diverse interests, perspectives, and expectations of these various constituencies are taken into account when priorities are set and decisions are made.

Thus, empowerment is both an individual and a collective phenomenon. It is the objective of demands from many individuals and groups — especially but not only women — for a greater voice in decisions that affect them. At the same time, it results in a call for not only individuals but also governments, institutions, the health and education systems, and professionals to be accountable for what they do.

Empowerment has far-reaching implications for policy making. The number of voices at the table has increased, often making it more difficult to reach consensus, and potentially creating unrealistic expectations and heightening social conflict. Frustration with the complexity of trying to reach consensus has sometimes resulted in a backlash against empowerment, expressed as a desire to return to a time when decision making was simpler. Empowerment and participation do complicate the process of governing and of providing services. Nevertheless, equality is now entrenched as a constitutional principle, and Canada has accepted and institutionalized diversity and encouraged individual and group efforts to pursue autonomy, empowerment, and human dignity, even though their achievement is seldom uniform or easy. Pluralism is now enshrined in our constitution: multiculturalism, bilingualism, and the rights of certain groups — specifically women and Aboriginal peoples — are all recognized in the Charter. Society's institutions and decision-making processes must also recognize and incorporate it.

Medicalization

The term medicalization describes a social process — occurring over time — in which behaviours or conditions previously considered outside the realm of medicine became defined as medical concerns. Medicalization has eased suffering, cured disease, saved lives, and enabled couples to have healthy children. Increasing empowerment, however, has created resistance to what some perceive as excessive medicalization. Some think medicalization has contributed to a loss of autonomy by women over their bodies and their reproductive functions and that it has promoted a narrowly defined medical view of complex social problems. As scientific and technical knowledge about women's physiology and reproductive functions expands, so too does the pressure to define

> The medicalized nature of new reproductive technologies (NRTs) ... must be dismantled and reconstructed based on a [holistic] approach to health.
>
> *Brief to the Commission from Students, Women's Studies Course, University of Calgary, April 11, 1991.*

women's experiences in medical terms and to respond to their problems with technical solutions.

The phenomenon of medicalization is illustrated clearly in the evolution of social attitudes and medical practices with respect to women's reproductive experience. Appropriately or inappropriately, many aspects of women's reproductive lives — childbirth, contraception, abortion, premenstrual syndrome, and menopause — have moved into the medical domain. Certain communities are doubly affected by this shift — Aboriginal Canadians, for example, told Commissioners that the medicalization of reproduction has the potential to undermine traditional Aboriginal approaches to fertility, pregnancy, and childbirth.

As with the expansion of technology in other human endeavours, the application of medical technologies to reproduction raises questions about power relationships and who controls the technologies and their use. A key issue in the medicalization of women's reproductive lives is the unequal distribution of power inherent in the doctor/patient relationship. The patient has less technical and medical knowledge than the physician and may tend to surrender personal decision making. This power imbalance places a heavy responsibility on physicians to be aware of its potential consequences and of the need to make information available to patients and to support their decision making without directing it and without infringing on their dignity and autonomy. This is particularly relevant in situations where power imbalances are exacerbated by the fact that the patient is female and the doctor is male. The greater the vulnerability of the patient, the greater the physician's responsibility to use her or his power in the service of the patient.

Even though the goals espoused in the Hippocratic oath involve putting the interests of the patient first, the power imbalance is of concern because the best interests of the woman and what she values may not always be identical to the physician's interests and values. For example, studies have shown that when given full information on which to base a decision about treatment, patients tend to be much more averse to risk than clinicians are;[1] they also may value even the successful outcomes of intervention less than clinicians do.

There are also concerns that the increasingly routine use of some technologies will make it difficult to refuse their use and so will reduce women's scope for decision making and control over their own reproduction. For example, some types of prenatal tests, developed originally to detect disabling conditions in the children of high-risk couples, are now being used more generally and are becoming a routinely offered part of prenatal care. As discussed further in Part Two of our report, some women may feel pressure to have the testing once it becomes routine, despite having religious, cultural, ethical, or other reservations.

One challenge that lies ahead is to increase scientific understanding of reproductive concerns while situating issues of reproductive technology in a larger social context and safeguarding women's personal control over issues that affect them directly and significantly. In some cases of childlessness, the most appropriate response may be medical. In others, individuals and society may be served better by consciously pulling back from medical and technological approaches — we may need to "de-medicalize" our approach. Determining when and how to do this, based on the potential impact of technologies, is one of the issues that has occupied the Commission and should continue to occupy society in the future as existing technologies evolve and new ones develop.

Another fear is that medicalization tends to generate its own momentum — even to the point, some feel, of creating a technological imperative. Some witnesses argued, for example, that new reproductive technologies promote feelings of "obligatory fertility," making it difficult for women to refuse treatment or stop it once begun, and that the technologies are therefore limiting rather than expanding their choices. Alternative non-medical responses, such as adoption, foster parenting, or a decision to accept childlessness, may appear inadequate or unacceptable, they said, when compared to the resolution hoped for from the technologies.

On the other hand, testimony before the Commission also showed that medicalization and medical technology have given some women options that otherwise might not have been available. Many couples who are infertile who appeared before the Commission welcomed knowing there was a medical reason for their condition and said that the availability of the technologies helped them resolve their feelings about it, knowing that everything that could be done had been done. Other positive aspects of a medical approach to infertility include greater attention to the origins of infertility, including environmental causes; recognition of infertility as more than just a "woman's problem"; increased options and alternatives for people who are infertile; and earlier and more precise diagnosis and treatment of infertility problems, with greater likelihood of effective treatment for some causes.

Impact of New Reproductive Technologies on Canadian Society

The trends that have emerged in Canadian society all point to the need for a new approach to decision making about technology, including new reproductive technologies. In an increasingly diverse society, where the interests of more groups and individuals are recognized and attended to, it is becoming more difficult to reach consensus on the difficult issues that must be resolved in all areas of life. This includes decision making about the health care system and new reproductive technologies, as we discuss in Chapter 4. It also raises the issue of the impact of new reproductive technologies on individuals, on identifiable social groups, and on society as a whole. The increasing diversity of Canadian society means that we cannot make assumptions about the impact of new reproductive technologies on society as a whole. Different groups will be affected in different ways by the technologies, and in the remainder of this chapter we discuss the concerns that came to the attention of the Commission through our public hearings, consultations, and research program. In particular, we examine the concerns about the potential of the technologies to affect the health and well-being of women in Canadian society.

We were directed to examine the impact of the technologies on some groups, such as women, children, and families, by the terms of our mandate. Within these main groups, we also looked at other groups, such as people with disabilities and members of racial, ethnic, and cultural minorities, because the nature of their status in Canadian society may result in their being affected differently by the technologies. This section gives a brief overview of this impact. Because the technologies themselves differ as well, with diverse consequences for users and for society, this limits the generalizations that can be drawn. These effects will be examined in greater detail in our discussion of particular technologies in Part Two of our report.

> The social management of motherhood is characterized by a certain inconsistency. While the planet as a whole tries to cope with overpopulation, in Canada our governments continue to worry about falling birth rates. They encourage Canadian women to produce more Canadians and place limits on immigration. People who have the means to have children but are not prepared to pay the price and choose not to have any are often judged as selfish. Access to abortion is barred to women whose health is not at risk. At the same time as governments develop policies to encourage higher birth rates, they make cuts in the social programs on which more and more women and children depend.
>
> *Brief to the Commission from the New Brunswick Advisory Council on the Status of Women, October 19, 1990.*

Impact on Women

The diversity of women's views about new reproductive technologies reflects their various circumstances and experiences. Through the Commission's extensive communication channels, such as toll-free telephone lines, focus groups, roundtables, surveys, and other information vehicles, as well as in our public hearings, we heard the views of many women, sometimes speaking as individuals, sometimes speaking on behalf of their communities.

Women's Reproductive Health and Well-Being

Canadians are raising serious and thoughtful questions about the nature of reproductive technologies and their impact on women's health and well-being. As Commissioners, we had to consider the strong belief on the part of some Canadians that new reproductive technologies are needed to address important problems and that such technologies have opened up new choices for women. In this view, any attempts to curtail development of the technologies are unwarranted, because such an approach assumes that women are not the best judges of what is good for their own reproductive health and well-being. If use of these technologies is restricted "for women's own good," what other areas of women's health care or access to other kinds of services could be affected next?

As well, however, Commissioners had to consider the strong concerns of others about the harmful effects of the technologies on women, individually and collectively. These concerns take several forms. We heard from women that they have not been involved in decisions about the development of new reproductive technologies and the provision of services, and that women's interests have not been represented in the boardrooms and professional forums where these decisions are made. Some feel decisions have been made about technologies and services without considering their adverse consequences for women's autonomy as individuals and their status and value as members of society.

> We understand the urgency felt by women who suffer from infertility, but we also think that the technologies present such enormous questions for our society we have to look at [them] from a broad social perspective, and particularly from a collective perspective as women.
>
> *J. Rebick, National Action Committee on the Status of Women, Public Hearings Transcripts, Toronto, Ontario, October 29, 1990.*

Some of those testifying before the Commission believe that the technologies have not been developed to serve women or to improve their health and well-being; rather, the technologies have increased the ability of doctors and others to control reproduction (medicalization of reproduction). If technologies are to be used in a way that respects women's reproductive autonomy, it is argued, the entire approach to reproduction must change — infertility should be prevented in the first place where possible, and basic reproductive health care should be provided. Indeed, it was argued that greater priority should be given to improving the social and economic conditions of women generally, as only then could new reproductive technologies be used in a way that respects women's reproductive autonomy and sexual equality.

There was also debate about the impact of new reproductive technologies on reproductive choice. Some women believe that in the area of reproductive health, more choice is not necessarily better; they see the availability of such technologies as in fact limiting their choices by making it easier for people to judge women's behaviour and decisions. In this view, society has a collective responsibility to women, which may require limiting choices by individual women if these choices promote harmful social perceptions of womanhood or detrimental attitudes toward women as a group.

> I was struck by the discussion this morning of how difficult it is to get women talking about NRTs when the bread and butter issue is [the] economic situations of women in Newfoundland and Labrador — it seems to be the chief and overriding issue concerning our lives.
>
> *Roundtable Discussion, Public Hearings Transcripts, St. John's, Newfoundland, October 15, 1990.*

Some women think that because women's bodies and social status could be put at risk, women should have the primary role in determining whether new reproductive technologies are socially desirable and, if so, how they should be provided and regulated. Because of women's lack of involvement, they said, new reproductive technologies have been developed by exploiting the genuine desires of those who are infertile, as means by which physicians and researchers achieve career advancement and financial gain — all at the expense of women who experience adverse physical, emotional, or financial consequences as a result of the technologies.

Some women believe strongly that the development and use of new reproductive technologies is a consequence of women's unequal status in society. Just when women are making strides toward independence and equality, it is argued, the advent of new reproductive technologies serves to reinforce the image that women are mothers and nurturers first and foremost. Some analysts contend that new reproductive technologies contribute to devaluation of women in society because they emphasize the societal belief that women's primary role, and the only role for which they should be valued, is reproduction.

We heard that new reproductive technologies could also undermine a holistic view of women's health, if they are delivered in a way that deals only with body parts. This possibility was particularly evident in discussions of commercial preconception agreements, which could contribute to women being seen as "wombs for hire." Similar concerns were expressed about commodification of human reproductive tissues and processes — that is, treating women and children as objects or means to an end rather than as ends in themselves, thereby devaluing their humanity and dignity.

In discussions with Canadians we found concern that focussing public attention and resources on new reproductive technologies could divert attention from reproductive health concerns that affect the majority of women: research into prevention of sexually transmitted diseases (STDs), many of which can lead to infertility; research into and the availability of safe and effective contraception; the availability of safe and effective abortion; family planning services; elimination of workplace hazards to reproductive and general health; health promotion activities; and pre- and post-natal care. New reproductive technologies were seen to shift scarce research and health care dollars from these other health concerns.

This view emphasizes the need to focus public attention and resources on reproductive health care as a continuum. If assessed within the framework of women's reproductive health care needs as a whole (from puberty to post-menopause), new reproductive technologies could be seen as one of many reproductive health issues. Given that avoidance of reproductive dysfunction is one of the objectives of reproductive health care, society could seek to eliminate the preventable medical conditions that lead to infertility. In this view it would preclude the need for people to seek treatment in the form of new reproductive technologies.

Concerns from Particular Groups of Women

Many women from different groups expressed concern over access to both basic health care services and new reproductive technologies. These women had concerns specific to the personal and collective issues within their group.

Aboriginal women told us about the lack of basic health and education services and felt that these should take priority over new reproductive technologies. They also said that new reproductive technologies must be offered in ways that are culturally and linguistically appropriate to the communities being served. Aboriginal peoples have unique ways of viewing children in their communities, resulting in different ways of dealing with childlessness, such as custom adoption (where the child remains in the community and in contact with her or his family and cultural origins).

> I believe that there should be national standards but I would also make a fervent plea that those standards reflect the diversity of people in Canada. Those standards should not be used in my mind as a controlling mechanism but one that would respect the interests of people like the aboriginal people in Canada ... who are at this time and have always been very concerned about maintaining themselves as distinct national peoples in Canada.
>
> *M. Dion Stout, President, Indian and Inuit Nurses of Canada, Public Hearings Transcripts, Ottawa, Ontario, September 20, 1990.*

Some felt new reproductive technologies could undermine such traditional approaches.

Women from racial, ethnic, and linguistic minority groups told us they often have difficulty gaining access to basic health care services and information in culturally appropriate ways. Such basic services, they told us, should be the priority and are generally more important than access to new reproductive technologies. Where new reproductive technologies are provided, intervenors said, there should be equal access to the technologies, without either individual or systemic discrimination. They feared that they may be denied the benefits of these technologies and instead encouraged to control their fertility.

There were concerns throughout the country that access to new reproductive technologies is easier for affluent white couples, and that minority or low-income people are seen as less deserving of access. Indeed, for women who are economically disadvantaged, access to basic health care services is a priority, but we heard the view that if new reproductive technologies are to be made available there should be equal access regardless of income. Also, linguistic and cultural barriers often reduce access to the technologies for many. In fact, in focus groups, submissions, and presentations, many intervenors identified a need for culturally and linguistically appropriate counselling and information.

Intervenors also noted the disproportionately negative impact of judicial intervention in pregnancy on women from racial and ethnic minorities (discussed in Chapter 30). Some said that minority women are more vulnerable to judicial controls such as court-ordered sterilizations or other interventions. Some noted women's vulnerability to pressure from sex selection

New reproductive technologies have the potential to radically change the way we think about reproduction, sexuality and parenting. However, there are existing biases that are already operating and have determined the way in which NRTs are applied.

The values which presently make an impact on NRTs are largely those of the medical establishment, who are predominantly male, disability-phobic, white, middle class and heterosexual. For example, in vitro fertilization is presently accessible only to qualified women; that is, women under 40 who are in a stable, long-term heterosexual relationship and who can afford the expense.

IVF candidates must conform to stereotypical notions of what kind of woman makes a good mother. Women with disabilities, poor women, single women and lesbians do not quite fit this conception of the ideal wife and mother.

B. Van't Slot, Women's Network, Public Hearings Transcripts, Charlottetown, Prince Edward Island, October 16, 1990.

in some cultural communities (discussed in Chapter 28). Still others underlined the danger of exploitation of women of lower socioeconomic status through preconception arrangements (Chapter 23) or through financial incentives for reproductive functions such as egg donation (see Chapter 21), emphasizing the potential for dual exploitation because of both socioeconomic status and minority status. These particular concerns were accompanied by broader concerns about the difficulty of assessing the implications of the technologies for groups or communities in the absence of more extensive public knowledge and discussion about them.

Single women and lesbians fear that restrictive access to assisted insemination may deny them the opportunity to have children by this means. Medicalization of assisted insemination and restrictions against self-insemination are seen as unnecessary impediments to access to safe sperm for self-insemination.

Women in rural and remote areas are concerned about geographic distances and travel costs. They are also concerned that devoting scarce resources to new reproductive technologies may divert them from more urgent health care requirements. We discuss these and other issues of equitable access to services in greater detail in Part Two in the context of our examination of specific technologies.

Women who have had negative experiences with reproductive interventions sounded warnings about unexpected consequences of technology. They cautioned that reproductive interventions used today may have negative health repercussions in future and emphasized the need for data about the short- and long-term psychological and physical health risks of new reproductive technologies and their overall safety and efficacy.

At the same time, women with fertility problems and women at risk of passing on a genetic disease emphasized their needs and their ability to make decisions in their own best interests, provided they have complete and accurate information about associated risks and expected outcomes. Women with fertility problems talked about the importance to their lives in the long term of having children, and stressed their desire for more public awareness of the emotional and societal issues related to infertility and its prevention and possible treatment. Reproductive freedom, they asserted, was dependent upon equal access to the technologies as well as information and counselling for those who are infertile. They identified difficulties in access due to cost of treatment and availability of services.

As is clear from this brief review of testimony before the Commission, not all women see the development and use of new reproductive technologies in the same way. This is not surprising, given the diversity of women's backgrounds, experiences, and life circumstances. From one perspective, the existence of the technologies offers women who are infertile, families at risk of congenital anomalies or genetic disease in their children, or individuals suffering from Parkinson disease some hope and an opportunity to improve their well-being.

From another perspective, however, discussions of new reproductive technologies should focus on broad societal concerns and the interests of women as a social group. In this view, the good of society as a whole rather than the choices of individuals should guide the assessment of such technologies. The collective interests of women as a social group should take precedence over the interests of individual women, the argument continues, the interests of society as a whole over the interests of families at risk. Consequently, the criteria to evaluate the use of new reproductive technologies should be the probable effects on women's autonomy, equality, and status in society. Still others argued for evaluation of new reproductive technologies with the best interests of the resulting child and families in general as the paramount consideration.

On reflection, it is clear that these are not separable alternatives: both individual and collective interests must be taken seriously in a humane and caring society. We have sought to demonstrate this in the chapters that follow.

Impact on Children

Children born as a result of reproductive technologies were the second group identified in the Commission's mandate. Technologies using donated gametes (eggs, sperm, or both) are creating new kinds of family and social relationships. Traditional notions of biological and kinship ties are called into question as a result, because the concept of family has never before included the situations that are emerging through the use of new technologies.

In addition to social relationships, we are concerned about the possible impact of these technologies on the health, emotional well-being, legal status, and economic circumstances of children and their families. These effects will differ from technology to technology and with the circumstances under which a given technology is used. Each of these areas is considered more fully in Part Two.

The other groups that must be taken into account in considering the impact of the use or non-use of new reproductive

> Historically, the family unit has been premised on the "traditional" family form existing as a result of a legally sanctioned marriage. The principles and definitions governing the law of filiation assume that reproduction occurs within either a marital relationship or a stable heterosexual relationship and it usually perpetuates this bias. In addition, the rules of law reflect an assumption that reproduction occurs only through sexual intercourse, an assumption greatly challenged by the various forms of assisted reproduction.
>
> *E. Sloss and R. Mykitiuk, "The Challenge of the New Reproductive Technologies to Family Law," in Research Volumes of the Commission, 1993.*

technologies include couples who are infertile; couples at risk of congenital anomalies or a genetic disease in their children; and donors of sperm, eggs, and embryos and their families. The consequences for these individuals may be physical, psychological, financial, and legal; these effects vary significantly with the type of technology used, yet significant gaps remain in our knowledge of the exact nature and extent of these consequences.

There is a dearth of information about, for instance, the direct outcomes of being conceived through assisted reproduction. Physical outcomes are important to monitor, but there may also be emotional and psychological outcomes to being born through the use of assisted methods of conception. For instance, we know very little about the effect on a child's sense of identity and belonging of being born through assisted insemination using donor sperm or following *in vitro* fertilization using donated eggs. Very often, these practices are surrounded by secrecy, with many parents not wanting to tell their children about their biological origins.

Little is known about the long-term outcomes of being born through donor insemination (DI) — a Commission study of donor insemination found only one published follow-up study (carried out in Japan in 1968) of children conceived through DI. Other reports about the long-term outcomes tend to be based on case studies or very small samples. Once again, without concrete information, all we can do is infer from what we know about children in analogous situations — adoptees. We know now, for example, that adopted children often experience a powerful urge to seek information about their biological parents and to know about their genetic and cultural heritage — "genealogical bewilderment" was a term coined as long ago as 1952 to describe the adjustment problems experienced by a substantial proportion of adopted children who had no information about their biological origins.

Impact on Family Structure

Many of the recent changes in society converge in a single social structure: the family. The "traditional" family (two parents and a child or children) was for many generations the most common family structure in Canada. However, an array of new family forms has emerged during this century. Family forms that were once rare or socially unacceptable — one-parent families, common-law unions, blended families, same-sex couples, childless couples — are becoming more common. It has become more common and widely accepted for both parents to work outside the home. The increasing diversity of Canadian society means that the Eurocentric notion of the nuclear family is less dominant than it once was. Perceptions about the importance and nature of family relationships are changing. These new family forms are the result of emerging trends in family formation. Factors in these changes include a trend toward marrying at a later age; a decline in the total number of marriages; and rising rates of divorce and remarriage — all of which have implications for fertility and therefore for new reproductive technologies.

In the Commission's national survey of values and attitudes, we explored some attitudes toward these various family forms. Results of the focus groups conducted in preparation for the survey indicated that a heterosexual married couple with children was what most participants considered to be a family; other family structures were acknowledged, but what was fundamental to most participants' perceptions of a family was the presence of children.

We are particularly concerned about the family, which is the main building block of our society. Any society for that matter. If Canada is to be strong we must build strong families. The family is now facing new and confusing pressures. The breakdown of the family unit is a significant reason in our view for the disorder we are witnessing in our nation at the present time.

H. Hilsden, Pentecostal Assemblies of Canada, Public Hearings Transcripts, Toronto, Ontario, November 20, 1990.

For example, when asked whether a man and a woman living common law without children constitutes a family, in the national survey 47 percent said it does not, while 24 percent said it depends, and 25 percent said it does. A homosexual couple without children was considered a family by 13 percent of respondents, whereas a homosexual couple with children was considered a family by 37 percent of respondents. Our survey found that, overall, women are more accepting than men of a wider range of family forms. A single man or woman with children was considered a family by 65 percent of those surveyed. These responses suggest the importance of the presence of children in defining a family. Further, our survey of ethnocultural communities revealed that children were seen as important in carrying on cultural and ethnic heritage.

Although the traditional family is still considered the social norm, this perception is changing gradually. Research has demonstrated little support for the contention that any one family structure is essential for the well-being of children. In fact, studies point to other factors — such as the environment of the family (its economic and emotional well-being), the quality of relationships within the family, the time and energy family members have to devote to family life, and the availability of support systems in the form of extended family and networks of friends — as being more important to a child's well-being than any particular family structure.

In discussions with members of visible minorities, Aboriginal communities, and the general public, the consensus was that no one single type of family structure was ideal for the well-being of children. As one participant noted, "What is important is how you bring them [the children] up ... and the morals you teach them." There was a sense that the family is the vehicle through which values are passed on to children. Examples we heard of specific values that should be communicated and learned through the family included respect for others, self-respect, decency, how to work hard, and religion.

If "traditional" families continue to be seen as the norm, however, society may decide to restrict access to new reproductive technologies to those who conform to this view, despite the fact that non-traditional families are increasingly common. New reproductive technologies could play a role in facilitating the addition of children to non-traditional families as well as to traditional families.

> Aboriginal children were perceived as the greatest gifts given to aboriginal women by the Creator. Children were always given privileged and special status in the North American aboriginal family. They were showered with affection, kindness and attention not only by their biological parents, but by all clan members, siblings, and members of the extended family.
>
> *M. Dion Stout, President, Indian and Inuit Nurses of Canada, Public Hearings Transcripts, Ottawa, Ontario, September 20, 1990.*

Impact on People with Disabilities

People with disabilities are also concerned that the use of such technologies may heighten negative societal attitudes toward disability generally. In particular, they think the use of prenatal diagnosis to identify fetuses with anomalies, possibly leading to abortion, creates a dangerous environment for people with disabilities. As testing becomes more common, will parents face societal disapproval if they knowingly bring a child with disabilities into the world? There are also concerns that the focus on prenatal diagnosis may divert resources from providing support to people with disabilities and their families. These issues are examined in greater detail throughout our discussion of prenatal diagnosis in Part Two.

> Will disabled women who are the poorest of the poor be able to gain access to the infertility clinics? Are the clinics even wheelchair accessible? What if a deaf woman came in and needed sign language? Would a doctor [look] at the same old stereotypes of disabled women and feel that they should not even try to have a baby? And many people feel that way when disabled women even think of getting pregnant.
>
> *P. Israel, DisAbled Women's Network Canada, Public Hearings Transcripts, Toronto, Ontario, October 31, 1990.*

For women with disabilities, new reproductive technologies raise two main concerns: access to services, and the effects of prenatal diagnosis on society's attitudes toward disability. Many women with disabilities have the same desire to bear children as others and argue that they should have equal access to technologies where they are provided. Indeed, the very nature of some disabilities may mean that women will require assistance in order to have children. Thus, they said, disability should not be a factor used to screen out potential candidates for services involving new reproductive technologies.

Impact on Society

In light of the potential for new reproductive technologies to affect society as a whole, certain questions arise. How will they change our understanding of how to relate to each other as members of society? How will we define social relationships such as families, parents, siblings, and generations? The Commission is concerned with these questions not only as they affect current relationships in society but also as they affect how our society evolves. Our assessments of the potential harms and benefits of new reproductive technologies covered a broad range of considerations, including, among others, the need to avoid harm to future generations from either using or failing to pursue a given technology or practice. This is particularly relevant, for example, when we consider the potential of some of the technologies, such as research involving the use of fetal tissue to treat diseases that affect many Canadians.

> The scope and magnitude of the issues before this Commission [are] truly staggering. What you are attempting to examine goes to the heart of what we are as humans. The questions raised by these new technologies [challenge] each of us in very fundamental ways about our views of life, ethics and morality. The solutions we find will define us as individuals and as a society.
>
> *A. Lie-Nielsen, Executive Director, Prince Edward Island Council of the Disabled, Public Hearings Transcripts, Charlottetown, Prince Edward Island, October 16, 1990.*

Although the individuals on whom new reproductive technologies have a direct impact remain a minority in society, their collective experiences still have the capacity to influence broader societal values and norms, just as the collective experiences of any identifiable social group can influence how society perceives and responds to a particular issue. For example, how society views and values adoption has been affected by the collective experience of those involved in it. Adoption was once shrouded in secrecy, with a certain social stigma attached — for the adoptive parents, for the adoptee, and for the woman who "gave up" or "surrendered" a child for adoption. Increasingly, however, public calls by adoptees for access to information about their biological parents, as well as media stories about how adoptees have re-established relationships with biological parents — often encouraged by their adoptive parents — have expanded our understanding of the social circumstances that lead to adoption.

Similarly, the increasing number of children born through assisted insemination or *in vitro* fertilization has created greater awareness of these ways of having children and is influencing how society sees these children; it may also result in different views on the technologies that brought them into being. We need to consider what impact, if any, there will be on the demographics of the family. Is it likely that the number of single-parent families or non-traditional two-parent families will increase because of increased availability of donor gametes? How would children be affected as a result? Various individuals and groups are bound to see these issues in different ways, depending on their position or status in society, their values, their knowledge of the technologies, their interests in the use of the technologies, and a host of other factors.

In the absence of specific laws and regulations — which are society's concrete expression of collective decisions — decision making by individuals, practitioners, and public policy makers will be shaped by an interplay of individual and group views and perceptions about technology in general. This interplay also will affect how specific laws and regulations are eventually made. But experience shows that laws and regulations tend to lag behind knowledge and knowledge-based developments by a decade or more, just as the process of change in social institutions lags behind changes in social realities. Furthermore, by the time change in law occurs, new developments may well have rendered it obsolete.

Thus, there is an ongoing iterative process — the origins and use of new reproductive technologies have implications for society, which in turn shape decisions about provision of and access to the technologies. As these decisions are implemented, a fresh set of social conditions evolves in which new or modified technologies may develop, and new societal responses will be required.

We are filled with compassion for the infertile couple who wants to have a child and cannot give birth through the normal, natural process. These couples should have recourse to alternative methods of reproduction.

We have outlined our concerns in this brief, as we are apprehensive about the speed with which these new techniques are evolving.

The Committee is focusing on the consequences, both good and bad, of NRTs on future generations. We wanted to bring up concerns in connection with a social issue. Even though, because of our age, we are not directly affected by NRTs, we believe that they will have an impact on the family structure. [Translation]

Brief to the Commission from Le comité "Vieillir au féminin" de l'Université du troisième âge de l'Université de Moncton, January 18, 1991.

A New Approach to Decisions About Technology

As we have seen throughout this chapter, new reproductive technologies have a varying impact on different sectors of society; members of some sectors are affected much more directly and profoundly than others, but some changes will affect all of society. Depending on whether and how some technologies are used, they could contribute to making Canada a more caring or a less caring society. Public policy should be developed with these implications in mind; this is the perspective that informed the Commission's approach to assessing the technologies and developing our recommendations.

Society does not have to be driven by technological change; we have choices about how to control technologies to ensure that, if they are used, it is in beneficial ways and in ways that avoid or minimize their adverse consequences. It is society's responsibility to see to it that knowledge gained from science develops in a way that is beneficent, along directions most likely to have humane and advantageous consequences.[2]

New reproductive technologies are a specific instance of this general position — that society has a responsibility to determine the place and uses of technology. From the Commission's perspective, society's approach to technology must be balanced in its orientation and solidly grounded in experience and identified needs. Despite growing unease about technology, particularly when it touches on the life sciences and medicine, and deep concern that new powers to intervene in human lives yield the potential for abuse or inappropriate application, it is possible to approach these issues based on careful examination and weighing of the evidence.

This approach identifies several considerations: first, society's need and responsibility to control the development and use or non-use of technologies in light of broader ethical, social, economic, and other concerns; second, within this context of societal control, the need for individuals to be able to make informed choices with respect to their own use or non-use of a technology. Dealing with technology effectively and appropriately means taking the broad view (all of society) and the long view (over more than one generation) without losing sight of the individual. This suggests that more voices and perspectives than before need to be involved in making decisions about technology — among others, members of the public, experts, and those experiencing or affected by the technologies.

Between the extremes of unquestioning acceptance and outright rejection of new reproductive technologies is an approach based on a step-by-step examination of evidence regarding the origins, current practices, outcomes, and implications of, and alternatives to, specific technologies. The result may be that some technologies are encouraged, others are regulated or restricted, and some are banned altogether. This evidence-based evaluation must be done in the context of the technologies' broader implications for individuals and for society as a whole. If we ignore their implications, or allow them to proceed without discussion of their positive and negative aspects, new reproductive technologies could bring about changes that contradict or clash with society's values and beliefs, and we will become a less tolerant and caring society as a result.

The Commission intends to contribute to the social debate about the implications of new reproductive technologies by promoting public discussion of their social impact that is well informed and based on accurate information. We have tried to ensure that the needs and interests of all groups and individuals in society have been taken into account in our discussions and thinking about new reproductive technologies to minimize, whenever possible, any inadvertent negative consequences. We frame the discussion in terms of our guiding principles, with the ethic of care as a context, as we set out in Chapter 3, and have focussed on evidence-based medicine, as discussed in Chapter 4. We intend to provide a policy-oriented approach to new reproductive technologies that can also be used as a framework for developing public policy on other emerging technologies. We are confident that this approach can increase the likelihood that new reproductive technologies are provided and used only in ways that coincide with the values and priorities of Canadian society and that, where they are used, they are used responsibly and with care.

Specific References

1. Wennberg, J.E. "Sounding Board: Outcomes Research, Cost Containment, and the Fear of Health Care Rationing." *New England Journal of Medicine* 323 (October 25, 1990), p. 1203.

2. Polanyi, J. "The Responsible Scientist." *Oyez*[3] 4 (2)(Fall 1992): 12-14.

What Guided Our Deliberations: Ethical Framework and Guiding Principles

♦

Given the range and complexity of the issues before us, it was vital to develop a way for Commissioners with varying backgrounds and life experiences to approach the technologies — to establish a framework for decision making. How new reproductive technologies are controlled and regulated will affect the way people think about their rights and responsibilities to each other and to future generations. It was therefore necessary for Commissioners to develop an explicit and consistent ethical approach to examining these implications and making decisions; it would also enable us to make clear to others the reasoning and basis for our recommendations.

The process through which we developed this approach and the shape it took are the subject of this chapter, which describes the ethical framework and guiding principles that informed and infused our deliberations as we worked toward our recommendations. Our goal is to ensure that the reasoning behind our recommendations is clear to policy makers, to those working in the field, and to Canadians generally. As we examine individual technologies and the issues they raise in Part Two of our report, the relationship between the ethical principles described here and the real-life dilemmas facing individuals and society as we consider the use or non-use of technologies will also become clear.

We considered two basic approaches. One approach involves choosing an overarching ethical theory, such as utilitarianism, natural law, or contractarianism. These theories, which are examined in greater detail in research studies and background papers prepared for the Commission (see research volume, *New Reproductive Technologies: Ethical Aspects*), postulate a single overarching rule or ideal that can be used to resolve moral debates. A second approach uses a broader ethical orientation —

called the ethic of care — and, within that orientation, a set of guiding principles to serve as a prism for moral deliberations.

We adopted the second approach. Three factors influenced our decision. First, adopting a single overarching theory generally requires rejecting the others when in fact they have substantial areas of agreement — for example, as we discuss later, a commitment to a moral point of view. In addition, the relative merits of these theories have been the subject of philosophical debate for centuries — there is no reason to think that this can be resolved in the near future, and certainly not by this Commission.

Second, there are immense difficulties in applying general theories to the complex issues raised by new reproductive technologies. It is often extremely difficult to draw a direct, clear, and uncontroversial line from the very general concepts found in a given ethical theory to the specific circumstances of particular ethical decisions. The long distance from theory to application can often create irresolvable differences. Indeed, the level of disagreement *within* each of these schools of thought on particular issues of reproductive technology is often as great as the level of disagreement *between* the various schools.

Finally, overarching ethical frameworks like utilitarianism or social contract theory often are premised, in one way or another, on an understanding of human nature that sees people as individuals first and foremost, protecting their own interests against the encroachment of others. Yet human beings are connected to one another in families, communities, and social bonds of all sorts. People connected in these ways care for one another and seek one another's welfare, knowing that people cannot enjoy rights and interests by themselves. In our view, an ethical perspective that gives priority to this mutual care and connectedness and tries to foster it is particularly helpful. The ethic of care means that a large part of ethical deliberation is concerned with how to build relationships and prevent conflict, rather than being concerned only with resolving conflicts that have already occurred.

Obviously, conflict cannot be prevented entirely; no ethical stance could ensure that. It is therefore important to have not only an ethical perspective that fosters care and community but also guiding principles to cast light on issues when conflicts do arise. Each principle sheds a different kind of light on the options available. Reaching moral decisions often involves considering more than one of these principles, as usually more than one will be relevant to the situation. Moral reasoning requires consideration of whether and how each of the principles applies, all within the overall perspective of the ethic of care. This approach seeks to prevent adversarial situations whenever possible; yet the guiding principles are in place to act as a sort of bottom line of social justice when all else fails. The reasons that led the Commission to adopt this approach are discussed in more detail in this chapter.

One of the difficulties we saw with adopting one traditional overarching ethical theory was that it would focus attention on the differences between the various theories. We thought it was more useful to focus on what these theories have in common, including a commitment to a moral point of view. All the traditional overarching theories agree that there is such a thing as a moral perspective on issues — a perspective that is distinct from a self-interested or economic perspective — and that it is defined by some notion of equal respect for persons.

From a narrowly self-interested or economic point of view, some people's lives may not matter to others, because they are unable to harm or benefit them. From a moral point of view, all people matter in and of themselves. It matters how well their lives go, and if our decisions affect their well-being, then we must take that into account. Adopting a moral point of view thus requires sympathetic attention to people's interests and circumstances, understanding how things look from their perspective, and taking account of their well-being. The ethic of care resonates with the moral point of view common to all these ethical theories.

The Ethic of Care and the Guiding Principles Approach

Commissioners believe that the approach offered by the ethic of care and our guiding principles gives the most insight into the particular issues the Commission is examining. It provides the greatest opportunity for preventing adversarial situations and offers the possibility of finding agreement on specific issues, even among those who adhere to different overarching ethical theories. The theoretical development of the ethic of care is taking place in many different contexts: in secular mainstream ethics, in feminist theory, and in religious thinking. We have drawn on all these sources to enrich our understanding. Of course, promoting the ethic of care is not entirely new — to a degree it has been reflected over the centuries in various formulations of medical ethics and the duty of physicians.

> The Commission should commit itself to a stated set of guiding principles and use these principles in its ethical deliberations. If there is a broad consensus in favour of each of these principles, then this approach will add considerable credibility to the Commission's conclusions, since these will be seen as neither ad hoc nor merely the result of logrolling among competing interests.
>
> *L.W. Sumner, reviewer, research volumes of the Commission, 1992.*

The Ethic of Care

Although there are differences of emphasis among the ethical thinkers from whose work we have drawn, the ethic of care holds, broadly speaking, that moral reasoning is not solely, or even primarily, a matter of finding rules to arbitrate between conflicting interests. Rather, moral wisdom and sensitivity consist, in the first instance, in focussing on how our interests are often interdependent. And moral reasoning involves trying to find creative solutions that can remove or reduce conflict, rather than simply subordinating one person's interests to another. The priority, therefore, is on helping human relationships to flourish by seeking to foster the dignity of the individual and the welfare of the community.

Where intervention is necessary, its aim should be creative empowerment so that, as far as possible, everyone is served and adversarial situations do not arise. At the very least, intervention must, in this view, avoid causing harm to human relationships. The traditional first principle of medicine, non-maleficence (do no harm), is thus applicable not only to medical practice but to intervention in society generally and is made into a positive commitment to empowerment. The concept of non-maleficence goes beyond simply avoiding actions that might cause harm, to taking steps to prevent harm and create conditions in which harm is less likely to occur and beneficial results are the more likely outcome.

The Guiding Principles

Although most would agree with the goals of the ethic of care, it is less than immediately obvious how these goals can be implemented in practice. Without some further development, the theory remains vague — benign but ineffectual. This is widely recognized by its proponents, who therefore adopt basic principles of justice — often those developed within traditional ethical theories — as a means of applying an ethic of care.

Accordingly, while adopting the ethic of care as an orienting ideal, the Commission found it useful to identify eight principles of special relevance to our mandate that enable decisions to be made that give concrete expression to the ideal of care. The principles are to be found in ethical theory generally and

> We live in a scientific and technological culture. Our lives are not only filled with the products of science and technology but both pervade our society as ways of making sense of the world. We see things as problems according to a certain rationale and we expect technology to fix them. Our approach lacks vision and guiding principles, sensibility and accountability.
>
> *A. Burfoot, private citizen, Public Hearings Transcripts, Montreal, Quebec, November 21, 1990.*

biomedical ethics in particular. They are also consistent with what we heard in testimony and submissions from Canadians and with the values and principles implicit in the reports of inquiries in other countries. The eight principles are individual autonomy, equality, respect for human life and dignity, protection of the vulnerable, non-commercialization of reproduction, appropriate use of resources, accountability, and balancing of individual and collective interests.

There is some overlap among these eight principles. For example, the principle of non-commercialization of human beings and human reproduction is largely a conclusion from the other principles, such as equality, protection of the vulnerable, and respect for human life and dignity. Similarly, the appropriate use of resources is often connected to the principle of accountability, and the promotion of autonomy is often seen as requiring equality of access to health care. It may be possible to combine these related principles, although perhaps at the price of losing sight of important issues. Conversely, it may be possible to divide up some of these principles into even finer categories. However, the eight principles seem to capture ethical considerations that are both important and relatively distinct. Since these principles informed our deliberations and infuse our reasoning in the rest of our report, we give a brief account of each of them in the following pages. Moreover, there is no hierarchy here; no principle automatically trumps any other. Different principles are considered as they apply to specific issues.

Individual Autonomy

By individual autonomy we mean that people are free to choose how to lead their lives, particularly with respect to their bodies and their fundamental commitments, such as health, family, sexuality, and work. Clearly, this is not an unqualified principle. Individual autonomy does not include the freedom to harm others, to use force to coerce them, or to undermine social stability. Moreover, restrictions are sometimes placed on people's freedom of action in cir-

> Any decision on the regulation of new reproductive technologies must endeavour to balance the interest of all members of society at the same time though the council believes that any policies which are developed must be grounded on the principle that women have the absolute right to decide what happens to our body and to determine our own choices with respect to reproduction and reproductive health care.
>
> *W. Williams, The Provincial Advisory Council on the Status of Women, Newfoundland and Labrador, Public Hearings Transcripts, St. John's, Newfoundland, October 15, 1990.*

cumstances if it is determined that they lack the competence necessary to make reasonable decisions. However, a defining feature of modern culture is that individuals are seen as having the right (and the responsibility) to decide what kind of life they want to lead. From this principle it follows, for example, that actions or decisions that affect people's health, bodily integrity, security, and identity require informed consent.

Equality

The principle of equality means that every member of the community is entitled to equal concern and respect. The view that the well-being of each person matters and matters equally precludes any social practice that reflects or perpetuates the assumption that some people's lives are worth less than others. Adopting the principle of equality keeps this tenet in view.

The principle of equality forms the basis for our particular concern with ensuring that the interests and concerns of Canadians in all their diversity are taken into account in decisions about new reproductive technologies. This is why we have examined specifically how the technologies affect women, members of racial and ethnic minorities, people with disabilities, Aboriginal people, and lesbians. We recognize that achieving equality sometimes requires special steps to ensure that groups that have experienced discrimination in the past are placed on an equal footing with other members of society. This is particularly relevant in discussions of access to services, because services must be not only accessible but also designed to take into account the diversity of needs, expectations, and abilities in the populations they are intended to serve.

> Our interpretation of the principles governing human rights in Canada and the current thinking of the leaders in Canadian family law lead us to the following conclusion: all citizens should be equally eligible for medically assisted reproduction services.
>
> Any legitimate restrictions, relating to economic factors or the distribution of scarce resources, should not be used as an excuse for discrimination on the basis of marital status or sexual orientation, but should be implemented in a manner that respects human rights and the basic principles of justice. [Translation]
>
> *G. Létourneau, Président, Commission de réforme du droit du Canada, Public Hearings Transcripts, Montreal, Quebec, November 21, 1990.*

Equitable access to public services such as health care and education is based on this principle. We heard from many Canadians that they believe treating people with equal respect requires equitable access to basic services. Non-discrimination in access to these services has also become part of Canada's constitutional and legal environment through prohibition of discrimination on the basis of sex, race, and other grounds in the *Canadian Charter of Rights and Freedoms* and in human rights legislation.

Respect for Human Life and Dignity

All forms of human life (and indeed human tissue in general) should be treated with sensitivity and respect, not callousness or indifference. Although the law does not treat zygotes, embryos, and fetuses as persons, they are connected to the community by virtue of their origins (having been generated by members of the community) and their possible future (their potential to become members of the community). Not only all persons but also zygotes, embryos, and fetuses should be treated with appropriate respect because of this. In Part Two of our report we discuss more specifically how this principle applies to zygotes, embryos, and fetuses (see Chapters 22, 30, and 31).

Protection of the Vulnerable

Vulnerability relates to power imbalances, and this principle requires that the welfare of those who are less capable of looking after themselves or who are open to exploitation for various reasons be given special consideration. The most common example concerns the welfare of children. Since children cannot look after all their own needs, parents have the authority to make decisions for them. However, this authority is a trust, to be exercised for the benefit of the children, and the state is responsible for ensuring that this trust is kept. Vulnerability to exploitation may also arise from a person's socioeconomic status, membership in a minority group, or disability. Safeguards exist to ensure that adults who are temporarily or permanently unable to make competent decisions are not ignored or taken advantage of; someone is appointed to make decisions on their behalf and must act in their best interests. Society also has a responsibility to ensure that vulnerability is reduced where possible and that those who are vulnerable are not manipulated or controlled by those in positions of power and authority.

Non-Commercialization of Reproduction

Two concepts are relevant to our discussion of this principle: commercialization and commodification. By commercialization we mean activities involving the exchange of money or goods and intended to generate a profit or benefit for those engaging in this exchange. By commodification we mean the treatment of human beings or body tissues and substances as commodities — as means to an end, not as ends in themselves. Thus, commercialization necessarily includes commodification, but commodification need not entail a profit motive.

Commissioners believe it is fundamentally wrong for decisions about human reproduction to be determined by a profit motive — introducing a profit motive to the sphere of reproduction is contrary to basic values and disregards the importance of the role of reproduction and its significance in our lives as human beings. Commodifying human beings and their bodies for commercial gain is unacceptable because this instrumentalization is injurious to human dignity and ultimately dehumanizing. We therefore consider commercialization of reproductive materials and reproductive services to be inappropriate.

However, as we discuss in Part Two of our report, there may be a legitimate role for commercial interests in certain aspects of reproductive health care — for example, in the development of drugs and medical devices or in certain ancillary services such as storage and transportation. But, for the reasons just discussed, it is important to place strict limits on the extent of commercial involvement in this field and particularly to guard against inappropriate commodification of human tissues, products, and processes. It may sometimes be

> First, we strongly believe that neither bodies, nor gametes, nor human embryos, nor any part of our reproductive potential, should be considered fungible or marketable commodities. Permitting the exploitation, conditioning and distribution of the seeds of life, human embryos and infants, in accordance with market forces, ignores the principles of human dignity and individuality.
>
> We demand that the principle of no charge for services that has always guided Canadian law and policy on blood and organ donations be upheld, and we recommend that marketing of gamete and embryo transfers be prohibited. [Translation]
>
> *G. Létourneau, Président, Commission de réforme du droit du Canada, Public Hearings Transcripts, Montreal, Quebec, November 21, 1990.*

appropriate to treat human tissues, including reproductive tissues, as means to an end — as in research or therapy intended to benefit people — provided this occurs under strictly defined conditions that ensure respect for the source of the materials or tissues. But it is never appropriate to treat human reproductive tissues or substances as objects of commerce or commodities on which there is a profit to be made.

Appropriate Use of Resources

The principle of appropriate use of resources recognizes the existence of diverse needs and finite resources, which requires that resources be used wisely and effectively. Resources used to help some people in one way become unavailable to help other people in other ways. Decisions about the provision of programs, procedures, or technologies must therefore be made in accordance with clearly defined public policy priorities. Society must establish its health care priorities, for example, and strive to maintain them in difficult political and economic times. As we discuss in Chapter 4, this will require a shift in attitudes on the part of Canadians, a new orientation in the health care system, and a new approach to medical treatment. Our recommendations concerning the importance of evidence-based medicine, the need for assessment and evaluation of uses of technology in medical practice, and the appropriate roles for prevention and acute care are premised in part on this fundamental principle of making the most appropriate use of available resources.

Accountability

The principle of accountability means that those who hold power, whether in government, medicine, technology, or other fields, are responsible for the way they use that power. This entails the conviction that Canadian society has a right — and a responsibility — to regulate and monitor how reproductive technologies are used to ensure that our values, principles, and priorities are being respected. In the past, these functions have been assumed through the self-regulation of the professions. But as we will see in subsequent chapters, there is increasing dissatisfaction with self-regulation as the sole method of ensuring accountability, because it is seen as an approach in which people from outside the professions have little role in the development or enforcement of policies and codes of practice. The implications of new reproductive technologies are so profound that demands for more active public participation in their regulation are clearly legitimate. Although medical self-regulation does oblige professional organizations to act in the public interest, a self-regulating profession is not necessarily best equipped to assess the social, ethical, and economic implications of the technologies and may be insufficiently accountable to those whose needs they are meant to serve, particularly in the absence of a broader regulatory system.

Balancing Individual and Collective Interests

This principle reflects our belief that both individual and collective interests are worthy of protection, and that individual interests do not automatically take precedence over collective interests, or vice versa. The individual interests with which we are concerned include those of women or couples seeking assisted conception or prenatal diagnosis services, those of gamete donors, and those of children born as a result of a new reproductive technology. The

Here in the Northwest Territories where Dene and Inuit peoples predominate, community life is built around family life. Child bearing is considered a gift and a privilege. Infertility is indeed a tragedy for many childless couples, and we affirm the right of such couples to pursue methods of child bearing which do not jeopardize the inherent value, rights and dignity of the persons involved.

L. Hudson, Tawow Society, Fort Smith, Public Hearings Transcripts, Yellowknife, Northwest Territories, September 12, 1990.

collective interests include those of society as a whole, as well as those of identifiable groups within society, such as women, children, people with disabilities, and members of racial and ethnic minorities. We discuss the application of this principle later in this chapter.

What We Heard: Support for This Approach

Ethical issues were the focus of many of the interventions and submissions we received during our consultation process. There was a widespread public perception that the ethical implications of reproductive technologies require greater attention and a more systematic response than they have received to date.

Some of the individuals and groups we heard from presented their ethical reasoning in the form of specific principles. These principles varied from sector to sector and, to a lesser extent, within each sector. No social grouping had a single approach to ethical issues — their priorities, applications, and belief systems varied. However, we saw evidence of extensive support for the guiding principles we adopted. Although different groups focussed on different principles, the principles are complementary rather than competing; the eight principles we identified thus reflect widespread consensus in Canadian society on the ethical basis that should guide decision making.

Indeed, these principles were endorsed by a very broad range of groups — professionals and laypeople, women and men, religious and secular groups, members of racial and ethnic minorities, people with disabilities, doctors, and patients. That these principles were endorsed by groups with diverse experiences and interests confirms our belief that they capture important ethical considerations. Moreover, principles similar to those we adopted have been found useful in other inquiries regarding new reproductive technologies. Many of the international inquiries we examined appeal to principles of

> We must bear in mind that the principle of respect for individuals is proclaimed in the Universal Declaration of Human Rights and the constitutions of most countries. It is recognized as a key principle.
>
> Its theoretical grounds are the same as the basic principles of bioethics:
>
> 1.   the principle of respect for individuals and their autonomy;
> 2.   the principle of compassion;
> 3.   the principle of justice or equity.
>
> These three principles are the basis of the right to privacy, to free and informed consent, to confidentiality, and to justice. [Translation]
>
> *Y. Grenier, private citizen, Public Hearings Transcripts, Montreal, Quebec, November 21, 1990.*

autonomy, respect for human life and dignity, and protection of the vulnerable. There was also considerable support for principles of non-commercialization and equitable access.

Finally, there is a growing trend in the bioethics literature to the guiding principles approach. Our review of the literature revealed the following principles at the core of bioethics: beneficence (and non-maleficence), justice, informed consent, respect for human life and dignity, honesty, and confidentiality. The differences between these principles and our own stem from the fact that bioethics developed originally to deal with the relationship between doctor and patient, whereas our principles are intended to deal with broader issues of public policy as well.

Given this level of consensus, we believe that the guiding principles we adopted provide concrete and constructive guidance with respect to the issues raised by new reproductive technologies.

Applying the Guiding Principles

Setting out the guiding principles is only the first step; many questions of priority setting and application remain. Each principle points to a legitimate concern that may be applicable to groups that are affected by new reproductive technologies. To apply the principles, therefore, we also need to identify the individuals and groups that are potentially affected by the use or non-use of these technologies. How each decision and recommendation will affect them needs to be considered explicitly. Moreover, as we discussed in Chapter 2, all of society is affected indirectly, whether by the social and ethical precedents that are established or by the fact that resources are directed here rather than elsewhere. Identifying the range of groups to be considered, in conjunction with the guiding principles, enabled us to take a comprehensive and consistent approach to decision making. Ensuring that we have given proper consideration to all those affected by the technologies provides the basis for morally responsible recommendations.

There is, of course, a danger of oversimplification in describing the guiding principles approach in this way; it is not a magic formula for resolving all moral disputes. There will be disagreements about the interpretation of the guiding principles and about the extent to which one or another applies in particular cases. Some of these disputes may not be resolvable. Although there is consensus on the principle of respect for human life and dignity, for example, Canadians are deeply and seemingly irresolvably divided over how to interpret that principle. Where we encountered such differences in preparing our report, we used our guiding principles to help identify and explain the nature of the disagreement as clearly as possible.

We believe, however, that many disputes are resolvable by a variety of means. First, many of the ethical concerns that arise about the use of reproductive technologies do so because some people believe that the use of these technologies will lead, over time, to disastrous social consequences for women, families, and people with disabilities, among others. Others believe that these negative effects will not occur because society is capable of preventing abuse through regulation. This is an important dispute, but it is a dispute more about facts than about values. To some extent, the dispute can be resolved by generating and disseminating better information and by establishing a system of public accountability that gives all groups in society a say in the future development of these technologies. The development of the Commission itself is a step in this direction.

Some debates can be left for future decision-making bodies. Given that the technologies are changing constantly and that not all have reached a stage of development where we know enough about them to make informed decisions, some decisions about future development or use cannot be made at this time. Establishing decision-making bodies with clear mandates and responsibilities for making and reviewing decisions in light of the latest available evidence has worked well in other jurisdictions.

Finally, some options will be more appropriate or feasible than others in light of Canada's legal, political, economic, and cultural context, existing institutions and practices, as well as our obligations as a member of the international community. Although ethical arguments are of fundamental importance, public policy must also recognize the existence of social and economic constraints, and these may help narrow the range of feasible options. Adopting a guiding principles approach does not guarantee a satisfactory resolution of all moral issues. It does, however, illuminate the ethical implications of new reproductive technologies and provide a clear and constructive approach for evaluating these implications and establishing public policy in light of them.

Individual and Collective Interests

The need to balance individual and collective interests arises in all areas of public policy. But the conflict can be especially poignant in the area of reproductive technologies, and in this we faced some of our most difficult decisions.

Defining the Problem

On one hand, the interests of people who are infertile, people at risk of having children with a genetic disease or severe anomalies, or people with diseases that may be treatable using knowledge from zygote or fetal tissue research are important and deeply felt human concerns. On the other hand, we cannot ignore the obligation of society to weigh the broader implications of making available medical services in these areas, to allocate scarce resources in an appropriate manner, and to monitor and regulate health care so as to assure the safety of the population and future generations.

We do not accept the view, sometimes expressed, that liberal democracy differs from some other forms of government because individual rights always take precedence over the interests of the collectivity. Canada's constitutional history demonstrates unequivocally that in a liberal democracy, individual rights can be limited when the aim is to protect important societal interests. Indeed, we believe that framing a need or desire in the language of "rights" may not be the most helpful way of approaching this issue.

The ethic of care involves an outlook premised on seeking creative ways to accommodate diverse interests. It requires balancing individual and collective interests to forestall, as much as possible, competitive or adversary stances. We believe that weighing individual and collective interests in this way (facilitated by our guiding principles and considering the range of individuals and groups affected) may lead to more humane and caring policies.

We uphold the value of rights. There are many examples of how rights can promote people's self-respect and mobilize them to remedy injustices — the women's movement, the civil rights movement, and the development of human rights instruments through bodies such as the United Nations are among the prime examples. But it is also important to recognize that different people's rights overlap, that rights are subject to various limitations, and that rights usually come with responsibilities attached. To claim a right does not by itself resolve policy issues — or resolve how to assess whether a given claim is indeed a right. Moreover, although rights are important, they can be understood only within a larger context of societal limitations and individual responsibilities. And this leads us back to questions about the proper relationship between individual and collective interests.

Throughout our deliberations and in formulating our recommendations, Commissioners have sought to understand the nature of individual rights, interests, and responsibilities, as well as the interests and responsibilities of society as a whole. We have also sought to understand, as part of the balancing process, the rights, interests, and responsibilities of various groups in Canadian society. Finally, we have sought to reflect on these issues from the general perspective of the ethic of care.

The Role of the Charter

The *Canadian Charter of Rights and Freedoms* sets out a range of individual rights, including the right to life, liberty, and security of the person, the right to equality, and the right to freedom of expression and association, among others. These represent and protect the legitimate aspirations of individuals and groups, and the Supreme Court is empowered to strike down government legislation and policies that violate these aspirations.

Individual rights are qualified by other sections of the Charter, reflecting Canada's approach to the continuing tension between individual and collective. For instance, section 1 of the Charter says that any right in the Charter can be limited in ways that are "demonstrably justified in a free and democratic society." But to be demonstrably justified, these limits cannot be based on mere convenience or prejudice. Where there is a legitimate social objective, and where reasonable limits on individual rights are necessary to achieve that societal goal, then the good of the collective can be held to limit the rights of the individual. Similarly, section 33 of the Charter, the notwithstanding clause, allows governments, as the elected representatives and the expression of the will of the collective, to limit individual rights for the good of society. Any decision on the part of a government to limit individual rights in a particular piece of legislation is temporary, however, and subject to review after five years.

Individual rights are also qualified by the existence of a third category of rights: the rights of specific groups within Canadian society. The rights of Aboriginal and multicultural communities are protected (sections 25, 27, and 35), as are the rights of linguistic and religious groups (sections 23 and 29). There is also constitutional protection for programs that may limit the rights of the individual in order to redress collective wrongs to historically disadvantaged groups.

These sections of the Charter provide some protection to government policies that are aimed at promoting the interests of specific groups from a rigid insistence on individual rights. In these and other ways, the Charter both affirms and limits individual rights. It insists that individual rights cannot be limited for reasons of convenience or prejudice, but it recognizes that valid societal interests can justify some limitation on them. Thus, the Charter both expresses and reflects a uniquely Canadian framework for relations between individuals and the state. Its introduction both was based on and accelerated a trend toward acknowledging pluralism and rights-based participation in Canadian society. We believe that an interpretation of rights that balances individual and collective interests remains deeply rooted in Canada's political culture and is applicable to public policy decisions in the areas covered by our mandate.

Given its significant impact on the relationship between governments and citizens, it is not surprising that the Charter raises various issues in relation to the regulation of new reproductive technologies. For example, section 7 (which guarantees "life, liberty, and security of the person") has implications for the right to informed consent before medical treatment, including the right of pregnant women to refuse unwanted medical treatment; for issues surrounding gamete donors' rights to privacy and the locus of control of the use of their gametes; and for the right of children born through the use of new reproductive technologies to learn about their social and medical histories. Section 15 raises the issue of the permissibility of restrictions on access to new reproductive technologies based on an individual's age, marital status, sexual orientation, economic status, or other prohibited grounds of discrimination. This does not necessarily mean that courts would find that discrimination had occurred — in the case of age, for example, medical grounds may make this appropriate.

As well as providing a benchmark against which government policies and legislation can be tested and challenged, the existence of the Charter has altered the way some Canadians think about government policy. As a result, law is seen by some as an agent of social policy, rather than a technical tool for administering government policy; legal judgements are seen as the way to resolve conflicts between individual and collective interests.

> The legislation [should] include underlying principles and establish a framework and process for assessing the appropriateness of new technologies as well as ongoing research. The principles would include, the rights of women to control their own reproductive destiny; the rights of individuals to make their own decisions based on all information; the right to accessibility of treatment for everyone; the non-commercialization of reproductive services, and an assurance of compliance with equality guarantees and the *Charter of Rights and Freedoms*.
>
> *B. Suek, Charter of Rights Coalition/ Manitoba, Public Hearings Transcripts, Winnipeg, Manitoba, October 23, 1990.*

Situations Where Individual and Collective Interests May Differ

There is no inherent conflict between individual and collective interests. On the contrary, a community can flourish only when its individual members are flourishing, and individuals can flourish only within a larger social context. It is important for society to care for its members, to ensure that it is a society worth belonging to. In some situations, however, protecting the interests of some individuals would be harmful or prohibitively costly for the rest of society.

In some cases, the pursuit of an individual's objective may be inherently detrimental to collective values or requirements for public health and safety. In other cases, an individual activity may be tolerable if it occurs rarely but harmful to society if it crosses a certain threshold and becomes more commonplace. In yet other cases, solving the legitimate problems of an individual may require so great an investment of societal time, energy, and resources as to affect our ability to meet other societal needs. For example, some people think that heart/lung transplants should not be publicly funded because there are other more pressing unmet medical needs, and they think the cost of these operations is so high for the likelihood of benefit that society could spend the money more effectively elsewhere, providing greater benefit to a greater number of people.

There is an important distinction between the third and the first two cases, specifically that there is nothing socially harmful about the individual's desire for the surgery. On the contrary, the operation is good from both an individual and a collective point of view, and so society would provide it if possible. Unfortunately, it may not be possible, given the full range of health priorities. Fulfilling the individual desire would not harm the collective good, but it would not contribute much compared to other possible uses of scarce resources — thus, its "opportunity cost" may be too high. Some have argued that the Charter can be interpreted as imposing an affirmative duty on the state to make new reproductive technologies available, so that those who are unable to become parents in the usual way can enjoy the same reproductive "rights" as other members of society. It is highly unlikely, however, that the courts would uphold such claims, given the broader social interest in providing basic health care for all Canadians and the existence of finite resources with which to do so.

It is not always easy to distinguish among the situations in which individual and collective interests may differ, because the three categories (inherently detrimental, threshold situations, opportunity costs too high) are often connected in the context of a particular reproductive technology and are sometimes mixed together in the public debate. Furthermore, full information on the cost and likelihood of success of particular procedures may not be available initially, making decisions more difficult. But it remains important to distinguish among these different objections, because the appropriateness of a particular policy depends in large part on the category of situation it is intended to address.

Individual Rights and Social Interests

Individual and group rights claims made under the Charter must be taken into consideration as well as societal interests. As the discussion throughout our report makes clear, the impact of new reproductive technologies extends well beyond the individuals directly involved in their use. The research, development, and application of new reproductive technologies affect not only the prospective biological and social parents, but the children born as a result of their use, women as a group, and society as a whole. The presence of group and societal interests may well qualify the right to become a parent through the use of new reproductive technologies and condition the other individual rights involved.

It is impossible to formulate a rule about whether the interests of individuals or society are more important. Rather than subordinating one to the other, it would be more appropriate to say that each qualifies and shapes the other and that a delicate balance is required. Thus, a strategy that encompasses both individual and social interests should always be the first and preferred approach. Moreover, it is potentially misleading to talk about "individual versus collective" conflicts, as if all uses of reproductive technologies could be lumped together or resolved in the same manner.

There is no single formula for weighing individual and collective interests that would allow us to resolve all these issues. Rather, we need to look at given situations on their merits and consider how individual interests affect society's values, norms, and resources, and vice versa. As we deliberated, we were acutely aware of the need to take individual, group, and societal interests into account, in line with both our ethical principles and the requirements of the Charter. Our thinking and recommendations with respect to the individual technologies and the ethical issues they raise are discussed in Part Two.

Conclusion

The Commission saw one of its responsibilities as promoting informed public debate on new reproductive technologies. In deciding how to approach our ethical deliberations, therefore, we felt it was important to adopt a perspective that draws upon the language and principles of Canadian public debate. Our aim was neither to mirror the existing views of Canadians nor to transcend them radically. Rather, we hope to improve public understanding and the capacity to engage in social debate by identifying

The Commission saw one of its responsibilities as promoting informed public debate on new reproductive technologies. In deciding how to approach our ethical deliberations, therefore, we felt it was important to adopt a perspective that draws upon the language and principles of Canadian public debate.

shared ethical principles in a considered approach that can help to guide future public policy making. We hope that our approach will help Canadians see how profound the implications of reproductive technologies are and why it is so important to ensure that, if they are used, they are used in an ethical manner. Nor need this approach be limited to the new reproductive technologies — it offers a perspective that society could apply to other emerging technologies and other social policy issues.

Setting public policy also requires careful attention to and consideration of the values and attitudes of Canadians. Many of these values and attitudes are embodied in the Constitution, particularly in the Charter. At the same time, the opinions Canadians hold may sometimes differ from how the Charter is applied in particular cases. This is sometimes the case with equality issues, for example, where public opinion on a given question may differ from the values entrenched in section 15 of the Charter. The legitimacy of public policies is therefore a function of both their consistency with constitutionally entrenched values and their congruity with the values and attitudes of a broad range of Canadians.

This brief sketch of the Commission's guiding principles conveys our ethical stance in somewhat general and abstract terms.   Their full dimensions and nuances and how the principles apply will become clearer as we explain our reasoning and recommendations with respect to specific technologies and the real-life decisions to which they give rise in Part Two of our report.

Just as important as the ethical basis for individual and societal decisions about the use or non-use of new reproductive technologies is society's capacity to implement our collective decisions. How are Canadian systems and institutions structured to implement society's decisions? How are priorities set, policies established, and services designed and delivered? Do they currently have the capacity to respond to the demands of public policy making in an increasingly diverse, knowledge-based society on the verge of the twenty-first century? What changes, if any, are needed? Understanding Canadian systems and institutions was an important part of the context for our study of new reproductive technologies. Among all the systems that will be affected by our recommendations, the health care system is the central one. This is where ethical dilemmas, medical decision making, and service delivery converge. The next chapter of this part of our report is devoted to an overview of the health care system as the context within which the provision of reproductive technologies is possible.

General Sources

Beauchamp, T.L., and J.F. Childress. *Principles of Biomedical Ethics*. 3d ed. New York: Oxford University Press, 1989.

Coward, H. "World Religions and New Reproductive Technologies." In Research Volumes of the Royal Commission on New Reproductive Technologies, 1993.

Francoeur, R. *Biomedical Ethics: A Guide to Decision-Making*. New York: John Wiley and Sons, 1983.

Gilligan, C. *In a Different Voice: Psychological Theory and Women's Development*. Cambridge: Harvard University Press, 1982.

Glendon, M.A. *Rights Talk: The Impoverishment of Political Discourse*. Toronto: Collier MacMillan, 1991.

Jantzen, G.M. "Connection or Competition: Identity and Personhood in Feminist Ethics." *Studies in Christian Ethics* 5 (1)(1992): 1-20.

Kymlicka, W. "Approaches to the Ethical Issues Raised by the Royal Commission's Mandate." In Research Volumes of the Royal Commission on New Reproductive Technologies, 1993.

Lockwood, M. "Warnock Versus Powell (and Harradine): When Does Potentiality Count?" *Bioethics* 2 (3)(1988): 187-213.

Mappes, T.A., and J.S. Zembaty. *Biomedical Ethics.* 3d ed. New York: McGraw-Hill, 1991.

Marcus, I., et al. "Feminist Discourse, Moral Values, and the Law — A Conversation." *Buffalo Law Review* 34 (1985): 11-87.

Noddings, N. *Caring: A Feminine Approach to Ethics & Moral Education.* Los Angeles: University of California Press, 1984.

Schenker, J.G. "Religious Views Regarding Treatment of Infertility by Assisted Reproductive Technologies." *Journal of Assisted Reproduction and Genetics* 9 (1)(1992): 3-8.

Thomas, J.E., and W.J. Waluchow. *Well and Good: Case Studies in Biomedical Ethics.* 2d ed. Peterborough: Broadview Press, 1990.

4

New Reproductive Technologies and the Health Care System

The state of Canada's health care system and what the place of new reproductive technologies should be within it were the subjects of extensive and detailed debate before the Commission in our public hearing and consultation processes. Much of this debate centred on whether reproductive technologies should be offered within the health care system, whether offering them would place an unwarranted burden on an already overburdened system, and whether attention to these technologies would divert health care resources from other pressing needs, whether in reproductive health or other areas. While sharing many of the concerns we heard, Commissioners approached the issues from a somewhat different perspective, asking how we could reconcile the great importance people attach to having children with the need to manage the health care system responsibly, given the many legitimate claims on its resources, without overburdening it.

The importance of the health care system to Canadians was abundantly clear from our consultations and research: the system is a source of national pride, it is an important factor in people's lives, and it is a tangible way in which our society expresses mutual support and caring for its members. The health care

> The importance of the health care system to Canadians was abundantly clear from our consultations and research: the system is a source of national pride, it is an important factor in people's lives, and it is a tangible way in which our society expresses mutual support and caring for its members.

system is a symbol of strongly held Canadian values, reflecting the fact that we think individuals should be treated equally in the face of disease or injury. In many ways, the health care system helps to define Canadians and how we see ourselves, and it evolved as it did only because of the values we hold collectively — hence the importance of managing the system responsibly and not overburdening it with functions or responsibilities that should lie elsewhere. At the same time, the evidence before the Commission is that Canadians attach great importance to having children; not only people who are infertile but the vast majority of Canadians want to have children and anticipate having them in their lives. How should we reconcile these two goals if, as in the case of new reproductive technologies, one might have the potential to undermine the other?

Commissioners concluded that Canada has the capacity to develop a response that reconciles these two goals. If having children is important to most Canadians, as we have found it is, and if safe and effective means exist to help people who would otherwise not be able to have children to do so, then the ethic of care directs us to take this into account in societal decisions about how our collective resources are allocated, including those allocated to the health care system.

It would be unethical, however, to offer services or assistance in the form of unproven procedures or treatments. It would be irresponsible to devote public resources to such procedures in the absence of knowledge about their risks and effectiveness, and about their costs and benefits relative to other approaches to solving the problem and other calls on the available resources. A rational framework is needed as the basis for making such decisions.

What was required, therefore, was a means of determining whether these procedures could be provided ethically — with reasonable assurance about their risks and effectiveness — and whether doing so represented an appropriate use of public resources. Our approach was to adopt the concept of evidence-based medicine.

Evidence-Based Medicine

The evidence before the Commission suggests that a significant proportion of medical care is ineffective, inefficient, or unevaluated. (Similarly, much of the care provided by dentists, chiropractors, nurses, social workers, and many others practising in the general field of health care has not been evaluated.) This situation has clear implications for the quality of care people receive and for inefficient or less than maximal use of limited resources. Evidence-based medicine — that is, medical practice and management of the health care system based on knowledge gained from appropriate evaluation of treatments and their results — offers a way to correct this situation. To date, however, the massive investment of time and resources in new medical technologies and treatments has not been balanced by an equal commitment of resources for their assessment and evaluation. We know a great deal about the inputs to the system — the resources used, number of beds, numbers of patients treated — but relatively little about results — the health status of patients following treatment.

New reproductive technologies in particular have brought these concerns to the forefront. Individuals and groups representing a broad range of interests told the Commission about their concerns that reproductive technologies are being introduced without adequate research into their effectiveness, the risks associated with them, and their short- and long-term effects on health. Some of women's previous experiences with reproductive health care have fuelled concerns about safety, particularly with respect to the potential for unanticipated consequences. For example, when technologies and drugs such as the Dalkon

> Decisions regarding technology are made daily by practitioners, administrators, and policy makers. Ideally, decisions regarding health technology should be based on evidence from comprehensive assessment — that is, information on the safety, effectiveness, costs, and ethical, legal, and social implications of the particular technology under consideration. Reality proves otherwise; the large majority of technological innovations in health care are in use long before any systematic assessment has taken place. Sometimes, at the second- or third-generation level, technologies are found to be ineffective, or even unsafe, after belated assessment.
>
> *A. Kazanjian and K. Cardiff, "Framework for Technology Decisions: Literature Review," in Research Volumes of the Commission, 1993.*

Shield®, diethylstilbestrol (DES), and thalidomide were first introduced, researchers and physicians alike believed they were effective and did not involve high risks. As we know now, however, there were unexpected and devastating consequences for women and their children. These experiences offer hard-learned lessons about the need for evaluation before wide dissemination of medical treatments, for full disclosure to patients about known or potential risks, and for the continuing collection of data on the results of treatment.

When these concerns are added to broader concerns about the potential of new reproductive technologies to affect human relationships and society generally, it is clear that Canadians are demanding a systematic and rational approach to decisions about whether the use of new reproductive technologies is acceptable and, if so, whether and under what conditions their provision should occur within the health care system. In the Commission's view, evidence-based medicine is the first component of a rational approach to decisions about the funding of medical care. As the health care system is currently structured, however, there are barriers to implementing this approach. Moreover, increasing financial and other pressures on the system have created a situation where change — even change generally agreed to be necessary — is difficult to effect.

Commissioners therefore recognized that we had a social responsibility to ensure that our recommendations contribute to developing effective and equitable health policy while maintaining the integrity of that system and, indeed, improving its capacity to deliver services if possible. At the very least, we felt a responsibility not to erode a system that is meeting Canadians' medical needs and generally fulfilling our expectations about its role in our collective life.

In devoting a chapter to the health care system the Commission is acknowledging that our recommendations will not be implemented in a vacuum. If new reproductive technologies are to be made available, it will be in the

> **Evidence-Based Medicine:** Medical practice based on data and assessment of whether procedures or treatments are of benefit for their intended purpose.

context of a health care system that is already under considerable pressure. Given the cost of providing new reproductive technologies and associated services and programs, we must consider the issues in light of these pressures, asking ourselves questions about outcomes, priorities, and equity in allocating public health dollars and delivering services. Decisions about providing new reproductive technologies must clearly be part of this broader process of deciding what the health care system should or should not be called upon to do. Evidence-based medicine offers a way to establish the effectiveness and risks of procedures or medications before they are made available generally; if effectiveness and risks have not been established, treatment should be provided only in the context of research until this information can be generated. The long-established practice is that those receiving procedures that are in the category of research must be fully informed of their experimental nature and consent to the procedures in knowledge of

> Evidence-based medicine offers a way to establish the effectiveness and risks of procedures or medications before they are made available generally; if effectiveness and risks have not been established, treatment should be provided only in the context of research until this information can be generated.

this. Evidence-based medicine also offers a more rational and equitable way of allocating public health dollars by suggesting which treatments are beneficial to people at what cost to the system and which are ineffective or overly costly given their likely benefits.

Thus, like the ethical framework created by our guiding principles and the ethic of care, evidence-based medicine shaped the Commission's approach to assessing the various forms of infertility treatment. It too provided a prism through which to view the technologies and to determine whether their provision within the health care system was ethically acceptable and constituted an appropriate use of resources.

Beyond this, however, it became clear as our work proceeded that the ethical and practical approaches we were developing as a basis for assessing new reproductive technologies have broader application in the health care system. Our approach would make it possible for Canada's response to new reproductive technologies not only to avoid being part of a problem — in the sense of overburdening, distorting, or undermining the system — but to be part of a solution by contributing to the system's capacity to continue to deliver effective health care services in a fair, rational, and cost-effective way. Strategies to achieve these goals are the common threads running through Part Two of our report as we examine the various technologies and recommend approaches to dealing with them.

On this issue, we must rethink our methods of evaluating technology. Our "technology assessment" usually covers only a few features, and does not, for example, look into how subsequent users of a technique will change it. And usually, our assessment is carried out by people who are already favourably disposed toward the technique. [Translation]

H. Doucet, Faculté de Théologie, Université Saint-Paul, Public Hearings Transcripts, Ottawa, Ontario, September 18, 1990.

In the remainder of this chapter, we examine the current state of Canada's health care system as an important part of the context for our inquiry and for implementation of our recommendations. The approach inherent in evidence-based medicine is evident already in many of the issues and proposed solutions emerging in the health care field, as pressures on the system create incentives for policy makers and other decision makers to look at what the system is doing, whether it is doing the right things, whether it is doing things well, and how to alter patterns of resource allocation in light of the answers to these questions.

Health Care and Health

Most Canadians equate medical care and treatment with better health; we tend to place great faith in the power of surgery, drugs, and medical technology and believe that having more health care services will result in healthier people. Medical care may be critical and even life-saving for those who are acutely ill, and some treatments of chronic illness are of clear benefit; however, the capacity of medical care to produce a healthy population is, in fact, relatively limited. Medical treatment is important and even essential in certain situations, but it is only one of the determinants of overall health.

We know this for at least two reasons. First, research in Canada and elsewhere shows clearly that there is a direct relationship between health status and income. The higher the income, the longer and healthier the life, despite the fact that medical treatment is available and used throughout the country, and even when smoking, nutrition, and other

Medical care is available to and used by people in all segments of Canadian society; therefore, it is clear that most of the difference in health status between groups of people is not attributable to the medical care system. These facts, coupled with current pressures on the health care system, make it timely to reassess the contribution and limits of medicine.

factors are taken into account. In the aggregate, low socioeconomic status, not lack of health care, is the greatest correlate of poor health. Second, research in Canada, the United States, and elsewhere shows that the rate of use of certain medical procedures, including certain types of surgery, varies very widely between similar communities, yet high use makes no appreciable difference to health status. Medical care is available to and used by people in all segments of Canadian society; therefore, it is clear that most of the difference in health status between groups of people is not attributable to the medical care system. These facts, coupled with current pressures on the health care system, make it timely to reassess the contribution and limits of medicine.

Notwithstanding the facts about health care and health status, the prevalent belief that the availability and use of medical care are central to health has led to massive amounts of our collective resources being allocated to the medical system. Yet money spent to provide medical care is then unavailable for purposes such as affordable housing, education, income security, and environmental protection, which also have a great potential impact on the overall health of the population. Allowing these other determinants of health to deteriorate by devoting insufficient resources to them is risky. We have reached the point where, paradoxically, the further allocation of dollars to health services could actually have detrimental effects on health.

What is an informed society willing to pay? How much spending on health care is "enough"? The fact is that under the current method of allocating resources to health care, we simply have no accurate way of knowing. There may be enough resources already allocated to the health care system to continue to provide effective existing treatments, as well as to accommodate effective new technologies, provided we can identify and stop providing the minimally effective or demonstrably ineffective interventions now being funded. At present, however, we have little evidence on which to base this determination, because much of medical care has never been evaluated, and resource allocation decisions have not been made on the basis of the evaluation information that does exist.

The role of medical care is vital and, if used appropriately, of great value in our lives. But not all medical care is of equal value in achieving health. As evidence and awareness of these facts expand, there are increasing calls within the health care system and in the broader community to recognize the limitations of medicine and to acknowledge and support other ways of achieving health. To do this, we need to discover whether and under what conditions treatments work — that is, to demonstrate their effects on health — and then to manage the health care system in light of this evidence.

As we will see, while generally applicable throughout the health care system, this approach is particularly relevant to new reproductive technologies. It would be useful to know, for example, the relative effectiveness — in terms of both individual health and cost to the health care system — of a chlamydia prevention program and an *in vitro* fertilization program. (Chlamydia, the most common sexually transmitted disease among women in their late teens and early 20s, can lead to pelvic inflammatory disease [PID], which in turn may lead to fallopian tube blockage — a principal reason for the use of *in vitro* fertilization.) The urgency of adopting an evidence-based approach has become particularly evident as pressures on the health care system have mounted in the past decade.

Pressures on the Health Care System

Canadians are generally satisfied with the quality of our medical care system, but concern is surfacing about whether the system can continue to respond to current pressures on it without buckling under the strain. These pressures include the rising costs of care and the tendency to expand the boundaries of the system — in response to both practitioners' treatment patterns and patients' expectations — as new technologies become available or as medical solutions are sought to problems once considered outside the system's purview. In

> Canada's health care system is therefore at an important crossroads. If we can learn to manage it better, it can continue to play an important and respected role in Canadian life. If we do not, we run the danger of allowing the system to be eroded by these pressures, with deteriorating standards, less access, and social inequities the likely results.

the absence of evidence on the effectiveness of treatments, the health care system is vulnerable to pressure groups; politically astute patients and service providers, in alliance, not only may be making the system responsive to real needs, but also may be pushing the system in directions that are not sustainable and that society collectively does not want.

Canada's health care system is therefore at an important crossroads. If we can learn to manage it better, it can continue to play an important and respected role in Canadian life. If we do not, we run the danger of allowing the system to be eroded by these pressures, with deteriorating standards, less access, and social inequities the likely results.

Growing Use and Costs

Several factors have generated rising costs for the health care system. The number of older Canadians, for example, has increased steadily in the past two decades; moreover, there has been an increase in per capita use of health care services and medications by elderly Canadians. This greater use is attributable in part to the absence of more appropriate community-based supports; many residents currently in nursing homes and many patients in acute care hospitals, whatever their age, could be released tomorrow if a system of home care and community-based day programs were in place.

Another factor that has created pressure on the health care system is the disproportionate increase in the number of physicians relative to the increase in the general population. Between 1981 and 1991, the number of doctors practising in Canada rose by 38 percent, while the population grew by just 12 percent. Recognizing the pressures this creates on the system, provincial ministers of health agreed recently to reduce enrolment at the country's medical schools by 10 percent as part of a nation-wide agreement. The aim of this policy is not just to contain costs but to use our collective resources more appropriately and effectively. There is no good evidence that the increase in number of physicians per capita is a good use of resources and results in better care for patients.

Fee-for-service reimbursement, which is the way most doctors are paid, has also contributed to rising costs. As gatekeepers of the health care system, physicians control access to diagnostic testing and hospital and medical services; in fact, service providers (physicians), not consumers,

> Along an alternative line of questioning, there would appear to be a relatively high level of pessimism about the presence of potentially costly situations facing the health care system. For example, over 80% of respondents surveyed agreed that many use health services unnecessarily and 70% felt that doctors often prescribe unnecessary medication. It would appear that a majority (69%) also feel that hospitals are overutilized and that home care approaches are sufficient for many individuals.
>
> M. de Groh, "Reproductive Technologies, Adoption, and Issues on the Cost of Health Care: Summary of Canada Health Monitor Results," in Research Volumes of the Commission, 1993.

largely determine the extent of use. The fee-for-service arrangement can lead to an increase in the number of services provided or create an incentive for physicians to select hospital or medical services over other forms of care. This is an extremely complex issue of system design, and one that simplistic solutions will not resolve. Putting physicians on salary, for example, would not necessarily ensure greater levels of evaluation and accountability in the system or a more rational allocation of resources within it.

The fact remains, however, that under the current system physicians are not accountable for the cost implications of their treatment decisions; they respond rationally to a system that does not ask or expect them to consider the cost of various approaches to treatment or the alternatives offered by non-medical approaches. This tendency is reinforced when patients expect more diagnostic and treatment services and equate expensive and technology-dependent approaches with "better" medicine. The news media and word of mouth also play a role in expanding public knowledge and hence the potential demand for treatment, especially the newer and more technology-intensive forms of care.

The technologies themselves are not responsible for rising costs, however. Rather, it is their application and patterns of use that lead to spiralling costs. Some technologies may in fact have the capacity to reduce costs in specific areas of medical care, provided they are used only where they have been demonstrated effective for the purpose in question.

Indeed, the proliferation of new medical technologies has been seen as another source of rising health care costs. It is true that these technologies have developed and spread rapidly in recent decades — new imaging technology, transplant technology, and intensive life support, as well as the technologies that are the subject of the Commission's mandate. Diagnostic procedures have also proliferated. Some of them are technology-based, and some of them are used routinely without evidence that they make any difference to health outcomes. In addition, tests and services are sometimes provided to enable physicians to defend against subsequent litigation, although "defensive" medicine remains less of a problem in Canada than in the United States. The technologies themselves are not responsible for rising costs, however. Rather, it is their application and patterns of use that lead to spiralling costs. Some technologies may in fact have the capacity to reduce costs in specific areas of medical care, provided they are used only where they have been demonstrated effective for the purpose in question.

In summary, patterns of medical treatment and technology use, the disproportionate increase in the number of physicians, and the lack of accountability in the fee-for-service reimbursement system — all have contributed to cost pressures in the health care system. The problem is compounded by declining economic growth. Although health care spending by governments rose during the expansionary 1970s, relative to overall growth in the economy it remained steady or increased only slightly.   Financing the expansion of the health care system during the 1970s did not create cost pressures because the economy was expanding — health care spending and gross domestic product rose in tandem and at

> The technology of monitoring of pregnancy and birth may at first glance be simple, but in fact it involves the complex field of medical practice and hospital organization.
>
> *Brief to the Commission from the Toronto Birth Centre, March 31, 1992.*

roughly comparable rates.   By the 1980s, however, with slower overall economic growth, the same rates of increase in health care spending that had been acceptable in the 1970s became unmanageable; the question of how to finance health care in an economy with little or no growth began to create serious and mounting pressures to contain costs.

Government Expenditures on Health Care

The cost to governments is only part of the cost of health care in Canada. Health care costs also include what Canadians spend on dental care, eyeglasses, prescription and non-prescription drugs, chiropractors and other alternative caregivers, supplementary health insurance, and other health-related expenses, as well as health insurance premiums (in those provinces that still have them) and health levies or taxes on employers.   Many of the solutions proposed to ease resource pressures involve attempting to reduce the cost to governments. These solutions include off-loading some of the

> Increasing the proportion of health care costs borne by these private payers is a dangerously simplistic response. The issue is not how much the health care system costs governments, but how much it costs our economy as a whole. The other issue here is that most cost shifting — for example, through user fees — goes against the ethos of distributing health care resources according to need rather than ability to pay.

cost to governments by requiring others — patients, employers, or insurance companies — to pay more. Increasing the proportion of health care costs borne by these private payers is a dangerously simplistic response.   The issue is not how much the health care system costs governments, but how much it costs our economy as a whole. Resources devoted to health care — whether they come from the pockets of taxpayers, employers, insurance companies, or governments — are resources unavailable for allocation to other social priorities or investment in other parts of the economy. The other issue here is that most cost shifting — for example, through user fees — goes against the ethos of distributing health care resources according to need rather than ability to pay. Simply shifting the burden from one group of payers to another, then, will not solve the problem; other remedies are needed.

Federal and Provincial Responsibilities for Health Care

In practice, responsibility for the health and well-being of Canadians is shared by the federal and provincial governments. Under its peace, order, and good government power, the federal government can regulate aspects of health and welfare that are of national concern. Pursuant to its criminal law power, the federal government can prohibit practices and products that are dangerous to health. The federal government is responsible for health, safety, and environmental regulation in areas of federal jurisdiction, such as interprovincial transportation and telecommunications. It delivers health services to status Indian and Inuit persons, to members of the Canadian armed forces, and to people in federal institutions, such as penitentiaries. Through its spending power, the federal government conducts health research and public education and significantly subsidizes provincial health care services. Finally, the federal government has the power to ratify international treaties and to participate in other international health and welfare initiatives.

Health care delivery is a matter of provincial responsibility, pursuant to provincial jurisdiction over hospitals and health professions, and matters of local or private concern. The provinces and territories administer the costs of medical and hospital care through health insurance plans and through their general budgets and regulation. They also finance a range of other health care services, including home care, community health centres, and non-physician services, such as physiotherapy and occupational therapy, delivered in health care settings. The provinces and territories are also involved in public health promotion. Pursuant to their jurisdiction over property and civil rights, the provinces are responsible for occupational health and safety, environmental regulation, and the regulation and licensing of health care facilities and health care professionals, including nurses and physicians.

In the midst of these developments, provincial governments are grappling with a new pressure: declining federal cash contributions to health care costs. Provincial and federal governments have shared the cost of health care through various formulas and arrangements negotiated periodically since the late 1950s. Initially, the federal contribution was determined by what the provinces actually spent to provide health care services. This arrangement proved unsatisfactory both for the federal government, which wanted a greater degree of predictability in the amount of transfers to the provinces, and for the provinces, which wanted greater flexibility to set their own spending priorities and to determine how the federal contribution would be spent.

The formula was therefore changed in 1977 with the passage of the *Federal-Provincial Fiscal Arrangements and Established Programs Financing Act*. Since 1977, then, federal contributions to health and post-secondary education have been in the form of "block funding," with no link to

---

The *Canada Health Act*

Although health care services are administered and delivered by the provinces and territories, they are subsidized by the federal government under various federal laws and according to criteria set out in the *Canada Health Act*. The act, which came into effect in 1984, confirms the criteria and conditions that must be in place for provincial and territorial health care systems to be eligible for federal funding. These criteria are public administration, comprehensiveness, universality, portability, and accessibility.

Public administration means that the health care plan in the province or territory must be administered on a non-profit basis and by a public authority. *Comprehensiveness* refers to the fact that most services provided by hospitals and medical practitioners are insured. *Universality* means all residents of a province or territory are entitled to insured health care services. *Portability* means that Canadians moving from one province or territory to another or visiting temporarily continue to be protected by health insurance. *Accessibility* refers to the provision of insured health care services without financial impediments.

Under the act the federal health minister has the authority to penalize any province that fails to comply with the criteria, the most severe sanction being to reduce or withhold federal transfer payments to the province.

Although the national health care law is based on the fundamental principle of public funding for "medically necessary" services, a survey conducted for the Commission found that no province or territory has defined this term operationally.

Health care services are referred to collectively as a "system," a term that implies an integrated whole, but in fact most provinces' systems are composed of many diverse parts with few formal links among them. In effect, most provincial "systems" represent the sum total of many individual decisions made by diverse groups of practitioners in a range of health care settings.

---

provinces' actual spending patterns. The provinces and territories receive per capita grants from the federal government in the form of transfers of tax points (that is, they are given a percentage of tax revenues), with the remainder made up in cash. The proportion of the transfer that consists of cash varies from province to province, depending on the tax points they receive. The federal minister of health can enforce compliance with the five principles of the *Canada Health Act*, the ultimate penalty being the withholding of the federal cash contribution until the province breaching the act corrects the situation.

As part of its strategy to reduce the deficit, the federal government introduced the *Government Expenditures Restraint Act*, which became law in February 1991. The *Restraint Act* limits annual growth in federal transfers to the provinces under the *Contributions Act* by a formula — growth in gross national product (GNP) less 3 percent (with adjustments for changes in a province's population). Because the tax revenue percentage portion of the transfer is calculated first, the remaining cash portion declines if income tax revenues rise more quickly than GNP growth less 3 percent. Income tax revenues have generally risen more quickly than this; as a result, it has been estimated that within 10 to 15 years under the current formula, the cash portion of federal transfers will disappear entirely (sooner in some provinces than in others, because of the relative proportion of tax points and cash in their transfer arrangements).

Dwindling federal cash transfers for health care (and post-secondary education, which is covered by the same legislation) have the same effect on provincial treasuries as any other decline in revenues. Provinces have to decide whether to respond by cutting back, either in the health care system (for example, by de-insuring some services or closing facilities) or in other programs; financing spending through borrowing; or raising additional revenues through taxation or other means.

Importantly, the cash transfers are virtually the only tool available to the federal government to exert influence over provinces' compliance with the five criteria set out in the *Canada Health Act*. This means that phasing out these transfers through the current formula makes it more difficult — some would argue impossible — for the federal government to maintain a strong presence in the health care system and ensure compliance with the *Canada Health Act*. Either there will be no federal contribution to hold back, or the amount will be so minimal as to provide no incentive for provinces to adhere to the *Canada Health Act* criteria with respect to such issues as user fees. The federal government has stated that it intends to maintain its leverage through other funding mechanisms, but it is difficult to see what mechanisms will remain at its disposal once the full effects of the *Restraint Act* are felt. This is of great concern to Canadians — who showed a high level of commitment to the five principles in the *Canada Health Act* in surveys conducted for the Commission.

This collapse of a strong central cohesive force, coupled with the other pressures on the health care system described earlier in this chapter, raises fears that universality and accessibility will be eroded, leading to development of a two-tier system — one publicly funded, and one available to those who can pay for it. We think it very important, therefore, that the federal government consider how to maintain its capacity to require provincial compliance with the criteria of the *Canada Health Act* and to introduce the mechanism necessary to do so.

> We think it very important, therefore, that the federal government consider how to maintain its capacity to require provincial compliance with the criteria of the *Canada Health Act* and to introduce the mechanism necessary to do so.

Concern about the pressures on the system has also led to debate about what the boundaries or limits of the health care system should be if we are to keep universality intact so that all Canadians can continue to benefit.

The Limits of the System

We heard extensive testimony reflecting growing recognition that there are limits to what the health care system can achieve and limits on the demands to which the system is capable of responding. Two major types of boundaries are being discussed in current debates about the health care system: its external limits and its internal limits.

In reproductive technologies, as in other health fields, the external limits of the system are generally defined by provincial health insurance programs. As legally defined in the *Canada Health Act*, the health care system includes only medically necessary hospital and physician services. But in reality, provincial systems include both medical care and health care. Defining the external limits of the medical care system means determining what kinds of problems are appropriate for it to treat. For example, is alcoholism a problem that requires medical treatment? Are learning disabilities? Is smoking cessation?

Services considered to be "medically necessary" are covered by provincial and territorial health insurance plans, which vary across the country; the types of problems deemed appropriate for medical attention are determined by what the province or territory (and tradition) considers to be medically required. In a way, these plans set the external limits of the health care system, but they differ slightly by jurisdiction — thus, there is no universally applicable definition of the external limits of the health care system. In Ontario, for example, provincial health insurance covers the cost of *in vitro* fertilization, whereas other provinces' plans do not; that is, Ontario's policy is to include IVF within the boundaries of the health care system. Provinces that do not insure IVF have made the decision to keep this procedure outside the boundaries of their health care systems. This means it is available in those provinces only to those able to pay for it.

Several questions arise when we try to define external limits. What can the medical care system realistically be expected to accomplish? Do such services represent the most appropriate strategy to deal with a given problem? What is more properly the responsibility of other systems — such as education, social services, income support, or health promotion?

Unless the issue of external limits is addressed, the boundaries of the medical care system could expand indefinitely. This is unrealistic, not only financially but conceptually. Expecting it to respond to all problems not only places unreasonable burdens on that system but, importantly, detracts from its ability to deal properly with the issues that are clearly within its mandate — to provide effective treatment for medical conditions.

Once a decision has been made to insure a service, the internal limits of the system — who receives treatment and under what circumstances — are defined by practitioners and institutions. If it is agreed that a specific problem is medical in nature and therefore should come within the ambit of the medical care system, the next decision is whether treatment should be offered to all those affected by the problem, or whether there should be limits or criteria for determining who gets treatment. It may be generally agreed, for example, that blocked arteries to the heart constitute a medical problem and should be treated within the health care system. But what should the internal limit be? Should all persons with this diagnosis have surgery? Or should it be limited to those for whom there will be an appreciable increase in length and quality of life? Similarly, should everyone diagnosed with infertility receive *in vitro* fertilization? Or should it be limited to those cases where medical history, diagnosis, and other relevant considerations suggest that the likelihood of a live birth is greater?

> The concept of health has expanded tremendously, far beyond the capacity of the public sector to undertake responsibility for it. The public sector has undertaken responsibility for health *care*, fairly narrowly defined. The more you expand the definition of health and then go from there to say that anything that contributes to health is in some way a public responsibility, the more you load up the state with responsibilities that it *can't* fulfill; that many of its citizens do not think are legitimate for it to fulfill ... The state can't take responsibility for all the things that contribute to health. And that's especially important it seems to me for the area of new reproductive technologies.
>
> *R.G. Evans, reviewer, research volumes of the Commission, 1992.*

Decisions about the system's boundaries have significant implications for the cost of medical care. This has been recognized by many jurisdictions, and one, Oregon, has attempted to respond to this issue. In order to extend Medicaid coverage to most state residents below the federal poverty line, the state decided to narrow the boundaries of what treatments and services would be covered. More people will be covered for medically high priority services, rather than covering more procedures for fewer people. A commission consisting of physicians, consumers, and representatives from the public health and social services sectors undertook the task of ranking more than 700 services in order of importance, with the understanding that, if funding is insufficient, services will be eliminated, starting at the bottom of the list. The value attached to each procedure was determined using research into effectiveness, a formula considering cost and benefit, public hearings, and survey data.

Although IVF was one of the treatments ranked, as we explain in Chapter 20, there were methodological problems that meant it may have been given a falsely low ranking. Nevertheless, the general approach is one that many people feel will lead to a more stable, humane, and effective way of distributing health care resources, while reducing the provision of services that are medically ineffective and are not valued highly by the community. They say that it is only a matter of time before Canada is forced to adopt a similar approach to providing health care services. Others have said, however, that the project rations health care only for some of the population — those who are poor — and will have a disproportionately negative impact on poor women and children, because people who can afford private insurance are not affected. They say that because of this, prioritization is an unfair and inappropriate method for distributing health care, which could lead to a distortion of the doctor/patient relationship and to poor care.

There are important differences between Canada's health care system and the system in Oregon. Nevertheless, it is clear that we need to use resources effectively to avoid, for as long as possible, a rationing approach to cost containment. A better approach to relieving pressure on the health care system is to reorient it to obtain better value for money — value in this situation being defined as the health achieved through the expenditure of dollars on the medical care system. This is an approach the Commission endorses — not only because it offers a means of using resources wisely while maintaining services of the quality Canadians have come to expect, but also because reorienting the system to reflect principles such as effectiveness and value for money is a way to manage the system to withstand the pressures that might otherwise cause it to break down. Reorienting the system in this way will not remove the need to make tough choices — but the fiscal boundary at which choices occur will be farther out.

The System's Limits and New Reproductive Technologies: The Issues of Access

Decisions about the external and internal limits of the health care system are clearly relevant, then, to new reproductive technologies. For instance, should infertility be considered a condition that requires medical attention? If so, who should have access to treatments made available within the system? The complex issue of access to new reproductive technology services has two components — availability and accessibility.

Availability concerns the external limits of the health care system — whether services are provided at all through Canada's publicly funded system. Ethical issues and questions about the broad allocation of resources to and within the health care system often figure in availability debates. Decisions about whether a given service should be made available must necessarily be made in light of how delivery can be effected, but for the most part availability decisions revolve around whether, in principle, it is appropriate to provide the service at all.

Accessibility of services deals with the issues of to whom they are available and what the limitations are. These wide-ranging issues of organization and delivery include who can deliver the service, where it is delivered (both geographically and in which health facilities), what quantity of services is provided, how a service is paid for, the medical conditions for which it is provided (the internal limits previously discussed), and any other operational factors influencing whether or how a person obtains the service.

The Commission's research showed that the provision of new reproductive technology-related services in Canada is not uniform with respect to either aspect of access. Services are available in some regions but not in others. Eligibility criteria vary from place to place, resulting in differential access to such services as do exist. Testimony before the Commission showed how this unevenness is affecting Canadians seeking treatment.

As the Commission's deliberations proceeded, it became clear that access to new reproductive technologies is one of the broad issues touching several aspects of our mandate and one that must be resolved with reference to Canadian values and health care priorities. It raises questions about the boundaries of the health care system — and hence the demands on it and the cost of sus-

> One basic thing is that the health care system is not immune to the kinds of biases reflected in the general society. In fact, those social biases have worked their way right through the system.
>
> *Discussion with Health Economists, Transcript, Vancouver, British Columbia, April 25, 1991.*

taining it — but also issues of social justice, equality, and fairness. It also raises questions of the relationship between the need for standards of care and provincial jurisdiction in setting these standards. We believe, however, that these health care issues are primarily national in nature because of their profound social implications. We therefore return to these questions of access in the context of our examination of each of the technologies in Part Two. Here we present our overall conclusions and how we arrived at them.

Coming to recommendations about access to reproductive technologies involved several inter-related considerations for the Commission that necessitated a step-by-step approach. First, the Commission considered whether the technologies should be available at all in Canada: this involved individual assessments specific to each technique or procedure that factored in our guiding principles, what Canadians told us about the significance of the technology in their lives and its implications for them individually or as members of a particular segment of society, and our findings about safety and efficacy. If we determined on this basis that a technology should be available, the next consideration was whether it should be offered as a medical treatment through the publicly funded health care system and, if so, under what conditions. We made this determination through an evidence-based assessment of whether the procedure was actually of benefit for its intended purpose, whether it could be provided at acceptable levels of risk and within a framework of appropriate regulation, and whether its inclusion in the health care system represented a wise use of public resources in and of itself and relative to other public health priorities.

Finally, if we determined that a procedure should in fact be offered as a medical treatment within the medical care system, we looked at the factors that determine access to procedures within that system. This means examining such issues as equitable access, as defined by both the *Canadian Charter of Rights and Freedoms* and the *Canada Health Act*, and the kinds of barriers to access that could arise — for example, geographical distance, linguistic or cultural factors, financial considerations, and so on.

Our conclusions, as will become evident in Part Two of our report, are that

- if safe, ethical, and effective means are available to help Canadians achieve the goal of having a healthy child, then as a caring society we should consider how to devote our collective resources to doing so;

> If safe, ethical, and effective means are available to help Canadians achieve the goal of having a healthy child, then as a caring society we should consider how to devote our collective resources to doing so.

- if procedures have been demonstrated to be safe and effective, and if we have determined as a society that they should be available, then we must be prepared to commit public resources to their provision through the health care system; to do otherwise would be to ignore Canadians' values with respect to non-commercialization of reproduction and equity and fairness in access to treatment, and, as we will show in subsequent chapters, to undermine the publicly funded health care system by imposing uncontrollable burdens on it; and

- if a procedure is to be provided through the public health system, access to it must be determined by medical criteria and in accordance with the principles established in the *Canada Health Act*, the *Canadian Charter of Rights and Freedoms*, and human rights legislation.

Emerging Issues in Health Care

Among the responses to pressures on the health care system are several with relevance to new reproductive technologies. These issues — which have been gaining prominence in recent debates about the dimensions and goals of the system — include quality control in medical care, the appropriate allocation of resources for acute care relative to prevention, increased information and choice for users of the health care system, privacy and confidentiality, and greater opportunities for participation in individual and collective decisions about health care.

Quality Control

Evidence-based medicine is essential to the concept of quality control in the provision of medical services. The Hippocratic oath directs the physician to work for the benefit of the patient and not to do harm; this means both refraining from actions that are likely to harm and seeking actively to avoid harm or prevent it from occurring. To avoid or prevent harm, it is essential to ensure quality control, a broad concept encompassing the need to "do the right things" as well as the need to "do things right." Yet serious problems with respect to quality control have been identified in the health care field. We discuss how issues of quality control relate to new reproductive technologies and make recommendations regarding them throughout Part Two of our report.

Quality control is an issue for Canadians not only in relation to reproductive technologies but also with regard to medical care generally. Canadians told us they are concerned both about the safety of drugs and procedures and about the long-term health effects on technology users and their children.

A first element of quality control, sometimes referred to as quality assurance, is setting standards for appropriate care, comparing current practice to these standards and, if necessary, adjusting practices to bring them into line with standards, then adapting or adjusting standards as knowledge evolves. There is a need for clear guidelines in this area. As we will see, physicians' use of treatments varies, and there is inconsistency in how and why individual reproductive technologies are used. Nor is responsibility for developing and monitoring adherence to guidelines clearly established.

A second important element of quality control is making sure that only effective treatments — treatments that work — are used. Preventing harm requires finding out how well a treatment works and what its potential risks and side effects are before using it widely. Techniques used to evaluate treatments range from randomized clinical trials to the informal methods of individual physicians. No technique is universally applicable for every medical technology — sometimes simpler approaches are sufficient, and frequently it is best to derive evidence from several techniques. The crucial point is that some sort of systematic evaluation needs to be in place. Unfortunately, this is often not the case.

Moreover, the results of evaluation may not always be used appropriately. For example, clinical trials to test effectiveness and identify risks may result in a treatment being approved for use for a clearly defined set of indications — that is, the specific medical circumstances in which its use was tested. Once a treatment has been approved for use and becomes more widely known, however, often it is used to treat an expanding range of people with other indications — without any evidence that it will do any good. When this happens, the benefits of the treatment in terms of overall health improvement in the population decline. Further, the safety and effectiveness that were established for the treatment's original use may not apply to these new and wider uses. Similarly, once drugs have been tested for safety and effectiveness and approved for use, there is no monitoring to ensure that the drugs are being used in the way and for the purposes for which they were tested and approved.

As we have seen, however, a more serious problem than limited evaluation is no evaluation at all. It is estimated that between 30 and 80 percent of all medical therapies, including surgeries, have never been rigorously evaluated. This is not to say that conducting such evaluations is easy — on the contrary, the design and

> Once a treatment has been approved for use and becomes more widely known, however, often it is used to treat an expanding range of people with other indications — without any evidence that it will do any good. When this happens, the benefits of the treatment in terms of overall health improvement in the population decline.

execution of needed evaluations may be very difficult, but they must be done. Moreover, management of the health care system must be based on these efforts: information from evaluations must be reflected in clinical practice and in resource allocation decisions.

The Commission saw several examples of the benefits of this approach. The Canadian Collaborative CVS-Amniocentesis Clinical Trial Group, for example, conducted multicentre randomized control trials in the introduction of two different techniques for prenatal diagnosis — amniocentesis and chorionic villus sampling. These were international pioneering initiatives that have helped set the standard for introducing and assessing prenatal diagnosis technology and controlling its further dissemination on the basis of study findings (see Chapter 26).

Apart from examples such as these, which are the exception rather than the rule, the far more common sequence is for medical treatments or technologies to be introduced and disseminated through a gradual process. First, promising reports appear in the medical literature. Then, professionals adopt the innovation and the public begins to expect it as media reports and word of mouth make it more widely known. Next, the innovation tends to become a standard part of the care offered by many practitioners. Only then are large-scale clinical trials of some innovations conducted and the results disseminated. Critical evaluations of these studies may or may not result in further discussion of the potential risks and benefits of using the technology or procedure. Finally, medical consensus develops, either discrediting the procedure or generally accepting it. Such a process is precisely how many forms of pregnancy and childbirth care were introduced, with scientists only now conducting extensive evaluations of the results of these practices and discovering that significant numbers of them either should be discontinued or need more investigation before their benefits (or lack of them) can be determined.

Decisions about which services are publicly supported through provincial health insurance coverage have been influenced historically not by evaluation results but by lobbying, media coverage, and emotional appeals. Many Canadians continue to believe, however, that funding and diffusion of health care technology are rational, consistent across provinces, facilities, and practitioners, and closely related to effectiveness. In fact, analysis of patterns of technology use shows that the inherent attributes of a given health technology (effectiveness, safety) are not related in any consistent way to its diffusion. Moreover, health care technology diffusion is not related consistently to the prevalence of disease. Not surprisingly, this situation is of great concern to governments, which now want to be able to make empirical, evidence-based decisions about how much of which technologies or procedures should be provided.

> Decisions about which services are publicly supported through provincial health insurance coverage have been influenced historically not by evaluation results but by lobbying, media coverage, and emotional appeals. Many Canadians continue to believe, however, that funding and diffusion of health care technology are rational, consistent across provinces, facilities, and practitioners, and closely related to effectiveness.

Support for a more rational approach is growing, accelerated in part by recognition of the need to make most effective use of finite resources. Two provinces, for example, have established health technology assessment offices, and a joint federal/provincial/territorial body, the Canadian Coordinating Office for Health Technology Assessment (CCOHTA), was instituted by the country's health ministers in 1989. The Quebec government set up the Conseil d'évaluation des technologies de la santé in 1988, while the government of British Columbia established the Office of Health Technology Assessment through a grant to the University of British Columbia in 1990. The University of Manitoba also has a unit within the Department of Community Health Sciences devoted to health services research and

> Appropriateness of technology including the provision of health promotion and illness prevention programs must be a major concern given the country's pre-occupation with quality care, cost effectiveness and health care ethics.
>
> *A. Baumgart, National President, Canadian Nurses Association, Public Hearings Transcripts, Ottawa, Ontario, September 20, 1990.*

analysis, the Manitoba Centre for Health Policy and Evaluation. Then, in January 1992, the Conference of Deputy Ministers of Health adopted an eight-point set of policy directions that is tantamount to a national health strategy. One of the eight points is the development of national clinical guidelines to reduce the provision of unnecessary medical treatments. CCOHTA also reports annually to the Conference of Deputy Ministers of Health on its work. In addition, the Ontario Ministry of Health and the Ontario Medical Association recently established (1992) the Institute for Clinical Evaluative Sciences to conduct research on the accessibility, quality, and efficiency of medical services in the province.

All medical interventions involve a weighing of the potential risks and benefits; there are no risk-free situations. It is clear, nevertheless, that appropriate medical care can be provided only if evidence collected through clinical trials and other appropriate forms of evaluation is available to guideline setters, practitioners, and funders. Evidence alone is not sufficient, however; it must be translated into funding decisions, guidelines, behaviour, and practice.

The Commission's approach to examining reproductive technologies rested on the premise that safety and efficacy must be demonstrated before judgements can be made about the appropriateness of providing or not providing treatment. Before such a judgement is made, treatment provided in the absence of evidence should be considered research, not therapy. This raises questions about when medical technologies cease being experimental procedures and become therapeutic treatments, as well as who is qualified to make this distinction and how such decisions should be made. This gap is being filled by a new term — "innovative therapy" — the practice of which requires no scrutiny by research ethics boards. Because borders of innovative therapy are not clear, the possibility arises that this rubric could be used to circumvent the structures, regulations, ethical oversight, and protections that apply to research involving human subjects.

> Treatment provided in the absence of evidence should be considered research, not therapy.

The protections afforded by categorizing a procedure as research include (1) review and approval by the research ethics committee of the institution (hospital, university) where the research is being conducted; (2) specific requirements for obtaining informed consent from participants; and (3) inability to charge participants for services received as research. Relevant concerns that are dealt with in this way include certain ethical aspects, such as the information needed by people before they give their consent to participate in research, and how the privacy and the confidentiality of information about them generated by the research will be protected. Thus, whether a procedure is designated "research" or "treatment" has very important practical implications. Research is important — it is irresponsible to provide treatment if it is not also accompanied by research aimed at assessing the results of treatment and improving practices. However, in this field we see no useful place for the category "innovative therapy" — in fact, people consenting to such procedures should have the protections afforded by categorizing the procedures as research.

One of the issues that arises inevitably in discussions of quality control is the cost of evaluations, particularly when techniques such as clinical trials are involved. In the Commission's view, it is reasonable to recommend that provincial ministries of health fund such trials, mainly because it is the responsibility of these ministries to manage the health care system on behalf of taxpayers, making wise use of resources and appropriate decisions about which services should be included in the system. It is from their budgets that treatments, if demonstrated effective, will eventually be paid for, and such trials will provide evidence on which to base rational resource allocation. It is the view of Commissioners that ministries of health should demand rigorous technology assessment before agreeing to fund services through the publicly supported health system and should be prepared to fund such assessments in the interests of providing better medical care and a better managed health care system.

> It is the view of Commissioners that ministries of health should demand rigorous technology assessment before agreeing to fund services through the publicly supported health system and should be prepared to fund such assessments in the interests of providing better medical care and a better managed health care system.

Provinces might well be able to share the cost of such trials and avoid duplication by coordinating their efforts. In addition, we believe that the federal government, through our proposed National Reproductive Technologies Commission, should fund some of the most urgent clinical trials and work with the provinces to identify areas where sharing of cost and information would contribute to the rapid assembly of sufficient data on which to base health care service and funding decisions.

Over the years, ministries of health have made decisions to include specific procedures or services within the health care system before they were assessed properly, relying on the various professional colleges and professional associations to set guidelines for practice and on the cooperation and discipline of individual practitioners to refrain from using them in unproven ways. In the past, ministries may not have seen much benefit in investing in technology assessment (for example, funding trials), largely because they saw little indication that the evidence produced by such research actually influenced or changed medical practice. However, under the licensing system we propose for assisted conception services and other reproductive technologies, the structure and mechanisms will be in place to ensure that the evidence produced by clinical trials does lead to changes in practice and to control of inappropriate use of technologies and procedures. This is a cogent reason for ministries of health to fund both initial assessment and continuing evaluation of technologies in the reproductive sphere.

A quality control question separate from whether the technologies work is whether they have short- or long-term health effects that should determine the evolution of practice — for example, whether the circumstances or conditions under which a treatment is provided should change in light of knowledge gained by providing the treatment to large numbers of people over a significant period of time. Assembling this knowledge requires various monitoring and follow-up techniques, such as the reporting system and the record linkage approach we suggest with respect to the long-term health effects on women and children of assisted conception techniques (see, for example, Chapter 18, where we explain the concept of record linkage as a means of tracking long-term health effects of technology use in greater detail). Monitoring and follow-up of this type provide a way to close the quality control loop, by ensuring that knowledge gained through practice is fed back into the process of revising, adapting, and updating guidelines and standards of practice.

Acute Care and Prevention

How the health care system values and allocates resources between medical care and preventive efforts is another emerging issue. Consensus is emerging on the need for a shift in resource allocation between illness care on the one hand and illness prevention and health promotion on the other, but the appropriate dimensions and timing of such a shift are not yet entirely clear. The use of new reproductive technologies illustrates some aspects of this issue because it raises questions about why such treatment is needed in the first place and whether infertility could be prevented. What should be the relative roles of prevention and acute care (that is, medical treatment) with regard to infertility?

Preventing harm is inherent in the ethic of care. In addition, if prevention is demonstrated to be more effective in terms of health outcomes and cost than treating a problem after it has occurred, it is obviously the more desirable option as well as the more ethical approach. The issue is complex, however, because the line between prevention and treatment may be hard to establish. For example, some aspects of the current practices of physicians and dentists relate to prevention, even though their services are usually considered to be in the treatment sphere. Without systematic evaluation against established standards or criteria, it is impossible to know whether prevention programs are achieving the preventive effects intended. As we have seen, many treatments and medical services are also unevaluated and of unproven value in terms of producing health. These situations make it very difficult to judge whether the current distribution of health care resources between medical care and preventive approaches makes most sense. However, this does not mean we should take no action for change — in fact, it is crucial that we do act, as we discuss in Part Two.

One apparent roadblock to greater emphasis on illness prevention and health promotion is the shortage of reliable data about the effectiveness of prevention and promotion strategies. We agree that evaluations of effectiveness should be an integral part of prevention strategies to provide a basis for policy and program adjustments and resource allocation decisions.   At the same time, we note that many medical treatments and drug therapies have been introduced and funded without being demonstrated effective through appropriate evaluation and assessment. A double standard appears to be at work, with a greater burden of proof being required for prevention than for medical treatment: preventive efforts have often been required to demonstrate their effectiveness *before* they are supported, while medical treatments have been introduced and paid for through the health care system without good evidence of effectiveness.

> Evaluations of effectiveness should be an integral part of prevention strategies to provide a basis for policy and program adjustments and resource allocation decisions ... A double standard appears to be at work, with a greater burden of proof being required for prevention than for medical treatment.

The debate about the appropriate roles for prevention and acute care has important implications for new reproductive technologies. The lessons learned from the general debate have been instructive in our deliberations regarding the appropriate roles for prevention and acute care in relation to infertility and how resources should be apportioned between them. How can we determine, for example, the relative cost-effectiveness of efforts to reduce exposure to risk factors for infertility — such as sexually transmitted diseases, smoking, and aging/delayed childbearing — and efforts to treat infertility once it has occurred? We return to these questions in Part Two, where we discuss infertility, its prevalence, and associated risk factors.

The Role of the Patient: Informed Choice

The third emerging issue in health care involves the concept of informed choice. Today's health care users want comprehensive information and greater involvement in both individual and collective decisions about health and medical care. Information is one essential component of informed decision making; the other involves the skills and opportunities needed to weigh information and make judgements in light of identified values and priorities. Fully informed choice offers potential benefits for both individuals and the health care system.

Physicians are required to obtain the informed consent of competent patients before providing any treatment offered in the health care system. There is a growing perception, however, that the current informed consent standard is insufficient, particularly in the context of new reproductive technologies. A new concept — informed choice — is emerging not as an alternative to informed consent (which will remain a requirement of the law and medical profession guidelines), but as an essential supplement and complement to it.

People have a legal right to decide what is done to their bodies; it is a denial of the inviolability of the person for someone to be touched without consent. The current informed consent standard, developed by the courts in response to litigation over the years, clarifies what information physicians must disclose to patients and acquire from them to avoid violating patients' legal rights. The standard requires that doctors obtain patients' consent by providing sufficient information about the treatment to ensure that patients know what they are agreeing to before beginning treatment. The informed consent standard thus arose in response to the question of what physicians must do to respect the physical and psychological integrity of their patients. Many people inside and outside the medical profession now believe that this approach is too narrow, given the complexity of medical problems and the range of ways to resolve them, and given growing recognition of the importance of involving people in decisions about their own health.

The concept of "informed choice" represents this broader approach. Physicians are still under a legal obligation to respect the patient's inviolability and autonomy and thus to obtain informed consent to treatment. But informed choice involves in addition the presentation of other available options, including non-medical ones, and support for patients in making choices from among these options.

The approach represented by informed choice is based in part on growing recognition that patients tend, quite understandably, to be more concerned about risks than clinicians are. When fully informed about the potential risks surrounding various approaches to treating prostate cancer, for example, men have been found to prefer less invasive treatments, particularly given great uncertainty about the benefits of more aggressive approaches. In other words, when patients have precisely the same information as clinicians about the probable results of treatment, their

> Are the women who turn to the NRTs told from the outset about the real success rates of the various reproductive technologies? ...
>
> Women should know what price they will have to pay, not only in financial terms for the procedure itself, but in terms of risks to their physical and mental health and in terms of availability and time.
>
> *Brief to the Commission from the New Brunswick Advisory Council on the Status of Women, October 19, 1990.*

choices differ considerably from those clinicians might make, because patients weigh the information differently and are generally more averse to risk. Instructions in the form of living wills and advance medical directives are other examples of how patients may be less open than physicians to intervention.

Researchers have concluded that the amount of invasive medical technology now being provided may actually exceed the amount patients would choose to have if they were fully informed and left to decide according to their own priorities and preferences. These findings may well be applicable more widely throughout the health care system and could have cost advantages for the system, but, just as important, this approach means that treatment would be offered in ways that are more consistent with patients' values and priorities.

As we discuss in greater detail with respect to specific

> Our experience with physicians is that the training is more focussed on informed consent as opposed to informed choice, and there's an important distinction there.
>
> Informed consent is very much a legal concept ... It involves a physician having ascertained the course of treatment that he/she would like to administer and then getting the person to understand it sufficiently that the physician can feel as if the patient is going along with it. [On the other hand,] informed choice, as we practise it in our clinic, is outlining to the consumer the various options, with their upsides and the downsides. That's the education component, following which the support necessary to allow them to make the choice is provided.
>
> *Theme Conference on the Impact of New Reproductive Technologies on Women's Reproductive Health and Well-Being, Transcript, Vancouver, British Columbia, July 31, 1990.*

technologies, informed choice means providing relevant and understandable information about the options and the possible implications of various decisions. It means supporting individual decision making by helping people identify what is important to them and how various decisions would coincide with their priorities, given their values and circumstances. Informed choice also entails allowing as much time as possible for discussion and reflection. The concept does not mean that doctors are abdicating responsibility for recommending certain treatments or courses of action; nor is the physician always required to give the patient every piece of information available. But the concept of informed choice does entail providing information and support to enable people to reach decisions, building on the relationship of confidence and trust between the patient and the physician to create a sense of partnership in treatment decisions. The advent of medical procedures using highly complex technological procedures can make confidence and trust more difficult to maintain, but it does not eliminate the need to exercise them.

The call for informed choice is tied closely to other issues of importance to the Commission that we introduced in Chapter 2, such as the principle of autonomy, individual empowerment, and the need for accountability of people providing services or making decisions about the health care system to those who use it. We examine the implications of informed choice in the context of new reproductive technologies throughout Part Two of our report.

Privacy and Confidentiality

Privacy — the right to control information about oneself — is a fundamental value in our society, and one the Commission respects. The practice of medicine and the use of medical technologies generate large amounts of personal information in physicians' records, provincial health insurance plan records, and the records of clinics, hospitals, and other facilities. We want to ensure that our recommendations do not add to the list of intrusions into people's private lives. Therefore, we have made recommendations throughout our examination of individual technologies to ensure that privacy is respected in the collection and use of information regarding the use of reproductive technologies, which can generate intensely private information about the people involved. The loss of privacy is a risk associated with the technologies if personal information relating to their use is not safeguarded.

Individual patients clearly have an interest in ensuring that information about themselves remains confidential. People who make use of services such as assisted insemination or *in vitro* fertilization may not want that information disclosed to anyone. At the same time, others may have an interest in obtaining access to the information for various reasons. For example, researchers and policy makers could use information on the results of *in vitro* fertilization and other treatments as the basis for record linkage studies to determine long-term health effects and for decisions on health policy and public health protection. An individual born as a result of egg or sperm donation may want to learn the identity of the gamete

> While the women described many health professionals as caring, attentive, and sometimes highly compassionate, they also described a medical system that they perceived as fragmented and uncoordinated, and that isolated clients. Whatever a women's background and circumstances, she perceived a need for support and advocacy to deal with some aspects of the medical system ... The settings and nuances of care made them feel vulnerable. This was equally true of the nurses in the study who talked about needing considerable emotional resources to deal with the medical system as clients.
>
> S. Tudiver, "Manitoba Voices: A Qualitative Study of Women's Experiences with Technology in Pregnancy," in Research Volumes of the Commission, 1993.

donor or donors. Employers or insurers may want information about an individual's health history or genetic make-up.

The Commission recognizes the inherent tension between an individual patient's interest in privacy and the interests of other individuals and society as a whole in making information available for specified purposes. The challenge, therefore, is to ensure that information is collected, used, and disclosed only in appropriate circumstances and under clearly defined conditions.

> I think there are two rights involved here: the right to confidentiality that was guaranteed at some point in the contract, and the right of the child to know his genetic origins. [Translation]
>
> *A. Klotz, private citizen, Public Hearings Transcripts, Montreal, Quebec, November 21, 1990.*

One important distinction in this regard is the difference between information that reveals the identity of a specific individual and coded information, which does not reveal an individual's identity. Coded medical data may contain information on an individual's diagnosis, treatment, and the results of treatment, as well as information about some personal characteristics (for example, age, sex, income, and general geographic location), but none of this information would permit the specific identity of the patient to be known — the data are identified only by code number, not by the patient's name. Although the data include personal information, it is known as *non-identifying* information.

Non-identifying information is the type used most often for research and policy making. For these purposes, the specific identity of people receiving treatment is not of concern; what matters is analysis of the aggregate results of many cases, which permits researchers to draw conclusions and policy makers to make informed decisions. By contrast, employers and insurers, as well as children born as a result of gamete donations, may be interested in *identifying* information — that is, named information that is linked to a specific individual.

The Commission considered how society's interest in using the information in medical records for research into patterns of illness or disability and the outcomes of treatment can be served while also satisfying people's legitimate interest in keeping information about themselves private. Research results are needed so that the use of harmful procedures or

> The Commission considered how society's interest in using the information in medical records for research into patterns of illness or disability and the outcomes of treatment can be served while also satisfying people's legitimate interest in keeping information about themselves private.

drugs can be stopped and improvements in medical treatment can be made. Citizens rely on governments to protect their safety, but governments can do this only if sufficient relevant knowledge can be accumulated to guide policy. Access to information about the nature and results of treatment is thus an integral part of evidence-based medicine; it is one of the essential components permitting safe care and the responsible use of health care resources.

This is of particular interest in the field of new reproductive technologies because many of the drugs, devices, and procedures used in assisted conception have yet to be assessed for effectiveness or to determine the nature and scope of the potential risks associated with them. Many of our recommendations concerning these technologies will depend on the results of such assessments being made available to policy makers and technology users alike.

New technological developments raise a host of questions. What measures exist (or need to exist) to protect disclosure of information about an individual's health or genetic make-up derived from prenatal testing to organizations or government agencies that may have a commercial or political interest in it? What protections exist (or should exist) regarding the collection, use, or disclosure of information (including samples of genetic material) relating to new reproductive technologies? Are there in fact any circumstances in which life insurance companies or employers should be permitted to gain access to information without the individual's explicit consent?

No single law regulates or protects privacy and confidentiality. Canadian law in this area is extensive and complex; rights and obligations have evolved from a complex web of international law and codes, constitutional documents, federal and provincial laws, court decisions, and professional guidelines, codes of conduct, and codes of ethics. The conflict between sometimes disparate laws adds to the complexity. At the international level, Canada has ratified human rights agreements that assert the right to protection against arbitrary interference with privacy. Canada has also adhered to international data protection principles covering both the public and the private sector in the collection, use, and disclosure of personal information. However, adherence to these latter guidelines is not mandatory.

Domestically, the courts have interpreted the *Canadian Charter of Rights and Freedoms* as protecting certain privacy rights. The federal government and three provinces have enacted general privacy legislation regulating the collection, use, and disclosure of personal information by government institutions. As well, specific pieces of legislation, such as the *Income Tax Act* and the *Statistics Act*, have incorporated privacy protections with regard to information collected in administering them. In addition, numerous laws and court decisions establish obligations of confidentiality, as do professional codes of conduct and ethics.

When it comes to individual medical records, it is the law that personal information collected by health care facilities and practitioners is confidential. Confidentiality is the duty owed by one person not to disclose information given by or about another. These laws imposing obligations of confidentiality contain exceptions: for example, the law in most provinces requires health professionals to report certain communicable diseases or cases of suspected child abuse, even if this means disclosing confidential information. This recognizes that the interests of the individual must be balanced with the interests of others. However, any increase in the number of exceptions to obligations of confidentiality — such as mandatory reporting requirements imposed on physicians — erodes privacy, and thus there is a need to demonstrate a legitimate public or social need before access is given without the individual's permission.

> When it comes to individual medical records, it is the law that personal information collected by health care facilities and practitioners is confidential. New ways of protecting privacy will need to be put in place to deal with these new situations.

Increasingly, new ways of protecting privacy are called for because of new developments. Technology has permitted new forms of surveillance, such as cameras on street corners and in stores and telecommunications monitoring devices. Biotechnology has made possible testing for genetic traits and testing for the use of illegal drugs. New ways of protecting privacy will need to be put in place to deal with these new situations. In this report we are concerned mainly with how the legal and philosophical principles embodied in privacy law can be respected in the practices of facilities and practitioners offering new reproductive technologies, at the same time allowing record linkage studies and other research techniques in support of evidence-based medicine and public policy and resource allocation decisions.

New Reproductive Technologies and the Health Care System

The issues facing the health care system generally — growing expectations of patients and providers, rising costs, the internal and external limits of health care, the appropriate roles for prevention and acute care, the need for more systematic quality control, increasing demands for information and participation in decision making — are all demonstrated in the field of new reproductive technologies. By the same token, much of what the Commission has learned about new reproductive technologies has broader lessons for the health care system. Because the technologies evoke highly sensitive issues and have profound personal and social implications, the field requires the highest possible professional standards, combining excellent medical practice with concern for the potential psychological, social, ethical, legal, and financial impact of the technologies. If we can find a way to achieve a high performance standard in new reproductive technologies, this field could provide a model for high-quality, evidence-based medical practice in general.

The increasing recognition that a significant proportion of medical care either makes very little difference to health status or has never been evaluated could prompt the beginning of a new approach to health care. New reproductive technologies offer ideal conditions in which to begin such an approach — it is a well-defined field with an identifiable set of practitioners and in Canada operates within a single-payer health care system. It must be emphasized that new reproductive technologies are applied — and can only be applied — within the broader health care system. It is the health care system that makes available trained personnel and the necessary facilities and equipment; it is through the health care system that many of the preparatory and follow-up services surrounding use of the technologies will have to be provided; and it is through the publicly funded health care system that a measure of quality control and accountability can be established to safeguard the health and safety of Canadians and ensure the wise use of collective resources.

> New reproductive technologies offer ideal conditions in which to begin a new approach to health care — it is a well-defined field with an identifiable set of practitioners and in Canada operates within a single-payer health care system.

Infertility and new reproductive technologies are also fields that demonstrate the importance of involving systems other than health care — including social services, education, and legal systems — in addressing health-related problems. Our recommendations about new reproductive technologies therefore will also be relevant as a model for other similarly complex health-related problems.

The debate about new reproductive technologies has raised questions concerning what services should be considered medically necessary, who should have access, and who should pay the costs. These discussions, in turn, have helped open up the broader public debate about the future of health care in our country. There are significant difficulties inherent in attempts to reorient the health care system, as our discussion of its external and internal limits makes clear. The system is under constant pressure to find a sensible balance between ready and equitable access and cost containment. It will likely always be difficult to determine which situations and conditions should be considered medical problems. But this does not negate the need or responsibility to tackle the issue. In fact, the future of Canada's health care system depends on it.

Despite the current pressures on Canada's health care system, its great strengths should not be overlooked. The United States does not have a publicly funded system — and 37 million people have no health insurance.[1] Perhaps an equal number are underinsured and face financial catastrophe if they have a serious illness or accident. Many more are at a wholly unpredictable risk of having their coverage reduced or withdrawn, depending on the financial health of their employers. Moreover, a mixed public and private system also has inherent structural problems that result in inequities for people seeking treatment and in distortion of publicly supported health care priorities (see Chapter 20).

What Commissioners learned during our consultations and research reinforced our strong support for the values of social equity and access that are embodied in our health care system. In addition, what we observed in other countries confirmed our belief in the importance of maintaining the integrity of a publicly funded health care system. It is clear, however, that the health care system can maintain its integrity only if both its capacities and its limitations are clearly defined and respected.

Fortunately, because Canada has the appropriate structures in place — including a single-payer health care system and responsible professional organizations with a history of country-wide co-operation and collaboration — we have the opportunity in this country to organize this area of medical practice in a way that would enable new reproductive technologies to serve as a model for other areas of medical care. Openness on the part of the professionals involved, health ministries, and other interested parties will be required to apply the lessons about evidence-based practice to new reproductive technologies. We have an unusual opportunity to achieve this; it would be regrettable if we did not seize it.

> Fortunately, because Canada has the appropriate structures in place — including a single-payer health care system and responsible professional organizations with a history of country-wide cooperation and collaboration — we have the opportunity in this country to organize this area of medical practice in a way that would enable new reproductive technologies to serve as a model for other areas of medical care. We have an unusual opportunity to achieve this; it would be regrettable if we did not seize it.

We are not alone in reaching these conclusions about Canada's health care system — they reflect the assessment of a growing number of people within and outside the system. By almost any measure, that assessment is a positive one — the development of our universal single-payer system is a success story about which Canadians are justifiably proud. At the same time, health care is at a crossroads and presents Canadians with crucial questions about the future of a system we all value highly. Unless we find ways to deal with current pressures on the system in a way that maximizes the health of citizens, we run the risk of overloading it to the point of breakdown.

The crux of these choices lies in the balance between what Canadians are willing to put into the system and what we want to get out of it — questions, in other words, about resources and results. Until now, directions in health care have been determined largely by the efforts of many groups, both within and outside the system, struggling to push or pull it toward serving one interest or another. Allowing this situation to continue risks straining the system to the point where its survival is threatened. In our view, the survival of the health care system depends on sufficient numbers of Canadians agreeing on the need to preserve the collective benefits of a universal health care system, agreeing on what we want from the health care system, and agreeing, through our governments, to take the steps necessary to achieve those results.

This is the context in which the Commission's study of new reproductive technologies took place. As we have seen in this chapter, investing more resources in acute care and medical treatment does not necessarily contribute to improved health. Moreover, because the system has a virtually unlimited capacity to absorb resources, that investment could go on expanding indefinitely.   The case of new reproductive technologies provides a good example; part of the debate about new reproductive technologies turns on whether and to what extent the health care system can respond to all demands for the new technologies and related services.

Unless we decide soon to adopt a new direction in managing the health care system, such debates will continue to buffet the system, and it will inevitably be eroded. If we continue along the current path, once the existence of a new medical technology becomes known, the demand by physicians and consumers for it will prove irresistible, and once again an already overburdened system will expand to meet their demands. At some point society is bound to react by simply

> If we continue along the current path, once the existence of a new medical technology becomes known, the demand by physicians and consumers for it will prove irresistible, and once again an already overburdened system will expand to meet their demands ... The result would be a two-tiered system, with access to services determined by ability to pay — a system that would cost the country's economy far more than the current system, even if some of the cost was not borne by the public purse.

refusing to invest any more. At that point decision makers would seize upon extra billing, user charges, and similar ways to obtain additional resources — the only possible responses if we continue to focus solely on the resources we put into the system. If that occurs, the system will inevitably be changed to introduce other payers, thus altering it in ways most Canadians would find totally unacceptable, as well as causing it to be more costly and inefficient. The result would be a two-tiered system, with access to services determined by ability to pay — a system that would cost the country's economy far more than the current system, even if some of the cost was not borne by the public purse.

Before that happens, we have another choice. We can choose to focus instead on *results* — on what we get out of the system in which we have invested so heavily. By results we mean not only doing things right but also doing the right things. It means evaluating the results of treatment and agreeing not to provide those that are ineffective. But it also means agreeing collectively on which of the effective treatments we as a society are willing to provide within the health care system.

This is not the easiest choice, but it is the right choice. It will require a concerted response and a concerted commitment to change. In the view of Commissioners, we should begin the process of change with a comprehensive, coordinated response to new reproductive technologies along the lines we recommend in the remainder of this report. Change will involve difficult decisions about the external and internal limits of the system — which services should be part of the system's mandate and which should not, and what conditions should govern the provision of services. It will also require fundamental shifts in system orientation, bringing into the health care mainstream concepts and practices that are given lip service but are now operating on its margins: evidence-based medicine, technology assessment, prevention, and health promotion.

The choices that are necessary must be based on more than scientific data, however. Although they must be informed by the evidence, they must also involve thorough and principled analysis of the ethical, social, and other implications of various courses of action. This is what the Commission has attempted to do with respect to new reproductive technologies. After wide consultation, evaluation of the evidence, and ethical analysis, we have made recommendations about which technologies can be considered effective and that Canadians should be willing, collectively, to pay for. Governments will have to decide whether they agree.

Despite the difficulty of embarking on change of this magnitude, and even though the shift may take years to complete, focussing on results will produce indisputable benefits: better medicine, better resource management, and preservation of a system Canadians consider essential to our way of life. Making this choice now will ensure that our children and grandchildren continue to enjoy the standard of health care and the overall health status we have come to expect. It is the choice that will allow us to maintain the advantages of a system Canadians prize so highly: quality care and equitable access for all Canadians, regardless of income.

General Sources

Barer, M.L., and G.L. Stoddart. *Toward Integrated Medical Resource Policies for Canada.* Report presented to the Federal/Provincial/Territorial Conference of Deputy Ministers of Health. Banff: Alberta Health, Health Strategy & Evaluation Division, 1992.

Barer, M.L., et al. "Trends in Use of Medical Services by the Elderly in British Columbia." *Canadian Medical Association Journal* 141 (July 1, 1989): 39-45.

British Columbia Royal Commission on Health Care and Costs. *Closer to Home.* Victoria: Crown Publishing Inc., 1991.

Callahan, D. *What Kind of Life: The Limits of Medical Progress.* New York: Simon & Schuster, 1990.

Canada. Health and Welfare Canada. *National Health Expenditures in Canada: 1975-1987.* Ottawa: Minister of Supply and Services Canada, 1990.

Canada. National Council of Welfare. *Health, Health Care & Medicare.* Ottawa: Minister of Supply and Services Canada, 1990.

Canadian Institute for Advanced Research. *The Health of Populations and the Program in Population Health.* Toronto: The Institute, 1989.

Detsky, A.S. "Northern Exposure — Can the United States Learn from Canada." *New England Journal of Medicine* 328 (11)(March 18, 1993): 805-807.

Evans, R.G. *Accessible, Acceptable and Affordable: Financing Health Care in Canada.* Vancouver: Health Policy Research Unit, University of British Columbia, 1990.

Evans, R.G., et al. "Controlling Health Expenditures — The Canadian Reality." *New England Journal of Medicine* 320 (9)(March 2, 1989): 571-77.

Hamerton, J.L., and J.A. Evans. "Prenatal Diagnosis in Canada — 1990: A Review of Genetics Centres." In Research Volumes of the Royal Commission on New Reproductive Technologies, 1993.

Hyndman, B., et al. "The Integration of Theoretical Approaches to Prevention: A Proposed Framework for Reducing the Incidence of Infertility." In Research Volumes of the Royal Commission on New Reproductive Technologies, 1993.

Lomas, J. *Finding Audiences, Changing Beliefs: The Structure of Research Use in Canadian Health Policy.* Working Paper Series #90-10. Hamilton: Centre for Health Economics and Policy Analysis, McMaster University, 1990.

Madore, O. *Established Programs Financing for Health Care.* Ottawa: Research Branch, Library of Parliament, 1991.

Marmot, M.G., M. Kogevinas, and M. Elston. "Social Economic Status and Disease." *Annual Review of Public Health* 8 (1987): 129.

McKeown, T. *The Role of Medicine: Dream, Mirage or Nemesis?* Princeton: Princeton University Press, 1979.

McKinlay, J.B. "From 'Promising Report' to 'Standard Procedure': Seven Stages in the Career of a Medical Innovation." *Milbank Memorial Fund Quarterly* 59 (3)(1981): 374-411.

Ontario. Premier's Council on Health, Well-Being and Social Justice. *Nurturing Health: A New Understanding of What Makes People Healthy.* Toronto: Queen's Printer for Ontario, 1993.

Organisation for Economic Co-operation and Development. *Health Care Systems in Transition: The Search for Efficiency.* Social Policy Studies No. 7. Paris: OECD, 1990.

Quebec. Commission d'enquête sur les services de santé et les services sociaux. *Rapport de la Commission d'enquête sur les services de santé et les services sociaux.* Quebec: Government of Quebec, 1988.

Quebec. Conseil des affaires sociales et de la famille. *Objective: A Health Concept in Quebec: A Report of the Task Force on Health Promotion.* Translated by M.S. Gayk. Ottawa: Canadian Hospital Association, 1986.

Quebec. Ministry of Health and Social Services. *Improving Health and Well-Being in Quebec: Orientations.* Quebec: Government of Quebec, 1989.

Rachlis, M., and C. Kushner. *Second Opinion: What's Wrong with Canada's Health-Care System and How to Fix It.* Toronto: Collins Publishers, 1989.

Rachlis, M.M. "The Canadian Health Care System." In Research Volumes of the Royal Commission on New Reproductive Technologies, 1993.

Ronald, A.R., and R.W. Peeling. "Sexually Transmitted Infections: Their Manifestations and Links to Infertility and Reproductive Illness." In Research Volumes of the Royal Commission on New Reproductive Technologies, 1993.

Shapiro, E. *Manitoba Health Care Studies and Their Policy Implications.* Winnipeg: Faculty of Medicine, University of Manitoba, 1991.

Torjman, S. "Social Welfare and New Reproductive Technologies: An Overview." In Research Volumes of the Royal Commission on New Reproductive Technologies, 1993.

Tugwell, P., et al. "A Framework for the Evaluation of Technology: The Technology Assessment Iterative Loop." In *Health Care Technology: Effectiveness, Efficiency & Public Policy,* ed. D. Feeny, G. Guyatt, and P. Tugwell. Montreal: Institute for Research on Public Policy, 1986.

United Nations Development Programme. *Human Development Report 1992.* Oxford: Oxford University Press, 1992.

Wennberg, J.E. *The Evaluation Sciences and the Strategies for Health Care Reform.* Paper presented at the Second Annual David L. Everhart Lecture, May 7, 1992. Hanover: Dartmouth-Hitchcock Medical Center, 1992.

Specific References

1. Davis, K. "National Health Insurance: A Proposal." *American Economics Review* 79 (1989): 349-52. This figure is based on unpublished data from the U.S. Congressional Budget Office.

Achieving Responsible Regulation of New Reproductive Technologies

We developed the ethical framework and evidence-based approach, described in the two preceding chapters, as tools to illuminate and orient our review of the elements of our mandate. This permitted us to assess reproductive technologies, make judgements about them, and develop recommendations. Our conclusion, based on this ethical and evidence-based review, is that decisive, timely, and comprehensive national action is required with respect to the regulation of new reproductive technologies. In light of this belief, and in conformity with the federal government's constitutional responsibilities and the expectations of Canadians, Commissioners strongly recommend several major federal initiatives in the field of new reproductive technologies to provide the national framework that we believe is urgently required. The broad outlines of this national framework are sketched in this chapter; how they will apply in detail with respect to the individual technologies enumerated in our mandate is discussed in greater depth throughout Part Two of our report.

Before proceeding with this discussion, we consider it important to emphasize that although the national framework (for which Commissioners heard calls time and again in testimony and submissions) is necessary, it is not sufficient. Strong provincial and professional leadership in specific

> Our conclusion, based on this ethical and evidence-based review, is that decisive, timely, and comprehensive national action is required with respect to the regulation of new reproductive technologies.

areas referred to throughout Part Two of our report is also essential. Indeed, the success of the broad national approach we recommend will also depend on provincial and professional action and involvement in a wide range of new reproductive technology-related issues in the years to come. Concerted action and cooperation by the provinces, the professions, and other key participants in the context of the proposed national framework are the only way to ensure ethical and accountable use of new reproductive technologies in Canada — for now and for the future.

Federal Legislation: Establishing Boundaries and Setting Limits

As the discussion throughout our report makes clear, certain aspects of the research, development, and use of new reproductive technologies have particular social significance and raise particularly pressing issues for Canadians as individuals and as a society. Our analysis of the extensive data and research gathered during the course of our mandate leads us to conclude that public concerns about the need for effective social control of the use of these technologies are justified.

Consistent with the federal government's responsibility to legislate for the peace, order, and good government of Canada in matters of national interest, including in relation to the national health and welfare of Canadians, and in light of Parliament's extensive powers to protect public health, public security, and the public interest by means of the criminal law, we conclude that certain technologies and practices should be subject to the most stringent form of control available: outright prohibition under threat of criminal prosecution under the Canadian *Criminal Code*. This form of control will, in effect, establish clear boundaries around new reproductive technologies, excluding those practices that are, because of their unsafe or unethical character, considered unacceptable under any circumstances. In particular, the Commission recommends that the Parliament of Canada legislate to ensure that

- for-profit activities in connection with the creation, exchange, and use of human reproductive materials, including sperm, eggs, zygotes, embryos, fetuses, and fetal tissue, are prohibited (see Chapters 19, 20, 22, and 31);

- advertising for, making payment for, or acting as an intermediary in order to derive financial or commercial benefit from preconception arrangements, are prohibited (see Chapter 23);

- research involving human zygotes or embryos directed toward development of ectogenesis, cloning, the creation of human/animal hybrids, and the maturing and fertilization of eggs from fetuses is prohibited (see Chapter 22); and

- unwanted medical treatment and other interferences, or threatened interferences, with the physical autonomy of pregnant women are prohibited (see Chapter 30).

In our view, these legislative prohibitions fall squarely within the federal government's constitutional mandate to protect public health, public security, and the public interest, and to promote constitutional values of human dignity and equality. These measures would place clear limits on practices that Canadians consider unacceptable and would help to ensure that the future evolution of new reproductive technologies reflects the public interest.

The criminal law approach, while essential for establishing boundaries with respect to some uses of new reproductive technologies, provides less flexibility than is desirable for continuing regulation and management of other, more acceptable, aspects of the technologies. A second kind of response is therefore required in addition to these criminal law measures, to ensure that the technologies and practices deemed acceptable, provided they are subject to appropriate limits, receive the continuing monitoring and the public debate required by their profound implications.

These other areas require a more dynamic and responsive approach, one capable of adapting to new medical and scientific knowledge, responding to the results of technology assessment, and accommodating changes in Canada's social fabric. They also require an approach that can assure Canadians that appropriate attention is being paid to broader issues as well — including the protection and advancement of the public interest, the individual and collective interests of women, and the well-being of parents and children in the formation of families.

In the next section we outline our proposals for implementing the regulation of the technologies and practices we consider acceptable — provided they are assessed and delivered in an appropriate way — and to ensuring their continuing congruence with Canadians' values and priorities.

> The lack of a federal regulatory or informational presence in NRTs is all the more serious because of the paucity of provincial/territorial and professional standards guiding research and monitoring ... Thus, Canada needs a national body to review and approve research proposals, set ethical standards, set national standards of informed consent for NRT research and therapy, standardize data collection on NRTs, and monitor access and service provision.
>
> *Brief to the Commission from the Canadian Advisory Council on the Status of Women, March 1991.*

Calls for a National Reproductive Technologies Commission

Throughout our public hearings and in the many briefs we received, one of the clearest themes that emerged was the need for a national body to establish standards and to oversee activities and developments in the field of new reproductive technologies within the overall boundaries set by federal legislation. Near unanimous concern was expressed that without such national standards and control, the current patchwork of standards and services would persist. As one group appearing before the Commission expressed it, "it is simply unacceptable for us to think of such matters that are so fundamental to the very essence of life differing greatly across the country" (*Women's Rights Committee of the Nova Scotia New Democrats, Public Hearings Transcripts, Halifax, Nova Scotia, October 17, 1990*).

The call for an independent national body came not only from national, regional, and local women's groups, but from groups representing legal, health care, religious, and scientific bodies. As the Charter of Rights Coalition Manitoba stated in their testimony before the Commission:

> A national council on reproductive technologies [should have] a mandate to assess the medical and ethical implications of ongoing research on reproductive technologies and the appropriateness of new technologies; foster links among researchers, decision-makers and consumers of reproductive technologies; instigate public education and discussion on reproductive technologies in all areas of the country and encompassing all groups; administer a research budget ...; [and] have the authority to develop regulations under [federal] legislation about each emerging technology. (*B. Suek, Charter of Rights Coalition Manitoba, Public Hearings Transcripts, Winnipeg, Manitoba, October 23, 1990.*)

Those appearing before the Commission proposed several functions for the national body, including setting and enforcing national standards and guidelines, standardizing data collection and analysis, licensing clinics and practitioners, monitoring research and services, and providing information and advice to governments regarding policy, legislation, and regulation.

We examined the extensive evidence on how new reproductive technologies are currently being researched, developed, and applied in Canada, we listened to Canadians talking

> We have concluded that an independent national body, charged with overseeing and controlling the development and application of research, technologies, and practices in this field, is urgently required. In our view, this is the only way to ensure that the appropriate mix of resources, skills, and experience is brought to bear on reproductive technologies in all their dimensions: ethical, social, legal, scientific, and medical.

about how they expect their governments to respond to these issues, and we considered the possible ways of achieving our goal of ensuring that only ethical, effective, and accountable use is made of reproductive technologies. We have concluded that an independent national body, charged with overseeing and controlling the development and application of research, technologies, and practices in this field, is urgently required. In our view, this is the only way to ensure that the appropriate mix of resources, skills, and experience is brought to bear on reproductive technologies in all their dimensions: ethical, social, legal, scientific, and medical.

The Need for a National Regulatory Commission

Throughout Part Two of our report we recommend numerous measures and safeguards that we have concluded are necessary to ensure that only technologies and services that are ethically acceptable and effective at tolerable levels of risk are offered and that they are offered in appropriate ways. Several requirements are common to all the areas the Commission examined: the need for adequate and reliable information to guide policy and practice; the need for standards and guidelines for the organization and provision of services; the need for effective means to ensure compliance; and the need for accountability.

Efforts with respect to specific technologies have been made to meet some of these needs. However, we found that levels of self-regulation and accountability vary enormously from one area of practice to another. It is clearly important, in contemplating coherent regulatory intervention with respect to new reproductive technologies, to build upon previous efforts and to enlist the skills and cooperation of relevant professionals and communities of expertise and experience.   Because it is so fundamental to the future of our society and to us as individuals, however, primary responsibility

> A government body should be established with responsibility for approving proposals to apply new knowledge and procedures in new reproductive technologies in clinical practice. This body should also have the authority to accredit infertility centres and the people in them. [Translation]
>
> *G. Bleau, Centre de recherche en reproduction humaine de l'Université de Montréal, Public Hearings Transcripts, Montreal, Quebec, November 22, 1990.*

for regulating research and technology relating to human reproduction cannot be left entirely to self-regulating professional and other bodies, but must be assumed by government.

At the same time, we believe that existing legislation, government structures, and self-regulation mechanisms are not adequate to meet the demands of regulating this complex and rapidly evolving area of technology. This is because, for the most part, their mandates are too narrow and too focussed on one isolated facet of the technologies — be it the health services delivery, the medical, the scientific, or the research aspect — to provide the comprehensive overview and integrated approach we see as essential.

Thus, we conclude that a new, federally funded, independent body should be established by Parliament to assume comprehensive regulatory responsibility in this area. As we have already argued, such regulatory responsibility is consistent with Parliament's power and responsibility to intervene in the interests of national health and welfare pursuant to the federal peace, order, and good government, criminal law, trade and commerce, and related federal powers. In light of these considerations, the Royal Commission on New Reproductive Technologies recommends that

> A regulatory body must be formally established to set and enforce standards, principles and regulations under which NRT research is carried out ...
>
> We believe the body must not be composed merely of scientists, doctors or academic ethicists, but must be representative of the community as a whole.
>
> *N. Riche, Executive Vice-President, Canadian Labour Congress, Public Hearings Transcripts, Toronto, Ontario, October 31, 1990.*

> **1. The federal government establish an independent National Reproductive Technologies Commission charged with the primary responsibility of ensuring that new reproductive technologies are developed and applied in the national public interest.**

Creation of a National Commission to provide national regulatory oversight and control in the field of new reproductive technologies is needed on several grounds. The rapid pace at which reproductive technologies and practices are being introduced and disseminated dictates an immediate regulatory response. A National Commission could be established and put into operation within a relatively short time frame. This is a crucial consideration. In Commissioners' assessment, the time that would be required to enhance current mechanisms or develop new mechanisms for interprovincial regulatory and policy harmonization, and to adapt them to the complex area of new reproductive technologies, goes far beyond what is acceptable, given the urgency of action to deal with these issues while there is still time to contain and control current practices and future developments.

A National Commission would permit the creation and implementation of coherent, comprehensive, and effective nation-wide standards and monitoring devices. This is in contrast to what could realistically be achieved through piecemeal federal reform on a department-by-department basis, through individual responses by each province and territory, or through non-governmental or self-regulatory initiatives.

Just as this Royal Commission did in its work, a National Commission could apply an ethical framework in decision making and ensure that the interests of all concerned groups and individuals are considered in setting policy and standards and assuring adherence to them in practice. This is in contrast to the relatively narrow range of interests that has been involved in the past in decision making in this area. Because of the multiple dimensions of reproductive technologies, a mechanism is needed to ensure that the strengths, skills, experience, and values of all interested systems and communities are integrated and taken into account in decisions about the technologies. A body such as the one we recommend, with a comprehensive mandate and inclusive membership, would provide such a mechanism.

Like this Royal Commission, a National Commission would be highly visible and would generate significant levels of public awareness about the technologies and their application, as well as other developments in the field of reproductive health and research. Appropriately structured, the National Commission would provide an important avenue for airing and evaluating public concerns about specific issues and practices. As an independent body, established at arm's length from existing institutions

> [A] national organism for implementing reforms ... might be charged with such responsibilities as establishing national IVF reporting standards and a national registry, advising government, encouraging studies on the long-term medical and psychological effects, [and] overseeing the licensing of clinics [and] gametes and embryo banks ... [W]e believe that both the consuming public and health service providers have particular reasons for supporting national government standards.
>
> Consumers seem likely to welcome initiatives that enhance public safety and that simplify and make accurate the technical information they need to make informed health decisions.
>
> G. Létourneau, President, Law Reform Commission of Canada, Public Hearings Transcripts, Montreal, Quebec, November 21, 1990.

and reporting directly to Parliament, a National Commission would enable the public to have confidence that the control and monitoring of new reproductive technologies was not subject to manipulation from political, commercial, scientific, bureaucratic, or other interests and that the technologies were being regulated in the interests of Canadians in all their diversity, not only for the present but for future generations as well.

As a single and identifiable source of regulatory authority, a National Commission could provide maximum opportunities for public input and participation and could be held to a high standard of public accountability. A National Commission of the type we envisage would respond to the need for public participation, visibility, and accountability identified by intervenors throughout our mandate.

By establishing policies and standards for reproductive technologies and services provided in Canada, a National Commission could minimize interprovincial disparities in services and standards, promote equal treatment across the country, and reduce duplication of effort, thereby making more responsible use of available resources. In particular, a National Commission could ensure greater standardization of practices relating to patient referrals, counselling, consent, treatment, reporting, and evaluation,

> We ask that governments inform the public in a timely and appropriate way about the implications and consequences inherent in the use of new reproductive technologies and then to introduce laws to regulate their use. [Translation]
>
> *Brief to the Commission from the Association féminine d'éducation et d'action sociale, November 1990.*

among other matters, through its licensing and monitoring functions. By harmonizing the existing patchwork of standards and practices and ensuring consistency and equity in how individuals across the country are dealt with, the National Commission would respond to one of the major concerns expressed by those who appeared before the Commission.

In summary, we reject a piecemeal and incremental response to new reproductive technologies on both conceptual and practical grounds. As discussed in Chapter 1, we are of the view that the federal government has the necessary constitutional jurisdiction to establish the National Commission we recommend. We recognize that there has been a clear trend, in recent federal policy, away from the commission model as a choice of regulatory instrument, and toward an amalgamation of agency functions and an overall reduction of federal intervention and spending in the interests of cutting federal government costs. We consider, however, that the immediate and long-term cost of establishing and funding a National Commission along the model we propose represents a reasonable financial commitment, given the federal government's constitutional responsibilities in this area and the importance of the functions the National Commission will assume. Such expenditure is also more than warranted, in view of the short- and long-term savings in direct costs to the Canadian health care system, and the overall societal benefits.

We note that existing federal agencies such as the National Transportation Agency and the Canadian Radio-Television and Telecommunications Commission, among others, are performing comparable licensing, monitoring, and advisory functions, on a vastly greater scale than we envision for the National Reproductive Technologies Commission. We are convinced by what we heard from Canadians, and by what we learned from our own investigations and study during the course of our mandate, that the expenditures that would be entailed by our recommendations are equally, if not more, justified in relation to new reproductive technologies. We believe that for the federal government to reject our recommendations for a National Reproductive Technologies Commission in the name of fiscal restraint would be not only politically irresponsible, but false economy, and that a majority of Canadians will share this assessment.

> We must establish a commission to provide factual and unbiased information for the public on new reproductive technology; to provide a network to generate communication between peoples for understanding and respect; to monitor and ensure strict adherence to codes of ethics; to establish a national policy of ethics for IVF and other related clinics; to establish licensing standards and ensure a registry or record of their success and problems.
>
> *M. McWaters, private citizen, Public Hearings Transcripts, Vancouver, British Columbia, November 27, 1990.*

In short, for all the reasons outlined above — the need for a holistic approach to a rapidly evolving technological field, the urgency of action, the need for comprehensiveness and uniformity, and the need for public visibility and accountability — Commissioners are strongly of the view that a National Reproductive Technologies Commission of the type we propose must be put in place as an immediate federal priority.

> The field of new reproductive technologies is developing too rapidly, and the potential for harm to citizens is too great, for Canada's response to be delayed, fragmented, or tentative.

We believe that the National Commission we recommend presents not only the most effective, but the only feasible response to the urgent need and justified public demand for coherent, effective, and appropriate national regulation of new reproductive technologies. The field is developing too rapidly, and the potential for harm to citizens is too great, for Canada's response to be delayed, fragmented, or tentative.

Functions of the National Regulatory Commission

The major functions we propose for the National Commission are licensing and monitoring; guideline and standard setting; information collection, evaluation, and dissemination; records storage; consultation, coordination, and intergovernmental cooperation; and monitoring of future technologies and practices. We propose that the National Commission establish six sub-committees to assume these functions in specific areas of its mandate.

In particular, we recommend that the National Commission establish five permanent sub-committees with responsibility for developing standards and guidelines and for regulatory oversight in the following areas of activity and service: sperm collection, sperm storage and distribution, and the provision of assisted insemination services; assisted conception services; prenatal diagnosis; human zygote/embryo research; and the provision of fetal tissue for research.

In addition we recommend that the National Commission establish a sixth sub-committee with primary responsibility in the field of infertility prevention. This sub-committee would have as its major mandate the compilation and evaluation of data pertaining to the causes of infertility, and the regulatory, public education, and other options available for reducing its incidence or for preventing it.

> We recommend that ... the criteria and effectiveness evaluation methods used by fertility clinics be standardized, so that clinic users can exercise more informed choices about where to seek treatment. [Translation]
>
> *M. Lopez, Association Québécoise pour la Fertilité Inc., Public Hearings Transcripts, Montreal, Quebec, November 22, 1990.*

We also recommend that the National Commission be empowered to create temporary or ad hoc sub-committees, with expert participation from outside the National Commission, to report to and advise the permanent sub-committees on issues raising particular difficulties or warranting special attention.

Licensing and Monitoring

In light of the regulatory shortcomings we identify in our discussion of specific technologies later in the report, the Commission recommends that a primary focus of activity of the National Commission be the licensing and monitoring of practices and services related to new reproductive technologies. In particular, we recommend that the following five areas be subject to compulsory licensing by the National Commission through its sub-committees:

- sperm collection; sperm storage and distribution; and the provision of assisted insemination services;
- assisted conception services, including egg retrieval and use;
- prenatal diagnosis;
- research involving human zygotes; and

- the provision of human fetal tissue for research or other specified purposes.

Engaging in any of these activities or providing services that are subject to regulation without a licence, or without complying with the National Commission's licensing requirements, would constitute an offence subject to fine and/or imprisonment.

Individuals or facilities seeking to engage in the activities that we recommend be subject to licensing would be required to apply to the National Commission in a prescribed form, and to provide the Commission with all information necessary for it to assess whether the applicable standards and conditions of licence had been met.

> We believe that the National Commission we recommend presents not only the most effective, but the only feasible response to the urgent need and justified public demand for coherent, effective, and appropriate national regulation of new reproductive technologies.

Provided they met such conditions, applicants could be eligible for licences to provide services in more than one licensing category. A facility providing assisted conception services might, for example, also seek a licence to collect or to store and distribute sperm.

Licence applications would be heard by a panel of at least three members of the National Commission, in an oral hearing, open to the public. In addition to submissions from the applicant, the panel could also hear submissions from interested third parties with relevant information.

Following the licence hearing, the panel would issue a written decision to grant or deny the application, subject to any relevant conditions of licence. The National Commission's decision to approve or deny a licence would be subject to appeal to the Federal Court of Canada on matters of jurisdiction. Licence holders would be subject to continuing monitoring and review through the requirement, among other conditions of licence, that they report to the National Commission on their activities annually. They would also be required to inform the Commission in the event of staff or other changes substantially affecting the conditions of licence. Licences would be subject to renewal every five years, and would be revocable by the National Commission at any time for breach of conditions of licence.

Guideline and Standard Setting

As an essential aspect of its licensing function, we propose that the National Commission be responsible for developing national guidelines and standards of practice applicable to the development and delivery of new reproductive technologies. We recommend that these standards and guidelines be developed by the permanent sub-committees on the basis of the recommendations detailed in Part Two of this report and in conjunction with relevant professional bodies and other interested parties. The guidelines and standards developed by the sub-committees would be used to assess the merits of individual licence applications during the licence hearing process. These guidelines and standards would also apply as ongoing conditions of licence for service providers and activities subject to compulsory licensing. As outlined above, licence compliance would be subject to continuing review, and failure to respect any conditions of licence imposed would be grounds for revocation of licence, upon recommendation by the relevant sub-committee.

In addition to their role in the actual licensing process, the guidelines and standards developed by the sub-committees could provide important direction for providers and activities that are not subject to direct regulation by the National Commission. As discussed in Chapter 26, for example, such standards could furnish guidance for individual physicians providing services, such as prenatal ultrasound or MSAFP screening, outside licensed prenatal diagnosis facilities. Such guidelines could also provide important direction to individual practitioners in prescribing fertility drugs for women having difficulty conceiving.

Information Collection, Evaluation, and Dissemination

As a necessary complement to its licensing function, we recommend that the National Commission be responsible for tabulating, analyzing, and evaluating data about the technologies and their use collected by practitioners and facilities providing licensed services across the country. We also recommend that the National Commission work to remain abreast of new information and findings that become available internationally. Continuing analysis and evaluation of incoming data would enable the National Commission and its sub-committees to modify and adapt guidelines, such as those relating to treatments that can be offered safely and effectively, as technologies and practices evolve and as new information becomes available. Such activities by the National Commission have at least two major benefits to provincial ministries of health in their management of health care. First, they will enable more rapid gathering of sufficient data on which to base timely and reliable conclusions about the benefits and harms of technology uses in this evolving field than would be possible for any individual province working in isolation. Second, this national approach would permit efficient and effective use of public resources by reducing duplication of effort and enabling the benefits of country-wide technology assessment to be shared by all provincial health care systems.

In keeping with the objective of open and accountable regulation, we recommend that the research and analysis compiled by the National Commission and all of its sub-committees be available to interested researchers and members of the general public. We also recommend that the National Commission submit and publish an annual report to

Parliament as a means of keeping Canadians apprised of what is occurring in practice in Canada and of new directions and developments in this field. By presenting data and an analysis of what is happening in the field of new reproductive technologies in an accessible language and format, the National Commission's annual report can promote public awareness and inform public debate on issues requiring public discussion and policy consideration. In addition, the collection of information on use of the technologies will allow evaluation of longer-term outcomes in a way that has not been possible to date. By increasing the volume and accessibility of objective information about new reproductive technologies, such publication will also help Canadians make informed decisions about whether and under what circumstances to consider using these technologies.

Records Storage

The National Commission would collect and store two major categories of records and data provided by the various categories of licence holders as part of their conditions of licence. The first category would include records on donors of gametes (eggs and sperm) and zygotes, and on children born as a result of gamete or zygote donations. The second category would include data to enable the evaluation of the outcomes and longer-term implications of infertility treatments for women and for the ongoing health of children born as a result of reproductive technologies. These data would be collected in standardized formats established by the National Commission to enable country-wide comparisons and record linkage with other data bases for research purposes.

For both categories of records and data, systems would be put in place to ensure secure storage of the data and protection of confidentiality of information on individuals. As outlined in greater depth in Chapters 19 and 20, in the case of records involving gamete and zygote donations, only non-identifying information about donors would be available to parents and children, except in the event of court-ordered release of identifying information.

As discussed in Chapter 18, data would be available only in coded form (so that individuals could not be identified) and only to bona fide researchers working on research projects evaluated and approved by the National Commission.

Consultation, Coordination, and Intergovernmental Cooperation

We recommend that the National Commission provide advice to, and assist in the coordination of, governmental and non-governmental initiatives in relation to new reproductive technologies, including providing information to the Government of Canada about international developments and assuring an international presence on these issues. This would be among the subjects the National Commission should address in its annual report to Parliament. We recommend that the National Commission promote cooperation in health and public education and other efforts in relation to new reproductive technologies, and between governments, health practitioners, researchers, and others involved in the development and application of new reproductive technologies. All are essential partners in the efforts that will be needed to protect and promote the interests of technology users and of Canadians generally.

We recommend in particular that the National Commission work closely with the provinces on issues related to access to and funding of services and technologies. Throughout our report, we have remained acutely conscious of the fundamental relationship between technology use and provincial health care funding policies. For example, the use of some services of unproven benefit has grown rapidly, in part as a result of funding decisions regarding this service under provincial health insurance plans, while other interventions of proven benefit have not been funded; we examine several such examples in Part Two of our report. Provincial health plan funding decisions thus have had a direct impact on access to and use of technologies, irrespective of the merits of such technologies in treating or overcoming reproductive problems or conditions.

We are strongly aware of the substantial implications of many of our recommendations for provincial health care policies and

> The Commission [should] strongly recommend the establishment of:
>
> - a National Review Board on Medical and Bioethical Issues which would provide ongoing study and evaluation of advances in technology,
> - in order to advise the government of Canada and the provincial governments on needed legislation or regulation,
> - to assist in the development of national standards for that purpose, and
> - to provide direction with regard to research grants. Such a Board would include medical researchers, practitioners and nurses, representatives of the disciplines of law, philosophy, ethics, religion and an equal number of lay persons and should be at least fifty per cent women.
>
> *Brief to the Commission from the United Church of Canada, Division of Mission in Canada, January 17, 1991.*

funding choices. We recognize the need for the National Commission's decision-making processes to take into account provincial interests and to reflect provincial priorities and preoccupations. There is a clear need to work together on these issues. We address these provincial health-related issues in greater depth as they arise with respect to particular technologies and practices in the chapters that follow. In addition, we recommend that the provinces and the National Commission establish a regular forum for the mutual exchange of information and concerns — for example, through the Conference of Deputy Ministers of Health, an existing body that has successfully promoted collaborative action on issues of national importance and mutual concern to federal and provincial/territorial governments.

Monitoring of Future Technologies and Practices

As knowledge in the field of new reproductive technologies increases, the issues facing governments and the public will continue to evolve. The decision-making structures and processes we propose for the National Commission must therefore be capable of adapting over time, to meet emerging and unanticipated needs and regulatory demands. For example, many of the concerns we heard from Canadians related to procedures that are, for the moment, projected possibilities rather than actual practice. As time passes, however, this situation may change, so that new controls and guidelines may become imperative.   We have identified these areas throughout Part Two of our report and have recommended that the National Commission monitor developments closely, so that it can react in a timely way as the need arises.

Because of the rapid evolution of reproductive technologies, we recommend that the National Commission be empowered to set and modify its policies, priorities, and procedures to meet the changes in the regulatory environment that are sure to arise. At the same time, we believe that the licensing and policy-making structures we propose will permit the National Commission and its sub-committees to maintain a rigorous level of oversight across the spectrum of reproductive technologies.

Continuing interaction with those directly engaged in the research, development, and application of reproductive technologies will assist the National Commission in this objective. Equally important, the National Commission must work to promote informed public discussion and debate of new reproductive technology issues as they emerge, in Canada and elsewhere. For example, it would be open to the National Commission to develop and publish discussion papers setting out the issues and policy options in various fields, with the aim of provoking broad public discussion and promoting the development of consensus on areas in which the National Commission is considering or is intending to introduce policies or regulations.   In our view, such efforts will enhance the National Commission's ability to provide sound advice to governments on domestic and international policy matters related to new reproductive technologies in a forward-looking and prescriptive way, rather than merely a reactive way. Promoting a high level of public dialogue in relation to emerging issues will also ensure greater levels of public accountability and public trust, without which effective and responsible regulation cannot occur.

Composition of the National Regulatory Commission

We recommend that the National Commission be composed of 12 members, appointed by the Governor in Council, at least 6 of whom, including the president, are appointed on a full-time basis. We recommend that National Commission members be appointed for an initial five-year term, with a possible one-, two-, or three-year renewal of their terms, to allow for the staggering of new appointments. We are of the view that this number and term of appointment will permit the development of a high level of expertise while allowing for sufficiently diverse representation of interests and a close working relationship among National Commission members.

Human reproduction and the issues surrounding it are of equal importance and interest to women and men. They both have a role in reproduction, but they bring different experiences and perspectives to these issues. Moreover, women more often undergo the treatments and other procedures related to new reproductive technologies. Commissioners want to ensure, therefore, that the perspectives of both women and men are applied to the specific sorts of decisions and advice that the National Commission will be called upon to provide. We were reminded many times by intervenors and in submissions of the particular impact of new reproductive technologies on women, and of the clear need for women to be integrally involved in deliberations about new reproductive technologies. For these reasons we believe that women should make up a substantial proportion of the National Commission's members, normally at least half. In addition, membership of the National Commission should always include persons knowledgeable about the interests and perspectives of those with disabilities, those who are infertile, and those who are members of racial minority, Aboriginal, and economically disadvantaged communities. A range of expertise should also be represented, including reproductive medicine, ethics, law, and social

> The selection of community representatives should not be in the hands of NRT service providers. The CACSW agrees with the World Health Organization, which advises that committees overseeing service systems for infertility should consist of a group of informed laypeople from the community, at least 50% of whom should be women. The proceedings and deliberations of these committees should be available to the public. Although the WHO directive was intended to apply only to infertility services, the CACSW believes the committees should be mandated to oversee all aspects of reproductive health services.
>
> *Brief to the Commission from the Canadian Advisory Council on the Status of Women, March 1991.*

sciences. In other words, Commissioners see the need for a broad mix of views in the membership of the National Commission and are confident that there are many Canadians, both women and men, who are fully qualified to take on these responsibilities and from among whom such appointments can be made.

As discussed in greater detail in the chapters that follow, we recommend that the National Commission's six permanent sub-committees include both National Commission and non-National Commission membership, and that outside (non-National Commission) members include people representing the views and interests of governments, professional bodies, consumers, and other groups with particular interest in the area of sub-committee activity in question. Like National Commission members themselves, we recommend that at least half of sub-committee members be women, and that all members be chosen with a view to ensuring that they have a background and demonstrated experience in dealing with a multidisciplinary approach to issues, as well as an ability to work together to find solutions and recommend policies to address the difficult issues raised by new reproductive technologies in a way that meets the concerns of Canadian society as a whole.

> We urge the Commission to recommend the setting up of an independent body which is representative of our multi-cultural and multi-racial society. This body should be mandated with the monitoring of the developments that are taking place in the research and practice of NRTs. We further urge that as it is women whose bodies and lives are most strongly affected by reproduction, this body be made up of women. It is only through such participation that we can begin to address the present patriarchal biases being reflected in NRTs.
>
> *S. Thobani, Immigrant and Visible Minority Women of British Columbia, Public Hearings Transcripts, Vancouver, British Columbia, November 26, 1990.*

Other Federal Policy and Program Initiatives

In Part Two of our report, we recommend other measures that would fall within the responsibilities of the federal departments of Health, Human Resources and Labour, the Environment, and Industry and Science, as well as the Medical Research Council of Canada (MRC). These recommendations fall into several broad categories:

- recommendations directed to infertility prevention and reproductive health promotion through steps to address sexually transmitted diseases, smoking, delayed childbearing, alcohol use, and other aspects of sexual health education, as well as exposure to factors in the workplace and the environment that may pose risks to fertility (Chapters 10 to 15);

- recommendations directed to reform of the current process for approval and post-marketing surveillance of prescription drugs (Chapter 18);

- recommendations concerning the funding of medical research in such areas as sexual and reproductive health (Chapters 10 and 13) and human embryo research (Chapter 22);

- recommendations about the current state of the adoption system in Canada (Chapter 16); and

- recommendations about patenting in the context of reproductive technologies (Chapter 24).

Ensuring That Future Development Is in the Public Interest

Taken together, the comprehensive initiatives we propose — legislation creating boundaries around acceptable practices and establishing a National Reproductive Technologies Commission to regulate and monitor activities and developments in this field — are essential to the future welfare of individual Canadians and for Canadian society as a whole. The regulation we recommend will ensure that new reproductive technologies are dealt with in a timely, comprehensive, coherent, and effective way. It will help ensure that Canadians in all parts of the country are dealt with equally and protected equally, in conformity with the fundamental values set out in the *Canadian Charter of Rights and Freedoms* and congruent with the values and priorities of Canadians themselves.

In making these recommendations we are conscious, as we have stated, of the significant provincial interest in the field of new reproductive technologies. Over the course of our mandate, however, we were reminded repeatedly of the dangerous and inequitable situation created by the existing patchwork of laws, standards, programs, and services across Canada. During our public hearings, in oral and written briefs submitted by individuals and groups, and in public opinion surveys, inequitable interprovincial variation in levels of access to services and in the regulation and control of the technologies emerged as a major source of public dissatisfaction and concern.

As we examine specific technologies in Part Two of our report, we note that several provinces/territories have already focussed on the need for law reform to take account of developments in this field. Some have adopted legislation touching upon certain aspects of new reproductive technologies, such as the issue of the paternity of children born through the use of donor sperm, while others are awaiting our recommendations before deciding what action to take. We recognize that coherent and effective regulation in the best interests of all Canadians is impossible without the cooperation and support of the provinces and of non-governmental organizations and individuals involved in the research, development, and delivery of new reproductive technologies and services. We believe that this need is already widely recognized and that, given the tremendous importance of these issues for individual Canadians and for Canadian society as a whole, cooperation and support will be forthcoming.

As is evident in the development of our publicly supported health care system, Canadians have been able to work together when it was important for the well-being of all that we do so — this is among the achievements that make us proud to be Canadians. We believe that governments will see that the interests of citizens and society depend on our participation together in a response to the deeply important choices before us. If we want Canadians to continue to feel that the country's institutions and public policies express common values and promote a sense of our common humanity, decency, and caring, we must overcome difficulties of jurisdiction and boundaries and take a united approach. We need to set clear limits on what can and cannot be done with new reproductive technologies, then manage the use of the technologies within these boundaries in a caring, ethical, and responsible way. It is concern for the well-being of our fellow citizens that binds us together; the approach we recommend gives concrete expression to this concern.

> We need to set clear limits on what can and cannot be done with new reproductive technologies, then manage the use of the technologies within these boundaries in a caring, ethical, and responsible way.

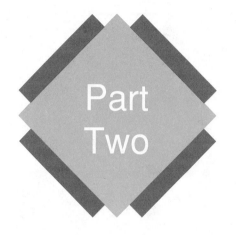

Part
Two

New Reproductive Technologies: Examination of Conditions, Technologies, and Practices

Developing a Comprehensive Picture of Technologies and Practices

Framework of Our Approach

Understanding reproductive technologies involves much more than a grasp of medical conditions, procedures, drugs, and devices. Also important are the decision-making processes that surround use of the technologies; the relationships between people who may wish to use a reproductive technology and health care providers; the new legal and social situations that arise from the use of technologies; the implications of the technologies for the health care system and other social institutions; and what it means for society, for example, to choose assisted conception rather than other ways of addressing involuntary childlessness or to embark on research involving the use of fetal tissue. The Commission therefore needed to develop a comprehensive picture not only of the people involved and the technologies available, but also of the environment and circumstances in which people interact with the technologies. This chapter describes how we went about assembling a comprehensive picture on which to base our assessment of the technologies.

Because the Commission was to examine not only specific conditions and technologies, but also their social, ethical, legal, economic, health, and research implications, we had to have an integrated approach to our work. Some parts of our inquiry were geared to specific health conditions or technologies; others looked at the origins or implications of the technologies. The bulk of our investigations, however, concerned both aspects — learning more about current technologies and understanding their broader implications — because they are inevitably intertwined. The understanding reached through these investigations, which involved fact finding and analysis, together with an understanding of the context for our work — the social conditions, attitudes, and values that will shape Canada's response to the technologies — was vital to the Commission's ability to make appropriate recommendations. To reach this understanding, we drew together information and data from richly diverse sources and a wide range of activities:

- literature and historical reviews and analysis to understand both how the state of knowledge about conditions and practices covered by our mandate has developed, and what it currently is,

- surveys of patients and practitioners,

- analyses of related Canadian inquiries conducted to date,

- analyses of other countries' decisions and experiences,

- studies of Canadians' views about the technologies generally as well as individual experiences with them,

- field studies and data gathering in Canadian infertility clinics, hospitals, and genetics centres,

- information on pivotal Canadian systems and institutions, such as the health care and legal systems,

- explorations of ethical, legal, psychosocial, and other issues and implications, and

- analyses of economic implications and feasibility studies.

In all, we commissioned an enormous volume of research, totalling approximately 130 studies, and developed a comprehensive body of information and analysis on which to base our recommendations, much of it available for the first time in Canada. This solid base of research findings allowed us to address the issues more knowledgeably and in a way likely to produce practical and useful recommendations based on the reality of the situation, not on speculation. This was a complex but necessary task, involving the melding of our assessment of values and social attitudes with our knowledge about the technologies and their possible implications.

Although the conditions and technologies are related and have similarities, they also differ from one another in significant ways. General statements about them seldom hold true; the impact of each is distinct for different individuals and groups. Although all deal with reproduction in one way or another, each must also be examined and assessed on the basis of its particular characteristics, impact, and implications, and detailed discussion of the Commission's findings is presented in the remaining chapters in this second part of our report. However, recognizing that there are certain aspects about all of them that we needed to bear in mind, we organized our inquiry in each of the principal areas of our mandate according to a nine-point framework, the elements of which are described below.

Origins and Historical Development

To understand the current situation with regard to new reproductive technologies, it is important to understand how they developed, the driving forces behind them, and the social context within which that development took place. The Commission examined the history and development of specific technologies, such as *in vitro* fertilization (IVF), assisted insemination (AI), and prenatal diagnostic techniques, as well as newer developments, such as research involving human zygotes and the use of fetal tissue. We also reviewed how perceptions of infertility and options for dealing with it — such as adoption or living without children — have evolved in Canadian society. Among the aspects of the technologies we examined were the roles that commercial and industrial interests have played and continue to play in their development and provision.

Current Practices

Until the Commission completed its research, no large-scale picture of the actual practice and results of new reproductive technologies in Canada was available. Yet this picture is essential to an understanding of whether and how the technologies should be used and in shaping public policy responses to them. To assemble the picture, the Commission gathered data and information from many sources, including field surveys of hospitals, clinics, institutions, patients, and practitioners. This original research created a new body of knowledge that provided the basis for our conclusions and recommendations, and remains as one of the Commission's legacies.

Results and Outcomes

Any reproductive activity, care, or treatment has the potential for short- and long-term effects, both physical and psychosocial. Our investigation recognized that results must therefore be considered in the broadest possible perspective. Certainly, the effects on users of the procedures or technologies must be taken into account — for example, the effect on the long-term health of a woman taking fertility drugs. Using an evidence-based approach, evaluations were carried out using meta-analysis, cost/benefit, and other analytic methods to determine which treatments are effective and the nature and extent of potential risks involved. Also important was investigation of the effects on other parties, particularly the children born as a result of technological intervention, as well as on society as a whole and on identifiable groups within it.

Costs and Benefits

A broad perspective on costs and benefits is necessary, so we examined not only how society allocates health care resources and funds medical technologies but also the non-financial costs involved in use of a given procedure or technology, including emotional or psychosocial costs and the impact on the quality of life of users and their families.

New reproductive technologies cannot be separated from economic questions, in part because they involve decisions about resource allocation within the health care system and outside it. The Commission also examined the economic aspects of various programs, treatments, and procedures, as well as ways to measure economic effectiveness as part of an overall approach to technology assessment.

Because society's resources are finite, one consideration in resource allocation is the financial cost of a particular course of action compared with the benefits expected from it. This applies not only to evaluating technologies such as *in vitro* fertilization but also to assessments of prevention programs.

Future Directions

The Commission's mandate directed us to consider the implications of technologies and procedures that may be developed in the future. It is impossible to predict exactly what developments might emerge in the coming years in a rapidly evolving field. It is possible, however, to make some predictions on the basis of current experience and trends, to identify desirable and undesirable directions for research and development, and to consider what social structures or mechanisms should be in place to monitor and manage that development. The issue of future developments is common to all technologies, not just those in medicine. Even if the precise course or nature of technological development cannot be predicted, it is possible for society to be alert to the prospects for change and to equip itself to anticipate and manage change in a manner consistent with social values and priorities.

Implications

As stated earlier, our mandate directed us to examine a broad range of implications, including ethical, social, research, economic, legal, and health. We examined the ethical and other questions raised by the existence of new reproductive technologies through a prism of guiding principles (discussed in Chapter 3) that informs our conclusions and recommendations.

Assessing implications is complex, because the relationship between society and technology is dynamic. Not only are society and technology evolving rapidly, but the sectors of society where change is being felt most strongly — for example, the role of women and the structure and composition of the family — are precisely those in which the impact of new reproductive technologies may be greatest. The relationship is also interactive; new reproductive technologies have implications for Canadian society, but they in turn are affected by changing social attitudes to reproduction, family, and technology, as well as by the values Canadians hold and the priorities we set as a society. The Commission examined both elements of this interaction; they are described more fully with regard to each aspect of our mandate later in this part of the report.

There is the potential for greater erosion of the value of human life and the dignity of the human person through the indiscriminate use of NRTs [new reproductive technologies] ... we do not oppose science, we do oppose scientism, which is a philosophical variety of idolatry which posits the justification for the implementation of a technology merely in its availability. We do not believe that because certain technologies are available that they should therefore be utilized. This ignores the social, ethical, and spiritual consequences of technological advance.

G. Gianello, Christians for Life, Public Hearings Transcripts, Toronto, Ontario, November 20, 1990.

As our detailed discussion of the technologies makes clear, health implications differ with the condition and technology being considered; the same is true for their legal implications. Several areas of law are affected by new reproductive technologies, ranging from constitutional and human rights law through family law to laws affecting privacy and intellectual property. Issues such as access to new reproductive technologies, for example, are affected by the *Canadian Charter of Rights and Freedoms*.

Alternatives

The Commission asked numerous questions about alternatives to the use of reproductive technologies, including the prevention of infertility and adoption as alternatives to the use of the more technologically oriented techniques of assisted conception. We looked at choices such as living without children and nurturing children other than through parenthood. We tried to discover the extent to which prospective technology users are informed and counselled about the availability of alternatives, and to what degree these are realistic. With respect to adoption, for example, which has been seen traditionally as an alternative for couples who are infertile, we found that it is now not feasible as an option for many people, because far fewer children are available for adoption. In fact, the number of children born through assisted conception currently exceeds the number of infants available and adopted in Canada each year. This has implications for how we look at alternatives such as donor insemination (DI) and *in vitro* fertilization.

In addition, it was important to examine the alternatives available to individuals within the range of technologies and what should determine choices among them. For example, factors such as invasiveness and expense may determine what is acceptable to some people; others may weigh more heavily the implications for family and interpersonal relationships or the ethical and social consequences of their decisions.

Options Considered

The Commission considered the options available to Canadian society for establishing boundaries around new reproductive technologies and managing the technologies within those limits. This involved making evidence-based assessments of the technologies; taking into account our understanding of Canadian values and attitudes in these areas; considering the nature and structure of the systems within which our recommendations must be implemented; and looking at all these considerations through the ethical prism formed by the guiding principles we adopted.

> This Commission has a mandate to study and make recommendations which might affect all of Canadian society. It is good to keep in mind that our society nowadays is secular and pluralistic; that is, multi-ethnic and multi-religious, with many groups espousing varying philosophies and lifestyles. It is a democratic society with the principle of freedom of religion and conscience enshrined in the Charter.
>
> Consequently, this Commission should not follow any particular religious point of view, and make its recommendations based on factual knowledge, the best interest of the population, the protection and respect of individual rights and the welfare of people, and the maximum freedom of persons to make responsible choices compatible with the common good.
>
> *H. Morgentaler, private citizen, Public Hearings Transcripts, Toronto, Ontario, November 20, 1990.*

Recommendations Made

After the range of options to deal with a technology was identified and Commissioners had considered them, we developed recommendations consistent with our guiding principles. Our specific recommendations are set out in the remaining chapters of our report.

As we weighed the evidence before us to reach conclusions and develop recommendations, our ethical principles and the interests of the individuals and groups affected were always borne in mind. In the narrative leading to our recommendations, we describe this process and the reasoning by which we reached our conclusions. Where Commissioners were unable to reach agreement on specific recommendations, an alternative view is presented in an annex.

Organization of the Commission's Work

The Commission organized its work around two major streams of activities: (1) consultations and communications, and (2) research and evaluation. The balance of this section offers a brief description of these activities and how they contributed to the Commission's findings and conclusions.

Consultations and Communications

The Commission used several approaches to solicit and gather opinions and concerns, including public hearings, calls for submissions, toll-free telephone lines, and an extensive publications program (see box). Participants in the public hearings represented Canadian society in all its complexity and diversity. We heard from women's groups, medical organizations, community groups, labour organizations, representatives of Aboriginal peoples and members of racial and ethnic minorities, and the academic and research communities. We also heard from these groups and others speaking from an ethical, religious, or legal perspective. By bringing together people from various disciplines and interests through events such as hearings and panel discussions, the Commission hoped to promote increased interaction and exchange on the issues at the community level.

The strong desire of Canadians for information about the issues and for opportunities to make their views known was evident in the number of people who communicated with the Commission to ask for or to impart information. Some 6 000 people called the Commission's toll-free telephone number. More than 2 000 took part in the hearings and in the lively debate at the public panel discussions the Commission organized. In all, more than 40 000 Canadians were involved in the Commission's work — in these ways and through submissions, surveys, and clinical studies.

To respond to this desire for information and to promote a more lively and informed debate and greater public participation, we used various outlets for information about the Commission, such as community newspapers, cable television broadcasts, and satellite transmission of panel discussions. We tried to ensure that all those with an interest in the issues had access to the information they needed and a way to participate in the Commission's work. In particular, we looked for ways to facilitate involvement by people living in rural or isolated areas and by women with both a job outside the home and family responsibilities, who might otherwise have found it impossible to participate in the Commission's consultations.

Consultations and Communications

Input from Canadians

Public and Private Hearings: more than 550 Canadians took part in and presented briefs to public hearings across the country.

Submissions and Letters of Opinion: 500 written submissions and opinions up to September 1993.

Personal Experiences and Private Sessions: 500 individuals wrote to the Commission about their personal experiences or participated in private sessions held across the country.

Information Meetings: to consult organizations such as public health associations, women's groups, religious organizations, groups representing people with disabilities, the legal and medical professions, the research community, and the pharmaceutical industry.

Search Conference: three-day session involving 32 experts in fields such as health, law, bioethics, and religion, as well as representatives of people with disabilities.

Public Opinion Research: more than 15 000 surveyed; surveys explored awareness, values, and attitudes.

Toll-Free Telephone Lines: to facilitate participation in the Commission's consultations for people who might have found it difficult or inconvenient to participate through hearings or submissions; to provide access to information about the Commission and its work; more than 6 000 calls received.

Informing Canadians

Research Reports Released: Commission released 14 research studies during its mandate.

Newsletter Published: 50 000 copies of semi-annual newsletter, *Update*, detailing our research and other activities, were distributed through mailing list and public events.

Distribution of Information: 250 000 pieces of information distributed during the life of the Commission, such as information kits, brochures on the public participation and research programs, newsletters, speeches; information for use by community newspapers, journals, and opinion and editorial page editors; and information distribution also by cable television and satellite networks.

Media Activities: more than 1 000 media interviews were given and more than 7 000 media articles appeared about the Commission and its work.

At the same time, we worked to enhance public awareness about the issues raised by new reproductive technologies.   The chairperson and commissioners participated in speaking engagements and other public forums, and we issued two dozen publications during our mandate, including a newsletter, pamphlets describing our public participation and research programs, and an analysis of our public hearings. In addition, the Commission sought and received permission to publish some of the research and analysis studies before we submitted our final report. (A list of these studies is provided in the Appendices.) These activities helped to raise Canadians' awareness of the nature and importance of new reproductive technologies and to promote public debate about them.

Research and Evaluation

The agenda for the research program was based on the Commission's mandate, on what we heard from Canadians, and on discussions among Commission members regarding the subjects on which information and analysis were needed. Also important were consultations with experts in disciplines ranging from ethics, law, and philosophy to medicine and the other life sciences.   The result was a broadly based, multidisciplinary research and evaluation program designed to ensure that our recommendations were informed by solid, timely, and in-depth information. Much of the research funded by the Commission in the numerous disciplines relevant to our mandate will act as a catalyst in these disciplines, inspiring additional work in the coming years and acting as a foundation for that research. The conclusions drawn from our research studies and surveys are set out in the remaining chapters of our report. The studies themselves are available in the 15 volumes of research being published along with our report.

In designing a research program to address the four specific areas of inquiry — the prevalence, risk factors, and prevention of infertility; methods of assisted reproduction; prenatal diagnosis (PND) and genetics; and research involving human zygotes and the use of fetal tissue — we used the framework described at the beginning of this chapter. We also recognized that some ethical, social, and legal issues could be common to more than one area and commissioned analyses to address these. In addition, several other activities helped us to understand the context within which new reproductive technologies are being developed and put into practice:

• The first was an analysis of the experience of other countries in studying the technologies and dealing with the issues they raise. How have other jurisdictions developed their approach to the technologies? What issues did they consider important? What kinds of solutions have been proposed? We analyzed the mandates, findings, and recommendations of more than 60 inquiries held in such countries as the United States, the United Kingdom, France, and Australia. Critiques of the reports helped to improve our understanding of their scope, strengths, and shortcomings, and their relevance to the work of this Commission. We review our findings later in this chapter.

- The second was to develop an understanding of the current situation in Canadian society, including values and attitudes of Canadians. We analyzed demographic trends relevant to the use of new reproductive technologies, as well as how these trends may be influenced by these technologies. We commissioned public opinion research to ascertain the level of awareness about new reproductive technologies and the issues surrounding them, and to understand the values and attitudes of Canadians in relation to the technologies. The two surveys, conducted in 1990 and 1992, involved a total of 9 167 people. We also analyzed results from two Canada Health Monitor surveys of 5 448 people concerning, among other issues, whether they thought they were infertile, their knowledge about how the human reproductive system works, and their attitudes toward adoption. We summarized our findings in Chapter 2 and refer to them again throughout this part of the report as they relate to specific technologies or practices.

- The third way of coming to understand the relevant context was an analysis of the current situation in Canadian systems and institutions. We commissioned descriptive and analytical papers to help us understand the organizational structures, responsibilities, powers, and resources of the systems within which the Commission's recommendations will have to be implemented: the health care system; the social welfare and education systems; the science and research system; and industry and government structures. The sectoral interests (for example, pharmaceutical) affecting the technologies and their use were examined and analyzed.

- Finally, the Commission examined relevant areas of law, such as

  (a)   occupational health and safety legislation, which has an impact on the risk factors associated with infertility;

  (b)   family law, which is basic to the issues raised by new reproductive technologies;

  (c)   legal trends related to judicial intervention in pregnancy and birth;

  (d)   property law and intellectual property law;

  (e)   aspects of criminal law;

  (f)   physician responsibility;

  (g)   rights of privacy relating to the collection, use, and disclosure of personal information, and obligations of confidentiality relating to personal information kept in records;

(h) Canadian common law and Quebec civil law approaches to reproductive issues; and

(i) Canada's obligations, under international law and international conventions and covenants, in such areas as human rights, the rights of women and children, and the right to the benefits of scientific progress.

In total, the Commission's research and analysis efforts involved more than 300 scholars and academics representing 70 disciplines — including ethics, law, the social sciences, humanities, medicine, genetics, life sciences, philosophy, and theology — at some 21 Canadian universities and 27 hospitals, clinics, and other institutions. In some cases — such as our surveys regarding 1 395 patients at fertility clinics and 22 222 women attending prenatal diagnosis clinics — the Commission's research provided national data for the first time in the research areas. The Commission was also able to call on the expertise of researchers in the United States, the United Kingdom, France, Australia, and other countries.

New Reproductive Technologies Inquiries Elsewhere

One of the lessons emerging from our review of inquiries in other jurisdictions in Canada and abroad is that new reproductive technologies must be examined in the broadest possible light. It would be inappropriate to criticize earlier reports for neglecting some of the broader issues; in many cases, inquiries were not asked to study them, or were not given the time and resources to examine them properly. This Commission's wider mandate and resources enabled us not only to consider the issues from an ethical and social perspective but also to explore their various dimensions in much greater detail through extensive public consultations and wide-ranging research.

Nevertheless, the work already done by other inquiries to grapple with the issues raised by new reproductive technologies remains a significant part of the domestic and international context for Canada's response to them. The fact that so many governments have established inquiries and passed legislation, all in the last 10 years, attests to the seriousness of these issues and to the speed with which they have become a subject of public concern and government activity. In Canada, several public inquiries and working groups have been established, both federal and provincial, to examine particular aspects of the technologies. However, there has been no previous comprehensive Canadian examination of new reproductive technologies and related issues such as research involving human zygotes/embryos and the use of fetal tissue. Moreover, few of the recommendations of these previous reports have been acted upon. Internationally, several countries have passed legislation to deal with some of the issues surrounding new reproductive technologies, often following public inquiries. No two inquiry reports or pieces of legislation take an identical approach, but certain trends are emerging. Although these trends were not necessarily evident in all inquiries, and the inquiries had different points of departure and brought varying perspectives to the issues, opinion appears to be converging on several broad conclusions apparent in the reports and legislation. Here we identify emerging areas of consensus among them, as well as areas of continuing disagreement and gaps that remain.

Emerging Consensus, Continuing Disagreement, and Unresolved Issues

We can divide the issues into four groups: issues on which there is broad agreement; issues on which there is substantial and persistent disagreement; issues on which opinion seems to be shifting and a new consensus emerging; and issues that have not been addressed at length to date.

Areas of Agreement

Virtually all inquiries and advisory bodies have concluded that

- *in vitro* fertilization and assisted insemination are legitimate medical responses to infertility; internationally, the trend has been to institutionalize this response through some form of national accreditation or licensing and record keeping for assisted conception research and treatment;

- informed consent is a precondition for all medical treatment and must be obtained for all uses of human gametes, zygotes/embryos, or fetal tissue in treatment or research;

- some forms of embryo research are clearly unacceptable (for example, cloning, human-animal hybrids); other forms of research are acceptable within the first 14 days of development *in vitro*, provided they are strictly regulated and approved by an ethics review committee and no attempt is made to establish the zygote *in utero* following research; no such research should ever be done for profit;

- internationally, there is general agreement that the use of donated gametes or zygotes is permissible; and

- the legal status of children conceived through the use of donated gametes or zygotes should be regularized.

In addition, the emerging international consensus is that a time limit should be placed on the storage of human gametes and zygotes/embryos. Decisions about the use or destiny of stored gametes and zygotes/embryos (for example, in the event of death or divorce of the donors) should be made in advance, either by law or by the donors at the time of donation. There is also agreement that commercial preconception agreements are unacceptable, as are financial inducements for gamete donors. Sex selection for non-medical reasons has also been prohibited in several countries or recommended for prohibition by a public inquiry.

Areas of Disagreement

In contrast with these common conclusions, in other areas differing policies or legislation, or both, have emerged, with no clear convergence in the conclusions reached. Several such issues are worth noting:

- Although most permit some embryo research up to 14 days of development, there is no agreement on the limits to such research. In particular, some allow research only on "excess" zygotes created for purposes of *in vitro* fertilization, while others allow researchers to create zygotes specifically for the purpose of research. There is also disagreement about the purposes for which such research is permissible; all agree that such research should never be done for profit, but some permit it only if it is intended to improve infertility treatments, while others allow research that offers new knowledge that could lead to health care benefits. Where legislation has been passed, the sanctions for inappropriate research vary as well.

- Although there is general agreement that assisted conception procedures are appropriate medical responses to infertility, there are differences of opinion on the criteria that should be used to determine who has access to these procedures. Most of the inquiries to date have recommended restrictions based on both social and medical grounds, and some governments abroad have introduced legislation imposing such restrictions. However, they differ on how these criteria should be defined and who should have the authority to apply them. In some cases, access would be restricted to married couples; in many, access would be open to unmarried heterosexual couples in stable relationships; and in a few, single women would have access. Opinion also differs on whether applicants should be assessed for their suitability as parents and what avenues of appeal should be available to those denied access.

- With the sole exception of the Ontario Law Reform Commission, Canadian inquiries and most jurisdictions abroad have firmly rejected the idea of commercial preconception arrangements. They differ, however, in their approach to discouraging or regulating non-commercial arrangements.

- There is general agreement that assisted insemination by donor (AID) is a legitimate medical treatment, but there is disagreement about whether it should be provided only by medical professionals. Some argue that AID should be deemed the practice of medicine, so that any non-professional who provides the service would be committing a criminal offence. Others argue that the provision of AID by women's self-help groups should not be prohibited.

Evolving Views

In some areas we can identify clear changes over time in the reasoning and recommendations advanced by public inquiries or advisory bodies. For example,

- Opinion seems to be shifting about whether children born of donated gametes should have access to biological and social information about the donor. The earliest Canadian inquiries strongly defended the principle of donor anonymity; indeed, some recommended that children not be told that they were conceived through the use of donor gametes and that records not be kept regarding the identity of the donor. More recent inquiries in Canada and abroad, however, suggest that children should be told the truth about the circumstances of their conception, accepting that the child has a legitimate interest in learning certain information about his or her biological parents, for both psychological and medical reasons. Hence, the reports insist that proper records about gamete donors be kept and that the child have the right to non-identifying information about the donor. Some reports also support the principle that access to identifying information should be possible as well, at least under certain conditions, such as medical necessity, when access is approved by a court, or (in a few reports) when the donor gives his consent. Countries' policies and laws differ regarding whose consent should be required in order for information to be disclosed and the age at which the child should have this information.

- There is increasing emphasis on the need for standardized and centralized record keeping on the use of assisted conception technologies and for some regulatory apparatus to ensure this. Earlier inquiries rejected the need for centralized record keeping or for a system of licensing. More recent inquiries have argued, however, that proper record keeping is essential for all such procedures. Indeed, some have recommended that some form of national accreditation or licensing be established for assisted conception clinics and that proper record keeping be a condition of acquiring the accreditation. In general, there is greater emphasis on the need for national standards, national registries, and a national agency to monitor new reproductive technologies.

Remaining Gaps

The Commission learned a great deal from the experience of other inquiries, many of which tackled difficult issues with rigour and insight, even if some lacked the mandate, time, or resources to engage in extensive public consultations or research. Our job was made easier by the excellent work that preceded ours in Canada and internationally, as well as by the resources that permitted us to adopt a broad social and ethical perspective. We also learned from the critics of the inquiries conducted in the past decade. The release of these reports invariably generated considerable debate among groups affected by new reproductive technologies and the general public. As this debate has evolved, and as the public has become more informed, certain gaps or issues not dealt with fully have become apparent in the way past inquiries approached the subject:

- the long-term social implications of reproductive technologies for particular groups in society (including women, children, people with disabilities, and members of racial and ethnic minorities);

- the implications of the diverse values and desires inherent in a multicultural population;

- the social meaning of infertility and the medicalization of reproduction;

- the prevention of infertility and alternatives to the use of technologies to treat infertility;

- technologies other than assisted conception (for example, prenatal diagnosis, research involving the use of fetal tissue);

- economic considerations and the relationship of new reproductive technologies to health care priorities (for example, should the procedures be publicly funded?);

- the role of commercial interests in new reproductive technologies; and

- the effects of globalization on new reproductive technologies.

In our own inquiry, some particular issues emerged that cut across the technologies and practices identified in our mandate; they relate to some of the clearest messages Commissioners heard from Canadians. These issues include access, safety, and effectiveness, the appropriate roles for prevention and acute care in dealing with infertility, the need to ensure informed consent and informed choice with respect to technology use, and the need to protect individual privacy by safeguarding the confidentiality of information gathered in the course of providing services related to reproductive technologies. Along with our review of the conclusions reached by public inquiries and advisory bodies in other jurisdictions, this input from Canadians provided an invaluable part of the context for our deliberations and of our integrated approach to the issues raised by use of the technologies.

Part of our integrated approach involved bringing together our moral reasoning with the values and attitudes of Canadians. There were a few occasions, however, when our moral reasoning led us to conclusions that were not strongly supported by the responses to some specific questions in our surveys of Canadians. This kind of situation usually arose when a value which Canadians strongly endorsed and said was important to them, such as equality, was not upheld in answer to a question on a specific situation, such as whether single women should have access to DI or whether people who are disabled should have access to IVF.

We gave great thought to this dilemma. We were guided by and took into consideration what Canadians said about both their fundamental values and their attitudes to specific questions, but they were not the only determinant of decision making in these complex areas. Where there was a divergence on specific policy questions, we decided that our moral reasoning should have greater weight if it was in line with fundamental values endorsed by Canadians, because we had spent much time weighing the evidence and thinking through the implications of different policies on such specific questions.

We turn now to the substance of our mandate — the conditions, technologies, and practices we were asked to examine. First, as background for understanding infertility and the technologies designed to overcome it, we provide a brief overview of the biology of human reproduction. Then, in the remaining chapters of the report, we apply our guiding principles, our weighing of the evidence we gathered, and our appreciation of the domestic and international context to reach conclusions and recommendations about the four main areas of our mandate: the prevalence, risk factors, and prevention of infertility; methods of assisted reproduction; prenatal diagnosis and genetics; and research involving human zygotes/embryos and the use of fetal tissue.

General Sources

Decima Research. "Social Values and Attitudes of Canadians Toward New Reproductive Technologies." In Research Volumes of the Royal Commission on New Reproductive Technologies, 1993.

Decima Research. "Social Values and Attitudes of Canadians Toward New Reproductive Technologies: Focus Group Findings." In Research Volumes of the Royal Commission on New Reproductive Technologies, 1993.

de Groh, M. "Key Findings from a National Survey Conducted by the Angus Reid Group: Infertility, Surrogacy, Fetal Tissue Research, and Reproductive Technologies." In Research Volumes of the Royal Commission on New Reproductive Technologies, 1993.

de Groh, M. "Reproductive Technologies, Adoption, and Issues on the Cost of Health Care: Summary of Canada Health Monitor Results." In Research Volumes of the Royal Commission on New Reproductive Technologies, 1993.

7

The Biology of Human Reproduction and Early Development

◆

Society's fascination with reproduction is reflected in intense public and media interest in new reproductive technologies. Yet few people are fully aware of the beauty and complexity of the process of human reproduction — the process in which new reproductive technologies can intervene. In this brief chapter we outline the biology — the anatomy and physiology — of human reproduction, from production and joining of egg and sperm to development of the zygote, embryo, and fetus.

Although scientific and medical research have steadily expanded knowledge of human reproduction, particularly in recent decades, much remains unexplained. We are, however, coming to understand with some precision why reproduction is natural and simple for some people and difficult or even unattainable for others. Although human reproduction cannot be understood solely in terms of biology, knowledge of this elaborate process is fundamental to any discussion of the technologies covered by our mandate: it is vital to any consideration of interventions in that process, whether before conception, as with infertility treatments, or after conception, as with prenatal diagnostic techniques. This account is intended to provide only the minimum information non-expert readers need to understand our analysis and recommendations regarding the risk factors for infertility, regarding the role of specific technologies in overcoming it, and regarding embryo research. Also provided are capsule definitions of reproductive conditions or structures that readers may find useful in understanding the discussion of infertility and technological intervention in subsequent chapters. Readers interested in pursuing this subject further can consult the general sources listed at the end of this chapter.

Human reproduction is a series of intricately connected and interactive steps. For reproduction to succeed, the anatomy of the people concerned, as well as their physiological, hormonal, and genetic systems, must all function normally and at the right time. The production and the delivery of eggs and sperm are vulnerable processes — anatomical, genetic, hormonal, or behavioural problems may interrupt them or prevent them from occurring at all.

Prenatal development is an equally elaborate and delicately balanced process. Both the embryo proper and the surrounding membranes and placenta develop from a single cell. The organs and body systems mature in a precisely regulated way — again, the physiological, hormonal, and genetic systems of the developing fetus and the pregnant woman must function in flawless coordination.

The complexity of reproduction and prenatal development creates risks of error — errors that are sometimes genetic in origin or caused by some agent, but also errors that occur by chance. Errors or dysfunction at any stage may act individually or in combination, with the result that the process does not lead to the birth of a healthy child. In fact, as explained later in this chapter, about half of all fertilized eggs do not develop in such a way as to result in live births.

The process of reproduction begins well before conception. The woman's hormonal system and reproductive organs must produce a mature egg for fertilization and must provide a hospitable environment for development of the resulting embryo. The man's hormonal system and reproductive organs must be functioning properly to produce sperm and permit sexual intercourse at the appropriate time in his partner's menstrual cycle. The steps between the production of egg and sperm and the birth of a child — as well as how the process can be interrupted and how technologies can be used to intervene if it is — are the subject of this chapter, where we set out the essential conditions that must be present and the developments that must occur for fertilization and pregnancy to result in the birth of a healthy child.

Egg Production

A healthy, fertile woman has some 400 000 immature eggs in her ovaries. Those eggs were in place even before the woman was born — originally, there were a million or more, but by puberty more than half have been lost through natural deterioration. From puberty until menopause, the woman's body goes through periodic cycles of physical and chemical change during which an egg matures and is released by the ovary in the process known as

> **Ovulation:** The maturation and release of an egg from the ovary.
>
> **Amenorrhea:** Absence of ovulation and menstruation in a woman of menstrual age.
>
> **Oligomenorrhea:** Scanty or irregular menstruation.

ovulation. After ovulation, the free-floating egg must be captured by the slender projections at the opening to the fallopian tube. The fallopian tubes — about 10 centimetres long and the diameter of a pencil — project from the uterus toward the ovaries. Just how the tiny egg crosses the gap between the ovary and the fallopian tube is still a mystery, but once it does, the egg can begin to travel down the tube toward the uterus.

All of these events and changes in the woman's body are stimulated and controlled by a delicately coordinated process of hormone production and feedback involving the pituitary gland, portions of the brain, and the reproductive system. Each event requires specific hormonal and physical conditions to be present before it can occur. In turn, each occurrence triggers further hormonal and physical changes without which the next steps in the process cannot take place.

Given that ovulation consists of several interdependent stages, the reasons for ovulation dysfunction are not always easy to determine. Ovulation may not occur because the hormones that stimulate it are produced in quantities that are too large or too small, or because the ovaries do not respond normally to the hormones produced. In addition, the cells that surrounded the maturing egg inside the ovary may fail to produce the hormones necessary for maturation of the egg to continue after the ovary releases it. These hormonal disorders could have their origins in the brain, in the pituitary or thyroid gland, or in the ovaries themselves; they can result from disease or exposure to harmful substances or conditions — or the cause may simply be unknown.

Other sources of potential problems with egg production are physical in nature. A woman's ovaries may be missing or damaged as a result of disease, premature menopause, or failure to develop properly in the first place. Failure to ovulate, disrupted ovulation, and other ovulation and menstrual disorders can be treated with drugs or hormone therapy, which can compensate for irregularities in a woman's own hormone production and feedback system. Drugs can be used singly, in combination, or in sequence to stimulate ovulation or to compensate for ovaries that do not function as they should. Drugs can also be used in procedures like *in vitro* fertilization to increase the likelihood of successful egg retrieval. In addition, technologies such as ultrasound scanning can be used to investigate the source of infertility if it is suspected that the problem lies in damaged, malformed, or absent ovaries, or damage to or blockage of the fallopian tubes.

Sperm Production

A healthy, fertile man produces 2.4 to 5 millilitres (one-half to one teaspoon) of semen containing between 200 million and 500 million sperm at each ejaculation. Only one sperm needs to join with an egg for fertilization to occur, but for this to happen, the sperm must be physically and functionally normal, active, and capable of swimming through the woman's reproductive tract, and be produced in sufficient numbers to ensure that at least one survives and reaches the egg. In addition, the man's hormonal system and reproductive organs must be free of anomalies and working correctly to ensure that he is capable of depositing the semen at his partner's cervix

> ### Stages of Development
>
> **Zygote:** The fertilized egg until two weeks after fertilization, when the embryo proper and the surrounding structures supporting it begin to form.
>
> **Embryo:** The developing entity from the third to the eighth week after fertilization.
>
> **Fetus:** The developing entity from the ninth week after fertilization until birth.

(the lower part of the uterus, opening into the vagina). The sperm must make their way through the opening of the cervix, through the uterus, and into the fallopian tube toward the maturing egg. The right hormones must be circulating in the body at the right time and in the correct amounts to promote normal sperm production and sexual function. This involves various brain structures and endocrine glands, as well as the reproductive organs, in finely coordinated feedback. Because it takes about three months for a man's body to manufacture sperm, factors such as illness, temperature changes, or exposure to drugs or chemicals during that period can affect sperm quality. The effects of some exposures are short-lived, but others may damage the sperm production system permanently. The reasons for scarce sperm or lack of sperm motility are usually difficult to determine, with the result that the condition often cannot be treated effectively.

Another problem arises if the man cannot deposit the sperm at the woman's cervix because of physical or psychological difficulties with sex drive, erection, or ejaculation; these may occur because of hormone disorders, physical causes such as disease or disability, or the influence of outside factors such as stress or exposure to harmful substances or conditions — or the cause may be unknown.

In addition, a woman's body may prove an inhospitable environment for her partner's sperm. For example, the cervix secretes a thick mucus that prevents bacteria, sperm, or other foreign substances from entering the uterus during all but a brief part of the menstrual cycle. Around the time of ovulation, however, the mucus normally becomes much thinner and more hospitable to sperm, facilitating their movement into the uterus and toward the newly released egg. Abnormalities in the cervical mucus, or physical or other anomalies, may prevent the sperm from getting through the opening of the cervix and moving up into the uterus and fallopian tubes, or the woman's body may even produce antibodies that destroy the sperm as they travel through her reproductive tract; the reasons for this "cervical factor" infertility are not known. Finally, sperm must be deposited at the right time in the woman's menstrual cycle, when an egg has been released from the ovary and is available for fertilization; these conditions are present for only a short time during each cycle.

> **Azoospermia:** Absence of living sperm in the semen.
>
> **Oligospermia:** Scarcity of sperm in the semen.
>
> **Motility (of sperm):** Movement; specifically, movement needed to traverse a woman's reproductive tract toward the egg; determined by observing a sample through a microscope.
>
> **Sperm morphology:** The form and structure of the sperm; abnormal sperm morphology may affect the ability of the sperm to fertilize an egg.

Most technological intervention for reduced fertility in men has involved the treatment of sperm to improve its capacity to fertilize an egg; no methods have been developed that can deal with male infertility problems such as failure to produce live sperm. Current methods of increasing the fertilizing capacity of sperm require the use of assisted insemination or IVF because a sperm sample has to be treated before being placed in the woman's reproductive tract or being brought into contact with an egg; these methods therefore involve treatment not only of the sperm, but of the woman as well. Drugs and hormone therapy have also been used to treat men who are infertile or subfertile to try to improve the fertilizing capacity of their sperm. In addition, cervical factor infertility is sometimes treated by depositing the sperm higher in the woman's reproductive tract (intrauterine insemination or IUI), thus bypassing any obstacles at the opening of the cervix.

Fertilization

The First 14 Days

If the egg encounters healthy, active sperm in the fallopian tube during the optimal time for fertilization (about 6 to 12 hours after ovulation), and if the chemistry and physiology of the egg and sperm are working normally, chances are the egg will be fertilized. For this to happen, the fallopian tube has to be unobstructed, and its lining has to be working properly to facilitate movement of the egg and sperm toward each other. If fertilization does occur, the lining of the tube must continue to function normally to move the egg to the uterus. If fertilization does not occur, the egg continues through the tube into the uterus and leaves the woman's body.

Fertilization is possible, though increasingly unlikely to occur, up to 36 hours after ovulation. Given the length of time sperm can survive in a woman's body (up to 72 hours) and the time that elapses between ovulation and the end of the egg's journey through the fallopian tube (12 to 24 hours), there is a regular though brief period in each cycle during which fertilization can occur. Sexual intercourse can be timed to coincide with ovulation — that is, during the woman's fertile period — but fertilization is not guaranteed. A fertile, sexually active couple not using contraception has an average monthly chance of having a pregnancy that leads to live birth of a child of about 20 to 25 percent.

> **Gamete:** The mature male or female reproductive cell — sperm or egg.
>
> **Genome:** The total genetic material contained in the chromosomes of an individual's cells. The human genome contains about 100 000 genes.
>
> **Syngamy:** The process through which the 23 chromosomes of an egg cell and the 23 chromosomes of a sperm cell combine so that the new cell has 46 chromosomes.

The subtle processes immediately following the sperm cell's entry into the egg are only partly understood. Penetration of the egg by a single sperm cell triggers a series of changes that include loss of permeability in the egg's outer covering (the zona pellucida), which blocks the entry of other sperm cells. Within the next 9 to 22 hours, the two nuclei (one from the egg and one from the sperm), now called pronuclei, are discernible inside the egg (see Figure 7.1). Also visible adjacent to the egg are two other nuclei — the first and second polar bodies — which are the non-functional remains of the egg's previous cell divisions. Each pronucleus now in the egg contains a discrete package of genetic information (23 chromosomes), one contributed by the woman and one by the man. After 22 to 24 hours, the nuclear membranes have disappeared, and the chromosomes of the sperm and egg have come together — this is referred to as syngamy.

To recapitulate, for fertilization to occur, a woman must have at least one intact and functioning ovary and one functioning fallopian tube; her hormone production and feedback system must stimulate maturation of the egg and the physiological and chemical changes that create a hospitable environment for fertilization and the egg's journey toward the uterus; intercourse must occur at the right time; and the viable egg and sperm must come together, preferably at the end of the fallopian tube nearest the ovary.

Damaged, blocked, or missing fallopian tubes — resulting from congenital anomalies, sexually transmitted and other diseases, or unknown reasons — are a frequent cause of infertility. Without functioning fallopian tubes, an essential factor in helping the egg and sperm come together is missing; there is no place for the egg and sperm to meet and no route for the fertilized egg to travel to the uterus.

Other reasons for fertilization failure involve anomalies in the physical structure or genetic make-up of the sperm or egg that inhibit their fertilization potential. For example, as the egg continues to mature after leaving the ovary, it must go through chemical and physical changes to make its outer wall ready for the chemical reaction through which sperm

Figure 7.1.   Summary of Fertilization

A sperm begins to enter the egg.

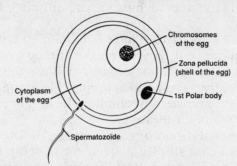

- Chromosomes of the egg
- Zona pellucida (shell of the egg)
- Cytoplasm of the egg
- 1st Polar body
- Spermatozoïde

After 9 to 12 hours
Two pronuclei are clearly visible within the egg - one containing the genetic material from the egg and one containing the genetic material from the sperm.

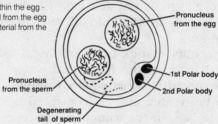

- Pronucleus from the egg
- Pronucleus from the sperm
- 1st Polar body
- 2nd Polar body
- Degenerating tail of sperm

After 10 to 22 hours
The chromosomes in each pronucleus are drawn together by microtubules in the protoplasm.

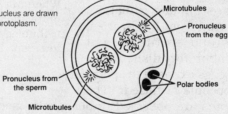

- Microtubules
- Pronucleus from the egg
- Pronucleus from the sperm
- Polar bodies
- Microtubules

After 22 to 24 hours
The chromosomes of the sperm and egg combine - referred to as syngamy.
Within 1 to 3 hours, the zygote will undergo the first cleavage division.

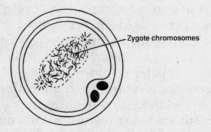

- Zygote chromosomes

and egg are joined in fertilization. If the egg's physiology or chemistry is abnormal, it is less amenable to fertilization. The substances accompanying the egg as it moves into the fallopian tube also have a role in attracting the approaching sperm, although how this works is not fully understood.

Just as eggs mature after ovulation, sperm also continue to mature after ejaculation. If they do not, or if they are physically, genetically, or chemically abnormal, they may not have the capacity to swim up the reproductive tract, respond appropriately to the lining of the fallopian tube and to the substances surrounding the egg, or reach the egg and take part in the process of fertilization.

The period beginning with entry of the sperm and ending with syngamy is being studied actively for insights into why fertilization fails. Sometimes, for example, more than one sperm penetrates the egg, resulting in a fertilized egg with three, not two sets of genetic information. Almost invariably, these eggs do not develop. Study of such eggs may, however, still provide researchers with valuable information about gene activity and early development.

When infertility results from problems with fertilization, technology has been used to intervene in several ways. For example, if the male partner's semen contains inadequate numbers of sperm or too few active sperm, it can be treated and concentrated before being used in assisted insemination or IVF. If the woman's damaged or blocked fallopian tubes cannot be repaired by surgery or other techniques, IVF can be used to circumvent this and bring the egg and sperm together. The woman is given drugs to stimulate ovulation, eggs are removed from her ovaries, and the eggs and sperm are put together in a laboratory dish. About 75 percent of eggs exposed to sperm in this way become fertilized. The resulting zygotes are observed under a microscope, and after one or two days' incubation, those that do not appear to be disintegrating, or that do not have extra nuclei because they have been fertilized by more than one sperm, can be placed in the woman's uterus in the hope that one or more will implant and development will begin.

> When infertility results from problems with fertilization, technology has been used to intervene in several ways.

The sperm used for IVF can be treated to improve their ability to fertilize. The techniques include sperm washing (which is used to separate viable sperm from other elements in the semen, thus concentrating viable sperm in a smaller volume of fluid) and sperm swim-up (a technique for isolating and concentrating the most active sperm). Sperm can also be treated with caffeine or other agents to make them more active. Among the newer methods being researched to compensate for sperm with reduced fertilizing capacity are zona drilling, where the outer covering of the egg is ruptured to improve the chances that sperm can penetrate it, and a technique called intracytoplasmic sperm injection. Further research is needed to show what consequences these treatments might have for the resulting fetus, although adverse consequences for the fetus have not been observed in the pregnancies that have resulted to date.

The Zygote and Its Genome

About 24 hours after the sperm penetrates the egg, the nuclear membranes of the two pronuclei dissolve and the chromosomes come together. This process (syngamy) takes about two hours, and in it the genetic contributions of the male and female gametes are fused into a single entity, the zygote, containing 46 chromosomes (see Figure 7.1).

Newly constituted, the zygote is remarkable in its theoretical potential to give rise to a distinct and unique member of the human community. This potential for development is both theoretical and statistical — according to the best available knowledge at this time, about 25 percent of eggs fertilized through sexual intercourse do not implant in the uterus, and about half of fertilized eggs do not result in a live birth (see Figure 7.2).

Although the genetic constitution (the genome) of the zygote is established at syngamy, the genes do not begin to function until the zygote has eight cells. Until then, the zygote is operating under genetically programmed instructions from the egg only. It is usually at the two- to eight-cell stage — about two days after the egg and sperm are first exposed to each other — that a zygote created *in vitro* is transferred to a woman's uterus in the hope it will implant and begin to develop. If all goes well, the information contained in the new genetic entity is replicated in each body cell in the developing embryo and fetus and in each cell of the human being that may result.

Some zygotes have chromosomal or genetic errors that mean they can never develop normally past an early stage. For example, a zygote may have too many or too few chromosomes, or its genetic make-up may not allow for normal development or for functioning of one of the processes essential for life. Other zygotes have a chromosome make-up that means they will develop into tumours (hydatidiform moles). Yet others have three sets of chromosomes, for example, because the egg was fertilized by two sperm. In fact, about 30 percent of human zygotes created *in vitro* have chromosomal abnormalities that mean they cannot survive. It is likely that a substantial proportion of zygotes resulting from intercourse have chromosomal abnormalities as well, given that in about 42 percent of cases, a fertilized egg does not reach the stage of a clinically recognized pregnancy (see Figure 7.2).

The 14-day period before implantation of a fertilized egg in the uterus is an important period of development for purposes of research. Research into fertilization and the early development of zygotes could contribute to our understanding of these processes and thus, for example, help

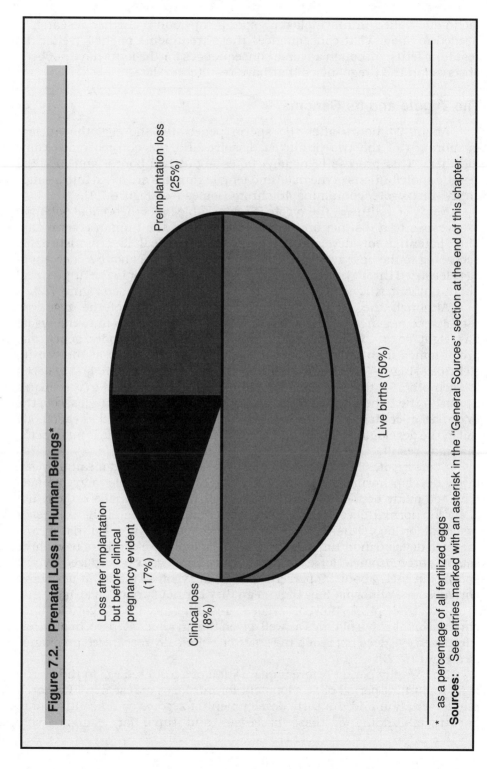

Figure 7.2.   Prenatal Loss in Human Beings*

Preimplantation loss (25%)

Loss after implantation but before clinical pregnancy evident (17%)

Clinical loss (8%)

Live births (50%)

* as a percentage of all fertilized eggs

Sources: See entries marked with an asterisk in the "General Sources" section at the end of this chapter.

workers in this field to improve the conditions in which zygotes develop following IVF and before transfer to the woman's uterus.   A better understanding of how fertilization works could also lead to the development of better forms of contraception for either men or women.   An important area of research involves the development of non-destructive viability tests that will enable clinicians to identify fertilized eggs that have a greater chance of implanting in the woman's uterus.   Similarly, research is revealing which observable cellular characteristics mean that zygotes are free of chromosomal or other anomalies and are more likely to develop, thus improving the chances that their transfer to the uterus will result in the birth of a healthy child.

Cleavage and the Blastomeres

Within a few hours of syngamy, the zygote begins a process of cell division called cleavage; the cell divides into two, then four, then eight cells, initially at about 18-hour intervals, eventually forming a clump of cells; each cell in the cleaving zygote is called a blastomere (see Figure 7.3).   Each successive division reduces the size of individual blastomeres by half, but the overall size of the clump remains nearly constant until implantation — at which time it is approximately the size of the period at the end of this sentence.

In summary, by about three days after fertilization, the zygote has become a tiny mass of cells.   A day or so later, having passed down the fallopian tube, the zygote reaches the uterus where, during the next two or three days, it develops a fluid-filled space within it, becoming a hollow ball of cells; it is then referred to as a blastocyst.

Some zygotes inexplicably stop cleaving — only slightly more than half the eggs fertilized *in vitro* reach the blastocyst stage. This failure to develop *in vitro* may be attributable in part to the hormones used to stimulate ovulation or to deficiencies in the culture medium in which the eggs and sperm are brought together, but a substantial proportion of zygotes resulting from intercourse also fail to develop (see Figure 7.2).

Cleavage is an area of active study. As part of the IVF procedure, pre-implantation zygotes are examined under a microscope; those that have stopped cleaving are not transferred to the woman's uterus. Study of their physical and chromosomal characteristics may help to understand what is going wrong.

Implantation and Differentiation

As the zygote moves down the fallopian tube toward the uterus, the corpus luteum — the empty nest of cells in which the egg developed in the

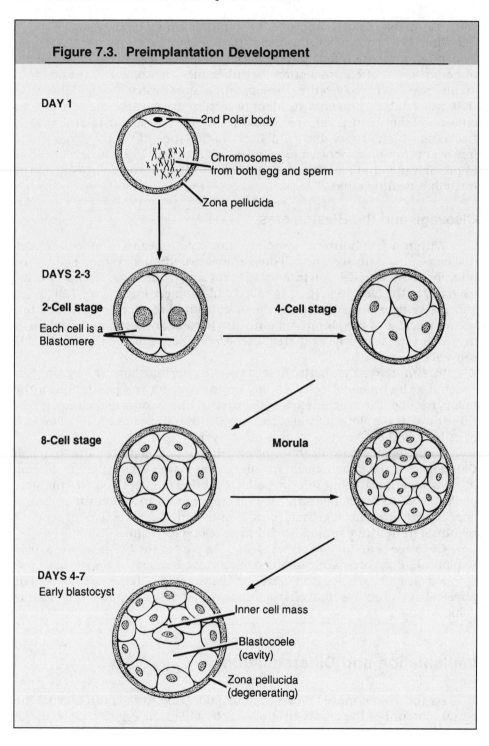

Figure 7.3. Preimplantation Development

Figure 7.4. Process of Implantation

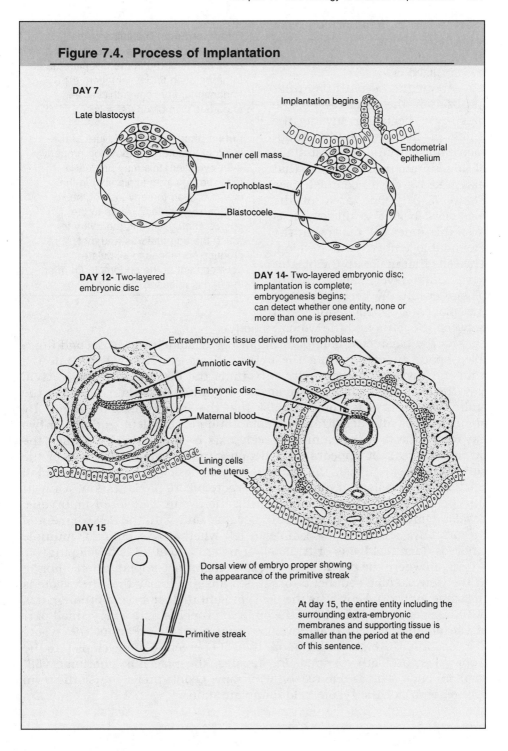

DAY 7

Late blastocyst

Implantation begins

Inner cell mass

Endometrial
epithelium

Trophoblast

Blastocoele

DAY 12- Two-layered
embryonic disc

DAY 14- Two-layered embryonic disc;
implantation is complete;
embryogenesis begins;
can detect whether one entity, none or
more than one is present.

Extraembryonic tissue derived from trophoblast

Amniotic cavity

Embryonic disc

Maternal blood

Lining cells
of the uterus

DAY 15

Dorsal view of embryo proper showing
the appearance of the primitive streak

At day 15, the entire entity including the
surrounding extra-embryonic
membranes and supporting tissue is
smaller than the period at the end
of this sentence.

Primitive streak

ovary — sends out a hormone that stimulates changes in the uterus lining, making it ready to receive the fertilized egg.

About the seventh day after fertilization, the outer cells of the blastocyst begin to invade the lining of the uterus (the endo-metrium), marking the first stage of implantation, a process that may take a week to complete (see Figure 7.4).   One area of the blastocyst begins to thicken; it is from this inner cell mass that the identifiable embryo will develop. The cells that make up the blasto-cyst's outer layer, called tropho-blasts, eventually become part of the placenta — the connection between the fetus and the woman's body.

> **Endometrium:** The lining of the uterus, which receives the egg after it has been fertilized in the fallopian tube. In preparation for implantation, the endometrium becomes thicker and engorged with blood vessels.
>
> **Luteal phase defect:** Failure of the lining of the uterus to develop properly after ovulation; this may prevent a fertilized egg from implanting in the uterus or lead to early loss of the pregnancy. "Luteal" refers to the *corpus luteum*, cells in the ovary in which the egg matures and that produce hormones to stimulate development of the endometrium after the egg is released.

As the blastocyst is implanting in the endometrium, a second fluid-filled space appears, within the inner cell mass. This will become the amniotic cavity that eventually surrounds the developing embryo itself. Now the blastocyst contains two spaces separated by a plate of cells — the embryonic disk. It is from this disk that the embryo itself develops. By about 14 days after fertilization, implantation is complete, and one or two days later the first indicator of a body axis becomes visible. Called the primitive streak, it appears as a heaping up of cells at one end of the embryonic disk.   Thus, the embryo proper develops from just a small fraction of the cells that make up the zygote before implantation. Only at this point, 15 or 16 days after fertilization, can *individual* embryonic development be said to have begun, because only with the development of the primitive streak is it possible to tell whether one embryo, multiple embryos (identical twins or triplets), or no embryo at all is developing.

Even where the zygote gives rise to a single post-implantation embryo, in the view of some commentators it is a mistake to say that the zygote is the same individual entity as the post-implantation embryo. Although it is of course genetically identical, the embryo proper is only a very small part of the organic system that develops from a zygote.   Part of the zygote develops into the embryo, but more than 99 percent of it develops into the trophoblast and other supporting tissues (the placenta, chorionic villi, amnion, etc.).   This is one reason why some people prefer to use the term "pre-embryo" for the zygote before implantation.

Failure of Zygotes to Develop

As mentioned, fertilization of an egg following sexual intercourse does not necessarily mean that pregnancy will result. As we have seen, not all zygotes implant, and of those that do implant a proportion are lost before a pregnancy becomes clinically recognizable. It is estimated that 25 percent are lost without implanting and a further 17 percent are lost after implantation but before a clinically recognized pregnancy; this means that in 42 percent of cases where an egg has been fertilized, no clinically recognized pregnancy results. There is also loss after this stage — at least 8 percent of clinically recognized pregnancies end in spontaneous loss, including about 1 percent that result in stillbirths (Figure 7.2).

Why zygotes fail to develop or implant in the uterus lining is understood only partly. Some losses result from problems in the zygote's functioning, while others could be the result of dysfunction in the hormone signalling and feedback system between the woman's brain, ovary, and uterus lining. Problems with zygote functioning could arise from genetic anomalies in the fertilized egg or damage to it. Dysfunction in the woman's hormone or central nervous system could arise spontaneously or result from exposure to harmful substances or conditions.

Research directed to finding out what inhibits or contributes to successful implantation, and thus how to promote it, is now going on in many parts of the world. If the problem is thought to lie in a hormone deficiency related to the corpus luteum, the woman can take hormones to promote a more favourable environment for implantation and early embryo development. Other research is looking at whether genetic factors could explain why some women are susceptible to pregnancy loss. For example, researchers working with mice have discovered that a defect in the genetic coding for a protein usually present in the uterus lining, resulting in a lack of the protein, may be preventing implantation. A similar mechanism may be at work in some women who have difficulty establishing a pregnancy.

In addition, as part of IVF procedures, zygotes are examined under a microscope to identify which are most likely to implant and develop successfully. Research into this process could help improve the effectiveness of IVF as well as promote successful implantation and embryo development in women who can conceive but have a history of miscarriage early in pregnancy.

Conclusion

Almost nine months of embryo and then fetal development follow the complex processes of ovulation, fertilization, development of the zygote, and implantation. The complexity of this process — as an entire human being develops from the joining of two cells — makes it open to the risk of errors and dysfunction. In fact, only half of all fertilized eggs survive embryo and fetal development and result in live births. The remainder are lost sometime between fertilization and the end of pregnancy, many of them before implantation and many within the first few weeks after implantation.

As we learn more about the human reproductive process, respect for its beauty and complexity increases. Studying human reproduction brings us into direct contact with the intricacy of our genetic make-up. Human development is the result of continuous interaction among more than 100 000 genes, many environmental factors, and many social and emotional experiences. Studying reproduction and the genetic mechanisms that shape the origins of life contributes to our understanding of the complexity of the human experience.

Even with the technologies and diagnostic capabilities developed since the 1970s, many aspects of human reproduction remain little understood. For example, some cases of infertility cannot be explained, even after investigation using the latest diagnostic tools. Another example is mutations, which can occur, for reasons not fully understood, when cells divide and expected replications of gene sequences do not occur. The examples are many but the point is the same: whatever our current level of knowledge about reproduction, many aspects are still understood imperfectly, incompletely, or not at all, and some may never be.

As this brief description has illustrated, human reproduction is intricate and unpredictable. Given everything that has to go right — at the right place and the right time — for fertilization to occur and then for fertilization to lead to the gestation and birth of a healthy child, the wonder is not that the process often fails but that it succeeds as often as it does. Even when all their systems are functioning normally, the chances that a healthy, fertile couple will conceive during any monthly cycle are only about 20 to 25 percent. For some 7 percent of Canadian couples, however, the chances are much lower. The many factors that can intervene to prevent conception and successful gestation are the subject of the next chapter, in which we examine the prevalence, risk factors, and prevention of infertility.

General Sources

Anthony, C.P., and G.A. Thibodeau. *Anatomy and Physiology.* 11th ed. St. Louis: Mosby Co., 1983.

Baylis, F. "Assisted Reproductive Technologies: Informed Choice." In Research Volumes of the Royal Commission on New Reproductive Technologies, 1993.

Chard, T. "Frequency of Implantation and Early Pregnancy Loss in Natural Cycles." *Baillière's Clinical Obstetrics and Gynaecology* 5 (1991): 179-89.

Cunningham, F.G., P.C. MacDonald, and N.F. Gant, eds. *William's Obstetrics.* 18th ed. Norwalk: Appleton & Lange, 1989.

Dawson, K. "Introduction: An Outline of Scientific Aspects of Human Embryo Research." In *Embryo Experimentation,* ed. P. Singer et al. Cambridge: Cambridge University Press, 1990.

Diedrich, K., et al. "The Intratubal Transfer of Pronucleus and Early Embryonic Stage Embryos." In *Advances in Assisted Reproductive Technologies,* ed. S. Mashiach et al. New York: Plenum Press, 1990.

Edmonds, D.K., et al. "Early Embryonic Mortality in Women." *Fertility and Sterility* 38 (4)(1982): 447-53.

Fédération CECOS, D. Schwartz, and M.J. Mayaux. "Female Fecundity as a Function of Age." *New England Journal of Medicine* 306 (7)(1982): 404-406.

Feichtinger, W., and P. Kemeter, eds. *Future Aspects in Human In Vitro Fertilization.* Berlin: Springer-Verlag, 1987.

*Hendrickx, A.G., and P.E. Binkerd. "Fetal Deaths in Nonhuman Primates." In *Human Embryonic and Fetal Death,* ed. I.H. Porter and E.B. Hook. New York: Academic Press, 1980.

Hertig, A.T., et al. "Thirty-Four Fertilized Human Ova, Good, Bad and Indifferent Recovered from 210 Women of Known Fertility: A Study of Biologic Wastage in Early Human Pregnancy." *Pediatrics* 23 (1)(Part 1)(1959): 202-11.

*Johanson, D.C., and M.A. Edey. *Lucy, the Beginnings of Human Kind.* New York: Simon & Schuster, 1981.

*Kline, J., Z. Stein, and M. Susser, eds. *Conception to Birth: Epidemiology of Prenatal Development.* New York: Oxford University Press, 1989.

*Leonard, A., Gh. Deknudt, and G. Linden. "Ovulation and Prenatal Losses in Different Strains of Mice." *expérimentation animale* 4 (1)(1971): 1-6.

*Lovejoy, C.O. "The Origin of Man." *Science* 211 (January 23, 1981): 341-50.

*MacArthur, R.H., and E.O. Wilson. *The Theory of Island Biogeography.* Princeton: Princeton University Press, 1967.

McLaren, A. "The IVF Conceptus: Research Today and Tomorrow." In *In Vitro Fertilization and Other Assisted Reproduction,* ed. H.W. Jones, Jr., and C. Schrader. New York: New York Academy of Sciences, 1988.

McLaren, A. "Why Study Early Development?" *New Scientist* 110 (April 24, 1988): 49-52.

Meldrum, D.R. "Female Reproductive Aging — Ovarian and Uterine Factors." *Fertility and Sterility* 59 (1)(January 1993): 1-5.

Menning, B.E. *Infertility: A Guide for the Childless Couple.* 2d ed. New York: Prentice-Hall Press, 1988.

Miller, J.F., et al. "Fetal Loss After Implantation: A Prospective Study." *Lancet* (September 13, 1980): 554-56.

---

* Sources marked with an asterisk were those used to compile the data for Figure 7.2.

Moore, K.L. *The Developing Human.* 2d ed. Toronto: W.B. Saunders Co., 1977.

Mullen, M.A. "The Use of Human Embryos and Fetal Tissues: A Research Architecture." In Research Volumes of the Royal Commission on New Reproductive Technologies, 1993.

Mullens, A. *Missed Conceptions: Overcoming Infertility.* Toronto: McGraw-Hill Ryerson, 1990.

Nora, J.J., and F.C. Fraser. *Medical Genetics: Principles and Practice.* 3d ed. Philadelphia: Lea & Febiger, 1989.

*Pianka, E.R. "On γ- and K-Selection." *The American Naturalist* 104 (940)(November-December 1970): 592-97.

Pullen, H., and J. Smith. *Making Babies: A Complete Guide to Fertility and Infertility.* Mississauga: Random House of Canada, 1990.

Rodin, J., and A. Collins, eds. *Women and New Reproductive Technologies: Medical, Psychological, Legal and Ethical Dilemmas.* Hillsdale: Lawrence Erlbaum Associates, Inc., 1991.

*Short, R.V. "Species Differences in Reproductive Mechanisms." In *Reproduction in Mammals.* 2d ed. *Book 4 — Reproductive Fitness*, ed. C.R. Austin and R.V. Short. Cambridge: Cambridge University Press, 1985.

Singer, P., et al., eds. *Embryo Experimentation.* Cambridge: Cambridge University Press, 1990.

Warburton, D., and F.C. Fraser. "Spontaneous Abortion Risks in Man: Data from Reproductive Histories Collected in a Medical Genetics Unit." *Human Genetics* 16 (1)(March 1964): 1-25.

Whittaker, P.G. "Recognition of Early Pregnancy: Human Chorionic Gonadotrophin." In *Implantation: Biological and Clinical Aspects*, ed. M. Chapman, G. Grudzinskas, and T. Chard. London: Springer-Verlag, 1988.

Whittaker, P.G., A. Taylor, and T. Lind. "Unsuspected Pregnancy Loss in Healthy Women." *Lancet* (May 21, 1983): 1126-27.

Wilcox, A.J., et al. "Incidence of Early Loss of Pregnancy." *New England Journal of Medicine* 319 (4)(July 28, 1988): 189-94.

Yovich, J., and A. Lower. "Implantation Failure: Clinical Aspects." *Baillière's Clinical Obstetrics and Gynaecology* 5 (1991): 211-52.

Infertility: Prevalence, Risk Factors, and Prevention — Introduction

The inability to have children is not a trivial matter. The Commission found a great deal of evidence of the value and importance Canadians attach to having children:

- In our survey of values and attitudes, we asked Canadians across the country to rank the importance of various aspects of their lives. They responded that their family and partner were by far the most important — more important than career, religion, ethnic background, or education, for eight out of ten people surveyed. So it is not only people who are infertile who think having a family is important.

- During our public hearings and private sessions, we heard from many individuals and couples who are infertile about how not having children has affected their lives. Participants in our private sessions explained eloquently how they felt without children. One woman said, "You have no future; nobody would know you were here," while another said, "You have lost your place in the chain of life." They talked of how infertility is not a one-time event or condition, something you adjust to and then move beyond. There are constant reminders throughout the life cycle, as the children of friends go to school, graduate from college, marry, and have their own children. So many landmarks and events in our lives together reflect connections to the next generation and a future from which many people who are infertile feel cut off.

Infertility touches the daily lives of many thousands of individual Canadians. Infertility has a strong collective aspect as well, however, and therefore requires a collective response from society. Given its importance to Canadians, the Commission concluded that a responsible and caring society should seek ways to recognize and support the desire of individuals and couples to have children. One way of doing so is to gain a better understanding of infertility in order to prevent it if possible.

At the same time, we cannot lose sight of the needs of those who are already infertile; this aspect is dealt with in the section on assisted conception (Chapters 18 to 20). Indeed, most attention to date has been given to those who are already infertile. The Commission heard time and again, however, that preventing infertility in the first place would be a more cost-effective and humane approach than using technology to circumvent it later. Consistent with the ethic of care, avoiding harm where possible is also the more ethical approach. Consistent with our guiding principles, prevention could also offer a means of making wiser use of public resources. The knowledge on which to base a greater emphasis on prevention, however, remains imperfect, incomplete, or in some respects absent altogether.

In Chapter 3, we showed how our ethical stance is predicated in part on preventing or avoiding crises where possible, instead of reacting after they occur. Embracing this perspective makes it imperative to reduce the proportion of individuals who become infertile in the first place, rather than relying on reproductive technologies to assist them after they have become infertile.

> We must, in Canada, prevent involuntary infertility in our youth and young adults rather than focusing exclusively on the provision of costly technologies to achieve a pregnancy.
>
> R. Grover, private citizen, Public Hearings Transcripts, Edmonton, Alberta, September 13, 1990.

We do not have the knowledge to prevent all infertility, but if policies and programs were in place to reduce exposure to factors known to jeopardize fertility, we could potentially reduce the proportion of people who find themselves unable to conceive, carry a pregnancy to term, or have a healthy child. Throughout the Commission's public hearings, it became evident that Canadians share this view and want more emphasis placed on a preventive approach to infertility.

Gaining a full understanding of infertility is challenging, and, as will be seen, the task is far from complete. What we found at the start of our work, however, was a daunting lack of available knowledge and data on the prevalence, incidence, and causes of infertility. No research had ever been conducted to determine the extent of infertility in the Canadian population: most studies that had been conducted focussed on fertility rather than infertility. Although there was some awareness of and some data were available on the role of some factors in causing infertility, there was much less concrete evidence on the role of other factors. Programs to prevent infertility, where they existed, had rarely been evaluated to see what strategies are in fact effective with various groups or categories of people.

Given the dearth of information, the Commission had to go back to the beginning, to assemble a knowledge base from which we could analyze the current situation and reach conclusions about the best course of action for individuals and for society. For the first time, then, the Commission developed an estimate of the prevalence of infertility in Canada. For the first time, we assembled a data base of research related to established

> In order to have a clear picture of the issue of reproductive technology, we must collect data on the incidence, prevalence, diagnosis, and treatment of infertility.
>
> *M. Joe, Minister Responsible for the Status of Women, Government of the Yukon, Public Hearings Transcripts, Whitehorse, Yukon, September 11, 1990.*

and emerging risk factors for infertility. For the first time, we linked specific risk factors with strategies for their prevention. And, for the first time, we developed a strategy for incorporating infertility prevention into the wider framework of disease prevention and health promotion programs in Canada.

As we outlined earlier, we took a broad, multidisciplinary approach to our work. Our understanding about infertility was informed by the research we commissioned, as well as the relevant literature. We gathered information from historical, legal, sociological, and economic sources and integrated our findings with research from the biomedical disciplines. Extensive research helped to broaden our understanding of the physiological aspects of infertility. At the same time, the testimony of the many people who spoke to us during the public hearings or in private sessions gave us an appreciation of the profound social and psychological impact of infertility. We were moved by, and are grateful to, the people who spoke to us about their infertility. For many, it was the first time they had spoken of it in public, and we recognize the tremendous courage this took.

Consistent with our commitment to viewing our mandate through the prism of Canadian social values and attitudes, a collective response to infertility requires an understanding of its social context. Because infertility has both individual and societal aspects, it must be responded to at a collective level. This response is conditioned by how widespread the problem is perceived to be; thus, Chapter 9 examines the prevalence of infertility in Canadian society.

The risk factors for infertility are numerous, and we examine the factors that place individuals at risk. One of the most striking aspects of our investigation into the causes of infertility was the lack of definitive knowledge in this area. The immediate physiological cause of infertility, such as an ovulation disorder in the woman or abnormal sperm characteristics in the man, can often be identified. The underlying reason for the disorder is very often difficult, or even impossible, to determine, however, because the factors that may lead to infertility are both complex and inter-related. The reproductive status of individuals is influenced by many considerations, such as their medical history, their everyday habits or choices — such as diet or use of tobacco, alcohol, or drugs — their age, or exposure to conditions or agents in the workplace or environment. Often these factors occur in combination. When two individuals come together to conceive a child, they bring with them their exposures to these various factors at different times over the course of their lives.

Risk factors are diverse and based on broader and often quite distinct areas of biomedical or sociological research and attendant research disciplines and methodologies. For example, the analysis of the relationship of weight, eating behaviours, and exercise as these concerns relate to fertility comes out of broader considerations about the very complex relationships between exercise, eating disorders, and weight control, an area of considerable research in its own right. Similarly, any examination of either environment- or workplace-related risks to fertility almost certainly moves into the field of toxicological research, an enormous area of biomedical research.

> Because of the scope of the problem, we must invest quickly in the search for new ways of treating and preventing infertility and for new effective means of contraception which are far less harmful to women's health. [Translation]
>
> L. Marquis, Fédération des femmes du Québec, Public Hearings Transcripts, Montreal, Quebec, November 21, 1990.

It became clear that what was required was an approach that attempted to take a global perspective on all relevant risk factors. Commissioners concluded that it would not make sense to advance knowledge on any one potential risk factor if this information were not placed in a context, namely, the attempt to understand infertility in a broadly encompassing fashion. Given the extraordinary scale of risk factors as a group requiring research attention, Commissioners were under no illusions about what could be accomplished during the mandate of the Commission. There is simply too much that is not known for this Commission to provide definitive answers about either the incidence or prevalence of specific risk factors or about the relative importance of these risk factors in relation to infertility. Commissioners believed, however, that a strong start could be made in the direction of approaching risk factors in a broadly encompassing fashion through the commissioning of analytic studies and overviews of existing research. In this connection, Commissioners recognized that adopting a deliberately global approach to risk factors potentially affecting fertility would encourage the integration of research now being pursued by various academic and medical disciplines on different risk factors, often in isolation from one another. The following chapters are the result of that determination to approach the risk factors affecting fertility in a comprehensive and integrated fashion.

Another issue for the Commission was the lack of scientific and medical attention to male infertility. Although researchers have made great strides in recent decades in extending what is known about male reproductive function and infertility, they continue to receive less emphasis than the female reproductive system. Yet a survey of fertility clinics conducted for the Commission showed that in about one-quarter (24 percent) of couples who seek infertility treatment, the male partner has a condition that makes conception difficult or impossible. It is difficult to attach exact figures to the proportion of infertility that is attributable to either the male or the female member of a couple, however, because in a substantial proportion of couples (26 percent) no abnormality is detected, even after thorough evaluation; these couples are "diagnosed" as having unexplained infertility. Nevertheless, the available data suggest that male infertility plays a substantial role in the inability of many couples who are infertile to conceive.

> The investigation of male infertility has lagged tremendously behind the investigation of female [infertility]. My personal viewpoint is that this has been the result of men believing the problem was always their wives.
>
> ... for years and years the wives were sent to the fertility clinics. That attitude has changed in the medical profession ... but I believe this is true in most infertility clinics ... we're not prepared to go on and do invasive investigations on the wife, unless the husband has been adequately investigated.
>
> R. Reid, Society of Obstetricians and Gynaecologists of Canada and Canadian Fertility and Andrology Society, Public Hearings Transcripts, Montreal, Quebec, November 22, 1990.

The Commission's objective was to gain an understanding of the range of factors that can make it difficult for people to have children. In general, data about the effects on men were much less available than information about the effects on women, primarily because of the greater emphasis on women's inability to conceive. A historical review conducted by the Commission found that, despite early recognition that some men were sterile, doctors focussed overwhelmingly on female infertility during the period between 1850 and 1950, neglecting the possible role of the man in the couple's inability to conceive.

From the data that were available, we found that there is a relatively clear relationship between infertility and the risk factors of sexually transmitted diseases (STDs), smoking, and aging. The association is less clear between infertility and factors such as most occupational or environmental exposures (although some specific exposures are clearly documented to be causal), medical interventions, diseases such as endometriosis, or personal factors such as alcohol or drug use, weight, exercise, and stress; however, there is enough evidence to warrant attention. The Commission is also aware that there is still a great deal to be learned about risk factors, so that new risk factors may emerge as our knowledge base broadens.

> Also in prevention there are a number of factors that have to be looked at. There has to be political will, there has to be professional will and there has to be funding, and in order for prevention policies, action plan strategies to be implemented there has to be compliance from the community.
>
> *J. Fontaine, Women's Health Directorate and Women's Directorate, Public Hearings Transcripts, Winnipeg, Manitoba, October 24, 1990.*

As part of our investigation the Commission also examined means of preventing exposure to these risk factors. Current efforts to reduce the prevalence of sexually transmitted diseases and of smoking among Canadians must be reinforced and extended, but programs and policies must also be developed to address the other risk factors we have identified.

The extent to which we are lacking a national infertility prevention policy or strategy in Canada soon became evident from our examination of prevention of specific risk factors. Current policies and programs to address reproductive health are fragmented and disjointed, reflecting decentralized roles and responsibilities of key participants such as provincial and federal governments, educators, and others with expertise and an interest in promoting reproductive health generally and preventing infertility in particular. It is evident that a national approach is needed if real progress is to be made in preventing infertility. In the final section of Chapter 15,

> In some areas such as prevention and promotion, Canada's current approach is a dismal failure. We put significant resources into treating infertility but we really make negligible efforts in areas such as sex education campaigns to decrease sexually transmitted diseases which we know heighten the risk of infertility. This is unconscionable in our view. We believe that a national priority must be given to health promotion and prevention programs to address the known causes of infertility.
>
> *A. Baumgart, Canadian Nurses Association, Public Hearings Transcripts, Ottawa, Ontario, September 20, 1990.*

therefore, we outline a national response to preventing infertility and highlight priority areas for action. We examine how an initiative at the federal level could be coordinated with existing federal initiatives such as programs to promote healthy lifestyles or to encourage youth not to smoke or use drugs. We show how such an approach would recognize and support other programs and address the need for coordination and involvement of federal and provincial governments, health care professionals, educators, and other key partners in prevention. A national response that makes a difference will require the participation of all of these partners.

Our findings with respect to infertility helped to inform our understanding of the possible place of new reproductive technologies in Canadian society. The discussion in this chapter therefore also provides a context for subsequent chapters dealing with specific technologies.

> Nevertheless, more consideration needs to be given to the causes and prevention of infertility. Some of the causes of infertility stem from our social and interpersonal practices. Therefore, preventative programs must emphasize the personal, social and biological causes and consequences of infertility.
>
> M. Gault, Manitoba Advisory Council on the Status of Women, Public Hearings Transcripts, Winnipeg, Manitoba, October 23, 1990.

The Social Context of Infertility

Human reproduction is among the most important and complex of human activities, both for individuals and for society as a whole. The process of reproducing ourselves is commonplace, yet it is biologically and socially complex. Any study of infertility has to begin with an understanding of the two aspects of reproduction — biological and sociological. These two aspects have always been intertwined, whether through perceptions and attitudes about parenthood and family, through social practices and taboos, or through public laws concerning, for example, marriage, adoption, homosexual relationships, filiation and legitimacy, abortion and contraception, prostitution, polygamy, and adultery.

As described previously, reproduction is at once a fragile and robust process. All species have a drive to reproduce; it is essential to their survival. Different species have evolved different reproductive strategies. Some species produce many young, increasing the odds of a few surviving to adulthood. Other species have evolved a different approach, with higher rates of loss before birth but relatively more invested after birth to ensure that those who are born do survive. Biologically, human beings fall into the second category; as we have shown, events can occur at many points in the reproductive process that preclude the possibility of a live birth. Thus, although reproduction is indeed "natural," it is increasingly clear that it cannot be taken for granted by individuals or by society. As we heard numerous times in our public hearings and private sessions with Canadians, what is natural and simple for some people can elude and frustrate others. Part of the frustration arises because of the social context within which reproduction takes place — one in which having children is considered a normal and desirable part of life. Before discussing the prevalence, risk factors, and prevention of infertility, then, we need to situate infertility within this social context, examine how this context affects our definition of infertility and what this means for people who are infertile.

The Social Meaning of a Biological Process

Our discussions with Canadians showed the drive to reproduce is no less complicated than the process itself. Responding to the Commission's national survey on values, for example, 77 percent of Canadians with children said they had felt a need to have children, even though most were unable to articulate just why. Overall, equal numbers of men and women reported a desire to have children, although women were more likely to report a "strong desire." At the time of the survey, 71 percent of respondents between the ages of 18 and 55 had children; 16 percent had no children but would like to have children in the future; and 10 percent had no children and did not intend to have any in the future. Three percent had no children and did not respond.

> We cannot over-emphasize how important we consider it that we dedicate sufficient collective resources to identifying and resolving the root causes of ... [infertility] ... rather than to treating the symptoms. We do know some of the causes that lead to infertility but we need to understand a lot more in order to be able to address them at their roots.
>
> *M. Eichler, Feminist Alliance on New Reproductive Technologies, Public Hearings Transcripts, Toronto, Ontario, November 20, 1990.*

The reproductive drive is likely innate, but in human beings this drive is socially shaped as well. The desire to become a parent is not well understood. How much of the deeply felt urge to bear children is inborn, and how much is created by societal expectations about appropriate roles and behaviours, are fundamental questions. It is obvious that social construction plays an important part in the desire to become a mother or a father. Regardless of its genesis, our survey showed that having children is of great importance to most Canadians. The three most important reasons for having children, according to respondents to our survey, are "It is a necessary part of life," "It's just something I expected to do," and "To help a child grow and learn."

It was also clear from our consultations that parenthood, and hence childlessness, have different implications for women and men. Women have been seen traditionally as mothers and nurturers of children; womanhood has been viewed in terms of being able to conceive, carry a pregnancy, and deliver a child. Society has expected women to become mothers and has relied on them to raise children. This definition of women's role — which often obscures their other roles and contributions to society — became more entrenched after the Industrial Revolution and the shift to a wage-based economy, where paid work was separated from the home. The home became defined largely as the place of family and the place of the woman, despite the continuing and increasing importance of women in the workforce. By contrast, men have usually been defined in terms of their other roles.

The availability of the first reliable contraception methods played a major role in showing that childbearing is not always inevitable. Today, the greater availability of contraception has enabled women to pursue new options and helped to highlight women's other roles. Even so, most people still consider having children part of the "natural" progression of adult life. Becoming a parent is usually deemed to be synonymous with growing up and acting responsibly. Some religious doctrines also emphasize openness to procreation as a vital part of the marriage commitment between husband and wife.

> Since infertility is defined as the inability to reproduce, it calls into question our very *raison d'être* as a person and as a couple. This phenomenon becomes apparent only when we confront it. Therefore, it should come as no surprise if infertility sparks emotional responses from couples, families, friends, colleagues, the medical profession and society in general. The vast majority of fertile people cannot begin to imagine the pain experienced by infertile couples and what drives them to seek treatment which offers them hope. [Translation]
>
> *Brief to the Commission from l'Association Québécoise pour la Fertilité Inc., November 22, 1990.*

Having children links generations within families and helps to ensure continuation of one's name, values, and genes. The Commission heard from childless couples who spoke eloquently about feeling cut off from the future. The effects of childlessness are felt strongly at all stages of life, not just during the childbearing years.

Given these attitudes toward having children, the inability to have children cannot be dismissed as inconsequential. For many people, the experience of not being able to have children triggers complex and powerful emotions. There is often a loss of self-esteem mixed with feelings of grief, anger, and sometimes guilt about the source of the infertility. Many also experience a sense of isolation from family members and friends. People told us that infertility is not something that is easy to deal with and move on from, because having children is so firmly embedded in the everyday social and family interactions in which most of us take part. As friends and siblings go through life, milestones in their children's lives — school events, graduations, weddings, the birth of grandchildren — continuously remind those without children of their childlessness. Coming to terms with the inability to have children is not something that can be dealt with once and then left behind.

A psychologist who counsels couples who are infertile explained to the Commission:

> One thing that I've learned through my work is that it is almost impossible to understand what it is like to be infertile, to grasp the profound impact of infertility, unless you personally have been in the position of wanting to conceive a child and have been unable to do so ... I have, since having worked with several hundred infertile couples, learned that loss of control, deteriorating relationships, increases in sick leave, inability to make career changes because of separation from the infertility clinic, lost friendships, depression, and marked deterioration in self-esteem are the hallmarks of the infertility experience. (*P. Gervaize, Reproductive Health Psychologist, Public Hearings Transcripts, Ottawa, Ontario, September 18, 1990.*)

The issue of how to define infertility — whether it should be viewed as a medical condition or as a social condition — continues to provoke considerable debate among Canadians, as it did during our public hearings. This is an important question; how we define infertility has implications for such issues as whether and how the problem can be prevented, whether the cost of medical treatment for infertility should be covered by provincial health insurance, and whether non-technological solutions to help people deal with infertility should be made available.

One view is that infertility has a physiological cause and should therefore be viewed as a medical condition. A representative from the Edmonton-based Fertility Management Services told us: "Infertility is not a disease insofar as it can be caught from somebody else who has it. But if a broken leg can be considered a disease, then infertility is a disease too, because it's something that's not functioning." A professor of medicine from the University of Alberta offered a similar view: "The reproductive system is part of the body. If you define disease as a malfunctioning of any system ... then clearly infertility is a disease."

Defining infertility as a medical problem suggests that medical treatment is the appropriate response. One woman who spoke to us during the public hearings explained: "I have viable ova and my husband has viable sperm. The difficulty is that one of the parts of the system, specifically the fallopian tubes, is not functioning properly. That is a physical disability. It is a medical problem that can be addressed by medical science."

Another way of looking at infertility is as a social condition. Some who see infertility as a social phenomenon argue that the need to have children is determined largely by social attitudes; in this view the painful consequences of childlessness result mainly from social pressures on couples to have children and from the lack of alternatives for those unable to have their own biological children. If childlessness were more acceptable, they suggest, or if adoption were an accessible alternative, people would find it easier to come to terms with being infertile and would be less likely to see childlessness as a problem.

Society does generate pressures to have children: for example, as we have noted, most Canadian couples see having children together as a necessary or highly desirable part of marriage. This attitude is communicated indirectly in many ways, ranging from the casual comments of friends and family to the images conveyed by the mass media and advertising. Our literature review and our survey of Canadians' values and attitudes confirmed that social perceptions — such as the belief that couples who choose not to have children are abnormal or selfish, that "they do not want to give things up" — make it more difficult for people who are infertile who have been trying to conceive for a long time without success to reconcile themselves to remaining childless. Nonetheless, the concern that pressure from spouses, family, and friends is an important factor in their desire for infertility treatment seems, from our survey results, to be unfounded. Indeed, many people who are infertile told us that those close to them do not consider infertility as serious a problem as they do, telling them that life without children is acceptable, when the couple themselves do not feel that way.

Defining infertility as a socially generated problem implies that we should look to social solutions. Those who see infertility this way believe that societal attitudes must change, for example, to be equally accepting of those who cannot have children or choose not to. From this perspective, remaining childless should be considered an equally acceptable and socially approved choice, so that couples feel free to choose that alternative and to decide, for example, not to seek a medical solution for their infertility.

The distinction between the innate need and societal expectations to have children remains unclear, however. Commissioners believe that both the physiological and the sociological dimensions of infertility must be

> I want to suggest that the stress felt by infertile women does not occur in a vacuum. It is societally formed. A married woman who doesn't have a child is pressured to feel less than a woman. But if a single woman wishes to have a child, that's a very different matter. If a lesbian woman wishes to have a child, she may be considered unhealthy for the very wish that would make her married sister appear healthier if she were successful in conceiving. This contradiction illustrates the extent to which these things have much less to do with physiology and much more to do with societal presuppositions.

> *Theme Conference on the Impact of New Reproductive Technologies on Women's Reproductive Health and Well-Being, Transcript, Vancouver, British Columbia, July 31, 1990.*

addressed, because both are important and they are often inter-related. In fact, medical treatment of infertility is used for social reasons quite frequently. For example, in a substantial proportion of cases, a woman is fertile but cannot conceive with her partner because he lacks viable sperm. If she is to be considered infertile, and thus eligible for medical assistance, it must be on the grounds that the couple, not the individual, is infertile. Yet this is in fact a social, not a medical, reason for providing a medical service — she has no fertile male partner; medical services provide sperm for her. It is evident, then, that social and medical considerations are very much intertwined.

In the Commission's view, therefore, it is important to deal with the social consequences as well as the impact on individuals; a caring society recognizes that both medical and social factors are at work and require both medical and social responses. A caring society that empathizes with the desire of people to have children, and recognizes the importance of children in most people's lives, will therefore take steps to prevent infertility where possible. At the same time, for those who face childlessness despite these efforts, a caring society will make other options available, either to help them have children, or to come to terms with childlessness.

The Commission heard from many individuals who have wrestled with these issues in making decisions about the kinds of lives they would lead. Some individuals and couples who are infertile told us of difficult and often deeply frustrating experiences. Others came forward to talk with great serenity about their decision to live without children.

A caring society also acknowledges the collective importance of children. The importance of children to society is emphasized in some concrete ways, such as universal public education. Although society encourages women to have children and it is the expectation that most women will have children, other social supports that would make child-rearing an easier choice — such as adequate and affordable child care — are not always in place. Thus, there is ambivalence about the importance of children and their role in society.

Social change, bringing with it greater acceptance of diverse choices in lifestyle, has made us more aware of how different people are affected by the societal norms surrounding childbearing. The pressures may be felt equally, though in different ways, by people who wish to have children but are infertile, those who choose not to have children, and those whose living arrangements society tends to regard as inappropriate for child-rearing — single people living alone and individuals living with a partner of the same sex.

Despite its social dimensions, understanding the physiological aspects of infertility — that is, the medical conditions that may impair the ability of men and women to have a healthy child — is necessary for two important reasons: to determine the appropriate role of medical treatment in helping people who are infertile to have children, and to identify and develop preventive measures. Understanding the social aspects of childbearing and infertility provides a context in which to understand how the prevalence of infertility may be defined in order to measure it, the factors that increase the risk of infertility, and how to prevent exposure to these risk factors with the goal of preventing infertility where possible. These issues are dealt with in Chapters 9 to 15.

The Underlying Causes of Infertility

Understanding the underlying causes of infertility is complex, because people's reproductive health is influenced by many factors, including their medical history, everyday habits and choices, their age, and exposure to conditions or agents in the workplace. Some of these factors can have immediate effects, while others may have consequences years later. Some factors may have effects that are compounded or exacerbated by the presence of other factors. Another difficulty is that although the effects of a particular factor may be quite evident in its most severe form, even with well-designed research it is difficult to determine the effects, if any, of mild or moderate exposure. A further complication is the fact that two individuals are involved in conceiving a child, and each may have been exposed to different factors at different times in their lives. Because of all these complexities, it is generally difficult to determine a linear sequence of cause and effect between an individual's exposure to a particular factor and infertility. For that reason, the term "risk factors" for infertility is often more appropriate than "causes of" infertility. It should also be remembered that not all infertility is preventable; for example, some women are born without fallopian tubes or a uterus, and men may also be born with anatomical anomalies that render them infertile.

To gain an understanding of risk factors for infertility, the Commission conducted an extensive investigation of the scientific literature published in Canada and internationally, to investigate the following list of factors:

- sexually transmitted diseases
- smoking
- delaying childbearing
- exposure to harmful agents
  - (a) in the workplace
  - (b) in the environment
- personal and medical factors
  - (a) alcohol and substance use
  - (b) weight, eating disorders, exercise, and stress

(c)   medical intervention

- •   unintended consequences of medical intervention
- •   sterilization
- •   contraception

(d)   endometriosis.

Our ranking of the risk factors is not definitive, but it indicates where we conclude, after weighing various aspects, that efforts to prevent infertility should be focussed. We believe, for instance, that sexually transmitted diseases and smoking should be highest priority, because of the risks they pose, the number of Canadians in their reproductive years who are exposed to these risk factors, and the feasibility of preventing or controlling exposure to them. At the other end of the list, although endometriosis, if severe, may cause infertility, its cause and how it could be prevented are unknown, and it is therefore not possible to develop strategies to prevent it.

We found there is evidence to show that all these factors may have adverse effects on female fertility given sufficient exposure, and thus they constitute risk factors. Data about the effects on male fertility were much less available than data about the effects on female fertility. This is disturbing in view of the proportion of couples whose fertility problems can be traced to the male partner.

One of the Commission's goals in this area was to assess the relative importance of each risk factor in terms of its contribution to infertility in Canada and the feasibility of preventing and controlling individual exposure to it. Such an assessment is needed to give policy makers a sense of where prevention priorities should lie. This proved impossible to do in a definitive way, however, primarily because information about many of the risk factors was inconclusive, incomplete, or absent entirely. We found little or no information, for example, on the extent of individual exposure to many of the thousands of chemical agents found in workplaces and the environment. In other cases, although we know that severe exposure to a particular risk factor poses a threat to fertility, the evidence is insufficient to determine whether the factor harms fertility in the far more common mild or moderate exposures.

Nevertheless, to give some direction for prevention policy, we considered four aspects of the evidence: the quality of research data and the strength of the evidence about each risk factor; the seriousness of the risks associated with exposure to it; the estimated size of the population exposed; and the feasibility of preventing exposure. The result was a list (see above) showing where we conclude efforts to prevent infertility can best be focussed. We believe prevention efforts should look at sexually transmitted diseases and smoking in the first instance. The impact of age on fertility is less clear than the impact of smoking and STDs, and, in addition, this risk factor is more difficult to address, since delayed childbearing may not be preventable, for example, in the case of partnerships formed later in life. Nevertheless, research suggests that women who delay childbearing until their later reproductive years face a moderate risk of infertility; this is something of which they should be aware as they make such decisions.

We believe that priority must be given to preventing infertility, rather than focussing only on medical interventions as a way to help individuals after they experience difficulties conceiving. Specifically, prevention efforts must focus on reducing the exposure of individuals to the risk factors we have identified, particularly when the means of accomplishing this are clear. Notwithstanding the complexities of the risk factors for infertility, the inter-relationships among them, and the diverse social, environmental, and occupational contexts within which they arise, this commitment to prevention must be an integral part of society's overall approach to dealing with infertility.

Strategies to address the risk factors for infertility will also have substantial spin-off benefits for other aspects of health, because factors that affect reproductive health rarely have an effect on the reproductive system alone — they have important effects on other parts of the body as well. For example, reducing the proportion of people who smoke not only could reduce the number of couples who have difficulty conceiving but would also reduce the incidence of heart disease and lung cancer.

> Specifically, prevention efforts must focus on reducing the exposure of individuals to the risk factors we have identified, particularly when the means of accomplishing this are clear.

Placing greater emphasis on preventing infertility requires that we develop programs and policies to address the different risk factors for infertility that we have identified. This can be done effectively only if other avenues in addition to the health care system are used to address the problem. Educators, health care professionals, policy makers, employers, parents, and many others are key partners in developing strategies and programs to protect the reproductive health of Canadians. Strategies must be diverse and multifaceted, reflecting the complexities of the risk factors they are designed to address and the diversity of the individuals and population groups they are intended to reach.

In Chapters 10 to 14, we describe how exposure to each of the risk factors we have listed can affect the ability to conceive, to carry a pregnancy to term, or to have a healthy child. We also recommend a range of initiatives to prevent individuals from being exposed to factors that may put their fertility at risk.

Prevalence of Infertility

♦

One of the principal tasks facing the Commission was to establish how common infertility is in Canada. Because there has been no Canadian research designed specifically to measure the prevalence of infertility — that is, the proportion of all individuals or couples who are infertile at a specific point in time — we did not know what the rate of infertility is in this country, or whether it has been rising, declining, or remaining stable.

Many Canadians believe that infertility affects a substantial proportion of the population. This perception may result in part from the fact that there is less secrecy surrounding reproduction and fertility than in the past, with people becoming more open about their infertility. A national survey conducted for the Commission found that 43 percent of those surveyed knew someone in their immediate family or among their friends who had experienced an infertility problem. This tells us little about the actual prevalence of infertility, but it does show why Canadians believe the problem is widespread. On the other hand, we also heard the view that infertility has not increased significantly over time. These contrasting views clearly underscore the importance of knowing what proportion of couples in Canada is affected by infertility and whether this is changing.

> Planned Parenthood Alberta wishes to make the following recommendation ... that research be undertaken to determine the actual incidence of infertility in Canadian couples of childbearing age, as well as of the causes of this infertility.
>
> *P. Webb, New Reproductive Committee, Planned Parenthood Alberta, Public Hearings Transcripts, Calgary, Alberta, September 14, 1990.*

This information is an essential basis for Canada's response to infertility. Policy and resource allocation decisions must be premised on the best available information about the prevalence of infertility, as a prerequisite for deciding what emphasis should be placed on understanding and preventing infertility as well as what resources should be devoted to these efforts and how health care resources should be allocated to treat people who are infertile. Thus, our findings on prevalence have an impact on our conclusions and recommendations with respect to infertility treatments in the next chapters.

We took up the challenge of assessing the prevalence of infertility in Canada in two ways. We developed a research approach that involved conducting three national surveys and synthesizing their results to generate a reliable estimate of infertility among Canadian couples. We reasoned that if there was congruence among the findings of the three surveys, it would be evidence that the figures were reliable. In addition to this original research, we conducted a secondary analysis of data from three surveys done for other purposes during the 1980s, comparing estimates of the prevalence of infertility derived from this secondary analysis with our own results.

As a result of our work, we know the prevalence of infertility in Canada for the first time: 8.5 percent of couples — some 300 000 couples — who were married or had been cohabiting for at least one year at the time of our survey, and who had not used contraception during that period, failed to have a pregnancy, while 7 percent of couples — some 250 000 couples — who had been married or cohabiting for at least two years, and who had not used contraception during that period, failed to have a pregnancy.

This information will remain one of the Commission's enduring legacies, not only for what it tells us about the number of people affected by infertility at a given point in time, but also because it provides a baseline against which future researchers can track the prevalence of infertility in the Canadian population. How we arrived at our definition of infertility for the purpose of estimating prevalence, as well as the methodology we used to establish this estimate, are presented in greater detail in later sections of this chapter.

Our estimate is considerably lower than the 15 percent figure commonly reported in the media. However, such media reports are based on a fundamental misinterpretation of the U.S. survey results that were the source of the 15 percent figure. Those surveys did not show that 15 percent of *all* couples are infertile, but that 15 percent of couples *who have not been surgically sterilized* are infertile. This difference is significant, because large numbers of Americans and Canadians choose surgical sterilization as their contraception method. As we discuss in this section, when the U.S. survey results are calculated appropriately — that is, *including* people who have been surgically sterilized — the U.S. infertility rate is close to the Commission's estimate for the infertility rate in Canada.

Commission Research

Until the Commission began its work, data measuring the prevalence of infertility in Canada were extremely limited. Periodic national surveys to gather information on reproductive issues such as infertility, sterilization, and contraceptive use have not been carried out as they have been in the United States. The first and only large-scale national survey devoted exclusively to the reproductive behaviour of women in Canada was the Canadian Fertility Survey, conducted in 1984. Since then, the only sources of data have been two surveys — the Ontario Health Survey (1990) and Canadian General Social Survey (1990) — which have focussed on other topics but included a few pertinent questions. Because these studies were not designed specifically to measure infertility, questions arise about the reliability of estimates based on them.

The Commission considered two ways of estimating the prevalence of infertility in Canada: conducting one large-scale national survey, or piggy-backing onto three smaller independent surveys that were already being conducted for the Commission by Canada Health Monitor and Decima Research. We chose the latter method, for several reasons. It was less expensive and more feasible in the time frame the Commission had available. In addition, if the three surveys gave similar results, we would have strong evidence that both the definition of infertility we had adopted and the results were highly reliable; we would have confirming evidence that the infertility rate generated by aggregating the results of the three studies was a valid estimate. A pivotal aspect of ensuring that the three surveys, taken together, would generate a reliable estimate of the prevalence of infertility was the development of an appropriate definition of infertility for this purpose.

How We Defined and Measured Infertility for the Population Surveys

As we have seen, views vary on how infertility should be defined. It is also evident that somewhat different definitions will be needed for different purposes. For example, the definition of infertility for purposes of conducting a population survey may differ legitimately from the definition used to determine eligibility for an *in vitro* fertilization program. Clearly, deciding who will be counted as infertile influences society's response to infertility: a narrow definition, encompassing fewer people, might mean that infertility is given a lower priority by policy makers, while a wider definition could result in higher priority and more resources being devoted to infertility.

The definition of infertility used to develop population estimates and to track changes in the prevalence of infertility over time must be both measurable and reproducible. For purposes of estimating the prevalence of infertility we considered three factors: (1) the endpoint to be measured (should we measure failure to conceive, failure to have a recognized pregnancy, failure to carry a pregnancy to term, or failure to give birth to a healthy child); (2) the period of time after which couples would be considered infertile; and (3) the population of interest.

Endpoint

For our population survey on infertility, we adopted the most commonly used endpoint — the absence of pregnancy — because using this standard definition would allow us to compare our findings with those of other studies. Alternative definitions of infertility are certainly useful for purposes other than population surveys; for example, in investigating the impact of various risk factors on the entire reproductive process, we broadened our definition to include failure to carry a pregnancy to term and to give birth to a healthy child. The birth of a healthy child is also a relevant endpoint for other research questions and for Canadians generally, who see the goal of infertility treatment as the birth of a healthy child. Similarly, the inability to conceive is a relevant endpoint in research into the causes of infertility. Such definitions are difficult or impossible to use, however, in estimating the prevalence of infertility in a population. For example, it is difficult to assess the ability to conceive, because miscarriages often take place before a woman knows she is pregnant, and miscarriages very early in pregnancy are usually not even recognized as such. Assessing infertility reliably when it is defined as failure to give birth to a healthy child also presents difficulties, because what constitutes a "healthy" birth is subject to varying interpretations, making it difficult to compare results. Given these factors, we chose as an endpoint whether pregnancy had occurred, as reported by respondents to the surveys.

Time Period

The next issue to be addressed was what time period to use in defining a couple as infertile. Infertility is not the inability to conceive at all (sterility), but rather the reduced ability to conceive over time. Couples in which one or both members have chosen a form of sterilization such as vasectomy or tubal ligation are referred to as voluntarily sterile. Some infertile couples will never conceive over their reproductive lifetimes (we refer to them as involuntarily sterile). Other couples, labelled as infertile, may eventually become pregnant without intervention. In other words, there is no specific point in time at which a couple trying to conceive ceases to be fertile and becomes infertile. To estimate the prevalence of infertility, researchers must therefore choose a time after which a couple who has not had a pregnancy will be considered infertile.

The time frame chosen, though in one sense arbitrary, is important, because it affects the number of individuals and couples included in the definition. The choice of different time frames is based on differing perceptions of how long it should take a couple to conceive. Research suggests that a normally fertile, sexually active couple not using contraception has an average monthly chance of conceiving of 20 to 25 percent (counting only pregnancies that result in live births).[1] This average involves wide variability among couples, because couples differ considerably in their ability to become pregnant. Those who conceive most easily do so during the first few months of trying, so that as time progresses these relatively fertile couples are no longer counted as being among those trying to conceive, while the chances of conceiving for those remaining decline.

Figure 9.1 shows the cumulative percentage over 24 months who will have begun a pregnancy that leads to live birth, if it is assumed that no couples in the population are sterile.

The time frame used most often by North American researchers assessing the prevalence of infertility — and the one commonly used by the medical profession — is one year because, as we have noted and as Figure 9.1 shows, the majority of couples will have conceived by this time. The one-year definition is not universally accepted, however, because some couples who have not conceived after one year have a pregnancy during the following year. The World Health Organization (WHO) has chosen two years as its time frame for defining infertility, on the basis that the failure to conceive naturally after two years generally indicates that there is a low chance of a couple conceiving without intervention.

Given that a significantly smaller proportion of couples has a pregnancy after two years than during the first two years, we chose to follow the example of the World Health Organization and adopt the two-year definition of infertility. We have also included one-year figures, however, because this is the measure used most often in other studies and allows our findings to be compared with those.

As with choosing endpoints, the appropriate period for defining infertility varies with the purpose. For demographic purposes, such as determining prevalence in the general population, it is important to have one consistent and widely used measure. To decide when to begin medical treatment, however, the period may differ according to the treatment being considered, the age of the participants, and their medical history. A less invasive and intrusive treatment might be started before two years have elapsed, for instance, while physicians might encourage a couple to continue trying to conceive for a longer period before attempting a more invasive treatment such as *in vitro* fertilization. By contrast, older couples in which the woman has fewer reproductive years remaining may be considered infertile and eligible for treatment before two years have elapsed (see Chapter 20).

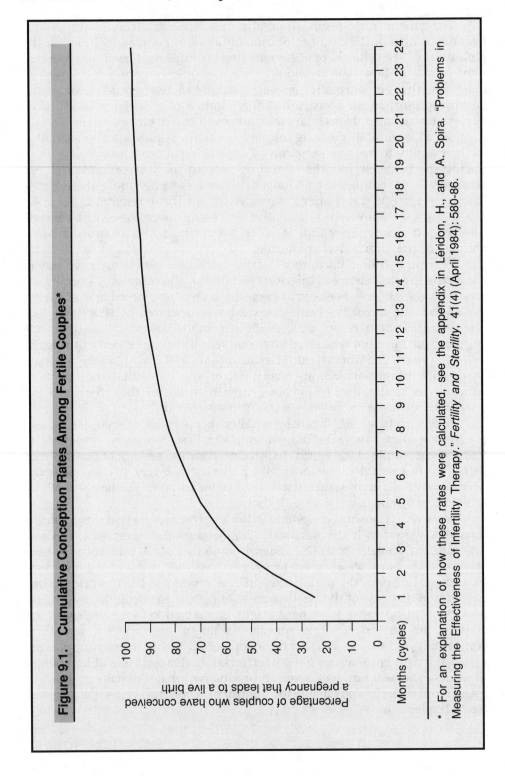

Figure 9.1. Cumulative Conception Rates Among Fertile Couples*

Percentage of couples who have conceived a pregnancy that leads to a live birth

Months (cycles)

* For an explanation of how these rates were calculated, see the appendix in Léridon, H., and A. Spira. "Problems in Measuring the Effectiveness of Infertility Therapy." *Fertility and Sterility*, 41(4) (April 1984): 580-86.

Population of Interest

The final element of our definition was the population of interest — in other words, who would be counted. Historically, infertility definitions have focussed on women, in part because pregnancy, the main indicator of fertility, happens in the woman's body. Unfortunately, this focus tends to perpetuate the myth that infertility is the woman's problem, when in fact it may well be the man's problem instead or as well.

We chose to focus on couples, because the reason or reasons why conception has not occurred may lie with either member of the couple or with both. There are also practical reasons for focussing on couples in a survey. Concerns about infertility arise most often in the context of a heterosexual couple who want to have a child. In addition, it can be assumed that couples living together, if they want to become pregnant, have sexual intercourse regularly and do not use contraception.

We narrowed the population of interest further by restricting our definition to couples who had been married or cohabiting* for at least a full year or two full years at the time of the survey. This is because couples *currently* cohabiting may not have been doing so for the one year (or two years) required to meet our definition. Couples cohabiting for less than that period might not have been sexually active for the full year (or two years) in question; therefore, including them in the population to be counted could have had a distorting effect on the number of couples found to be infertile.

We found that about 5 percent of the couples surveyed had not been cohabiting for at least one year. These couples were therefore excluded from our calculation of the one-year estimate of infertility. We also found that an additional 4 percent of those surveyed had not been cohabiting for at least two years; these couples were excluded from our calculation of the two-year estimate of infertility.

Some limitations are inherent in focussing on couples. One is that a significant segment of the population that is of reproductive age is omitted from the estimates. For example, approximately 40 percent of women aged 18 to 44 are not living with a male partner at present and would therefore not have been included in our survey. Methods have been devised in the United States to expand the population of interest to estimate infertility among all women of reproductive age. Researchers in Canada may want to look at these methods when conducting prevalence research in the future. After consulting the researchers in the U.S. survey, the Commission decided not to take this approach. As we will see, however, U.S. infertility estimates do not differ significantly from those reached by the Commission.

---

* For simplicity, all further references to cohabiting couples include both married and unmarried couples.

It should be noted that "couple," when used to define infertility, refers to heterosexual couples. We recognize that lesbians and single women might want to use reproductive technologies to pursue parenthood. By excluding them from the definition used for population studies we do not imply they should be excluded from access to services; these issues are dealt with in the next chapter on assisted human conception.

> For purposes of estimating the prevalence of infertility in Canada, the Commission adopted two definitions of **infertility**:
>
> The absence of pregnancy in a couple who have been cohabiting *for at least the past year* and who have not used contraception during that period.
>
> The absence of pregnancy in a couple who have been cohabiting *for at least the past two years* and who have not used contraception during that period.

Methodology

Three telephone surveys were conducted across Canada in late 1991 and early 1992, with a total of 1 412 randomly selected women who had been cohabiting with their partner for at least one year.* Despite the focus on couples, the Commission surveys were based on interviews only with women. This is the usual practice in data collection on this topic, as it has been shown that women tend to provide more accurate answers about contraceptive use and pregnancy, both for themselves and for their partners. In each of our three surveys, the method of identifying infertile couples was identical. We asked questions to establish the following:

- Whether the respondent was a woman aged 18 to 44 who is part of a couple that has been cohabiting for at least one year/two years.

- Whether the respondent used contraception in the past year/two years, or if she or her partner had been surgically sterilized.

- Whether the respondent had been pregnant in the past year/two years.

Answers to the first question provided the denominator, which is made up of all couples who have been cohabiting or married for at least one year/two years and in which the woman is between the ages of 18 and 44. The second question was used to identify couples using contraception and those in which one or both members had been sterilized, to distinguish

---

* See Appendix 1 of this chapter for a brief description. Readers interested in more detailed descriptions of the methodology, data collection, and analysis should refer to the study in our research volume entitled *The Prevalence of Infertility in Canada* accompanying this report: C.S. Dulberg and T. Stephens, "The Prevalence of Infertility in Canada, 1991-1992: Analysis of Three National Surveys."

them from the group that would be considered infertile. The third question (in combination with the second) identified all those couples who had *not* used contraception and were *not* pregnant during the previous year/two years. This established the number of couples to be included in the numerator, that is, the number of infertile couples. The numerator therefore consists of all couples cohabiting for at least one year (two years) who had not been using contraception for that period and who had not become pregnant.

Table 9.1. Classification of Couples Who Had Been Cohabiting for At Least One Year

	Number	Percentage
Contraceptive users	546	38.7
Contraceptively sterile (tubal ligation and/or vasectomy)	592	41.9
Non-contraceptively sterile (e.g., hysterectomy)	45	3.2
Pregnant women	75	5.3
Non-contraceptive users:		
• Fertile (miscarried, had abortion, delivered a child in past year)	34	2.4
• Infertile	120	8.5
Total	1 412	100.0

Source: Calculated using data from Dulberg, C.S., and T. Stephens, "The Prevalence of Infertility in Canada, 1991-1992: Analysis of Three National Surveys," in Research Volumes of the Royal Commission on New Reproductive Technologies, 1993.

Results

The combined results of these three surveys showed that the vast majority (80.6 percent) of couples who had been cohabiting for at least one year either were using contraception or were voluntarily sterile (the female partner had undergone a tubal ligation and/or the male partner had had a vasectomy). In approximately 3 percent of couples, one or both partners were sterile for other reasons; this group included, for example, women who had undergone hysterectomies. These findings highlight the fact that, at any given time, only a small percentage of couples is trying to become pregnant.

Prevalence of Infertility Among Canadian Couples

The combined results of the Commission's three surveys indicated that 8.5 percent of couples in Canada who had been cohabiting for *at least one year* did not become pregnant after one year of not using contraception. This represents approximately 300 000 couples.

About 7 percent of couples who had been cohabiting for *at least two years* were not pregnant after two years of not using contraception. This represents approximately 250 000 couples.

Approximately 5 percent of couples who had been cohabiting for at least one year were pregnant at the time they were surveyed. The remaining 11 percent of couples had been cohabiting for at least a year and had not used contraception during the past year (see Table 9.1). Some of these couples had conceived but were not classified as pregnant because they fell into one of the following groups: (1) they had had a miscarriage; (2) they had delivered a child; or (3) they had had an abortion during the past year. Couples in these categories were considered to be fertile, while the remaining couples were classified as infertile.

We were encouraged to find that the three surveys produced very similar results, suggesting that the one- and two-year estimates of infertility generated by the combined results of these studies are reliable (Table 9.2).

Table 9.2. Prevalence of Infertility Among Canadian Couples: Results of Primary Surveys

Survey	One year of cohabitation (%)	Two years of cohabitation (%)
Canada Health Monitor #6	7.7	6.0
Canada Health Monitor #7	8.6	7.2
Decima Research survey	8.7	7.3
Combined results	8.5	7.0

In our view the two-year estimate of the prevalence of infertility (7 percent) should be adopted because it is a more accurate assessment of the percentage of couples who have difficulty having a pregnancy. The difference between the two estimates suggests that approximately one couple in five that has not had a pregnancy after one year will go on to become pregnant in the second year.[2] In effect, this means that some couples who are considered infertile according to the one-year definition will simply take longer than a year to conceive.

Based on the two-year estimate of the prevalence of infertility (7 percent), approximately half a million Canadians (250 000 couples) in their reproductive years are currently affected by infertility.* This is not to say that all of these individuals are necessarily infertile; rather, they have difficulty having children with their current partner. The source of the infertility cannot be determined, nor can appropriate policy or programs be developed, solely on the basis of this estimate.

Another way of looking at the data is to consider that if 7 percent of couples have been infertile for two years, 1 couple in 14 has difficulty having children. Given that their chances of conceiving are significantly lower after two years, these couples may seek some form of medical treatment.

Comparison of Canadian and U.S. Infertility Estimates

The results of our three surveys were highly similar to U.S. results when we recalculated our figures using the current approach of the American National Survey of Family Growth.[3] Using this method, the one-year figure was 8 percent in Canada in 1991-92, compared with 7.9 percent in the United States in 1988.

One-Year Estimate of the Prevalence of Infertility — Canadian and U.S. Results Compared

Canada, 1991-92: 8 percent of currently married/cohabiting couples aged 18 to 44.

United States, 1988: 7.9 percent of currently married couples only, aged 15 to 44.

The figure commonly reported in the media — that one couple in six is infertile — is based on a calculation method that was used in the 1982 American National Survey of Family Growth but is no longer used. That method excluded from the denominator all couples in which one or both members had been surgically sterilized. As can be seen in the following box, this is a very substantial proportion; although the same *number* of couples is defined as infertile, they form a larger *percentage* of the whole population of interest.

When we re-analyzed our data using this approach — not counting people who have been surgically sterilized — we found that the prevalence of infertility was 15.4 percent among couples who had been cohabiting for one year and 13.2 percent among couples cohabiting for two years (see

---

* See Appendix 2 of this chapter.

box). In other words, recalculating our results using the old U.S. methodology showed that our findings were again similar to the U.S. results.

We believe that this approach is inappropriate because it does not estimate the prevalence of infertility in the total population, but only in a segment of the population (that is, those who have not been sterilized). Moreover, figures generated by this approach are too often misinterpreted; they are used to support the claim that 15 percent of *all* couples are infertile, while the percentage in fact applies only to couples who have not been sterilized. This is why the U.S. National Survey of Family Growth is no longer using this method.

Estimating Infertility With and Without the Surgically Sterilized

Surgically sterilized included   1 year   2 years

all couples married or cohabiting one year/two years,
not using contraception, and have not had a pregnancy
————————————————————————————————————   =   8.5%   7.0%
all couples married or cohabiting for one year/two years

Surgically sterilized excluded   1 year   2 years

all couples married or cohabiting one year/two years,
not using contraception, and have not had a pregnancy
————————————————————————————————————   =   15.4%   13.2%
all couples married or cohabiting for one year/two years
minus those couples where one or both members have
been surgically sterilized

Prevalence of Infertility by Region, Age Group, and Childbearing Status

We also analyzed the data from our three surveys to see whether they showed any differences in the prevalence of infertility between regions, age groups, or women with different childbearing histories. The data showed no difference in the prevalence of infertility from one part of the country to another. The reliability of this finding is limited, however, by the small sample sizes in each region. The data also showed no statistically significant differences in rates of infertility between couples with younger and older female partners. The reliability of this finding is again limited, because of small sample sizes and because of the greater frequency of contraceptive use and sterilization among older women. This makes it difficult for population-based surveys such as ours to assess the relationship between age and infertility (older women who are infertile are harder to identify because fewer are trying to conceive). The relationship between age and infertility has been well documented in the scientific literature, however, and is discussed in Chapter 12.

We did find a statistically significant relationship between age and infertility among childless women, with those who were older (ages 30 to 44) almost twice as likely to be infertile as those who were younger (ages 18 to 29). These findings reflect the fact that the older age group is more likely to have "collected" women who are infertile over time — those who have been trying unsuccessfully for several years to conceive. They likely also reflect the fact that women who have delayed childbearing until they reached this age were not trying to conceive before they were 30.

Secondary Research

In addition to our national surveys, we also conducted a secondary analysis of three previous studies conducted in Canada: the Canadian Fertility Survey (1984), the General Social Survey (1990), and the Ontario Health Survey (1990).* The 1984 Canadian Fertility Survey was a large-scale national survey, designed to assess fertility and other reproductive behaviour, that also included a limited number of questions regarding infertility. The Commission conducted a secondary analysis of its findings on contraceptive use and length of couple relationships to try to estimate the prevalence of infertility. By calculating how long couples had not been using contraception, how long they had been in the relationship, and/or how long it had been since their last pregnancy, we were able to develop some projected estimates of the proportion of couples who are infertile.

We further analyzed the 1990 Ontario Health Survey to identify cohabiting women who had not used contraception in the year prior to the survey. The survey included questions about pregnancies over the five years prior to the survey, making it impossible to identify conclusively the number of pregnancies that had occurred in the year prior to the survey. In addition, the way the questions were phrased may have encouraged a non-response from people not using contraception, resulting in an underestimation of infertility.

The 1990 General Social Survey was a large-scale national survey devoted exclusively to assessing fertility and reproductive behaviour. It

---

* The following presents only the key findings of the Commission's analysis of these studies. Readers interested in more detailed descriptions of their methodology, data collection, and analysis should refer to the studies in the research volume entitled *The Prevalence of Infertility in Canada* accompanying this report: T.R. Balakrishnan and R. Fernando, "Infertility Among Canadians: An Analysis of Data from the Canadian Fertility Survey (1984) and General Social Survey (1990)"; T.R. Balakrishnan and P. Maxim, "Infertility, Sterilization, and Contraceptive Use in Ontario."

attempted to estimate infertility by asking all respondents whether they or their partner had ever been told that they could not have any, or any more, children. We consider such a question to be inadequate for estimating infertility reliably, as it depends on a medical diagnosis, which not all couples will seek.

Projected estimates of the prevalence of infertility from these three sources were somewhat lower than estimates generated by our primary studies. However, they contain complications that call into question the reliability and validity of infertility estimates derived from them. Thus, although secondary analysis of data from these surveys provided some information, our findings underscore the fact that estimating infertility is too complex a task to be undertaken using methods not designed specifically for the purpose.

Trends in Infertility

U.S. studies show no increase in infertility rates over time. We do not have sufficient data to state whether this is the case in Canada, but the Commission has now established a baseline that will enable future studies to track changes in infertility over time.

The perception that infertility is becoming more common may have arisen in part because of the increased use of effective contraception. The relative success of modern methods of contraception may have contributed to the notion that fertility is completely within our control. As a result, couples who have used contraception for years may be quicker to define themselves as infertile when they decide to have a child but do not conceive as soon as they discontinue contraception. This perception is no doubt heightened by widespread use of a one-year definition of infertility. When this is added to increasing publicity about and availability of technological means to assist conception, the perception of an "infertility epidemic" is understandable.

We know that this perception is incorrect in the United States, where infertility has been tracked through the National Surveys of Family Growth in 1973, 1976, 1982, and 1988: the number of infertile couples there as a percentage of the population of reproductive age has not been increasing.[4] The population of reproductive age has increased because large numbers of baby boomers are now in their childbearing years; the absolute number of infertile couples has therefore increased as well. It is anticipated that the number of infertile couples in the United States will decline in the coming years as the baby boomer population moves out of the reproductive years.

Because Canada's current infertility rate parallels that of the United States so closely, it is not unreasonable to expect that trends in Canada will be closely related to trends in the United States. It would be a mistake to conclude, however, that Canada can continue to rely on U.S. statistics in this area. For example, as we explain later in this chapter, the incidence of sexually transmitted diseases such as chlamydia observed in Canada among younger women may have negative implications for the fertility of this generation in the future unless treatment and prevention programs are put in place to address the problem. The existence of a publicly supported medical care system in Canada, with easier access to treatment of sexually transmitted diseases, is another factor that may affect the prevalence of infertility — a factor that is not at work in the United States.

Nevertheless, if more individuals are exposed to risk factors associated with infertility, the number of infertile couples may rise in the future. For example, scientists in Denmark recently reviewed 61 studies, published around the world between 1938 and 1991, measuring the semen quality of men who did not have a history of infertility. Their analysis revealed that there has been a 50 percent decline in average sperm counts worldwide over this period, and a threefold increase in the percentage of men who had sperm concentrations in the lowest range.[5] Since male fertility has been shown to be correlated, to some extent, with sperm density, the study suggests that the population of subfertile men has increased. Although changes in the methods used to determine sperm concentrations may have influenced the study results, these methodological changes alone would not explain the large discrepancy in sperm counts between early and later years. The fact that semen quality declined so significantly over a relatively short period of time, as well as the fact that the incidence of testicular cancer increased substantially over the same period, have caused researchers to question whether environmental factors may be affecting male reproductive function.

It is not known, however, what effect the documented decline in sperm counts may have had on infertility trends worldwide. Nor do we know whether sperm counts in Canadian men have declined over the past 50 years or, if they have, what impact this has had on the prevalence of infertility in our country. These findings do, however, point to the importance of understanding the risk factors associated with infertility and the extent of individual exposure to them. They also demonstrate the need for regular data collection on the prevalence of infertility.

Through our own original research and secondary analysis, we have provided a solid base for tracking infertility in Canada from now on. Because estimating infertility is such a complex matter, and because of the pitfalls associated with using surveys and sources not designed for that purpose, any survey that attempts to examine fertility and reproductive behaviour should involve careful design of the necessary questions and the methodology to measure infertility. It is also important that sample sizes be sufficiently large to allow for the data to be analyzed for differences between regions and age groups. Tracking changes in the rates of infertility among specific age groups or risk groups would provide valuable information about the possible impact of such factors as sexually transmitted diseases and biological aging. The Commission recommends that

> **2.** **Health Canada conduct surveys of reproductive behaviour every five years, and that these surveys include a measurement of the prevalence of infertility, using a standardized definition, so that infertility can be tracked over time.**

Implications of Prevalence Findings

It is clear that infertility affects the lives of many people in Canada. The human costs implicit in our finding that about 250 000 couples in Canada are experiencing infertility, in that they have failed to become pregnant after two years of unprotected intercourse, contain an important message for policy makers. Given what Canadians told us about the importance of children in their lives, we must take this message seriously. Our findings underscore the importance of allocating resources to reduce the prevalence of infertility and to help people to have the children they want.

Determining whether infertility can be prevented and, if so, how to prevent it requires a thorough understanding of the factors that place individuals at risk of becoming infertile. This information has important implications for the development and targeting of prevention programs. These issues are the subject of the next six chapters.

Appendix 1: The Prevalence of Infertility in Canada — Surveys Conducted for the Commission

Canada Health Monitor #6 (*Price Waterhouse*)

The Canada Health Monitor is an ongoing, semi-annual telephone survey of the Canadian population used to analyze health-related concerns. A total of 2 723 individuals participated in the Canada Health Monitor survey. Demographic information obtained in the survey was used to identify those women who were aged 18 to 44, married or cohabiting for at least one year. Of 2 723 individuals, 281 fit this description and were willing to be interviewed. Calls were made during the period December 9-14, 1991.

Canada Health Monitor #7 (*Price Waterhouse*)

Infertility-related questions were included in the seventh Canada Health Monitor survey in order to reach a second, independent sample. A total of 2 725 respondents were interviewed from December 1991 through February 1992, resulting in a subsample of 407 women who met the criteria for age and marital status.

Infertility Among Canadians (*Decima Research*)

Relevant data were collected from a third national survey, undertaken for the Commission by Decima Research. Selection of women from a pool of over 5 000 Decima respondents was completed with quotas to achieve a sample proportional to the Canadian population with respect to region and city size. A subsample of 725 women met the criteria for age and marital status. Interviews were conducted from March 1 to March 14, 1992.

Source: The data from Canada Health Monitor and Decima surveys were analyzed by C.S. Dulberg and T. Stephens as described in the research volume entitled *The Prevalence of Infertility in Canada*.

Appendix 2: One-Year and Two-Year Calculations of the Infertility Rate

The number of couples who have been married/cohabiting for *at least one year* who can be considered to be infertile can be calculated as follows:

- The study showed that 8.5 percent of couples married/cohabiting for at least one year did not use contraception and failed to become pregnant.

- In this study, 5 percent of couples in the sample were dropped from the analysis because they were married/cohabiting for less than one year. The actual size of the Canadian population of couples married/cohabiting for at least one year is not directly accessible. Therefore, the size of this population of interest in Canada was estimated, based on the following:

  (a) 1991 Canadian Census Data — 3 781 309 currently married/cohabiting couples (in which female partner is between the ages of 18 and 44).

  (b) Based on sample results, we can estimate that the number of couples married/cohabiting for at least one year is 5 percent smaller than the number of currently married/cohabiting couples.

(c)   Estimate: there are approximately 3 592 244 Canadian couples, in which the female partner is between 18 and 44, who have been married/cohabiting for at least one year.

• The 95 percent confidence interval for the one-year estimate of infertility (8.5 percent) is 7.0 percent to 9.9 percent. This means that there is a 95 percent chance that duplicating the research would generate a one-year estimate of the prevalence of infertility within this range. Therefore, it is estimated that between approximately 250 000 and 360 000* couples, married/cohabiting for at least one year, failed to become pregnant after one year of unprotected intercourse.

The number of couples who have been married/cohabiting for *at least two years* who can be considered to be infertile can be calculated as follows:

• Seven percent of couples married/cohabiting for at least two years did not use contraception and failed to become pregnant.

• In addition to the 5 percent of couples who had not cohabited for the past year, an additional 4.3 percent of couples in the sample were dropped from the analysis (9.3 percent in total) because they were married/cohabiting for less than two years. Again, the actual size of the Canadian population of couples married/cohabiting for at least two years is not directly accessible.   Therefore, the size of this population of interest in Canada was estimated, based on the following:

(a)   1991 Canadian Census Data — 3 781 309 currently married/ cohabiting couples (in which female partner is between the ages of 18 and 44).

(b)   Based on sample results, we can estimate that the number of couples married/cohabiting for at least two years is 9.3 percent smaller than the number of currently married/cohabiting couples.

(c)   Estimate: there are approximately 3 429 647 Canadian couples, in which the female partner is between 18 and 44, who have been married/cohabiting for at least two years.

• The 95 percent confidence interval for the two-year estimate of infertility (7.5 percent) is 5.6 percent to 8.4 percent. This means that there is a 95 percent chance that duplicating the research would generate a two-year estimate of the prevalence of infertility within this

---

* The exact figures were 251 457 and 355 637 respectively.

range. Therefore, it is estimated that between approximately 190 000 and 290 000* couples, married/cohabiting for at least two years, failed to become pregnant after two years of unprotected intercourse.

General Sources

Angus Reid Group Inc. "Reproductive Technologies — Qualitative Research: Summary of Observations." In Research Volumes of the Royal Commission on New Reproductive Technologies, 1993.

Balakrishnan, T.R., and R. Fernando. "Infertility Among Canadians: An Analysis of Data from the Canadian Fertility Survey (1984) and General Social Survey (1990)." In Research Volumes of the Royal Commission on New Reproductive Technologies, 1993.

Balakrishnan, T.R., and P. Maxim. "Infertility, Sterilization, and Contraceptive Use in Ontario." In Research Volumes of the Royal Commission on New Reproductive Technologies, 1993.

Dulberg, C.S., and T. Stephens. "The Prevalence of Infertility in Canada, 1991-1992: Analysis of Three National Surveys." In Research Volumes of the Royal Commission on New Reproductive Technologies, 1993.

Hull, M.G.R., et al. "Expectations of Assisted Conception for Infertility." *British Medical Journal* 304 (June 6, 1992): 1465-69.

Léridon, H., and A. Spira. "Problems in Measuring the Effectiveness of Infertility Therapy." *Fertility and Sterility* 41 (4)(April 1984): 580-86.

Specific References

1. Hull, M.G.R. "Infertility Treatment: Relative Effectiveness of Conventional and Assisted Conception Methods." *Human Reproduction* 7 (6)(1992): 785-96.

2. Calculated by dividing the difference between 8.5 and 7.0 (which is 1.5) by 8.5. This generates a figure of approximately 18 percent, or one in five.

3. It should be noted that the sample group used in the American survey was slightly different from the sample group in our surveys. The National Survey of Family Growth focussed on married couples only, whereas we included both married and cohabiting couples. As well, the National Survey of Family Growth sample included married couples in which the female partner was between the

---

* The exact figures were 192 060 and 288 090 respectively.

ages of 15 and 44, whereas our study focussed on cohabiting couples where the woman is aged 18 to 44.

4. Mosher, W.D., and W.F. Pratt. *Fecundity and Infertility in the United States, 1965-1988.* Advance Data from Vital and Health Statistics of the National Center for Health Statistics, No. 192 (Hyattsville: U.S. Department of Health and Human Services, 1990). Although the percentage of couples who are infertile appears to have decreased over the past two decades (from 11.2 percent in 1965 to 8.5 percent in 1982), this drop is entirely due to the rise in surgical sterilization. Excluding the surgically sterile, the percentage of couples who are infertile has changed only slightly, from 13.3 to 13.9 percent (United States Congress. Office of Technology Assessment. *Infertility: Medical and Social Choices.* Washington: U.S. Government Printing Office, 1988, p. 51).

5. Carlsen, E., et al. "Evidence for Decreasing Quality of Semen During Past 50 Years." *British Medical Journal* 305 (September 12, 1992): 609-13.

Sexually Transmitted Diseases and Infertility

◆

The future fertility of a proportion of today's generation of young women is at risk from chlamydia and gonorrhoea; many will be unaware of the silent effects of these sexually transmitted diseases until they want to have children and find they cannot. Preventing sexually transmitted diseases must become a greater priority if we are to reduce the future prevalence of infertility in Canada. Strong action and focussed leadership are required to ensure that this happens.

Sexually transmitted diseases are diseases that are transmitted primarily by sexual contact, including oral, genital, and anal contact, although they can also be transmitted by a woman to her child during a vaginal birth. They have long been identified as a national public health problem. Representatives of many groups voiced their concerns to the Commission about the prevalence of STDs, given the clear link between sexually transmitted diseases and infertility. The Commission examined the evidence on the relationship between sexually transmitted diseases and infertility and concluded that STDs are the single most important preventable cause of infertility among women. An estimated 20 percent of all infertility among couples can be traced to damage to the female partner's fallopian tubes that has resulted from pelvic inflammatory disease (PID) caused by a sexually transmitted infection. Moreover, this figure pertains only to difficulties with conception; still more women encounter difficulties with pregnancy and birth — including an increased risk of ectopic pregnancy, spontaneous abortion and stillbirth, premature delivery, and acute or chronic infections in infants born to infected mothers — because of the adverse effects of sexually transmitted diseases.

Significant numbers of Canadians are affected by STDs — one estimate is that perhaps as many as one Canadian in five contracts a sexually transmitted disease during the reproductive years. Young women between the ages of 15 and 19 are particularly at risk; they have the highest incidence of both gonorrhoea and chlamydia — the diseases identified as having the greatest impact on female fertility — of any group in Canada.[1] We discuss the prevalence of gonorrhoea and chlamydia in greater detail later in this section, but the Commission believes it is important to draw these facts to public attention. Many young women are engaging in unsafe practices, unaware that they may be harming their future fertility. Effective programs to encourage young people to prevent sexually transmitted diseases, by delaying sexual activity, reducing the number of partners, and using barrier methods of contraception, are vital to reducing the overall prevalence of infertility in Canada.

> [Of] major concern is the higher than average rate of sexually transmitted diseases found in the aboriginal population. In the Yukon documented statistical data demonstrates that gonorrhea is prevalent [at] five times the rate of the other population of this territory. Other STDs, notably the aforementioned and *Chlamydia trachomatis*, which can cause or add to the problem of infertility, are of serious concern in this country.
>
> *M. Dion Stout, Indian and Inuit Nurses of Canada, Public Hearings Transcripts, Ottawa, Ontario, September 20, 1990.*

The impact of chlamydia is particularly insidious, because women who contract this infection may lack noticeable symptoms and therefore may not seek medical treatment. Left untreated, or treated incorrectly, these chlamydial infections can progress to pelvic inflammatory disease, which can cause permanent scarring and damage to the fallopian tubes, rendering the woman infertile (if both tubes are completely blocked) or subfertile (if the blockage in one or both tubes is only partial). Some women are unaware that they have contracted chlamydia until tubal damage is diagnosed when they want to have a child and seek medical help for impaired fertility. Because it is a "silent" infection, identifying and treating chlamydia early would require a systematic screening program. This is among the range of options we examine in this section as we consider how to develop a coordinated strategy for preventing infertility linked to sexually transmitted diseases.

The Focus of Our Investigations

The viral or bacterial microbes that cause sexually transmitted diseases affect not only the male and female reproductive tracts but other organs as well. Just under a dozen of the infections that are sexually transmitted can have long-term effects on the reproductive health of women and, to a lesser extent, men (see research volume, *Understanding Infertility:*

Risk Factors Affecting Fertility). We focussed our investigations on chlamydia and gonorrhoea (both of which are caused by bacterial organisms) because of the evidence linking them to infertility in women. Infertility in the context of these diseases is defined as difficulty achieving conception; these diseases had greatest relevance to our mandate, because new reproductive technologies involving assisted conception techniques can be used to overcome their long-term consequences.

We placed secondary emphasis on investigating other STDs, such as human immunodeficiency virus (HIV) infection, syphilis, and mycoplasma infection, which may reduce a woman's ability to give birth to a healthy child but do not appear to have an effect on women or men in terms of the ability to conceive. Assisted conception techniques therefore have less relevance to these diseases, although they have very serious health effects.

> Sexually transmitted infections are endemic in Canada in 1992; however, many are not reported and their consequences not well documented. Perhaps as many as one in five Canadians become infected with one of these pathogens during their sexually active years. More than 30 pathogens are known to be transmitted sexually, about 10 of which are particularly important because they have significant long-term effects on the reproductive health of women and, to a lesser extent, men. Their impacts on reproductive health include acute and chronic pelvic inflammatory disease; difficulties with conception due to tubal factor infertility; pregnancy wastage due to ectopic pregnancy, spontaneous abortion, and stillbirth; premature delivery; and acute or chronic infections in infants born to infected mothers. In addition, sexually transmitted infections can interfere with sexual health due to psychological or physical factors that adversely alter sensory or emotional experiences.
>
> *A. Ronald and R. Peeling, "Sexually Transmitted Infections: Their Manifestations and Links to Infertility and Reproductive Illness," in Research Volumes of the Commission, 1993.*

The Incidence of Sexually Transmitted Diseases

Information about the incidence of sexually transmitted diseases in the population as a whole is limited. Existing data come mainly from reported cases collected by provincial governments and the Laboratory Centre for Disease Control at Health Canada; these data are considered to underestimate rates of STD infection, however, because not all cases are detected or reported. In addition, studies measuring the incidence of sexually transmitted diseases in certain sectors of the population provide an indication of the prevalence of STDs in higher-risk groups. One such study was the Canada Youth and AIDS Study, which found that 5.5 percent of university and college students had had at least one sexually transmitted disease. The proportion was larger among those who had had numerous partners: infection rates in males and females who had had one partner were 1 percent and 3 percent respectively; by contrast, those with ten or more partners had rates of 11 percent and 24 percent respectively. Certain subgroups within the younger population are also at higher risk. The study found that 9 percent of youth who have dropped out of school have had a sexually transmitted disease. Street youth are at even higher risk: 22 percent reported having had a sexually transmitted disease. Those who have engaged in prostitution and others with numerous sexual partners had substantially higher rates (see Table 10.1).

Table 10.1. History of Previous Sexually Transmitted Disease

	Overall (%)	Males (%)	Females (%)
College/university	5.5		
One partner		1	3
Ten or more partners		11	24
Dropouts	9		
Street youth	22	16	30
Prostitutes	58	45	68
More than 100 partners		— *	70

* Information not available.

Note: n = 38 000

Source: King, A.J.C., et al. *Canada Youth & AIDS Study*. Kingston: Queen's University, 1989; and Radford, J.L., A.J.C. King, and W.K. Warren. *Street Youth & AIDS*. Kingston: Queen's University, 1989.

Gonorrhoeal Infections

Sexually transmitted diseases have been associated historically with population disruptions resulting from war, famine, and other factors that cause substantial population migration. As shown in Figure 10.1, an examination of the annual incidence of gonorrhoeal infections between 1940 and 1991 shows two periods of dramatic increase. The first was in the late 1940s, following the Second World War. The second period was during the 1970s when Canada, like other industrialized countries, experienced widespread changes in contraceptive practices and sexual behaviour. A large part of this second documented major increase also

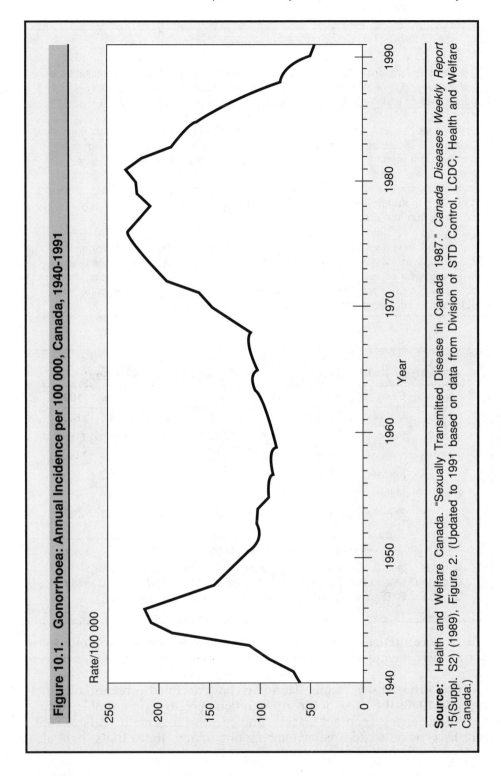

Figure 10.1.   Gonorrhoea: Annual Incidence per 100 000, Canada, 1940-1991

Source: Health and Welfare Canada. "Sexually Transmitted Disease in Canada 1987." *Canada Diseases Weekly Report* 15(Suppl. S2) (1989), Figure 2. (Updated to 1991 based on data from Division of STD Control, LCDC, Health and Welfare Canada.)

Gonorrhoea

The *Neisseria gonorrhoeae* bacterium can survive for only a short time outside the human body. This means that intimate physical contact with the mucous membranes of an infected individual is necessary to become infected.

Gonorrhoea has an incubation period (the time before symptoms may become apparent) of two to seven days. In women, the most common symptoms of the disease are a burning sensation during urination, increased vaginal discharge, and/or redness or swelling around the vulva. For most women (70 to 80 percent), however, symptoms may be so mild as to go unnoticed. Symptoms of gonorrhoea in men are more apparent; all but 10 percent have visible symptoms, usually a discharge from the urethra.

If untreated, the period of communicability for gonorrhoea may extend for months. This is of particular concern, as asymptomatic individuals may transmit the disease unknowingly for an extended period before the appearance of symptoms or another medical problem causes them to seek treatment. Drug therapy is highly effective and ends an infected person's communicability within hours.

Table 10.2. Rates of Gonorrhoea in Canada by Age and Sex*

Age	Sex	1980	1985	1988	1989	1990	1991
15-19	Male	331.4	277.5	166.4	156.2	119.5	60.1
	Female	539.4	566.0	357.5	337.6	239.1	118.9
20-24	Male	969.8	704.2	345.2	324.1	233.4	115.8
	Female	656.4	546.0	325.7	283.2	194.7	98.1
25-29	Male	711.3	436.3	207.7	196.8	150.5	75.9
	Female	309.6	227.3	132.4	121.0	77.1	38.1

* Rate per 100 000 population in that age group.

Source: *Canada Diseases Weekly Report* 15-50 (December 16, 1989); *Canada Diseases Weekly Report* 17-21 (May 25, 1991); and Health Canada. Division of STD Control/Laboratory Centre for Disease Control (LCDC).

reflects more intensive screening and detection of asymptomatic gonorrhoea (particularly among women) and more complete reporting of gonorrhoea cases.

Gonorrhoea rates among Canadians have declined substantially since the early 1980s, because of the introduction of control programs involving diagnostic services, contact tracing, and effective treatment. It is possible that less risky sexual behaviour among many individuals has also contributed to the decline. The downward trend shown in Figure 10.1 is very encouraging overall. Nevertheless, as may be expected, teenage girls and men in their early 20s continue to show the highest rates compared to other age groups (see Table 10.2). This finding may reflect more intensive screening as well as sexual activity in this group and the greater vulnerability of the female reproductive system.   The incidence of gonorrhoea among young women is of particular concern because of the implications for their future fertility.

Chlamydial Infections

Chlamydia is now the most prevalent STD in Canada. It is three to five times more prevalent than gonorrhoeal infections, depending on the population studied.[2] An estimated 100 000 cases of chlamydial infection occur in Canada each year.[3]   The available data are believed to underestimate the prevalence of this disease significantly for several reasons. Reporting requirements for chlamydia vary between provinces; most require that laboratories report all confirmed cases, but this is still not mandatory in some provinces. Even where mandatory reporting exists, testing procedures may not result in accurate results: many laboratories use tests that are not sensitive enough to detect all cases, while some newer tests may actually result in false positives. Moreover, chlamydial infections that are diagnosed clinically (without laboratory confirmation) often are not reported by physicians.

Younger people bear the major burden of chlamydial infections; two-thirds of identified cases are in individuals aged 15 to 24 years. Young women in this age group have the highest rates of chlamydial infections, at about 1.6 percent (see Table 10.3 for reported cases and rates).

Chlamydia

Chlamydial infections are caused by a bacterium called *Chlamydia trachomatis*, which can reproduce only inside cells of its host. The bacterium is an "energy" parasite in that it depends largely on the host cell for energy to fuel its metabolism and growth.

Treatment involves a 7- to 10-day course of antibiotic. If left untreated, chlamydia has been shown to persist for as long as four years.

Rates of chlamydia among sexually active youth are substantially higher than in the general population. A survey of studies published over the last 10 years in Canada shows that the prevalence of chlamydia has ranged from 5 to 7 percent in student health clinics; to 14 percent in family planning clinics; and to more than 25 percent of patients at STD clinics.[4] Most important to remember, however, is the fact that many individuals are asymptomatic and do not come for testing, so their cases are not reported;

50 to 60 percent of women and an estimated 7 percent of men with chlamydial infections are asymptomatic. Because of the reporting problems discussed above, it is not known whether rates are increasing or decreasing. Chlamydial infections became nationally notifiable in 1990; with these data it will be possible to analyze trends.

Table 10.3. Reported Cases and Rates of Chlamydial Infection by Age and Sex, Canada,* 1989-1990

Age	Male		Female		Total	
	Cases	Rate	Cases	Rate	Cases	Rate**
0-4	39	4.6	67	8.3	106	6.4
5-9	8	1.0	16	2.0	24	1.5
10-14	24	2.9	550	69.9	574	35.5
15-19	2 008	236.4	12 728	1 578.6	14 736	890.1
20-24	4 732	520.5	13 412	1 525.8	18 144	1 014.7
25-29	2 574	243.8	5 622	532.7	8 196	388.2
30-39	1 579	80.1	3 040	152.0	4 619	116.3
40-59	392	15.1	619	23.6	1 011	19.4
60+	27	1.7	48	2.3	75	2.1
Age not specified	326		1 107		1 433	
Sex and age not specified					1 466	
Total cases	11 709	102.3	37 209	315.6	50 384	216.8

*   Excludes British Columbia and the Northwest Territories.
**   Per 100 000.

Note: Since not all provinces/territories had 1990 data available, cases and rates were based on the most recent data available (1989 or 1990) for each province/territory, to provide an estimate of chlamydial infection for the period 1989-1990.

Source: Adapted from Health and Welfare Canada. "Chlamydial Infection in Canada." *Canada Diseases Weekly Report* 17-51 (December 21, 1991), Table 2.

Factors That Increase the Risk of Acquiring a STD

Being Female

Women are at higher risk than men of acquiring a sexually transmitted disease for several reasons, the main one being that the female reproductive tract seems to be more vulnerable to organisms transmitted during unprotected sexual intercourse. This is demonstrated by the difference in rates of transmission between the two sexes. A man with a gonorrhoeal infection will infect about half the female partners with whom he has unprotected intercourse, whereas an infected woman will infect about 25 percent of her male partners. Another factor relates to attitudes and inequalities that influence the degree of control women have over their choice of sexual partners and the use of barrier methods of contraception to protect against STDs.

Women's fertility is particularly vulnerable because they are more likely to harbour asymptomatic infections for prolonged periods, during which time internal damage can occur. Without treatment, women are likely to suffer serious long-term consequences such as pelvic inflammatory disease, chronic pelvic pain, ectopic pregnancy, and infertility related to blockage of the fallopian tubes. In contrast, men are less likely to suffer long-term consequences from most sexually transmitted diseases, and their fertility is unlikely to be affected.

Sexual Behaviour

Although sexually transmitted diseases can and do afflict sexually active individuals across all age and socioeconomic groups, research has shown that certain behaviours increase an individual's risk of acquiring a STD.   These include younger age at first sexual intercourse (which increases the number of years of sexual activity and the probability of exposure to a greater number of partners), multiple partners, or a relationship with a partner who has a history of multiple partners, and lack of appropriately protective contraception.   Barrier methods such as condoms and spermicides have been shown to prevent transmission of organisms, whereas oral contraceptives and intrauterine devices (IUDs), while effective in preventing pregnancy, do not protect against STDs. (Oral contraceptives have been shown to reduce the progress of a sexually transmitted disease into the upper reproductive tract, but they do not prevent women from acquiring the disease in the first place.)

These behavioural factors help to explain why STD rates are highest among young people. The Canada Youth and AIDS Study found that approximately one-quarter of grade 9 students (31 percent of boys/21 percent of girls) and half of all grade 11 students (49 percent of boys/46 percent of girls) have had sexual intercourse at least once. By the time they reach university or college age, three-quarters of Canadian students will have had sexual intercourse. These results are in line with Canada's Health Promotion Survey (1990), which found that nearly two-thirds (60 percent) of all those aged 15 to 19 have had sexual intercourse.[5] We note, however, that both surveys were based on self-reported data; actual rates of sexual activity may in fact be higher.

The reported level of sexual activity would not necessarily produce high rates of sexually transmitted diseases if young people had a good understanding of what constitutes safe sexual behaviour and if they accepted the necessity of and practised these behaviours. These include, first and foremost, using barrier forms of contraception, as well as delaying sexual intercourse until a later age and minimizing the number of partners. While media coverage and acquired immuno-deficiency syndrome (AIDS) education programs in schools have increased young people's awareness of the risk of HIV infection and, to some extent, other sexually transmitted diseases, there are data that suggest such knowledge is not translating into actual behaviour and safer sexual practices. The Canada Youth and AIDS Study found that only one-quarter of female college students who had had one partner use a condom consistently. Other studies have confirmed the low rate of condom use among those who are sexually active; the 1992 Santé Québec study reported that many individuals in the 15 to 29 age group were not using condoms, and the Ontario Health Survey reported that most of those with multiple partners do not use condoms, or they use them infrequently.

> Over the last three, four years, I have had the opportunity to go into many schools to talk about sexually transmitted diseases, to grade school students, junior high and senior high kids, and it is very sad to see how woefully misinformed they are. They just don't know what is going on. And accordingly, they are very much at risk for getting infected and for being candidates for these technologies later.
>
> *S. Genuis, private citizen, Public Hearings Transcripts, Edmonton, Alberta, September 13, 1990.*

What is particularly striking is that less than 10 percent of women with 10 or more partners use a condom. Women who are sexually active with more partners tend to rely exclusively on oral contraceptives, which are very effective in preventing pregnancy but provide no protection against contracting a sexually transmitted disease. In the absence of barrier contraceptives that are as effective as oral contraceptives in preventing pregnancy, it is not surprising that women choose the pill, given that they see pregnancy as the immediate risk and that they may have difficulty persuading a partner to use a condom. The challenge, then, is to convince young women that they need both forms of protection — one for pregnancy protection and a second for STD protection.

Marginalization from Health Care Services

Reduced access to health care services and health education is associated with other risk factors that place sexually active individuals at higher risk of acquiring a sexually transmitted disease — specifically being poor, adolescent, and among those referred to as street youth. STD rates are higher among street youth, among youth who have dropped out of school, and especially among young women engaged in prostitution. Higher STD rates in these groups reflect not only sexual behaviours, but also a decreased likelihood of using health care services, whether because of language or cultural barriers or because of other factors in the design or delivery of services that make them inconvenient, uncomfortable, or "unfriendly" to use. Thus, young people in these groups are less likely to be screened and treated and may unknowingly prolong the lifespan of the disease and transmit the infection to others.

> In spite of the serious, costly consequences of unintended pregnancy and the spread of STDs, many Canadians cannot obtain the most basic health services needed to prevent sexual and reproductive health problems. Access to quality services is especially restricted among individuals in rural and isolated areas, adolescents, single adult women, members of cultural and linguistic minority groups, physically handicapped individuals, and others with distinct health and socioeconomic needs.
>
> *N. Barwin and W. Fisher, "Contraception: An Evaluation of Its Role in Relation to Infertility — Can It Protect?" in Research Volumes of the Commission, 1993.*

Sexually Transmitted Diseases and Infertility in Women

Understanding the link between sexually transmitted diseases and infertility in women requires an appreciation of a sequence of events. Gonorrhoea and chlamydia can lead to pelvic inflammatory disease, which in turn can lead to damaged or blocked fallopian tubes, making pregnancy difficult or impossible to achieve. As well, several STDs are associated with reduced chances of carrying a pregnancy to term and giving birth to a healthy child.

STDs and Pelvic Inflammatory Disease

Pelvic inflammatory disease is an infection of the upper reproductive tract in women that occurs when organisms ascend via the cervix into the uterus and fallopian tubes. This may happen if a sexually transmitted disease is left untreated, if treatment is delayed, or if an infection is treated incorrectly. PID also can result from other infections — for example, those that can occur after childbirth or surgery. It is estimated that between one-third and one-half of women who become infected with a STD (mostly gonorrhoea and chlamydia) will develop pelvic inflammatory disease and, further, that this group of women accounts for about 80 percent of all cases of pelvic inflammatory disease.[6]

Infections of the cervix, the lining of the uterus, fallopian tubes, and ovaries are included in the overall category of pelvic inflammatory disease. In the most severe cases, infection can spread into the pelvic tissues, where it may infect neighbouring organs, including the bladder, intestines, and liver. Even without treatment, however, most women with PID become symptom-free after an acute illness of 5 to 10 days. Pelvic inflammatory disease resulting from chlamydial infections causes more tubal damage than gonorrhoea because it often causes no symptoms and is therefore less likely to be treated.

In women who develop infection of the fallopian tubes, the disease initially causes acute inflammation; in the long term, it may result in permanent scarring of the fallopian tubes and other areas of the reproductive tract. In cases where scarring damage is severe, both tubes can be blocked completely (this condition is called bilateral tubal obstruction or occlusion), making natural conception impossible. Even if the fallopian tubes are left partially open, with some potential ability to function, the resulting scarring may impair their ability to transport a fertilized egg toward the uterus (see Chapter 20).

Having more than one STD at the same time increases the risk of developing pelvic inflammatory disease. In 30 to 50 percent of women with gonorrhoea, a chlamydial infection has also been detected (see research volume, *Prevention of Infertility*). When acting together, chlamydia and gonorrhoea organisms cause more damage to a woman's reproductive tract than either on its own; when both infections are present, they seem to invade the reproductive tract more rapidly, with more acute and lasting damage to the fallopian tubes. Together they also appear to break down the defences of the reproductive system to allow entry of other organisms that are naturally present in the vagina, and these organisms may cause further damage to the reproductive tract.

Women with symptomatic pelvic inflammatory disease account for less than half the total number of cases, because a woman is often unaware that she has had the disease until she has difficulty conceiving and seeks medical treatment. In one study, over 70 percent of women with blocked fallopian tubes reported no history of a previous episode of pelvic inflammatory disease, despite laboratory tests demonstrating that they have had a previous chlamydial infection.[7]

Determining the prevalence of pelvic inflammatory disease in Canada is difficult, because existing data are based on hospitalization records. These do not capture undetected cases, nor do they include cases treated without hospitalization. Records collected by Health Canada indicate that in 1988-89 the rate of hospitalization for pelvic inflammatory disease was 205 per 100 000 women[8] (see Table 10.4). As the table shows, pelvic inflammatory disease was on the increase until the early 1980s; since then it has fallen. Women aged 20 to 29 are affected most frequently. Because we know that pelvic inflammatory disease is linked to infertility, the rate of the disease among younger women has serious future implications for their fertility.

Table 10.4. Pelvic Inflammatory Disease, Age-Specific Rates,[1] by Age Group, Canada, Selected Years, 1972-1988/89*

| | Age group | | | | | | |
	15-19 years	20-24 years	25-29 years	30-34 years	35-39 years	40-44 years	Total
1972	202.9	328.8	323.8	295.9	242.8	153.8	259.8
1976	245.6	380.3	329.5	292.0	212.2	137.7	276.8
1980/81[2]	281.0	432.0	374.1	295.3	195.3	128.3	301.6
1983/84	275.7	404.7	381.5	279.1	188.5	116.2	289.6
1984/85	286.6	403.3	370.6	285.3	191.5	113.0	289.1
1987/88	255.4	343.3	337.3	263.2	171.9	111.5	254.1
1988/89	243.6	306.1	294.4	274.3	163.6	49.7	205.3

[1] Per 100 000 females.

[2] Since 1980-81, all hospital morbidity data have been reported by fiscal year.

* Figures based on hospital separations.

Source: Health and Welfare Canada. "Sexually Transmitted Disease in Canada 1987." *Canada Diseases Weekly Report* 15 (Suppl. 2)(1989), Table 15. Updated to 1988/89 based on data from Health Canada.

Pelvic Inflammatory Disease and Tubal Infertility

No data exist that would allow definitive evaluation of the relationship between PID and tubal infertility in Canada. We have attempted, however, to use data from the United States and Sweden, as well as Commission data on the prevalence of infertility in Canada, to infer the proportion of infertility that results from PID, almost all of which is caused by sexually transmitted diseases. Based on our calculations, we estimate that in roughly 20 percent of Canadian couples who are infertile, the woman has tubal infertility resulting from PID. (How we arrived at this figure is explained in the following box.)

Recent research shows that women who do not seek prompt treatment for PID (within two days of symptoms appearing) are at increased risk of infertility.   One study showed that women who waited for three days or longer before seeking treatment for pelvic inflammatory disease caused by gonorrhoea or chlamydia had twice (2.6 times) the risk of impaired fertility as women who received treatment in the first two days.[9]   Unfortunately, because many women have no apparent symptoms, particularly with chlamydia-induced PID, they do not seek treatment this quickly.

Estimating the Impact of Pelvic Inflammatory Disease on Tubal Infertility

Although not a rigorous or ideal approach, the following calculation helps to show what the approximate effect of STDs on infertility might be. The calculation is not precise and relies on several assumptions (for example, it does not factor in aspects such as multiple infections); however, it is the best approximation available.

The U.S. National Survey of Family Growth, conducted in 1988, showed that 11 percent of women of reproductive age had reported a previous episode of pelvic inflammatory disease. The 1980 Lund study conducted in Sweden found that 15.2 percent of women had tubal infertility after one PID episode. It has been suggested, therefore, that 1.7 percent (15.2 percent of 11) of all U.S. women of reproductive age were infertile because of an episode of pelvic inflammatory disease.

Commission research showed that 8.5 percent of couples who had been cohabiting for at least one year at the time of the study were infertile. If we assume that the proportion of women who have had PID in Canada is the same as in the United States (1.7 percent), then this condition is the cause of infertility in 20 percent of all couples who are infertile. Twenty percent is considered to underestimate the contribution of PID to infertility because it assumes that all of the American women who reported a previous episode of PID had only one episode. In fact, we know that the risk of tubal infertility is higher with subsequent episodes.

Women with severe episodes of pelvic inflammatory disease have tubal infertility at five times the rate of women who have had mild episodes. Among 900 women studied, the risk of infertility because of blocked fallopian tubes after one episode of pelvic inflammatory disease was found to be 6 percent for mild infections, 13 percent for moderate infections, and 30 percent for severe infections. These rates also seem to hold true for chlamydia-induced PID, despite antibiotic treatment.

Pelvic Inflammatory Disease and Ectopic Pregnancy

Ectopic pregnancy is a life-threatening condition that occurs when a fertilized egg implants and begins development outside the uterus — most often in a fallopian tube. In industrialized countries, about half of all ectopic pregnancies are attributed to previous pelvic inflammatory disease.[10] (Scarring of the fallopian tubes, which can prevent a fertilized egg from travelling normally to the uterus, increases ectopic pregnancy risk.) In fact, an ectopic pregnancy is 7 to 10 times more likely in women who have had PID than in women who have not. (The rate of ectopic pregnancy is about 1 in 16 for women who have had pelvic inflammatory disease, compared to 1 in 147 for all women.[11])

This increased risk of ectopic pregnancy is important for several reasons: it constitutes a failure of reproduction; it is potentially life-threatening to the woman; and having had an ectopic pregnancy places a woman at further increased risk of tubal infertility in the future (because of damage to the fallopian tube if it ruptures or if the fetus has to be removed surgically). Among women who have had an ectopic pregnancy, an estimated one-third will become infertile, one-third will have a subsequent normal pregnancy, and one-third will have a subsequent ectopic pregnancy or miscarriage.

Disturbingly, the rate of ectopic pregnancies in Canada approximately tripled — from 5.7 to 16 per 1 000 reported pregnancies — between 1971 and 1988. (Reported pregnancies include all pregnancies: live births, stillbirths, abortions, ectopic pregnancies.) These rates also are likely to indicate rates of tubal infertility.[12]

STDs and Adverse Pregnancy and Birth Outcomes

Some sexually transmitted organisms can cause complications during pregnancy that lead to spontaneous abortion, stillbirth, or premature delivery. Sexually transmitted diseases can also be passed from the woman to the fetus during pregnancy and birth. Among the relevant findings are the following:

- Chlamydial infection during pregnancy may be associated with second-trimester spontaneous abortion, stillbirth, neonatal death, prematurity, and low birth weight.

- Gonorrhoea can be transmitted to the fetus through the placenta or birth canal and can cause corneal damage, pharyngitis, meningitis, and arthritis. The routine use of silver nitrate at birth has reduced the risk of eye infection (which can lead to blindness), from 30 percent to 0.5 percent in children born to infected mothers.[13]

- Women infected with syphilis are more likely to have pregnancy complications (for example, spontaneous abortion) and may have pregnancies that result in the birth of an affected child. The risk of prematurity, perinatal death, and congenital syphilis in the newborn is related directly to the stage of the disease in the pregnant woman. Infected children may be born with mental disability, chronic meningitis, blindness, and/or deafness; therefore, pregnant women are always tested for this treatable disease.

- A strain of mycoplasma that may be sexually transmitted (*Mycoplasma hominis*) has been found to be associated with premature delivery. There is some suggestion that the disease may also be associated with spontaneous abortion, stillbirth, and low birth weight.

This brief overview is intended to highlight the range of sexually transmitted diseases that can affect pregnancy and birth outcomes adversely; the effects of many are still not clearly understood, and this list is by no means comprehensive. Readers can refer to the research paper entitled "Sexually Transmitted Infections: Their Manifestations and Links to Infertility and Reproductive Illness" by A.R. Ronald and R.W. Peeling, published in our research volume *Understanding Infertility: Risk Factors Affecting Fertility*, for a more complete review of the subject.

Sexually Transmitted Diseases and Male Fertility

The contribution of sexually transmitted diseases to overall levels of male infertility is thought to be quite small, but our knowledge of the causes of male infertility is limited at present.

Acute infections with chlamydia, gonorrhoea, and other organisms in the prostate gland or genital tract can reduce a man's fertility by temporarily lowering his sperm count. For example, chlamydia can cause epididymitis, an infection of the seminal tubes — the rough equivalent of pelvic inflammatory disease in women. Scarring from epididymitis can obstruct semen flow. However, because it is rare for obstruction of both tubes to occur, it is thought to be very rare for a sexually transmitted infection to be a cause of male sterility.

Preventing Sexually Transmitted Diseases*

Preventing sexually transmitted diseases must become a priority if we are to reduce the prevalence of infertility among Canadian couples in the future. The evidence is clear that chlamydia and gonorrhoea can lead to tubal infertility in women. The incidence of these diseases among young women means that the future fertility of a significant percentage of this generation is at stake. Unfortunately, many will be unaware of the effects of these diseases until they want to have children and find they are unable to do so.

> Preventing sexually transmitted diseases must become a priority if we are to reduce the prevalence of infertility among Canadian couples in the future ... Commissioners believe that a country-wide strategy is necessary to combat this public health problem.

---

* See Annex for dissenting opinion.

Commissioners believe that a country-wide strategy is necessary to combat this public health problem. It would build on existing programs to prevent STDs and involve their coordination at a national level. The plan should be broad-based and multifaceted, involving sexual health education professionals, physicians, public health professionals, and the public.

There is evidence of strong public support for national action on this issue. Canada's Health Promotion Survey 1990 found that 68 percent of men and women believe it is very important for the government to take action regarding sexually transmitted diseases. Reflecting their concern about STDs, 80 percent of young people aged 15 to 19 years believe strong government intervention is required.

Quite apart from the personal suffering involved, STDs are a substantial cost to the health care system. One study has estimated that the direct and indirect costs of pelvic inflammatory disease are more than $140 million annually.[14] This figure is in line with findings of a study conducted for the Commission that estimated the costs of chlamydial and gonorrhoeal infections to Canadian society to range from $71 million to $197 million. Thus, preventing STDs will create significant savings for society, even before the cost of infertility treatments for couples unable to conceive because of a STD is considered. Cutting back on STD prevention, then, or failing to provide funding for screening and

> The current approach in Canada focuses on treatment, not prevention. Primary preventive strategies must be developed to reduce unwanted teenage pregnancy and parenthood and the need for abortion, post-abuse psychological treatment, investigation of infertility and resorting to in vitro fertilization or other attempts to restore fertility. The major hurdles to be cleared in achieving this objective appear to be the attitudes of a minority of Canadian society, who do not wish to publicly discuss or teach sexual responsibility, and the failure to utilize the effective approaches to sexuality education already at our disposal.
>
> *Brief to the Commission from the Expert Interdisciplinary Advisory Committee on Sexually Transmitted Diseases in Children and Youth, Health and Welfare Canada, November 26, 1990.*

> The prevention of pelvic inflammatory disease will significantly reduce the incidence and costs of infertility and the need for expensive new reproductive technologies in Canada ... The need for prevention and its effectiveness in reducing human and health care costs are evident. We now need a commitment to make prevention a reality.
>
> *Brief to the Commission from the Canadian Pelvic Inflammatory Disease Society, April 29, 1992.*

treatment programs, could very well represent a false economy that will cost society more in the long run.

There are two aspects to preventing sexually transmitted diseases. First, we need to prevent people from being exposed to the diseases in the first place. This can be accomplished by ensuring that sexual health education programs exist that equip individuals with the knowledge and skills to enable them to protect their reproductive health. Physicians must also incorporate preventive counselling into their practices. Second, individuals exposed to the diseases require access to early diagnosis and treatment, to minimize the chances of consequent fertility impairment. This requires routine screening of high-risk individuals and effective contact tracing procedures.

Sexual Health Education

As the evidence shows, 60 percent of 15- to 19-year-olds are sexually active, and many are engaging in practices that jeopardize their reproductive health. What knowledge youth do have about safe sexual practices is simply not translating to safe behaviours.

It is clear that we need to re-evaluate the sexual health programs currently being offered to young people to make them effective not only in imparting knowledge, but also in changing behaviours. Several studies have shown that prevention programs that use a variety of vehicles to deliver their messages and that include accessible health services are effective in reducing pregnancy rates among adolescents. Since the skills and knowledge required to prevent pregnancy are also relevant to STD prevention, these studies suggest that sexual health education, when delivered in conjunction with a supportive community environment, could help to reduce the prevalence of STDs.

For example, the Baltimore Pregnancy Prevention Program for Urban Teenagers combined school and clinic counselling to junior and senior high school students. School components included classroom presentations, informal discussion groups, and individual counselling delivered by a team consisting of a social worker, a nurse, and an educator with training in sex education. A clinic located across the street from the high school provided group education, individual counselling, and reproductive health care services. During the program's existence, pregnancy rates declined by 30 percent in program schools but increased by 58 percent in comparison schools without the program. In addition, program recipients were more likely to delay the onset of sexual intercourse.[15]

Another program, conducted in South Carolina, involved the extensive use of a range of sources, including parents, teachers, church representatives, community leaders, and the media, to deliver messages about pregnancy prevention to adolescents. The rate of pregnancy among females aged 14 to 17 years declined over the course of the program, and the decrease was statistically significant when compared with three other comparable areas without the program.[16]

In Canada, a study conducted for Planned Parenthood showed that teenage pregnancy rates in Ontario declined most dramatically over the period 1976 to 1986 in areas where prevention programs were most accessible and among those young people who were most likely to receive the programs.[17]

These examples demonstrate that sexual health programs that include a variety of components, delivered in a comprehensive way, can have a positive impact on teenage pregnancy rates. We believe that messages about STD prevention should be included in such programs. Specifically, we need to encourage young people to delay the onset of sexual activity, or, if they decide to become sexually active, to minimize the number of sexual partners they have and to use dual forms of contraception to protect themselves against both STDs and pregnancy.

Schools can play a pivotal role in helping to ensure that adolescents receive adequate sexual health education, and we discuss this role later in this section. Schools should not be expected to shoulder all the responsibility, however, for providing sexual health education; parents, church representatives, health professionals, and other community members have important roles as well. In particular, parents who have trusting and supportive relationships with their children are in an ideal position to provide information on sexual health within a context of values and attitudes that emphasize the importance of committed, caring, and respectful relationships. Sexual health educators can recognize that parents are an important resource for positive sexual health education by ensuring they have access to a wide variety of opportunities for learning about sexuality and sexual health issues. The Commission therefore recommends that

> Schools can play a pivotal role in helping to ensure that adolescents receive adequate sexual health education ... Schools should not be expected to shoulder all the responsibility, however, for providing sexual health education; parents, church representatives, health professionals, and other community members have important roles as well.

3. **Agencies involved in adult education pursue effective methods to equip, support, and encourage parents to assume an active role in providing sexual health education to their children.**

Most schools currently offer some sexuality education; however, continuity, comprehensiveness, quality, and content of the instruction vary markedly between individual schools, school districts, and provinces. To address this problem, national guidelines for sexual health education have been developed in response to a recommendation by the Expert Interdisciplinary Advisory Committee on Sexually Transmitted Diseases in Youth and Children and the Federal/Provincial/Territorial Working Group on Adolescent Reproductive Health. The goal was to provide a clear statement of principles of sexual health education to guide and unify those working in this area.

The Guidelines for Sexual Health Education were extensively researched and prepared by a national working group whose membership included a cross section of professionals with expertise in various aspects of sexual health. They set minimum standards against which to assess existing sexuality education programs, develop new ones, and evaluate the overall network of programming and related services available to Canadians.

The Guidelines for Sexual Health Education suggest that sexual health education requires the integrated and collaborative effort of a range of sectors: family, education, medicine, public health, social services, and government. They set sexual health education within a broadly based, community-wide action plan that helps to focus the work of individuals and organizations from these different fields.

The guidelines recognize the diversity of values and perspectives relating to sexual health education and do not suggest that universal agreement is required on all aspects of the content, methodology, and philosophy of sexual health education. Instead, the document outlines common principles that should be used as guideposts in developing and assessing sexual health programs. These principles are accessibility; comprehensiveness; effectiveness and sensitivity of teaching methods and approaches; training and administrative support for educators; planning, evaluating, and updating program objectives; and development of a social environment conducive to sexual health.

The Guidelines for Sexual Health Education are currently being assessed by Health Canada; a release date has not yet been established. In our view, the guidelines are well written, comprehensive, and supported by existing (albeit limited) research. The Commission therefore recommends that

4.   **Sexual health education programs be based on the national Guidelines for Sexual Health Education.**

and that

> 5.   **The evaluation, revision, and distribution of**
>   **these guidelines occur at least once every five**
>   **years.**

These national guidelines should be based increasingly on research that measures the effects of different types of sexual health education programs on the knowledge, attitudes, and behaviours of program recipients. There is little or no Canadian outcome-based research on this subject at present; once designed and implemented, few sexual health education programs are evaluated. This makes it difficult to know which prevention programs are most effective. Accordingly, the Commission recommends that

> 6.   **Initial funding for sexual health education**
>   **programs include funding for an evaluation**
>   **component to assess if the stated objectives of**
>   **the program are being met and to guide**
>   **subsequent program development and**
>   **modification.**

Many schools provide only limited sexuality education in selected grades. Ideally, sexuality education should be offered at all grade levels to reinforce learning and build on the messages conveyed in previous grades in an age-appropriate manner. Individuals should acquire the necessary knowledge and life skills before they choose or feel pressured to become sexually active. The Commission therefore recommends that

> 7.   **Provincial/territorial ministries of education**
>   **mandate the provision of comprehensive sexual**
>   **health education sequentially from the beginning**
>   **of elementary school through to the end of high**
>   **school.**

A second problem with existing sexuality education programs is that many provide information without addressing underlying attitudes and behaviours or providing a supportive environment. Research shows clearly that programs focussing solely on knowledge acquisition fail to change risky sexual behaviour. Positive sexual health outcomes are more likely to occur when sexual health education effectively integrates knowledge, motivation, skills-building opportunities, and a supportive environment. Students must not only be given relevant information but also be motivated to change their behaviour and helped to develop the skills to do so successfully. Effective sexual health education depends on a life skills approach that strengthens self-esteem, personal insight, communication skills, assertiveness, and respect for others. These attitudes and skills, in combination with relevant knowledge, place individuals in a stronger position to avoid unsafe sexual behaviours. For example, increasing the self-esteem and assertiveness of young women would reinforce their ability to refuse to have sexual intercourse or to insist that partners use condoms, just as promoting respect for others would reduce peer pressure to become sexually active or to engage in risky sexual behaviours.

An example of a life skills-based program is the pregnancy prevention program offered by Student Health Services at the University of Western Ontario. The program has three elements: a pregnancy prevention videotape, a pregnancy prevention book, and dormitory-based talks. The program thus combines information with motivation and skills building. Evaluation of the program showed that pregnancy rates at the university dropped as each phase of the program was introduced, and lower pregnancy rates have been sustained throughout the years the program has been in place. The Commission therefore recommends that

> 8. **Effective approaches to sexual health education integrate four key components: acquisition of knowledge; development of motivation and insight; development of behaviour skills; and creation of a supportive environment.**

Consistent with the ethic of care, we believe that information about sexual health, pregnancy, and STD prevention should be presented in a context that emphasizes the value of respectful, supportive, and committed relationships. We acknowledge, moreover, that postponing sexual activity until a monogamous and long-term relationship has been established is still more effective than any other method of preventing STDs. We also recognize, however, that even if all sexual health education programs emphasize postponing sexual intercourse, many young people are still going to become sexually active in their middle or later teenage years. Their sexual health is just as important to a caring society as that of young people who choose abstinence or postponement.

Sexual health education programs must balance individual choices and the values and beliefs of the larger society. Programs that promote or give information on only a single approach to sexual health, such as abstinence, offer nothing to protect the sexual health of young people who do become sexually active. Programs should therefore reflect the reality that society is characterized by a range of sexual attitudes and behaviours. Notwithstanding concerns that introducing young people to a variety of options for maintaining sexual health encourages sexual activity or promiscuity, there is no evidence to support this belief. The evidence suggests the contrary, in fact; effective sexual health education can encourage young people to postpone sexual intercourse. Importantly, it also increases the likelihood that those who are sexually active use contraception. The Commission therefore recommends that

9.   **Sexual health education programs be designed and presented with the recognition that individuals engage in a range of sexual behaviours (including abstinence, delay, sexual activity in the context of a caring and respectful relationship) and that they need accurate information pertinent to all these choices.**

A third problem concerns the information being conveyed in sexuality education programs. Too often pregnancy prevention is taught separately from STD prevention; however, the most effective form of contraception to prevent pregnancy (oral contraceptives) does not protect against STDs. Sexuality education programs must emphasize that dual protection is needed — protection against STDs and against pregnancy, condoms in addition to oral contraceptives. Clearly this requires that schools teach prevention of pregnancy and STDs in an inter-related way. The Commission therefore recommends that

10.   **Sexual health education programs convey the message that young people who are sexually active need to protect themselves in two ways, that is, against both pregnancy and sexually transmitted diseases.**

Pharmaceutical companies can also play a role in helping to educate youth (especially young women), through their marketing efforts, about the need for protection against both pregnancy and STDs. This might include, for example, conveying appropriate messages in packages of oral contraceptives (for instance, that condoms should also be used) and providing literature to physicians for distribution to people who are sexually active.

The mass media play a major role in the sexual education of young Canadians; their portrayal of sexual behaviour, for example, is likely to have a strong influence on attitudes. Ideally, the media should convey messages that promote gender equality, encourage the postponement of sexual activity, and promote the need for dual protection for those who are sexually active. But often this is not the case. The Commission therefore recommends that

11.   **Sexual health education programs be designed to help individuals identify and evaluate the sexual messages conveyed by the media, to understand what these messages mean for individual and societal sexual health.**

Research suggests that providing accessible health services in conjunction with sexual health education is more likely to result in safe sex practices, because reluctance to obtain contraceptives from conventional sources (such as pharmacies) can pose a barrier to their use. For example, an Ontario study found that regions where sexuality education was offered in conjunction with public health family planning services had the greatest reductions in teenage pregnancy rates.[18]

Some school boards have placed condom dispensers in high school washrooms. Others have established health clinics within high schools to provide contraceptive counselling. Providing contraception to young people is controversial; some worry that it will encourage earlier sexual activity. We have shown, however, that the availability of health services does not lead to earlier sexual activity, but rather to safer sexual practices among those who are already or plan to become sexually active. The Commission therefore recommends that

> **12.   School boards consider the benefits of making contraception more accessible to young people who are sexually active, for example, through condom dispensers in high schools and referral to appropriate health services.**

The legal situation with respect to access to health services by teenagers varies across the country. In our view, laws related to the age of consent for medical treatment should not preclude teenagers from obtaining contraception on their own behalf.

Many teachers feel poorly equipped to teach sexuality education and to deal with the issues because their training in the area is limited. The Guidelines for Sexual Health Education outline criteria for the training and administrative support of professionals who teach sexual health education. The Commission recommends that

> **13.   Provincial/territorial ministries of education and local school boards ensure that requirements for teachers delivering sexual health education in schools are in accordance with the criteria outlined in the Guidelines for Sexual Health Education.**

Sexual health education programs are effective when they are tailored to the needs of specific populations and attuned to the particular realities of those they are trying to reach. Studies such as the Canada Youth and AIDS Study provide valuable data on the knowledge, attitudes, behaviour, and skills of young people; programs based on this type of research are more likely to be effective in changing behaviour. Given that the knowledge obtained through research is essential in enabling the development of effective sexual health education programs, the Commission recommends that

14. **National surveys and other research be
     undertaken at least every five years to document
     the knowledge, attitudes, and experience of
     youth and adults regarding sexual health and
     sexual behaviour. Surveys should be designed
     to ensure that they also reach segments of the
     population known to be at high risk of STDs
     and/or marginalized from mainstream health
     services and sexual health education programs.**

Youth who do not attend school regularly may miss out on sexual health education programs. This is an important omission, as street youth and young prostitutes constitute a subpopulation with very high rates of sexually transmitted diseases. This group therefore accounts for a significant reservoir of sexually transmitted infection, yet one that will be difficult to reduce if group members are marginalized from mainstream sexual health education and services. The Commission therefore recommends that

15. **Agencies involved in public health education
     develop sexual health programs and services
     designed specifically to target hard-to-reach
     populations such as street youth and
     prostitutes.**

Health Care Professionals and the Prevention, Diagnosis, and Treatment of STDs

Primary health care workers — for example, family physicians and nurses — are in a unique position to contribute to the prevention of sexually transmitted diseases. First, they see patients regularly, are aware of the health issues facing them, and have the opportunity to engage in one-on-one preventive counselling about how to reduce the risk of exposure to sexually transmitted diseases. Health care workers in specialized settings can counsel individuals who would otherwise be hard to reach, such as street youth and prostitutes. Second, health care professionals have the opportunity to screen patients who are at risk of acquiring a STD, thereby identifying individuals who may be asymptomatic and yet likely to transmit their infection to others. Third, health care professionals have the opportunity to treat sexually transmitted infections and thus reduce the risk of serious consequences to individuals.

There are several impediments, however, to a preventive counselling role for health professionals, in particular the limited time doctors have available for counselling because of pressure to provide treatment. This reflects the general orientation of the medical care system toward treatment rather than prevention; its structure, training programs, and reimbursement methods focus primarily on treatment. Current efforts to change this orientation are encouraging, with government reports at both the federal and provincial level supporting a greater emphasis on prevention. For example, a recently published federal document, "Enhancing the Provision of Prevention Services by Canadian Physicians," attests to the growing emphasis among both policy makers and health care providers on health promotion and disease prevention.

Training of Health Care Professionals

Surveys conducted in the United States show that physicians generally feel poorly trained and therefore ill-equipped to counsel patients about sexual behaviour. This probably holds true for Canadian physicians as well, with the result that many do not feel comfortable providing preventive STD counselling. Most Canadian medical schools offer only limited instruction to undergraduates and residents on the prevention of sexually transmitted diseases. One survey showed that they provided an average of six hours of classroom instruction and between two and eight hours of clinical experience in the treatment and management of STDs.[19] There are no established Canadian criteria for this type of training, but a U.S. advisory committee has recommended that all medical students and residents receive a minimum of 20 hours of supervised clinical experience in STD management. Most STD instruction in Canadian medical schools clearly falls short of this standard.

Nurses also receive little training in STD prevention. A 1988 survey of university and community college nursing schools conducted by the Canadian Nurses Association showed that nursing students receive an average of six hours of instruction related to sexually transmitted diseases.

Many public health nurses and public health physicians are sensitive, experienced, non-judgemental, and effective in dealing with individuals with sexually transmitted diseases. Other health care professionals need to develop these skills in their dealings with patients. Their training should emphasize that psychological and social issues need to be discussed in a tactful and sensitive way to ensure that patients have the information they need to deal with an infection and prevent a recurrence.

Professional associations should take a leadership role in ensuring that medical students, residents, and nursing students receive STD training. The quality and duration of STD training provided by medical schools for various levels of clinical practice (ranging from family physicians to infectious disease specialists) should be reviewed and standards recommended. Guidelines for the prevention, diagnosis, and treatment of sexually transmitted diseases were released recently by Health Canada and provide standards of care that should be reflected in course content. (The guidelines are discussed below.) Professional colleges should also ensure that physicians are adequately trained regarding sexually transmitted diseases. The Commission recommends that

> 16. **The Royal College of Physicians and Surgeons of Canada (for obstetricians/gynaecologists and infectious disease specialists), the College of Family Physicians of Canada (for general practitioners), and the Canadian Nurses Association (for nurses) propose standards for the content and duration of STD training provided by medical/nursing schools for various levels of clinical practice. Examining bodies of these organizations should examine candidates regarding the diagnosis, treatment, and management of STDs.**

Although improved training in medical and nursing schools will place future professionals in a better position to provide STD counselling, those already practising also need up-to-date knowledge and skills. Many physicians graduated well before the advent of AIDS and penicillin-resistant gonorrhoea, and treatment protocols and knowledge about sexually transmitted diseases are changing rapidly. Continuing medical education is essential to keep those already in the field current and knowledgeable about sexually transmitted diseases. The Commission therefore recommends that

> 17. **Continuing medical education courses be offered by faculties of medicine for obstetricians/gynaecologists and infectious disease specialists and for general practitioners, and by nursing faculties and community colleges for nurses, on the diagnosis, treatment, and counselling of individuals with sexually transmitted diseases.**

STD Guidelines for Health Professionals

In November 1992, the Laboratory Centre for Disease Control (Health and Welfare Canada) released the updated *Canadian Guidelines for the Prevention, Diagnosis, Management and Treatment of Sexually Transmitted Diseases in Neonates, Children, Adolescents and Adults.* The guidelines outline how physicians and nurses should diagnose and manage sexually transmitted diseases and incorporate prevention into their practices. For example, the guidelines recommend that a complete sexual health history be a routine part of practice, providing important information about the extent to which a patient may be at risk for STDs.

The guidelines also recommend that practitioners counsel patients about risky sexual behaviour. This is especially important when a physician prescribes oral contraception for a young woman. Without STD counselling, physicians may inadvertently promote unhealthy sexual behaviour. Strong messages need to be conveyed to young women who are prescribed oral contraceptives about the need for dual protection against pregnancy and sexually transmitted diseases.

Health and Welfare Canada provided 28 000 copies of the guidelines for distribution by the provinces and territories to family physicians and public health workers. Copies will not be distributed to specialists such as obstetricians/gynaecologists, who are presumed to have up-to-date information about the appropriate management and treatment of STDs, although they will be available for purchase. In our view, however, it would be desirable for the guidelines to be provided to all physicians likely to see patients with a STD.

> **18.** **The Commission endorses the 1992 *Canadian Guidelines for the Prevention, Diagnosis, Management and Treatment of Sexually Transmitted Diseases in Neonates, Children, Adolescents and Adults* prepared by the Laboratory Centre for Disease Control, Health Canada, and recommends that Health Canada ensure that a free copy of the guidelines is available to all primary care physicians, obstetricians/gynaecologists, urologists, STD clinics, provincial and territorial nurses, community care clinics, nurses in school settings, educators teaching STD management at nursing and medical schools, and nursing and medical students.**

We also recommend that

> **19.** **The guidelines be updated every five years.**

The availability of guidelines does not necessarily mean that all physicians will follow them. A recent study evaluated awareness and use of the 1988 STD guidelines by 153 staff physicians and residents at six hospital family practice teaching units in Toronto. The majority (70 percent) of physicians were unaware of the guidelines. Among those who were aware of the guidelines, 46 percent agreed with them but only 39 percent stated that they followed them routinely.[20] A 1992 study by the Laboratory Centre for Disease Control also found that some physicians are treating chlamydia and PID inappropriately.[21] These findings highlight the need to ensure that physicians are aware of the new STD guidelines and that they are encouraged to follow the recommended procedures for the diagnosis, prevention, and treatment of STDs. Research is also needed to discover why some recommended preventive practices are not being followed.

A final area of concern with respect to health professionals and the management of STDs is tracing the contacts of people diagnosed with STDs. In our view, it would be desirable if standards for contact tracing were included in future revisions to the 1992 *Canadian Guidelines for the Prevention, Diagnosis, Management and Treatment of Sexually Transmitted Diseases in Neonates, Children, Adolescents and Adults.*

Periodic Health Examination

One way to detect STDs early and offer treatment, so as to reduce the chances of untreated cases leading to infertility, would be through check-ups or periodic health examinations. The Canadian Task Force on the Periodic Health Examination (established in 1976) has developed a scientifically rigorous approach to assessing the efficacy and effectiveness of preventive activities routinely undertaken by clinical practitioners. The task force published its first report in 1979, and several updates have been published since then. The College of Family Physicians of Canada has supported the work of the task force and, in 1983, published a loose-leaf binder containing the preventive care recommendations of the Canadian Task Force on the Periodic Health Examination and, with the help of Health Canada, distributed one to every College member.

The United States Preventive Services Task Force was set up after the Canadian task force but has gone further in its work. In 1989, the U.S. task force published a guide on clinical preventive services that assesses the effectiveness of 169 interventions and provides a series of charts with clinical preventive measures recommended for patients in various age groups. It also developed recommendations for patient education and counselling on preventing transmission of HIV and other STDs.

A summary of proceedings of a joint Canadian and American symposium, "Implementing Preventive Services," held in 1987, called for the creation of an infrastructure to implement the recommendations of the Canadian and U.S. task forces. The Canadian task force does not have adequate funds, however, to update, compile, and distribute its recommendations on effective preventive services. Commissioners were impressed by the task force approach, which involved evaluating evidence and discarding procedures that did not make a difference to health. We believe that it is an appropriate way of ensuring that health care resources are used effectively. The Commission therefore recommends that

> **20. The federal government provide adequate funds to the Canadian Task Force on the Periodic Health Examination or a similar body to compile, update, and publish its findings in a practical guide for primary health care workers on useful preventive services and that the guide include STD prevention.**

Research Needs

The foundation of all work in the prevention of sexually transmitted diseases is accurate knowledge from well-designed research. This can be obtained only by supporting productive investigators, facilitating continuing research in this field, and providing training for future researchers.

Making the reporting of chlamydia cases mandatory could help to provide a more complete picture of the prevalence of the disease. Pelvic inflammatory disease is not reportable, however, and asymptomatic cases of STDs that are not detected will also continue to be unreported. One way to obtain a more accurate picture of the incidence of chlamydial and gonorrhoeal infections would be to piggyback on an existing approach, such as the National Sentinel Surveillance Program, a Health Canada program that collects demographic and risk factor information from nine health facilities that together serve 10 percent of the Canadian population. Physicians at these facilities could be trained to screen high-risk individuals for STDs, and the data collected would provide a more accurate understanding of the incidence of chlamydial and gonorrhoeal infection in Canada.

Apart from research on AIDS, little targeted funding is available for research in the field of sexual and reproductive health, including sexually transmitted diseases. No government research funding agency earmarks funds for work on infectious diseases other than AIDS, and no funding agency has a specific mandate for research on reproductive health. Given the importance of this research, and given that the objectives of the Medical Research Council (MRC) of Canada include promoting and supporting research that advances the application of scientific research to the prevention, diagnosis, and treatment of disease, the Commission recommends that

> **21. Federal research funding organizations, such as the Medical Research Council, consider making basic and applied research on sexual and reproductive health, including sexually transmitted diseases, a higher priority.**

There is a clear need for evaluation of prevention programs to guide future program development and implementation. To do this, more researchers with epidemiological and evaluation skills will be needed. At present only a handful of researchers is working on the collation of routinely collected data on sexually transmitted diseases, and an equally small number is involved in evaluating STD prevention programs. A concerted effort is therefore required to train researchers and prepare for epidemiological research of the type needed to assess preventive strategies. The Commission recommends that

> **22. Federal research funding organizations, such as the National Health Research and Development Program and the Medical Research Council, consider targeting funding to the training of epidemiological researchers as part of an overall approach to assigning higher priority to applied research on sexual and reproductive health.**

Preventing STD-Related Infertility: A Comprehensive Reproductive Health Strategy

The prevention of sexually transmitted diseases is just one aspect of sexual and reproductive health. The protection and promotion of sexual and reproductive health merit a comprehensive, coordinated response because they affect all Canadians.

As a public policy field, sexual and reproductive health and sexually transmitted diseases lack the degree of integration, coordination, and comprehensiveness needed for effectiveness. There is little internal coordination among government branches with regard to STD prevention, sexuality, and reproductive health. There is also no effective vehicle for maintaining a network of contacts among the various professionals concerned; reproductive and sexual health does not have a broad community network that would facilitate the development of coordinated strategies.

As a result, a piecemeal approach is often taken to addressing the issues, inhibiting advances in STD prevention and reproductive health promotion. Family planning, pregnancy care, and sexual health services, often isolated from one another, are fragmented within the health care system. Reproductive health care and counselling services designed specifically to meet the needs of women are in short supply or entirely absent.

Furthermore, programs and funding for STD and AIDS prevention are generally kept separate, potentially diluting their effectiveness and requiring greater human and financial resources than would be required for a single concerted effort. Federal AIDS prevention efforts have also failed to capitalize on existing expertise in dealing with STDs.

> Former Prime Minister Pierre Elliott Trudeau stated "government has no role in the bedrooms of its citizens." Although most Canadians would accept the truth of this dictum, it does not exempt federal and provincial governments from assuming a major responsibility for the control and prevention of STDs throughout Canadian society.
>
> A. Ronald and R. Peeling, "Sexually Transmitted Infections: Their Manifestations and Links to Infertility and Reproductive Illness," in Research Volumes of the Commission, 1993.

In the view of Commissioners, the most effective way to promote sexual and reproductive health is through integrated and coordinated efforts, with STD prevention pursued within a broader coordinated strategy to address sexual and reproductive health. A national body could be highly effective and efficient in creating, coordinating, and fostering networks and activity in sexual and reproductive health. The Expert Interdisciplinary Advisory Committee on Sexually Transmitted Diseases in Children and Youth, for example, did exemplary work in reproductive health during its mandate (1986-1991). In Chapter 15, we discuss the need for a comprehensive reproductive health strategy and present our recommendations for a body to develop the strategy and oversee its implementation.

General Sources

Brunham, R.C., et al. "*Chlamydia trachomatis* — Associated Ectopic Pregnancy: Serologic and Histologic Correlates." *Journal of Infectious Diseases* 154 (June 1992): 1076-81.

Canada. Health and Welfare Canada. "Canadian Guidelines for the Prevention, Diagnosis, Management and Treatment of Sexually Transmitted Diseases in Neonates, Children, Adolescents and Adults." *Canada Communicable Disease Report* 18 (Suppl. 1)(1992).

Canada. Health and Welfare Canada. *Guidelines for Sexual Health Education* (Draft). Ottawa: Minister of Supply and Services Canada, 1992.

Canada. Health and Welfare Canada, and Canadian Medical Association. *Enhancing the Provision of Prevention Services by Canadian Physicians: Report of a National Workshop, March 20-23, 1990, Ottawa.* Ottawa: Canadian Medical Association, 1990.

Dixon-Mueller, R., and J. Wasserheit. *The Culture of Silence: Reproductive Tract Infections in the Third World.* New York: International Women's Health Coalition, 1991.

Dulberg, C.S., and T. Stephens. "The Prevalence of Infertility in Canada, 1991-1992: Analysis of Three National Surveys." In Research Volumes of the Royal Commission on New Reproductive Technologies, 1993.

Expert Interdisciplinary Advisory Committee on Sexually Transmitted Diseases in Children and Youth. *Final Report and Recommendations* and *Appendices.* Ottawa: The Committee, 1991.

Goeree, R., and P. Gully. "The Burden of Chlamydial and Gonococcal Infection in Canada." In Research Volumes of the Royal Commission on New Reproductive Technologies, 1993.

Green, L.W., M.P. Eriksen, and E.L. Schor. "Preventive Practices by Physicians: Behavioural Determinants and Potential Interventions." In *Implementing Preventive Services*, ed. R.N. Bathsa and R.S. Lawrence. New York: American Journal of Preventive Medicine, 1988.

Gulens, M. "Two Fold Infertility Risk when PID Therapy Delayed." *Medical Post* (June 23, 1992).

Gully, P.R., and D.K. Rwetsiba. "Trends in Gonorrhea in Canada: 1980-1989." *Canada Diseases Weekly Report* (May 25, 1991): 17-21.

Hatcher, R.A., et al. *Contraceptive Technology 1990-1992.* 15th rev. ed. New York: Irvington Publishers Inc., 1990.

Hyndman, B., et al. "The Integration of Theoretical Approaches to Prevention: A Proposed Framework for Reducing the Incidence of Infertility." In Research Volumes of the Royal Commission on New Reproductive Technologies, 1993.

King, A.J.C., et al. *Canada Youth & AIDS Study.* Kingston: Queen's University, 1989.

Millson, P., and K. Maznyk. "Pilot Study on Determining the Relative Importance of Risk Factors for Infertility in Canada." In Research Volumes of the Royal Commission on New Reproductive Technologies, 1993.

Ontario Ministry of Health. *Ontario Health Survey: Highlights.* Toronto: The Ministry, 1992.

Quebec. Ministry of Health and Social Services. *Enquête québécoise sur les facteurs de risque associées au SIDA et aux autres MTS: la population des 15-29 ans.* Quebec: Government of Quebec, 1992.

Radford, J.L., A.J.C. King, and W.K. Warren. *Street Youth & AIDS.* Kingston: Queen's University, 1989.

Specific References

1. Canada. Health and Welfare Canada. "Trends in Gonorrhea in Canadians 15-24 Years of Age, 1981-1988." *Canada Diseases Weekly Report* 15-50 (December 16, 1989): 253-54; Canada. Health and Welfare Canada. "Chlamydial Infection in Canada." *Canada Diseases Weekly Report* 17-51 (December 21, 1991), Table 2; Canada. Health and Welfare Canada. "Sexually Transmitted Disease in Canada 1987." *Canada Diseases Weekly Report* 15 (Suppl. S2)(1989), Table 15.

2. Canada. Health and Welfare Canada, "Chlamydial Infection in Canada," 282-91.

3. Canada. Health and Welfare Canada. "1989 Canadian Guidelines for Screening for Chlamydia trachomatis Infection." *Canada Diseases Weekly Report* 15 (Suppl. 5)(1989), p. 2.

4. Ronald, A.R., and R.W. Peeling. "Sexually Transmitted Infections: Their Manifestations and Links to Infertility and Reproductive Illness." In Research Volumes of the Royal Commission on New Reproductive Technologies, 1993.

5. Canada. Health and Welfare Canada. *Canada's Health Promotion Survey 1990: Technical Report.* Ottawa: Minister of Supply and Services Canada, 1993.

6. Goeree, R., and P. Gully. "The Burden of Chlamydial and Gonococcal Infection in Canada." In Research Volumes of the Royal Commission on New Reproductive Technologies, 1993.

7. Ronald and Peeling, "Sexually Transmitted Infections."

8. Canada. Health and Welfare Canada, "Sexually Transmitted Disease in Canada 1987," Table 15.

9. "Papers Presented at the 25th Annual Meeting of the SER, Minneapolis, Minnesota, June 9-12, 1992." Special Issue, *American Journal of Epidemiology* 136 (8)(October 15, 1992).

10. Weström, L. "Incidence, Prevalence, and Trends of Acute Pelvic Inflammatory Disease and Its Consequences in Industrialized Countries." *American Journal of Obstetrics and Gynecology* 138 (7)(December 1, 1980): 880-92.

11. Ibid.

12. Rootman, I. "Prevention of Infertility: Literature Review of Applicable Theoretical Models." Report produced for the Royal Commission on New Reproductive Technologies, January 1992.

13. Ronald and Peeling, "Sexually Transmitted Infections."

14. Canada. Health and Welfare Canada. "Costs of Pelvic Inflammatory Disease and Associated Sequelae in Canada." *Canada Diseases Weekly Report* 14-45 (November 12, 1988): 206-208.

15. Zabin, L.S., et al. "The Baltimore Pregnancy Prevention Program for Urban Teenagers." *Family Planning Perspectives* 20 (4)(July/August 1988): 182-92.

16. Vincent, M.L., et al. "Reducing Adolescent Pregnancy Through School and Community-Based Education." *JAMA* 257 (24)(June 26, 1987): 3382-86.

17. Orton, M.J., and E. Rosenblatt. *Adolescent Pregnancy in Ontario 1976-1986: Extending Access to Prevention Reduces Abortions, and Births to the Unmarried.* Hamilton: McMaster University, 1991.

18. Orton, M.J., and E. Rosenblatt. *Adolescent Pregnancy in Ontario: Progress in Prevention.* Hamilton: McMaster University, 1986, p. 131.

19. Doherty, J.A., and A.G. Jessamine. "STD Training in Canadian Medical Schools." *Canadian Journal of Infectious Diseases* 3 (3)(1992): 118-221.

20. Weyman, K., and A.R. Lanning. *Screening Guidelines for* C. trachomatis *Infection: Evaluation of Physician Awareness, Agreement, and Use.* Toronto: University of Toronto, 1992.

21. Gully, P.R., et al. "Management of Sexually Transmitted Diseases by Family Physicians: A Descriptive Study." Poster presentation at the 10th International Meeting of the International Society of STD Research, Helsinki, Finland, 1993.

Smoking and Infertility

◆

There is mounting evidence that women who smoke heavily have a reduced ability to become pregnant. This relatively new finding comes in addition to the already well-accepted evidence that smoking during pregnancy is associated with risks for the fetus and eventual child, including higher rates of spontaneous abortions and low birth weight. An association has also been shown between a pregnant woman's exposure to second-hand smoke and the birth of a low birth weight infant.

Twenty-nine percent of Canadian women in their childbearing years (ages 20 to 44) smoke; exposure to tobacco smoke is even more widespread if we take into account women exposed to second-hand smoke in their homes or workplaces. Therefore, the high proportion of women for whom tobacco smoke may play a role in infertility distinguishes smoking as a major risk factor for infertility.

An association between smoking and reduced fertility is biologically plausible, given the hundreds of chemicals in tobacco smoke and what we know about the effects of some of those chemicals on pregnancy. Their effects on fertility in women are not well understood, but animal studies have shown various effects on the hormonal system, testes, ovaries, and uterus that might be expected to reduce reproductive capacity if they occurred in men and women. For example, rats injected with nicotine have been found to undergo hormonal changes and a reduction in ovulation. By-products of cigarette smoke have also been shown to affect ovarian blood flow in laboratory animals.

Analyzing the research data on smoking and infertility in human beings is complex, however, because other factors that can affect fertility must be taken into consideration. For example, smoking is associated with heavier consumption of alcohol and coffee and lower socioeconomic status. It is important but difficult to distinguish the influence of one factor from another. Despite these problems, the existing data, when taken together, show an association between smoking and a reduced ability to become pregnant. The association is quite clear for women who are heavy smokers; among lighter smokers, the relationship between smoking and the ability to conceive is less clear. In addition, however, the finding that quitting smoking is followed by a return to normal fertility, together with the feasibility of preventing smoking, led the Commission to recommend that smoking prevention should be a high priority for policy makers.

The impact of smoking on male fertility needs to be elucidated; to date, most research has focussed on the impact of smoking on women's reproductive health. An association between heavy smoking and reduced sperm quality and quantity has been shown, however. This area requires further research, but it seems probable that a man who smokes heavily may reduce the ability of his female partner to conceive, if only by exposing her to second-hand smoke.

In the following pages, we examine the impact of smoking on time to conception, pregnancy, birth outcomes, and other relevant factors such as age at menopause. We also discuss what is known about the relationship between smoking and male fertility. Finally, we examine how we can prevent reproductive harm caused by smoking.

Impact of Female Smoking on Fertility

Over the past decade, most studies that have examined the effects of smoking on fertility have found an association between female smoking and a reduced ability to become pregnant.[1] The evidence shows a "dose-response effect," meaning that the more cigarettes a woman smokes, the greater the effect on her fertility (see Table 11.1). As mentioned above, some studies have found that ex-smokers return to normal fertility, which provides further evidence of the relationship between smoking and the ability to conceive.

The exact mechanisms by which cigarette smoking affects female fertility are not clear. Evidence suggests that the presence of nicotine in a woman's bloodstream may affect the ability of the fallopian tubes to transport the egg to the uterus and the ability of the fertilized egg to implant.[2] This also may help explain why women who smoke have been found to be at higher risk of having an ectopic pregnancy.

A multinational study was conducted between 1978 and 1980 by the World Health Organization in 12 centres comparing 1 108 women with confirmed ectopic pregnancies to equal numbers of women with normal pregnancies and to non-pregnant women. For developing countries, the prevalence of smoking was significantly higher among women with ectopic pregnancies (17 percent) than among women with normal pregnancies (7 percent); the relevant figures for developed countries were 47 percent and 37 percent. Even after adjusting for known risk factors (history of PID or gonorrhoea, IUD use, tubal ligation, and prior ectopic pregnancy), the women with ectopic pregnancies were still found to be twice as likely to be smokers.[3] This provides further evidence of a link between smoking and tubal dysfunction.

Table 11.1. Probability of Achieving Live Birth Among Smokers and Non-Smokers

Cigarettes smoked	Relative fertility rate*
Never smoked	1.00
Ex-smoker	0.99
1-5 cigarettes/day	1.00
6-10 cigarettes/day	0.97
11-15 cigarettes/day	0.93
16-20 cigarettes/day	0.79
More than 20 cigarettes/day	0.78

* The number of months elapsed between stopping contraception and achieving a live birth was compared between groups. Women who had never smoked were used as the reference group, and all other groups were compared to this group.

Source: Howe, G., et al. "Effects of Age, Cigarette Smoking, and Other Factors on Fertility: Findings in a Large Prospective Study." *British Medical Journal* 290 (June 8, 1985): 1697-1700.

The biological effects of smoking on fertility require further research. It is essential to know more, as the subject has clear implications for public policy and programs to prevent infertility, and for individual women's decision making when they plan to have children.

Infertility Treatment Results and Smoking

Does smoking make it less likely that infertility treatment will be successful? Recently, researchers have begun to examine this question. At some infertility clinics a sizable proportion of patients are smokers; for example, in 1990-91, 27 percent of women undergoing *in vitro* fertilization at the McMaster IVF clinic were smokers.[4]

Evidence from a Canadian study[5] and a British study[6] suggests that smoking may have detrimental effects on the chances of a live birth occurring following IVF, but large studies with complete and careful data collection are necessary to define the precise nature and extent of these effects. Evaluating the effects of smoking on IVF outcomes is complex; in particular, the impact of variables such as socioeconomic status must be taken into account.

In summary, the available data on this question are too limited to be conclusive, but they are enough to suggest that women who smoke are less likely to have a live birth after undergoing *in vitro* fertilization than women who do not smoke. Given the evidence linking smoking to adverse effects on the ability to conceive and on pregnancy outcomes, together with the overwhelming evidence that smoking is detrimental to health in general, there are compelling reasons for women undergoing infertility treatment to quit smoking.

Smoking, Pregnancy, and Birth Outcomes

The evidence that smoking reduces the likelihood of having a healthy, full-term infant (that is, using our broader definition of fertility) has been clearly documented; it is well recognized that smoking during pregnancy poses risks to the woman, the fetus, and the eventual child. These include an increased risk of ectopic pregnancy, abruptio placenta (premature separation of the placenta prior to delivery), placenta previa (placental attachment covering the inner cervix), spontaneous abortion, stillbirth, and infant death during the first month of life. Infants born to smokers are more likely to have low birth weights (on average, weighing between 150 and 300 grams less than children born to non-smokers[7]), resulting from intrauterine growth retardation and/or premature delivery. Cigarette smoking has also been shown to have an adverse effect on breast milk; women who smoke produce significantly less milk per day than non-smokers, and their milk has lower concentrations of fat, which is crucial for a child's growth and development.[8] Children born to women who smoke during pregnancy are also more likely to succumb to sudden infant death syndrome or to suffer from childhood respiratory illnesses.[9]

Clearly, risks associated with smoking during pregnancy have considerable implications for public health. In the United States, it has been estimated that approximately 14.5 percent of low birth weight births and 10 percent of all fetal and infant deaths are attributable to smoking. Children of women who smoke may also have a somewhat greater chance of developing cancer during their childhood and subsequently in their adult years.[10]

Smoking and Age at Menopause

Several researchers have noted a relationship between smoking and the age at which menopause begins. The toxic effects of smoking may cause depletion in the number of eggs in a woman's ovaries, thus hastening the onset of menopause. Research has shown that women who smoke half a package of cigarettes per day have a median age at menopause about one year younger than that of non-smokers.[11] The average age at menopause of heavier smokers — those who smoke at least a pack a day — is about two years younger than that of non-smokers. These findings indicate clearly that smoking has an effect on the female reproductive system, influencing women's fertility by reducing the number of years during which they are capable of bearing children.

Male Smoking and Infertility

Relatively few studies have been undertaken to measure the relationship between male smoking and infertility as an outcome; most have been concerned with outcomes more easily measured, such as sperm quantity and quality. A review of 12 published studies found that heavier smoking is associated with declines in both the quantity and the quality of sperm.[12] Eleven of the 12 studies found a reduction in sperm density among smokers; the average sperm density of smokers was 22 percent lower than that of non-smokers. Eight of the studies also found a relationship between male smoking and reduced sperm motility, which may affect the sperm's ability to reach the egg. Ten of the studies also evaluated the proportion of normally shaped sperm in smokers compared to non-smokers, but it was not clear whether the proportion of normally shaped sperm was affected.

In summary, most of the studies reviewed found a relationship between male smoking and reduced sperm density and motility. However, the small number of subjects and the fact that most studies used volunteers from infertility clinics may have influenced the results. How changes in sperm quality/quantity resulting from smoking affect the likelihood of conception and pregnancy remains largely unaddressed. Some studies have investigated whether there is a relationship between the man's smoking habits and the results of fertility treatments. The limited data available provide no clear evidence that a man's smoking adversely affects the likelihood his partner will become pregnant. For example, a Canadian study of IVF patients found that although a male partner's smoking was associated with a significant reduction in sperm concentration in samples prepared for insemination, there was no statistically significant effect on pregnancy or birth outcomes following IVF;[13] however, the numbers in the study were small.

Further studies are required to determine whether a relationship exists between smoking and reduced fertility in men. However, evidence does exist showing that a man's smoking during his partner's pregnancy affects the fetus, especially with regard to low birth weight.[14] This information, together with what is known about the adverse effects of cigarette smoking on female fertility, pregnancy, the health of children, and general health, show clearly that men whose partners are trying to conceive should try to stop smoking or, at the very least, should avoid exposing their partners to second-hand smoke.

Preventing Reproductive Harm

Research linking smoking and infertility adds to what is already known about the serious health risks associated with tobacco consumption. Tobacco use is considered the single most important and preventable risk to the health of Canadians. It has been estimated that 30 000 Canadians die each year from tobacco-related illnesses, making it the number one public health problem. Given that some one-third of Canadians in their childbearing years (aged 20 to 44) are regular smokers, as well as documented effects of smoking on the full range of reproductive outcomes, smoking must be considered to be a major risk factor for infertility. Reducing smoking among Canadians, and in particular among young people who are about to enter or are now in their childbearing years, could help to reduce the number of couples who have difficulty conceiving. It could also reduce the number of miscarriages, the incidence of low birth weight, and the number of children who suffer long-term health and developmental problems as a result of pre- and post-natal exposure to cigarette smoke.

Our recommendations for preventing reproductive harm from smoking focus on two broad areas. First, continued efforts are needed to reduce and prevent tobacco consumption in the general population. Programs are required to reduce and eliminate tobacco use among Canadians who currently smoke; to help non-smokers to remain smoke-free; and to eliminate involuntary exposure of non-smokers to tobacco smoke. Women who are trying to conceive or who are already pregnant should ideally live and work in smoke-free environments. Second, people who want to have a child, including those seeking medical assistance to do so, must be informed of the effects of smoking on their fertility.

Reducing and Preventing Tobacco Consumption

Policies and programs to reduce smoking among Canadians have proved effective. High taxation and strong legislation to restrict cigarette advertising and smoking in public places, in combination with education and smoking cessation programs, have resulted in substantial declines in tobacco use. The decline in the proportion of regular smokers has been equally significant (see Figure 11.1). Canada is seen internationally as being in the forefront in developing strong measures to reduce tobacco consumption.

Efforts to reduce tobacco consumption have been driven by the federal government's adoption of a comprehensive approach to discourage smoking and the work of the Steering Committee of the National Strategy to Reduce Tobacco Use in Canada, whose membership includes federal, provincial, and territorial governments and eight national health organizations. Seven strategic directions were developed: legislation, access to information, availability of services/programs, message promotion, support for citizen action, intersectoral policy coordination, and research/knowledge development. Since these seven activities cannot be pursued by any single government or group on its own, this approach emphasizes the need for many organizations to work together and to coordinate their activities and make the best use of resources.

> **23. The Commission endorses the work of the Steering Committee of the National Strategy to Reduce Tobacco Use in Canada and encourages governments at all levels, major health organizations, and community groups to continue actively to seek ways to encourage and help those who smoke to quit, to prevent tobacco use among non-smokers, and to protect the health and rights of non-smokers.**

Of particular concern is the fact that one-fifth of teenaged girls and boys smoke. Special efforts are required to prevent and eliminate smoking among younger people, because research has shown that the vast majority of smokers become addicted in their teens; the average age at which regular smoking begins is between 12 and 14 years. Teenagers tend to underestimate the addictive powers of smoking; a recent U.S. study showed that 92 percent of teenagers who smoke say they do not plan to be smoking in another year, but only 1.5 percent of them manage to quit.[15] People who reach the age of 20 years as non-smokers are unlikely to become smokers; therefore, if young people can be prevented from smoking in the first place, they are more likely to remain non-smokers throughout their lives.

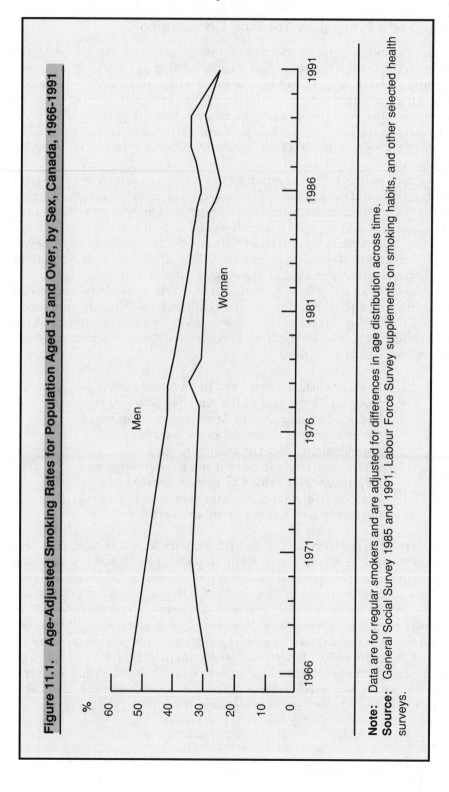

Figure 11.1.   Age-Adjusted Smoking Rates for Population Aged 15 and Over, by Sex, Canada, 1966-1991

Note: Data are for regular smokers and are adjusted for differences in age distribution across time.

Source: General Social Survey 1985 and 1991, Labour Force Survey supplements on smoking habits, and other selected health surveys.

Some provinces plan to introduce legislation to reduce tobacco consumption among young people.   For example, in 1992, the Chief Medical Officer of Health in Ontario released a report entitled *Opportunities for Health: A Report on Youth*, which emphasizes that "eliminating smoking by young people is the front line in the war against tobacco use."   In addition to educational efforts, the report recommends legislative measures to make tobacco less accessible to young people. In response to the report, the Ontario government is proposing the broadest measures in Canada to discourage smoking, particularly among young people.   They include raising the legal age for buying tobacco from 18 to 19 years, imposing fines on retailers who sell tobacco to under-age people, banning tobacco vending machines, outlawing the sale of tobacco in pharmacies, and including stronger health warnings on cigarette packages. Other provinces are also considering raising the legal age for purchasing tobacco.

Provincial efforts to reduce smoking among young people are encouraging; however, the effectiveness of the proposed measures will depend largely on whether and how well they are enforced. A 1992 study found that 93 percent of stores in four major cities in Ontario and Quebec would sell tobacco to minors.[16]

> **24. The Commission endorses provincial/territorial governments' plans to introduce legislative measures to restrict tobacco use among teenagers and urges them to ensure that these measures are enforced.**

Educational programs are also required to persuade young people to avoid or stop smoking. Such programs are not a mandatory part of health curricula in all provinces. In our view, all young people should receive health education that includes smoking prevention throughout elementary and high school grades. Therefore, the Commission recommends that

> **25. Provincial/territorial ministries of education mandate health education that includes smoking prevention for all young Canadians in elementary and high school grades.**

In the 1960s and '70s, school programs tended to focus on the health risks of smoking and did not address the social pressures on teens to smoke.   Since many young people see smoking as an avenue to peer acceptance, and many young women believe that smoking will help them control their weight, initiatives that address these underlying attitudes are needed. Approaches that promote the immediate and long-term physical and social benefits of non-smoking appear to be more meaningful to young people than approaches that emphasize the dangers of smoking.

Because smoking, alcohol abuse, and other high-risk behaviours tend to occur in tandem, and the strategies for preventing one high-risk behaviour apply to others, it makes sense to coordinate education about smoking with education about alcohol and drug use and the risks of unsafe sexual behaviours, all in the context of promoting healthy life choices. School efforts to prevent smoking among young people will have the greatest impact if they are coordinated with programs in the community. The Commission recommends that

> **26. Provincial/territorial ministries of education and health ensure that health curricula and school programs, in conjunction with community programs, focus on the benefits of a smoke-free life as a means of preventing and reducing smoking among young people.**

Health education can cause a short-term decline in smoking among young people, but changes in the long term are more difficult to sustain in a culture that still promotes tobacco use through such avenues as the sponsorship by tobacco companies of automobile racing, sports events, and concerts. Governments have already taken such steps as banning magazine, television, and radio advertising of cigarettes and tightening restrictions on tobacco purchases by minors. Commissioners strongly support such actions to reduce smoking among Canadians and believe that every additional step should be taken to discourage young people from smoking.

> Governments have already taken such steps as banning magazine, television and radio advertising of cigarettes and tightening restrictions on tobacco purchases by minors. Commissioners strongly support such actions to reduce smoking among Canadians and believe that every additional step should be taken to discourage young people from smoking.

Reducing and Preventing Smoking Among Couples Who Plan to Become Pregnant

As the evidence before the Commission shows, couples who want to become pregnant or who seek infertility treatment should be aware of the possible effects of smoking on their ability to conceive and have a healthy pregnancy. Smoking cessation is difficult for most people, however. Health care professionals should recognize this and when counselling them about the need to stop smoking should make their recommendations in a non-judgemental and supportive way. The effort to reduce and prevent smoking among couples who plan to become pregnant will need to be supported and carried out by several categories of individuals.   The Commission recommends that

> **27.   Public education efforts endorsed by the Steering Committee of the National Strategy to Reduce Tobacco Use in Canada include informing women of the evidence regarding the effect of cigarette smoking on ability to conceive, in addition to the adverse effects on their pregnancy and the health of the fetus.**

and that

> **28.   Public education efforts include messages that encourage men to stop smoking to maximize the chances that their female partner will be able to conceive and have a healthy pregnancy and birth.**

> **29.   Physicians and other health professionals (such as public health nurses) encourage women who smoke and who plan to become pregnant to quit smoking, and provide them with the support to do so.**

and that

> **30.   Prenatal classes (supported by provincial/ territorial ministries of health or municipal governments) include information and support with regard to the importance of smoking cessation.**

In infertility diagnosis and treatment, it is important that physicians (both general practitioners and those who evaluate couples at infertility clinics) carefully investigate whether factors such as smoking may be contributing to a couple's difficulty conceiving.   Both partners should always be asked whether they smoke, and men and women should be counselled about the importance of changing habits or practices that may jeopardize their ability to conceive and have a healthy pregnancy and birth. The Commission recommends that

> **31. Physicians determine whether either partner in a couple having difficulty conceiving is a smoker and recommend smoking cessation as the first approach before beginning fertility treatment for either partner.**

Given how common smoking is among people of reproductive age, it is important that research be undertaken in the future to clarify the relationship between smoking and fertility in women and men. Greater focus is needed on this ubiquitous and preventable risk factor. We believe that agencies such as the National Health Research and Development Program, the Medical Research Council, and provincial health research funding agencies should take this into account in their planning and funding decisions.

Preventing Smoking-Related Infertility

We have recommended a vigorous approach on several fronts, involving many groups and individuals, to prevent the onset of smoking among young people, to accelerate cessation among current smokers, and to reduce the exposure of non-smokers to tobacco smoke. By reducing the prevalence of smoking in the general population, these efforts could ultimately reduce the proportion of couples who are infertile in the future.

In addition to these broad strategies to reduce tobacco consumption among the general population, we have made specific recommendations about informing couples who wish to conceive about the adverse effects of smoking on their fertility. Public education is one route to increasing this awareness. Physicians and other health professionals who have regular contact with people in their reproductive years also have an essential role; they can provide counselling that includes information about the effects of smoking on the ability to conceive, to sustain a healthy pregnancy, and to promote the birth of a healthy child, as well as support to help people quit smoking and to make that decision a permanent one.

General Sources

Baird, D.D., and A.J. Wilcox. "Cigarette Smoking Associated with Delayed Conception." *JAMA* 253 (20)(May 24, 1985): 2979-83.

Boyer, H. "Effects of Licit and Illicit Drugs, Alcohol, Caffeine, and Nicotine on Infertility." In Research Volumes of the Royal Commission on New Reproductive Technologies, 1993.

Canada. Health and Welfare Canada. *Canada's Health Promotion Survey 1990: Technical Report,* ed. T. Stephens and D. Fowler Graham. Ottawa: Minister of Supply and Services Canada, 1993.

Consultation, Planning and Implementation Committee. *Break Free: Directional Paper of the National Program to Reduce Tobacco Use in Canada.* Ottawa: Health and Welfare Canada, 1987.

Feldman, P.R. "Smoking and Health Pregnancy: Now Is the Time to Quit." *Maryland Medical Journal* (October 1985): 982-86.

Laurent, S.L., et al. "An Epidemiological Study of Smoking and Primary Infertility in Women." *Fertility and Sterility* 57 (3)(March 1992): 565-72.

Millar, W. *A Trend to a Healthier Lifestyle.* Ottawa: Statistics Canada, 1991.

Ontario. Ministry of Health. *Opportunities for Health: A Report on Youth.* Toronto: Queen's Printer for Ontario, 1992.

Specific References

1. For a review of these studies, see Hughes, E.G., "Cigarette Smoking — Does It Reduce Fecundity?" *Journal of the Society of Obstetrics and Gynaecology of Canada* 14 (9)(November 1992): 27-30, 34-37.

2. United States. Department of Health and Human Services. *The Health Benefits of Smoking Cessation: A Report of the Surgeon General 1990.* Rockville: U.S. DHHS, 1990, p. 372.

3. Campbell, O.M., and R.H. Gray. "Smoking and Ectopic Pregnancy: A Multinational Case-Control Study." In *Smoking and Reproductive Health,* ed. M.J. Rosenberg. Littleton: PSG Publishers, 1987.

4. Hughes, E.G., E.V. YoungLai, and S.M. Ward. "Cigarette Smoking and Outcomes of In-Vitro Fertilization and Embryo Transfer: Prospective Cohort Study." *Human Reproduction* 7 (3)(1992): 358-61.

5. Pattinson, H.A., P.J. Taylor, and M.H. Pattinson. "The Effect of Cigarette Smoking on Ovarian Function and Early Pregnancy Outcome of In Vitro Fertilization Treatment." *Fertility and Sterility* 55 (4)(April 1991): 780-83.

6. Rosevear, S., et al. "Smoking and Decreased Fertilisation Rates In Vitro." *Lancet* (November 14, 1992): 1195-96.

7. Stillman, R.J., M.J. Rosenberg, and B.P. Sachs. "Smoking and Reproduction." *Fertility and Sterility* 46 (4)(October 1986): 545-60.

8. Hopkinson, J.M., et al. "Milk Production by Mothers of Premature Infants: Influence of Cigarette Smoking." *Pediatrics* 90 (6)(December 1992): 934-38.

9. Charlton, A. *Children and Passive Smoking.* Report commissioned by the Association for Non Smokers Rights (ANSR) and Union Européenne des Non-fumeurs (UEN). Edinburgh: ANSR, 1991.

10. Ashley, M.J. "Women and Smoking: The Health Consequences." In *Proceedings of National Workshop on Women and Tobacco.* Ottawa: Health and Welfare Canada, 1988.

11. Thomford, P.J., and D.R. Mattison. "The Effect of Cigarette Smoking on Female Reproduction." *Journal of the Arkansas Medical Society* 82 (12)(May 1986): 597-604.

12. Stillman, et al., "Smoking and Reproduction."

13. Hughes, et al., "Cigarette Smoking and Outcomes of In-Vitro Fertilization and Embryo Transfer."

14. Campbell, M.J., J. Lewry, and M. Wailoo. "Further Evidence for the Effect of Passive Smoking on Neonates." *Postgraduate Medical Journal* 64 (755)(1988): 663-65.

15. Moss, A.J., et al. "Recent Trends in Adolescent Smoking, Smoking-Uptake Correlates, and Expectations About the Future." Advance Data from Vital and Health Statistics 221 (December 2, 1992): 1-28.

16. Radecki, T.E., and C.D. Zdunich. "Tobacco Sales to Minors in 97 U.S. and Canadian Communities." Unpublished report from Doctors & Lawyers for a Drug Free Youth, Urbana, 1992.

Age and Infertility

♦

As women grow older, their fertility declines. This decline is inherent in human biology and the aging of the reproductive system; it is also related to cumulative exposure to risk factors such as those discussed in the chapters in this section. In addition, research has shown that women who have children in their later reproductive years (particularly after age 40) face an increased risk of adverse pregnancy and birth outcomes.

From a biological perspective, the ideal time for a woman to have children is when she is in her 20s. From a social perspective, however, for many women having children at this time is either not practical or not desirable. For some, obtaining an education and establishing a career occupy a portion of this time; others do not establish a long-term relationship until they are in their late 20s or 30s. For many women, the inadequacy of social supports makes it impossible for them to have their children earlier without paying a substantial penalty. And for some women a combination of all these factors is involved. Delaying childbearing for a few years may have positive consequences — those who begin parenting in their late 20s to early 30s are likely to have acquired more life skills, greater maturity, and financial stability, all of which may benefit their children.

Although many couples who delay childbearing may be better off as a result, and indeed society may benefit as well, some who delay may have to pay the unanticipated price of infertility. Women who try to conceive in their mid-30s or later are likely to be less fertile than they were in their 20s, and therefore they may have to wait longer before becoming pregnant. Once they have made a decision to have children, many couples who have postponed having children and have used contraception for many years are surprised when they do not conceive immediately, or at all, after discontinuing it. It is therefore important that couples make a decision about the best time to have children with full information about the impact of aging on a woman's fertility.

In this section, we examine the social context of childbearing, demographic trends in childbearing, and the potential implications for infertility of delaying childbearing. We go on to make recommendations for public education efforts to increase awareness of the impact of aging on fertility, as well as for programs and policies that would enable couples to have children earlier in their reproductive lives if they wish to and thus avoid some of the risks of infertility associated with aging.

The Social Context of Age and Infertility

The fact that women bear and are the primary caregivers of children remains the most profound factor defining women's role and society's expectations of them. But in the Canada of the 1990s, bearing and caring for children are far from being women's only roles. Most women today combine paid work with raising children and managing a household; indeed, one of the most significant shifts in society in the last three decades or so has been the influx of women into the labour force.

Over the past two decades, the number of women in Canada's paid labour force has almost doubled, and more and more women, representing a wider age range, are participating in paid work. Recent figures show that women account for 45 percent of all workers in Canada. Most of these women are combining paid work and raising children. In 1976, 31 percent of women with children under the age of six were in the paid labour force. By 1991, 57 percent of such women were working outside the home. When women with children aged 6 to 15 are included, the figure jumps to almost 70 percent.

Similar changes are evident in women's education. The percentage of women aged 15 years and over who obtained at least some post-secondary education rose from 25 percent in 1981 to 40 percent in 1991; women are also now earning more than half the bachelor and professional degrees awarded by Canadian universities.

Despite significant changes in women's lives in recent decades, and despite giving lip service to the importance of child-rearing, society has yet to accommodate these realities of women's lives; in particular, governments have taken few steps regarding adequate child care programs to accommodate women's dual roles as mothers and participants in the paid labour force, despite strengthening social consensus about the need to do so. Compared to several European countries, including France, the Netherlands, and the Scandinavian countries, Canada's lack of adequate policies on prenatal care, parental leave, child care, and workplace policies that accommodate family responsibilities is particularly evident. The shortage of social supports for those who bear and raise children has implications for the age at which women decide to have children.

Other factors related to family formation also have implications for the age at which women begin to have children. These include a trend toward marrying at a later age; a decline in the total number of marriages; and rising rates of divorce and remarriage.

A major consequence of these changes is that more women are delaying childbearing to pursue higher education, to achieve economic stability, and to establish a long-term relationship before having children.

Despite significant changes in women's lives in recent decades, and despite giving lip service to the importance of child-rearing, society has yet to accommodate these realities of women's lives; in particular, governments have taken few steps regarding adequate child care programs to accommodate women's dual roles as mothers and participants in the paid labour force, despite strengthening social consensus about the need to do so.

Although there has not been much Canadian research examining who is delaying childbearing, it is generally believed that women in this group are more likely to be career-oriented, live in urban centres, and have higher household incomes than those who bear children at an earlier age. This does not necessarily mean, however, that only upper-income couples are waiting longer to have children — as we will see in the next section, the overall shift is too marked to be attributable only to this segment of the population. Moreover, many of the social and financial factors that are influencing couples to delay childbearing apply to all socioeconomic groups. During the 1980s, for example, economic conditions and the uncertainty they generated, together with unchanged family incomes relative to rising living costs, likely influenced many couples to postpone having children.

Later marriages and changes in family structure are also affecting childbearing patterns; although not as strong an indicator as in the past, marriage is still a good predictor of childbearing in Canada. The average age of women at the time of their first marriage rose from 22.6 years in 1971 to 26 years in 1990. In many cases, couples who are marrying later are also having children later. Increasingly there are more blended families, single-parent families, and people who have never married, and these changes in family forms have implications for the timing of childbearing. For example, if a couple divorces before having children, childbearing may be delayed while they establish new relationships and start a family with a new partner.

Changes in women's education and occupations have also influenced childbearing patterns. In the past, women generally finished their education or were employed before marriage, then took several years off or left the workforce altogether to raise their children. In the 1990s, paid work is not a temporary activity before raising children; many women return to the workforce for financial reasons soon after having a child — their income is required to help support the family — and/or because they wish to pursue their careers.

Finally, access to effective contraception, sterilization, and abortion has given women greater control over their fertility than in the past. In the 1990s, women have a choice about whether to delay childbearing so they can achieve their financial, educational, career, or other goals.

Demographic Trends in Childbearing

The past two decades have seen a shift in the age at which women are having children (Figure 12.1). In that period many women in their 20s have postponed having children; this is evident in the downward trend in the birth rate among the 20- to 24-year-old age group, the stable birth rates among women in their mid- to late 20s, and the increased rates in women aged 30 to 34. The birth rate in the group aged 30 to 34 years has risen from 68 per 1 000 in 1981 to 86 per 1 000 in 1990.[1] Added to this is the fact that the "bulge" of baby boomers — those baby boomers born between 1953 and 1963 — are now in their 30s; these two things together have meant a substantial increase in the number of births to women aged 30 to 34 — 35 671 more in 1990 than in 1981.

The birth rate for women aged 35 to 39 has also risen — from 19 births per 1 000 women in 1981 to 28 in 1990; similarly, the number of births increased substantially, with 15 743 more in 1990 than in 1981. We can expect that the number of women bearing children in their 30s will remain high until the last baby boomers (those born in the early '60s) have moved beyond their prime childbearing years and entered their 40s — and this will occur in the early 2000s.

As a result of these trends, women over the age of 30 now account for a greater proportion of births than was the case a decade ago, while women in their early 20s account for a smaller proportion of births (see Figure 12.2).

Women having children in their 30s or even 40s is not a new phenomenon. During the baby boom, women in all age groups were more likely to be having children than in the early 1990s. In 1961, the birth rate for women aged 30 to 44 was more than twice what it was in 1990, reflecting the high fertility rate for all ages at that time. Strikingly, the 1961 rate for women aged 40 to 44 was more than seven times as high as the 1990 rate of 4.0.

These high birth rates during the 1950s and '60s were influenced not only by economic conditions but also by the fact that safe and reliable contraception was not as available as it is now. The average age at marriage and the birth of the first child was younger than it is today; most women were in their early 20s when they had their first child, and many continued childbearing into their 30s or even early 40s. This is a key difference between that period and the 1990s — many women are now

Figure 12.1.   Age-Specific Fertility Rates,[1] Canada,[2] 1921-1990

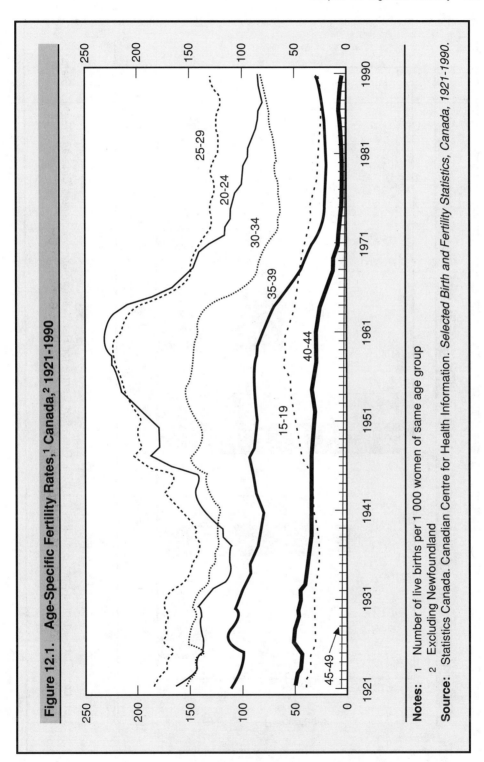

Notes: [1]   Number of live births per 1 000 women of same age group

         [2]   Excluding Newfoundland

Source: Statistics Canada. Canadian Centre for Health Information. *Selected Birth and Fertility Statistics, Canada, 1921-1990.*

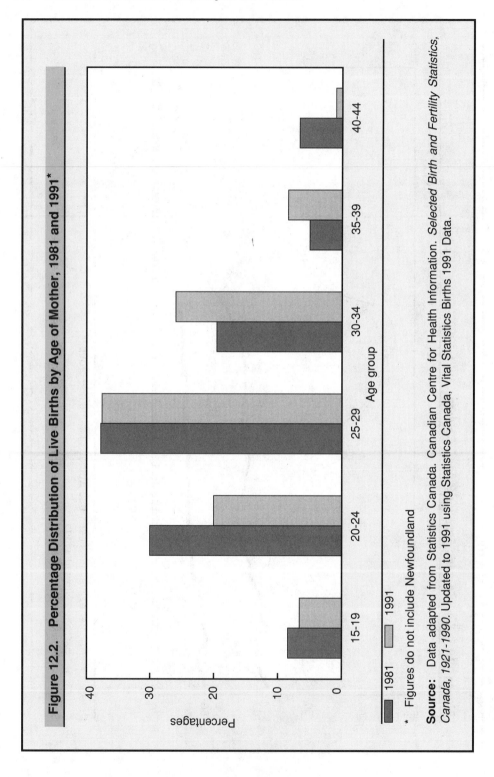

Figure 12.2.   Percentage Distribution of Live Births by Age of Mother, 1981 and 1991*

■ 1981   ▨ 1991

*   Figures do not include Newfoundland

Source: Data adapted from Statistics Canada. Canadian Centre for Health Information. *Selected Birth and Fertility Statistics, Canada, 1921-1990.* Updated to 1991 using Statistics Canada, Vital Statistics Births 1991 Data.

beginning their families in their early or even late 30s, whereas in the past, children born to women of that age were usually not their first.

As Figure 12.1 clearly shows, in the last half of the 1960s and into the '70s, the birth rate for all women, including older women, declined dramatically. The average family size declined as more effective contraceptive methods, better sterilization procedures, and legalized abortion became available, giving women greater control over the timing and number of their children. It is only in the past decade that birth rates have started to rise again in some age groups, particularly for women over the age of 30. This pattern of delayed childbearing is also evident in the United States and Europe. As we will see in the next section, this has implications for women's fertility and thus for society.

The Impact of Age on Female Fertility

Two kinds of factors contribute to reduced fertility as women age: (1) biological aging, that is, changes in the organs and tissues of the reproductive system and in the hormonal messages that govern its functioning; and (2) the cumulative effects of fertility risk factors that women may be exposed to over time.

With regard to the first, our understanding of the innate biological factors affecting reproduction is still limited. The maturation and release of eggs, embryo implantation, and the ability to carry a pregnancy to term are all known to be affected by aging, but the mechanisms and pathways by which this occurs have not been elucidated. Our survey of infertility clinics in Canada found that older women were more likely than younger women to have unexplained infertility, suggesting that there may be changes in women's reproductive systems as they age that are difficult to pinpoint.

> An increasing number of Canadian couples marry and start having children later in life ... The major question that this trend raises is whether couples — and women in particular — are compromising their ability to procreate by postponing childbearing. It is obvious that people expect to live well past their ability to reproduce. But what does the scientific literature say about the ending of ability to reproduce?
>
> *J. Jantz-Lee, "The Physiological Effects of Aging on Fertility Decline: A Literature Review," in Research Volumes of the Commission, 1993.*

The likelihood that fertilization of an egg will lead to pregnancy declines as a woman ages. For example, a recent study on *in vitro* fertilization in older women showed that the likelihood of pregnancy is greater when the eggs of younger women are used.[2] Moreover, a proportion of women stop ovulating before menopause;

one study showed that 10 percent of women have ceased to ovulate by the time they reach age 40.[3]

Apart from the effects of aging on the reproductive system, with the passage of time the various risk factors discussed in this and other chapters in this Part can also affect women's reproductive health. Cumulative exposure to these factors over time increases the risk of infertility, with implications for the fertility of older women. Moreover, the length of time between a woman's first sexual encounter and the onset of childbearing used to be quite short. This is no longer true; the period of time between first sexual activity and childbearing is now often a decade or more. As a result, the period for potential exposure to sexually transmitted diseases, and the consequent risk of pelvic inflammatory disease leading to tubal infertility, are greatly increased.

Separating the effects of biological aging on reproduction from the effects of other factors is difficult because they occur concurrently; the longer a woman lives, the greater her chances of being exposed to hazards and the older her reproductive system. The later the age at which a woman tries to conceive, the greater the chances that her fertility will have been reduced, either by aging or by the combined effects of biological aging and exposure to specific hazards on fertility over time.

Studies examining the effects of aging on female fertility have focussed on various aspects of reproduction, including the ability to conceive, to carry a viable fetus to term, and to give birth to a child without congenital anomalies. In addition, the effectiveness of various infertility treatments in older and younger women has been compared; such comparisons also help to shed some light on the relationship between age and fertility.

Conception

Although there are differing views on the specific ages and rates at which fertility declines, it is generally agreed that fertility declines as women age, beginning in their mid-20s through to the mid-30s, then more sharply in the mid- to late 30s. In the research, fertility is measured in terms of time to conception; in general, women in their mid- to late 30s take longer to conceive than women in their 20s.

Demographic studies of historical populations (using birth and marriage records) have been used to evaluate the length of time to conception and rates of sterility for different age groups of women. Such studies are useful because contraception and voluntary sterilization were not used to control fertility in these populations. However, these studies also have significant limitations; they do not take into account such factors as rates of miscarriage, marriage duration (with the possibility of reduced coital activity over time), the possible contribution of the male partner's age to infertility, medical histories, and reproductive impairment as a result of previous births, so exactly how applicable the results are to modern populations is not clear.

Despite such limitations, data from historical populations that did not practise contraception ("natural" populations) do provide a useful picture of the natural decline in female fertility that could be expected to occur in the absence of factors such as contraception. Figure 12.3 presents the fertility rates from seven populations — five natural populations, and the U.S. population in 1955 and in 1981. The data demonstrate that although the fertility rates vary significantly between the same age groups and time periods, the rate of fertility decline is similar among different natural populations.

The data from natural populations can also be used to give information on relative fertility rates; these are calculated by comparing the highest pregnancy rate observed within the population with the pregnancy rates observed in other age groups. Figure 12.4 demonstrates that fertility rates remain relatively stable until women are in their early 30s, beyond which the rate starts to decline. After the age of 40 years, the decline is more dramatic. For example, comparisons of fertility rates using data on women aged 20 to 24 years old as the baseline reveal a drop of 4 to 8 percent in the 25- to 29-year-old group, 15 to 19 percent in the 30- to 34-year-old group, 26 to 46 percent in the 35- to 39-year-old group, and as much as a 95 percent decline in the fertility rate of the 40- to 44-year-old group.

Data from natural populations (studies of 16 English parishes) also show that sterility rates rise with the woman's age.[4]

Another approach to assessing the effect of age on fertility is to study donor insemination of women whose husbands are azoospermic (not producing any sperm). These studies offer a way to overcome some of the major weaknesses of demographic studies, because the effects of coital frequency, the man's age, and the health of participants can be removed as influencing factors. The studies assume that the women are representative of the population, that they are healthy, and that the only obstacle to achieving pregnancy is lack of sperm.

One of the most widely cited of these studies, conducted in the early 1980s in France, reported on the results of donor insemination in 2 193 women who had not previously had a child. The probability of success after 12 insemination cycles using frozen sperm was 74 percent for women under 31 years of age, 61 percent for women aged 31 to 35, and 54 percent for women over 35 years of age.[5] This is not the only such study. A review of the four other studies available found that in the two largest studies[6,7] pregnancy rates (if compared to women aged 21 to 25 as the baseline) were similar for those aged 26 to 30, were stable or declined slightly among those who were 31 to 35 years old, and declined more precipitously after the age of 35. The remaining two studies[8,9] had very small sample sizes in the age group over 36, so the data were not as informative.

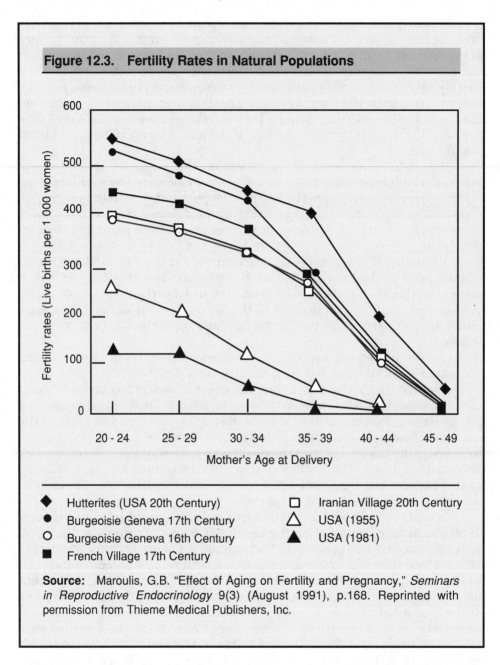

Figure 12.3. Fertility Rates in Natural Populations

◆ Hutterites (USA 20th Century)   ☐ Iranian Village 20th Century
● Burgeoisie Geneva 17th Century   △ USA (1955)
○ Burgeoisie Geneva 16th Century   ▲ USA (1981)
■ French Village 17th Century

Source: Maroulis, G.B. "Effect of Aging on Fertility and Pregnancy," *Seminars in Reproductive Endocrinology* 9(3) (August 1991), p.168. Reprinted with permission from Thieme Medical Publishers, Inc.

A Canadian study of 2 106 couples registered at 12 infertility clinics also showed the impact of the woman's age on the likelihood of achieving a pregnancy, finding that the woman's age is an important predictor of pregnancy success among infertile couples. If a woman was infertile for three years or more, each additional year in her age reduced the probability of pregnancy by 9 percent.[10]

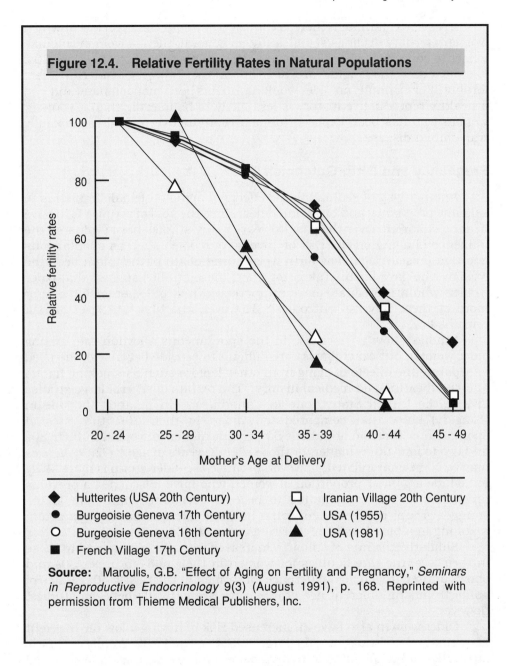

Figure 12.4. Relative Fertility Rates in Natural Populations

Mother's Age at Delivery

- ◆ Hutterites (USA 20th Century)
- ● Burgeoisie Geneva 17th Century
- ○ Burgeoisie Geneva 16th Century
- ■ French Village 17th Century
- □ Iranian Village 20th Century
- △ USA (1955)
- ▲ USA (1981)

Source: Maroulis, G.B. "Effect of Aging on Fertility and Pregnancy," *Seminars in Reproductive Endocrinology* 9(3) (August 1991), p. 168. Reprinted with permission from Thieme Medical Publishers, Inc.

The effectiveness of infertility treatments such as *in vitro* fertilization and gamete intrafallopian transfer (GIFT) has also been shown to be affected by the woman's age. After 40, pregnancy rates for GIFT decline greatly. As well, pregnancy after reversal of tubal ligation occurs less often in women over the age of 40 years (45 percent) compared to younger women (60 percent).

In essence, although there is controversy about the exact age at which women's fertility declines significantly, in general, then, a woman will take longer to conceive if she is in her mid- to late 30s than if she is in her 20s. Factors other than aging are also important, however, and can affect fertility. For example, an older woman who has been monogamous and had a healthy reproductive history is less likely to be infertile than a younger woman who has been exposed to such reproductive hazards as sexually transmitted diseases.

Pregnancy and Birth Outcomes

Another way of evaluating the effects of aging on female fertility is to examine pregnancy and birth outcomes, since the goal of couples is to have healthy children. Over the past 40 years many studies have evaluated the influence of aging on the risk of adverse outcomes such as spontaneous abortion (miscarriage), low birth weight, and death of the infant or of the woman who gave birth. Taken together, these studies suggest that older women who are pregnant have an increased risk of experiencing one or more of these adverse outcomes. However, the absolute level of risk remains low.

Studies show an increase in the spontaneous abortion rate among older women, but exact figures are difficult to provide because of the need to separate the effects of aging from other factors such as smoking habits and childbearing and medical history. The results of several large studies (five in the United States, one in Canada, one in Ireland, and one in Hungary) show that compared to women in their 20s, the rates of spontaneous abortion are about 50 percent higher in women in their 30s and two to four times higher for those over 40 years of age.[11] These figures may be somewhat inflated, however, because the older group is more likely to include a greater proportion of women who have miscarried a previous pregnancy and are attempting to become pregnant again than is the younger group; these women would be more likely to have a loss again, resulting in a bias toward higher rates among older women.

Similarly, the rate of stillbirth increases with age. Compared to those in their 20s, the rate doubles for women in their mid- to upper 30s and shows a three- to fourfold difference for women in their early 40s. Rates of stillbirth among different age groups vary dramatically between studies, however.

Older women also have an increased risk of having a low birth weight or premature infant or a very large infant (over 4 000 grams). This is attributed to higher rates of hypertension and pre-eclampsia (associated with pre-term infants and infants that are small for their gestational age) and diabetes (associated with large infants) among older pregnant women. Caesarian section is also more common in women over 30 years of age, especially those over 35.

In addition, studies have shown that rates of death resulting from pregnancy or birth complications rise with age. For example, U.K. data for 1985 to 1987 found that the mortality rate was 5.3 per 100 000 pregnancies in women aged 20 to 24, compared to 53.9 per 100 000 pregnancies in women aged 40 or over.[12] This still translates to a low absolute risk (one-twentieth of 1 percent), however, even for women over the age of 40. Also, recent studies have found that mortality does not increase with age if women receive excellent obstetrical care.

Finally, women who have children in their late 30s or early 40s also face a well-documented increased risk of having a child with a significant chromosomal disorder, such as Down syndrome (see Table 12.1).

Table 12.1. Estimated Risk of Giving Birth to a Child with a Significant Chromosomal Disorder, by Maternal Age		
Maternal age	**Any significant chromosomal disorder**	**Down syndrome**
30 years	1 in 380	1 in 900
35 years	1 in 180	1 in 310
40 years	1 in 60	1 in 90
45 years	1 in 20	1 in 25

Source: Adapted from Hook, E.B. "Rates of Chromosome Abnormalities at Different Maternal Ages." *Obstetrics and Gynecology* 58 (3) (September 1981): 282-85.

Taken together, these findings suggest that women over the age of 30 face a greater chance of experiencing a range of pregnancy and birth complications, although the absolute level of risk for most of these remains low until the woman reaches her late 30s. For women over the age of 40, the potential risks during pregnancy and birth increase substantially. Nevertheless, good obstetrical care means that the absolute risk remains small.

The Impact of Age on Male Fertility

Men do not have a biological end to their reproductive years and can continue to father children until late in life. Research into the impact of aging on male reproductive ability is limited, but such evidence as does exist suggests that there is a much less direct relationship between increasing age and declining fertility in men than in women.

To evaluate the effects of a man's age on conception rates, studies have been conducted using demographic data from polygamous societies where contraception is not used and where the norm is for a man to marry women of different ages. These studies have not shown a decrease in fertility attributable to the man's age.[13]

Other demographic studies have suggested that there may be a link between age and male fertility, although it is much less significant than for women. One study found that male fertility declined slowly and was still at 73 percent of the base rate of the early 20s when the men were 50 to 54 years old.[14]

Dominantly inherited genetic disorders are seen more frequently in the children of older fathers and are thought to be the result of new mutations occurring during the production of sperm (see Chapter 26). The nature of the sperm production process is such that there is a much higher chance of error in the copying of genetic material as cells divide and genetic material is replicated in the resulting sperm. For example, sperm produced by a man aged 28 will have undergone about 15 times more cell divisions than an egg ovulated by a woman of the same age. This is because sperm are produced continuously during adulthood, whereas all the eggs a woman will ever produce are present in her body even before she is born; each egg that matures during her childbearing years is ovulated and thus completes cell division only once. The incidence of mutation resulting from failure to copy a gene correctly at cell division is therefore much more likely to be related to the male partner's age than to the woman's, because the more times genetic material is copied, the greater the chance of an error occurring.

Down syndrome, on the other hand, does not result from gene mutation but from lack of proper chromosomal separation during cell division. The contribution of the male partner's age to the risk of having a child with this chromosomal anomaly is minor. By contrast, the egg may have been in "suspended" cell division — for up to 40 years or so — waiting to be ovulated; as mentioned above, the relationship between the woman's age and the risk of Down syndrome is very strong.

Implications

Current childbearing patterns have implications for the prevalence of infertility and the call for new reproductive technology services in the future. Women who wait to have children until they are in their mid-30s or older have a greater chance of having difficulty conceiving and complications during pregnancy; they also have a somewhat reduced chance of having a healthy child than women who have children in their 20s. These risks increase with the woman's age; a woman who tries to conceive at the age of 40 is more likely to experience difficulty than a woman who is 35.

Apart from the rise in the number and proportion of women who are having children in their late 30s or 40s, it is not known if infertility *rates* among older women are changing over time. The proportion of women aged 40 to 44 who have ever been married and who are childless declined slightly, from 10 percent in 1961 to 7 percent in 1981, then rose again to 11 percent by 1991. The data do not allow for an analysis of the proportion who are voluntarily childless; thus, we cannot determine whether infertility rates are stable, rising, or declining among older women. Future studies to track infertility rates over time will therefore need to be based on sample sizes large enough to allow for analysis of the incidence of infertility by age group.

> Professional and family life can be reconciled thanks to a host of measures such as paid parental leave, a universal network of daycares, and working conditions that are equal and respect the quality of life. As we know, more and more young women and couples are forced to give up the idea of, or postpone for some time, having a first or second child because of difficult living or working conditions. These young adults must enjoy better conditions in order to make the decision to have children. [Translation]
>
> *Brief to the Commission from Confédération des syndicats nationaux, November 22, 1990.*

Delaying childbearing to later ages in reproductive life could affect the demand for infertility treatment. However, couples in their mid- to late 30s or early 40s who find that they have a fertility problem will have less time to conceive or seek treatment than if they had attempted to become pregnant when they were in their 20s or early 30s.

In summary, healthy women who have not had a medical condition that could impair their fertility (such as pelvic inflammatory disease or endometriosis) have a reasonable chance of conceiving when they are in their late 30s and early 40s, although biological constraints mean conception is likely to take longer. Women's biology dictates a natural span of childbearing years; delaying childbearing reduces the amount of time available for a couple to conceive naturally. In addition, with increasing age, the risk of pregnancy and birth complications, while still low in absolute terms, will be greater than for women in their 20s.

Preventing Age-Related Infertility

People who want to have children should be aware of the normal decline in fertility as they age and consider this in their decisions about when to have children. Such decisions have to take many factors into consideration, but a knowledge of the biological realities of postponing childbearing should be part of the information couples have available when making this choice.

One approach is to provide the information in school biology and family life programs. Pregnancy-related public health programs, gynaecologists, and family physicians should also inform women of the impact of aging on their fertility. The curricula of nursing and medical schools should cover the subject in the context of maintaining and promoting reproductive health. Educating these professionals, who are an important source of health-related information for many Canadians, about this would help to make the information more widely available for couples who are deciding about whether and when to have children. Women (and men) can maximize their chances of having a healthy pregnancy if they consider factors that could affect their fertility (such as their age and whether they smoke) well before they actually try to conceive. Some physicians have begun to advocate getting pregnancy off to a healthy start by encouraging women to eat a balanced diet, not to smoke, and not to exercise excessively, even before they try to conceive.

Steps must also be taken to address the obstacles that contribute to the decision to delay childbearing. Interrupting a career to bear children is costly to women in terms of wages and status. Women who leave the workforce to have children tend to leave at a crucial time in their careers — between the ages of 25 and 35. When they do, they often pay an enormous lifetime price in terms of promotion, seniority, and skills acquisition. A study conducted for the federal departments of Justice and Status of Women found that a 25-year-old woman who leaves the workforce for two years to raise children will take 18 years to close the wage gap with a fellow worker who never left the workplace, at an estimated earnings loss of more than $30 000. The opportunity costs of having children — lost career opportunities, lost income during pregnancy and child care leave — together with the cost associated with raising children (which has been estimated conservatively at more than $150 000 to raise a child to the age of 18) and the shortage of high-quality, low-cost child care constitute major financial and social barriers that lead many women to delay the birth of their first child.

> Given the importance of children in our individual and collective lives, as well as what we know about the effects of age on fertility, having children earlier in their reproductive lives should be a realistic option for Canadian women, and one that is supported by social policies.

Policies to protect women who leave the labour force temporarily to bear and raise children are generally inadequate. This is especially true in non-unionized workplaces, settings in which a disproportionate number of women are employed. The lack of adequate leave provisions means that women must frequently sacrifice career opportunities, job security, pension vesting, and other work-related benefits when they leave the workforce to have children.

Moreover, few employers have programs or policies that provide assistance for employees trying to balance work and family responsibilities. Since the majority of women who work outside the home still assume most of the responsibility for child care and home management, reconciling childbearing with other responsibilities is much more difficult for women than for men.

The current imbalance in work and family responsibilities can be mitigated in part through work-related policies and programs that help both women and men balance their job and family requirements. Employers can be encouraged to support initiatives that recognize the needs of working parents. These initiatives do not necessarily involve high costs; they include approaches such as flexible work arrangements, job sharing, work at home, permanent part-time employment (with seniority rights, promotion opportunities, and pro-rated benefits), seasonal leave, information and referral to child care services, and paid leave for family responsibilities such as caring for an ill child. Work-related policies and programs must be designed not only to reduce the stress of family responsibilities on women, but also to encourage men to share those responsibilities.

Family-oriented work policies can also benefit employers. Employees who are relieved of the stresses associated with juggling work schedules and child care arrangements are generally able to work more productively and take less time off. Employers are becoming aware of the need to adopt policies that respond to family needs; some Canadian businesses have already introduced innovative workplace measures. However, despite increased interest and activity in such policies, relatively few employers have taken concrete actions to deal with work/family conflicts that may contribute to couples' decisions to postpone childbearing. In "Workplace Benefits and Flexibility," the authors of the Canadian National Child Care Study noted that despite employer awareness of work/family issues, many have been reluctant to implement policies that support workers in their dual roles.[15]

Employer initiatives are one route to flexibility for employees to handle work and family demands. Another option is to seek workplace changes through collective bargaining. Progress on this front, too, has been slow. The potential for change through collective bargaining is limited by the fact that only one-third of Canada's workforce is unionized and the fact that women tend to be under-represented in unionized workplaces and occupations.

The Women's Bureau of the federal Department of Labour has conducted research on the range of employers' policies and programs available for women and for dual-earner families in Canada. We support this activity. The Commission recommends that

> **32. The federal Department of Human Resources and Labour inform employers about and encourage them to adopt work-related policies and programs that help employees balance work and family responsibilities.**

and that

> **33. Federal, provincial, and territorial departments with responsibilities for labour-related issues review their legislation, policies, and programs to ensure that these provide adequate time for paid parental leave and that they protect employment opportunities, seniority, and work-related benefits for women who leave the workforce temporarily to have children.**

The lack of community supports, particularly child care services, may also be contributing to couples' decisions to postpone childbearing. In 1984, the federal government appointed a Task Force on Child Care to explore the issue of quality child care and adequate parental leave. This was followed in 1986 by a Special House of Commons Committee on Child Care. Both inquiries supported measures to address the problem — the demand for high-quality, affordable child care clearly outweighs the supply.

The special committee recommended that the federal government introduce a Family and Child Care Act that would complement the Canada Assistance Plan and provide federal funds to licensed child care centres and family day care homes. We support the intent of this proposal. The Commission recommends that

> **34. Health Canada, in conjunction with its provincial and territorial counterparts, introduce a comprehensive strategy for child care that addresses the need for licensed and affordable child care services.**

Child care may be the most pressing need for two-earner or single-parent families, but there is also a need to support women (or men) who choose to stay at home with their young children. Many Canadians recognize the need for public resources to be allocated in a way that supports people's choices about family formation and childbearing — suggesting, for example, that the value of child care provided by a parent who chooses to remain at home should be recognized through such measures as tax benefits for the income-earning member of the couple. Exploring the potential cost and other social implications of this proposal is beyond the mandate of this Commission. In our view, however, a caring society has a responsibility to consider the diverse needs of all its members and to support measures that offer families a degree of flexibility and choice in matters such as childbearing and child-rearing. Given the importance of children in our individual and collective lives, as well as what we know about the effects of age on fertility, having children earlier in their reproductive lives should be a realistic option for Canadian women, and one that is supported by social policies.

General Sources

Canada. Statistics Canada. Canadian Centre for Health Information. "Marriages 1990." Supplement No. 16. *Health Reports* 3 (4)(1991).

Canada. Statistics Canada. 1991 Census of Canada. *Fertility.* Cat. No. 93-321. Ottawa: Industry, Science and Technology Canada, 1993.

Canada. Statistics Canada. *Women in Canada. A Statistical Report.* Ottawa: Minister of Supply and Services Canada, 1990.

Canada. Status of Women Canada. *Report of the Task Force on Child Care.* Ottawa: Status of Women Canada, 1986.

Collins, J., E. Burrows, and A. Willan. "Infertile Couples and Their Treatment in Canadian Academic Infertility Clinics." In Research Volumes of the Royal Commission on New Reproductive Technologies, 1993.

Jantz-Lee, J. "The Physiological Effects of Aging on Fertility Decline: A Literature Review." In Research Volumes of the Royal Commission on New Reproductive Technologies, 1993.

Kerr, R. *An Economic Model to Assist in the Determination of Spousal Support.* Ottawa: Prepared for Status of Women Canada and Department of Justice, 1992.

Maroulis, G.B. "Effect of Aging on Fertility and Pregnancy." *Seminars in Reproductive Endocrinology* 9 (3)(August 1991): 165-75.

McFalls, J.A., Jr. "The Risks of Reproductive Impairment in the Later Years of Childbearing." *Annual Review of Sociology* 16 (1990): 491-519.

Touleman, L. "Historical Overview of Fertility and Age." *Maturitas* (Suppl. 1) (1988): 5-14.

Specific References

1. Canada. Statistics Canada. Canadian Centre for Health Information. *Selected Birth and Fertility Statistics, Canada, 1921-1990.* Cat. No. 82-553. Ottawa: Industry, Science and Technology Canada, 1993.

2. Sauer, M.V., et al. "A Preliminary Report on Oocyte Donation Extending Reproductive Potential to Women Over 40." *New England Journal of Medicine* 323 (17)(October 25, 1990): 1157-60.

3. Ibid.

4. Trussell, J., and C. Wilson. "Sterility in a Population with Natural Fertility." In *Population Studies: A Journal of Demography,* ed. E. Grebenik, J. Hobcraft, and R. Schofield. London, U.K.: Population Investigation Committee, 1985.

5. Fédération CECOS, D. Schwartz, and M.J. Mayaux. "Female Fecundity as a Function of Age: Results of Artificial Insemination in 2139 Nulliparous Women with Azoospermic Husbands." *New England Journal of Medicine* 306 (7) (February 18, 1982): 404-406.

6. van Noord-Zaadstra, B.M., et al. "Delaying Childbearing: Effect of Age on Fecundity and Outcome of Pregnancy." *British Medical Journal* 302 (June 8, 1991): 1361-65.

7. Virro, M.R., and A.B. Shewchuck. "Pregnancy Outcome in 242 Conceptions After Artificial Insemination with Donor Sperm and Effects of Maternal Age on the Prognosis for Successful Pregnancy." *American Journal of Obstetrics and Gynecology* 148 (5)(March 1, 1984): 518-24.

8. Stoval, D.W., et al. "The Effect of Age on Female Fecundity." *Obstetrics and Gynecology* 77 (1)(January 1991): 33-36.

9. Byrd, W., et al. "A Prospective Randomized Study of Pregnancy Rates Following Intrauterine and Intracervical Insemination Using Frozen Donor Sperm." *Fertility and Sterility* 53 (3)(March 1990): 521-27.

10. Collins, J.A., and T.C. Rowe. "Age of the Female Partner Is a Prognostic Factor in Prolonged Unexplained Infertility: A Multicenter Study." *Fertility and Sterility* 52 (1)(July 1989): 15-20.

11. Hansen, J.P. "Older Maternal Age and Pregnancy Outcome: A Review of the Literature." *Obstetrical and Gynecological Survey* 41 (11)(Suppl.)(1986): 734.

12. "Too Old to Have a Baby?" *Lancet* (February 6, 1993): 345.

13. Goldman, N., and M. Montgomery. "Fecundability and Husband's Age." *Social Biology* 36 (3-4)(Fall-Winter 1989): 146-66.

14. Menken, J., and U. Larsen. "Fertility Rates and Aging." In *Aging, Reproduction, and the Climacteric,* ed. L. Mastroianni, Jr. and C.A. Paulsen. New York: Plenum Publishing Corp., 1986.

15. Lero, D.S., et al. Canadian National Child Care Study. *Workplace Benefits and Flexibility: A Perspective on Parents' Experiences.* Ottawa: Health Canada (to be published November 1993).

Exposure to Harmful Agents in the Workplace and the Environment and Infertility

Research over the past few decades has demonstrated the dangers to the health of humans if they are exposed in sufficient dosage to various agents commonly encountered in the workplace and in the environment. When the Commission set out to investigate the impact of exposures in the workplace and environment on reproductive health, however, and in particular their effects on fertility, we found very little information. The actual contribution of most workplace and environmental agents to male and female infertility, or to reproductive problems such as miscarriage and congenital anomalies, is largely unknown: most have not been well researched.

Although the whole field of workplace and environmental hazards is characterized by a lack of information, data on the effects of workplace agents on male fertility are particularly scarce. Earlier, studies focussed almost exclusively on women's exposures, particularly during pregnancy, and on pregnancy losses or congenital anomalies. There are differing views on what underlies this emphasis. Some researchers attribute the research bias to society's traditional association of reproduction with women. Another view is that research on reproductive hazards has been used to justify discriminatory labour practices and policies that keep women out of the more highly paid jobs held mostly by men. Advocates of this view point to the fact that there has been less research about the effects of workplace hazards in female-dominated occupations. Whatever the reasons, the male contribution to infertility is only now beginning to be recognized and the effects of workplace and environmental hazards on it investigated.

The lack of both general and specific information meant that the Commission had to take a different approach to these risk factors than to others for which the evidence of an association with infertility is clearer. After examining what is known about the dangers that environmental and workplace hazards pose for various aspects of health, as well as the limited information that does exist on reproductive hazards, we concluded that this field will likely grow in importance as more information becomes available.

The Commission identified this area as a priority for further research and for expanded prevention efforts. Both must be planned and carried out within the broader context of occupational health and safety and environmental protection, and such efforts need to be harmonized across provinces and territories; a coordinated country-wide response at this early stage could help to avert future harm to the fertility of Canadian women and men. In addition, we believe that Canada should take a leading role in encouraging a major collaborative international effort to improve the state of knowledge about the effects of harmful agents in the workplace and the environment on human reproductive health.

> Canada should take a leading role in encouraging a major collaborative international effort to improve the state of knowledge about the effects of harmful agents in the workplace and the environment on human reproductive health.

Why So Little Is Known

There are several reasons why this field is characterized by so much uncertainty. The first is simply the magnitude of the problem. An estimated 67 000 chemicals and substances exist in the workplace, and we are all exposed to minute quantities of many of these chemicals in the environment. In 1983, the U.S. National Research Council identified 65 725 substances to which human beings are exposed, including 3 350 pesticides and 48 523 commercial chemicals. Testing every one of these substances to determine their impact on reproductive health would be virtually impossible, requiring vast human and financial resources.

Isolating the effect of specific agents is very difficult; multiple exposures are common in the workplace, and everyone is exposed to many chemicals in the environment, making it difficult to establish the effects of any one chemical on health or to find a comparison group of unexposed individuals. Moreover, the task involves evaluating not only the effects of individual substances but also their potential impact in combination with other chemicals with which they are likely to be found in the environment. For example, two chemical substances that have been found individually to have no adverse effect on human health may have a combined impact that is altogether different because their molecular structures could combine to form a harmful new compound.

The impact of other factors that may influence health must also be taken into account. For example, individuals exposed to chemicals in the workplace may also be exposed to physical factors such as cold or noise. Biological factors such as a worker's general health and social factors such as whether the person smokes or uses alcohol can also have a direct or indirect impact on reproductive health. Exposure to these other factors makes it difficult to isolate and assess the health effects of specific substances found in the workplace or the environment.

Another reason we lack information about the reproductive effects of workplace and environmental agents is that most studies have focussed on the acute or short-term effects of exposure to a substance or agent without assessing longer-term chronic effects such as reproductive impairment. Because acute effects are the easiest to assess, this is still the most commonly available information about most substances. Most of the studies that do address effects on the reproductive system equate "reproductive health impact" with "negative birth outcome" in the form of pregnancy loss or the birth of a child with congenital anomalies. Relatively few studies examine the effects of environmental or workplace hazards on reproductive health at earlier stages — such as irregular menstrual cycles or reduced production of sperm, delayed conception, or failure to conceive.

Several factors have contributed to the general lack of information on reproductive health effects [of exposures in the workplace and environment]. Traditionally, toxicological evaluations of chemicals seldom considered the effects on reproductive health. In some instances, pregnancy, miscarriage, and congenital birth defects were studied, but rarely did toxicological studies examine the effects of harmful agents on gametes, hormones, or, more generally, couple infertility ... This is also partly a reflection on our level of understanding of human reproduction.

There are many other reasons why information is lacking. For example, suitable methods to measure various reproductive outcomes and their associated health hazards have not been adequately developed. This has made it difficult to identify cause-effect relationships between suspected risk factors and adverse reproductive health outcomes. In some cases, this problem is compounded by a lag period of years or decades between the time of first exposure and the time the problem eventually arises. Further complications arise in the difficult, if not impossible, task of trying to sort out the effects of other influences on reproductive health, such as lifestyle or heredity.

P. Abeytunga and M. Tennassee, "Occupational and Environmental Exposure Data: Information Sources and Linkage Potential to Adverse Reproductive Outcomes Data in Canada," in Research Volumes of the Commission, 1993.

One way of evaluating the probable health effects of substances is by conducting laboratory tests on animals. These studies are valuable, but they have significant limitations that make it difficult to extrapolate their results to human beings. For example, the actual doses to which human beings are exposed in the course of everyday living are much lower than those usually used in animal experiments. Moreover, differences in the way species metabolize a substance may mean that what is harmful for one species is harmless for another. A third limitation of animal studies is that they tend to focus on the last stages of reproductive harm and do not deal adequately with damage to reproductive functioning that may occur earlier in the reproductive process.

In short, the existence of a large number of substances and the difficulty of testing them all rigorously mean that there are many potentially harmful materials in the workplace and environment whose health effects are largely unknown. In fact, no information on human health effects is available for the majority of chemicals now in commercial use in Canada and elsewhere. Even when data on a given substance exist, researchers may draw different conclusions about whether the substance represents a "suspected" or "proven" hazard to human health, or whether at "normal" levels of exposure it represents a health hazard at all. This is a complex field strewn with pitfalls; researchers must often overcome major hurdles and withstand criticism related to methodology, and research results are often subject to attack and reinterpretation by people with vested interests depending on whether the findings are "positive" or "negative."

> The existence of a large number of substances and the difficulty of testing them all rigorously mean that there are many potentially harmful materials in the workplace and environment whose health effects are largely unknown.

This brief review of the complexities facing researchers illustrates the difficulty of determining the reproductive health effects of substances and agents found in the workplace and environment. Since the data are so limited, the contribution of occupational and environmental exposures to existing levels of infertility in Canada is simply not known. Moreover, even for some substances or agents for which there are good quality data to show reproductive health effects in sufficient dosage (such as lead and nitrous oxide), information on the number of individuals who are exposed and the levels at which they are exposed is not available. Such major gaps in knowledge make it difficult to determine what preventive strategies are needed. Further, we do not know whether or what preventive strategies are needed with respect to many other exposures. Until we know more, we are not in a position to make good use of prevention or control strategies. This is no reason for lack of action, however.

There is an urgent need to mount a comprehensive research program, with funding and a long-term training strategy to develop new researchers, to address our lack of under-standing about occupational and environmental reproductive health effects. Canada is not the only country trying to deal with these issues in the face of major gaps in knowledge; this is an international problem with implications for the health of the human race. We believe that Canada should take the initiative in promoting a worldwide cooperative effort to assemble and analyze existing data, conduct new research, and draw conclusions about potential occupational and environmental hazards that face all of us.

> We believe that Canada should take the initiative in promoting a worldwide cooperative effort to assemble and analyze existing data, conduct new research, and draw conclusions about potential occupational and environmental hazards that face all of us.

Discussion here is divided into two sections, one dealing with workplace hazards and the second with environmental hazards. In each section we discuss the agents or substances that are known or suspected to be hazardous to reproductive health, together with strategies for preventing reproductive harm. In the final part of the chapter, we outline our recommendations for a major international cooperative research effort aimed at improving our understanding of this complex area.

Exposure to Harmful Agents in the Workplace

Agents that may harm reproductive health are known to exist in a wide variety of workplaces across Canada (see research volume, *Prevention of Infertility*) and the United States. The U.S. government has estimated that a potential 14 million workers are exposed each year to known or suspected reproductive hazards on the job — and this figure likely underestimates the situation because it is based on nine selected substances or con-ditions.[1] If the same level of exposures were occurring in Canada, an estimated 1.5 million workers would be exposed to potentially harmful agents in

> The lack of adequate research, the lack of thorough knowledge is often used as an argument against action. We don't think that inadequate knowledge or uncertainty should be a bar to preventive action. There is much that can be done even given incomplete levels of knowledge about reproductive hazards. That's the emphasis that we put because we approach this from the standpoint not of scientists but of representatives of the people that are affected.
>
> *J. Rose, Canadian Union of Public Employees, Public Hearings Transcripts, Toronto, Ontario, November 20, 1990.*

workplaces. Many Canadian workers employed in a diverse range of occupations are apprehensive about the possible effects of workplace factors on their fertility and their ability to have healthy children. The Canadian Union of Public Employees expressed its concerns to the Commission:

> Our members are speaking out because they *know* they are exposed to hazards at work. They read the newspaper stories ... [They] suspect they are exposed regularly to hazards that may cause infertility or adverse reproductive outcomes directly or indirectly. Unfortunately, since little is known about reproductive hazards at work, it is very frustrating looking for "proof" ... when workers suspect their reproductive health, or their children's health, is linked to their work. (*Brief to the Commission from the Canadian Union of Public Employees, November 20, 1990.*)

It is essential to acknowledge in this discussion that no work environment can ever be absolutely safe. There is always an element of risk to health or safety involved in work — whether it stems from the job itself, the circumstances under which it is performed, or the environment in which it is carried out. Reducing the risks to a very low level in many workplaces carries costs, but there are also costs (health, environmental, and financial) associated with failing to reduce the risks. Determining an acceptable level of risk involves consideration of both the costs and the benefits involved. This is a complex process, because not all costs of attaining very low exposure levels accrue to employers, nor do all the benefits accrue to employees. There may be costs to workers of setting exposure levels too low — for example if another process is substituted that is not believed to cause harm but does, or if the company becomes less competitive and unemployment results. No workplace can be made completely safe, but specific strategies can nevertheless minimize risks to the reproductive health of workers. The first step, however, is to establish what known or potential reproductive health hazards exist. As we have shown, this is a difficult and complex task.

> Employers have been more energetic in excluding workers at risk from the work site than they have been in reducing the hazards. Workers at risk has meant women of childbearing age, not just pregnant women. Industrial hazards that threaten reproductive capacity and foetal development and cause birth defects are not confined to the work place. Members of the community are also exposed.
>
> *C. Micklewright, British Columbia Federation of Labour, Public Hearings Transcripts, Vancouver, British Columbia, November 27, 1990.*

Current Knowledge

Reproductive hazards can be broadly defined as agents that cause reproductive impairment in adults or developmental impairment or death in the embryo/fetus or resulting children. Exposure to reproductive hazards may result in a range of adverse effects. These include delayed or prevented conception as a result of irregular menstrual cycles, sperm abnormalities, or reduced interest in sexual activity. Other potential effects include spontaneous abortion, pregnancy complications, prematurity, and damage to the developing embryo or fetus. Factors that may harm reproductive health generally fall into one of five categories — chemical, physical, biological, psychosocial, and ergonomic.

> Canadian employers are charged with the legal responsibility to protect the health and safety of their employees. They cannot do this effectively without adequate information on the possible hazards and how they can be prevented. We urge the Commission to recommend a massive education program about workplace reproductive hazards aimed at employers, workers, students, health professionals and the general public. At best, such information will lead to corrective measures. At worst, it will allow workers to make informed choices if they are exposed to known reproductive hazards on the job.
>
> *Brief to the Commission from the Public Service Alliance of Canada, Addendum II, "Workplace Reproductive Hazards," August 1991.*

Chemical Agents

Chemical substances can invade the body through inhalation, ingestion, or absorption through the skin. In women, a variety of chemical substances can cause menstrual disorders, affect the maturation and release of eggs, leading to infertility or sterility, prevent the implantation of the fertilized egg in the uterus, or interfere with the normal growth and development of the embryo and fetus. In men, chemical substances may reduce sperm count or affect sperm quality (for example, causing a greater number of misshapen sperm or reduced motility, making it less likely that sperm can reach and fertilize an egg).

Exposure to chemicals is not unique to workers in industrial worksites. Chemical hazards are also present in health care facilities (anaesthetic gases, solvents, medications), in offices (chemicals used in photocopy machines and other office equipment), in schools (cleaning solutions, laboratory supplies), in parks and other outdoor areas (pesticides, fertilizers), and many other work environments. In addition, as the discussion on environmental conditions later in this chapter shows, women who work in the home, and indeed all family members, can be exposed to toxic chemicals.

Among the chemicals or classes of chemicals known or suspected to cause reproductive impairment in men and/or women are the following: heavy metals; agricultural chemicals such as pesticides; polyhalogenated biphenyls; organic solvents; anaesthetic agents; epichlorohydrin; ethylene dibromide (EDB); ethylene oxide (EtO); formaldehyde; vinyl halides; and some hormones.   Metals that have been shown to cause adverse reproductive effects in human beings and animals in sufficient doses include lead, mercury, cadmium, arsenic, lithium, antimony, boron, and manganese.   Other metals that may occur in some workplaces, such as chromium, copper, nickel, and selenium, cause reproductive harm in animals, but their effects in human beings have not been examined.

In fact, relatively few chemicals — whether they are found in the workplace or in the home environment — have been investigated for their effects on reproductive function; the limited research has focussed for the most part on general health effects.   One chemical that has been investigated for its effect on female fertility is nitrous oxide, a gas administered with oxygen as a sedative for dental patients. In the 1970s, nitrous oxide came under suspicion as a reproductive toxin, but the studies that demonstrated this association were criticized for methodological weaknesses. A recent U.S. study, however, has provided good evidence that dental assistants exposed to high levels of nitrous oxide are less likely to conceive each month than those who are exposed to low levels of the gas.

Apart from isolated studies of this type, however, no information exists about the general human health effects of 70 percent of substances in the industrial environment, and even less is known about the effects of these substances on male and female reproduction. The National Institute for Occupational Safety and Health in the United States has records on more than 79 000 chemicals, but data on their reproductive effects are available for less than one-fifth of these chemicals. The quality and accuracy of most of the data have not been evaluated, which means that few conclusions can be drawn about whether they represent reproductive hazards.

Physical Agents

Contact with physical agents probably represents the most common form of exposure for most workers. Whether these agents have effects and, if so, what they are, are even less well understood than for chemical agents. The physical agent about which most is known is ionizing radiation (X-rays), which can impair reproductive function in human beings exposed at sufficient dosages; workers at risk of exposure include dental office workers, hospital employees, and scientists. Sufficient exposure to noise, temperature extremes, and vibration may also affect reproductive cycles, but it is not known what proportion of assembly line and construction workers, for example, are exposed to levels sufficient to have an effect or indeed what those levels are.   Although there is concern about the potentially negative general health effects of non-ionizing radiation and magnetic field exposure from electrical appliances and video display terminals (VDTs), there are no conclusive studies that show harmful reproductive effects.

Many studies have been carried out to evaluate any association between working with video display terminals and adverse effects on pregnancy. In most of these studies, no significant associations were found. However, the results of a recent study undertaken in Finland are worth noting. The purpose of the study was to investigate whether work with VDTs and exposure to low-frequency magnetic fields were related to spontaneous abortion. No relationship was found when VDT users were compared to non-VDT users. However, the study also measured the strength of the electromagnetic fields (EMFs) emitted by VDTs and found that the small subgroup of workers using VDTs that emit high levels of extremely low frequency magnetic fields were more likely to have spontaneous abortions than workers using VDTs that emitted low levels of these fields. The possible risk appears to apply to only a small proportion of users, then, namely those whose terminals emit high levels of low-frequency electromagnetic fields. It is difficult to determine the significance of these results in view of the fact that other electrical devices, including many found in the home, also emit this kind of electromagnetic field; some would estimate that women face greater risks of exposure in a well-equipped kitchen than in front of a VDT. It is clear that more research is required on the effects of low-frequency electromagnetic fields on pregnancy.

Biological Agents

Women and men who work in health care or scientific occupations with direct patient contact, laboratory exposure to infectious materials, or production of biological materials may be at risk of exposure to biological agents that can impair reproductive function. Some workers in non-health care occupations involving contact with animals or animal products, refuse collection, earth moving, and work or travel in areas where certain infectious diseases are present may also be at risk. Workers in some occupations (for example, teachers and nurses) have a greater chance of being exposed to diseases such as rubella, cytomegalovirus, and hepatitis B, which can cause intrauterine infections, produce teratogenic effects in offspring, infect the fetus, or cause spontaneous abortion. However, steps can be taken to prevent individual exposure to these diseases. Rubella immunization is offered to people, such as teachers of young children, who may be exposed in their work. Those who are at risk of hepatitis B through exposure to blood and body fluids can also be immunized to prevent infection. Cytomegalovirus can occur in individuals who work with young children, but several studies have indicated that women with such jobs are no more likely to have infants with problems than women not exposed; this is partly because their pre-pregnancy exposure may have already rendered them immune.

Psychosocial Factors

Psychosocial stress has been proposed as contributing to infertility in men and women for many years. Research has demonstrated clearly that stress can affect reproductive behaviour and function in animals. Psychosocial factors that can cause stress are found in every workplace; they include the number of hours worked, complexity of the task, the degree of supervision, and organizational structure. Their effects are very difficult to measure, however, because of the great range of individual behavioural responses to given conditions — what is stressful for one person may not be for another. Not only is occupational stress difficult to quantify, but the level of stress in people's personal lives also affects their perception of stress at work.

Studies on the influence of occupational stressors have tended to focus on male workers, examining health aspects such as the incidence of stomach ulcers, hypertension, and alcoholism but not reproductive effects. Only recently have studies included women and examined conditions such as job satisfaction, workload, and worker job control as stressors. Increasing attention is also being given to stress in women who put in a double workday — paid work outside the home combined with child-rearing and household management responsibilities.

In men, psychological stress can lower testosterone levels and has been associated with reduced sperm count. In women, stress can affect hormonal function, leading to temporary interruption of menstruation. Work-related psychological stress may also interfere with the sexual relationship between couples. A variety of sexual problems have been linked to psychological stress, including impotence and ejaculation difficulties in men, vaginismus in women, and reduced frequency of intercourse.

Job-Related Factors

"Ergonomics" refers to the study of the relationship between workers and their working environment, including such factors as the body position, types of movement required to perform a job, and forces exerted on various parts of the body when performing a job. Although the information base in this area is growing, there are relatively few studies of the effects of ergonomic factors on reproductive health. Heavy lifting and working in a confined position are known to pose potential risks to pregnant women, while shift work may interfere with women's menstrual cycles. For example, studies of female flight attendants have shown a high incidence of menstrual disorders (for example, cycles longer or shorter than normal), with jet lag and disrupted circadian rhythms as possible contributing factors.[2]

Preventing Reproductive Harm

The ability to have healthy children is fundamentally important to individuals and to society. Preventing reproductive harm must therefore be a fundamental part of society's approach to caring for its members. It is impossible, however, to separate reproductive health from overall health; workers' reproductive health cannot be protected in the absence of protection for their general health. This is not to say that if policy makers ensure that occupational health and safety regulations protect the overall health of workers, their reproductive health will necessarily be protected. In some situations, it may be necessary to develop special measures for particular reproductive hazards.

There is currently no coherent or consolidated public policy response to regulate occupational exposures that may affect reproductive health in any jurisdiction in Canada (see research volume, *Legal and Ethical Issues in New Reproductive Technologies: Pregnancy and Parenthood*). Rather, five discrete legal regimes involving occupational health and safety, labour and employment law, workers' compensation, human rights legislation, and tort law (civil actions in respect of a wrongful act or injury for which a designated party is deemed responsible) are in place at the federal and provincial levels to deal with workplace exposures. Of these legal regimes, occupational health and safety legislation is the major instrument through which provincial governments regulate exposures that may affect health in the workplace. These regulatory mechanisms were not designed originally to deal with exposures that may affect reproduction. They have been adapted on an ad hoc basis to address various aspects of the problem in response to scientific and medical findings as these become available and as specific cases arise.

> The ability to have healthy children is fundamentally important to individuals and to society. Preventing reproductive harm must therefore be a fundamental part of society's approach to caring for its members.

Given the number of agents present in workplaces, as well as the fact that reproductive dysfunction can occur in various ways that are difficult to measure, it is unlikely that policy makers will ever have complete information regarding the extent of reproductive impairment attributable to workplace conditions. This situation presents distinct difficulties in designing appropriate policies and targeted prevention strategies. Nonetheless, several preventive actions can help protect workers from exposure to potentially harmful substances, agents, and conditions.

The first approach involves eliminating from the workplace materials that have been identified as hazardous. For example, the use of certain substances identified as hazardous, such as the pesticide dichlorodiphenyl-trichloroethane (DDT), is prohibited under environmental laws.   This approach is limited, however, because very few substances have been identified with certainty as being hazardous.   It is evident that banning chemicals one by one after proof of toxicity will not be an effective or rational approach.

Although it would take decades to conduct scientific inquiries on the health effects of thousands of discrete substances, structural analysis can advance our knowledge base by considering information on classes of chemicals.   One of the methods currently used to identify adverse health effects is a process called "structure-activity relationship" analysis. Structure-activity relationship analysis compares the molecular structure and properties of a chemical with unknown effects to the molecular structure and properties of structurally similar chemicals with known toxic effects.   If we know that agents within certain classes of substances are hazardous to human health, then it is likely that any chemical within that family is potentially dangerous to reproductive health.   Although this approach has limitations, the use of this information could constitute a second approach for preventive action — namely, to ban particular families of chemicals.

A third approach is to introduce controls requiring specific steps in the design of manufacturing processes or workplaces to reduce worker exposure to known or suspected hazards.   This strategy attempts to minimize or eliminate the risk at source and is enforceable because design controls are visible — it is clear when they have not been implemented.

A fourth approach is to develop limits stipulating the maximum permissible level of exposure to substances identified as harmful at certain concentrations.   For example, radiology and laboratory technicians exposed to radiation in their work are monitored to gauge their individual exposure, and maximum allowable levels of exposure have been established, including for pregnant women.   However, this approach requires sufficient knowledge to establish what constitutes

> In our opinion, many infertility problems can be linked to conditions in the workplace. It is a fact that women are active labour force participants and that during their reproductive years, the vast majority of them are in the labour force and exposed on a daily basis to conditions and to an environment that can affect their reproductive capacity.
>
> Since our union also represents men, we wish to point out that certain conditions or elements in the workplace can affect the reproductive capacity of men as well. [Translation]
>
> *M. Simard, Confédération des syndicats nationaux, Public Hearings Transcripts, Montreal, Quebec, November 22, 1990.*

an acceptable level of exposure for most individuals, and, as we have shown, in many cases this information does not exist.

Each of these approaches has something to contribute; none is ideal or complete by itself. These approaches are not mutually exclusive — all are needed. The federal government has recognized the need to remedy the lack of adequate risk assessments. As we discuss later in this chapter, regulation of all new substances is expected to become more stringent as a result of the *Canadian Environmental Protection Act* (CEPA), which will create a national system for screening new substances introduced after January 1, 1987. This is discussed in the next section.

Although such an initiative has merit, we are concerned that the new provisions in the *Canadian Environmental Protection Act* may ignore the specific potential of workplace substances and processes to impair the reproductive health of women and men and the health of their children. Without adequate protection, there is potential for harm for all: workers and children could suffer the emotional and financial costs of reproductive harm; employers could also be affected, through either the workers' compensation system or tort liability; society could also have to bear the costs of medical and support services to help those affected. In line with our ethic of care and our goal of avoiding harm, we make recommendations later in this chapter with respect to these issues.

Design Controls, Exposure Standards, and Regulatory Measures

As alluded to above, design controls are one option after a determination that a hazardous substance, agent, condition, and/or process will be permitted in the workplace. Unlike exposure limits or performance regulations, which specify a measurable result that must be achieved while giving employers discretion about how to accomplish this, design controls specify the control measures that employers must adopt. These can include, for example, the isolation of hazardous agents, the physical enclosure of noisy equipment, or the use of specified measures such as ventilation equipment.

Design control regulations are easier to enforce than exposure limits because non-compliance can be detected visually. If these regulations remove the risk at source (for example, with ventilation equipment), they likely offer a higher level of protection than that achieved by setting exposure limits. This is particularly so since concerns have been expressed about the extent to which existing Canadian exposure standards actually represent "safe" levels for workers in general and for workers who may be particularly vulnerable to harm (such as pregnant women). In 1988, an estimated 2.2 million of the 12.6 million workers in Canada worked in jurisdictions where the exposure limits of the American Conference of Governmental Industrial Hygienists (ACGIH) have been incorporated into statutory provisions. The remaining 10.4 million workers worked in jurisdictions that either adopted ACGIH exposure limits initially and then began modifying them (for example, Saskatchewan, Manitoba, Alberta) or never legally adopted the standards and have been working to develop their own standard-setting procedure (for example, Ontario, Quebec). Of the made-in-Canada standards, only those for lead, radiation, and mercury take into account reproductive effects.

Where standards acknowledge the potential for reproductive harm, a two-tiered approach, establishing different exposure levels for men and for women of childbearing age, has generally been adopted. When health and safety officials have regulated substances deemed to be hazardous, they have done so to protect the fetus. Protection has been achieved by setting lower exposure levels for women who are pregnant or of childbearing age rather than for all workers. This approach raises equality concerns.

> Protection has been achieved by setting lower exposure levels for women who are pregnant or of childbearing age rather than for all workers. This approach raises equality concerns.

A recent U.S. court case with regard to lead is instructive about several aspects of the issues surrounding exposure to reproductive hazards in the workplace. At the Johnson Controls Inc. battery-making plant, the employer's policy barred all women, except those whose infertility or sterility was medically documented, from jobs involving actual or potential lead exposure exceeding the Occupational Safety and Health Administration standard. The issue was thus whether an employer could discriminate against women because of their ability to become pregnant. A lower court held that the employer could do so, but a 1991 U.S. Supreme Court decision reversed the lower court ruling. The Court held that an employer could not defend exclusionary policies directed at fertile women on the grounds that they are warranted as a form of fetal protection; it decided that such a policy violated the *Civil Rights Act* by discriminating against women on the basis of their sex, because it required only female employees to produce proof that they were not capable of reproducing, despite evidence of the debilitating effect of lead exposure on the male reproductive system.

The Court ruled further that the employer could not defend its policy on the basis of a "bona fide occupational qualification"; it was unable to establish that a woman's reproductive potential prevented her from performing the duties of her job. Further, the employer's professed concerns about the welfare of the next generation did not offer a defence, because those concerns could not be considered part of the "essence" of the business. According to the Court, it is the woman's right, and not her employer's, to balance her interest in employment against her concern for the well-being of future children.

Where exposure levels for reproductive hazards are lower for women of childbearing age, then, the employer may have an incentive not to hire women. For example, the employer could face potentially higher monitoring costs, or the employer might wish to avoid disrupting work arrangements by removing a female employee from a hazardous environment. Critics have also pointed out that focussing on the fetus reinforces the notion that it has interests distinct from those of the woman, as well as the perception that the state and employer should be able to intervene in the pregnant woman's conduct to protect the fetus. This approach diverts attention from the central issue — that exposure to a substance at a level that affects the fetus is probably harming the health and fertility of men and women as well. An approach that establishes different exposure limits for men and women ignores men's role in reproduction and the mounting evidence that the man's exposure to hazards in the workplace may result in reduced fertility and congenital anomalies in his children. The Commission therefore recommends that

> **35. Control of workplace hazards not be sought through discriminatory personnel policies, and that reduction of hazards be sought through the use of engineering and workplace design controls wherever feasible.**

Health and safety standards are effective only to the extent that they are respected. Because enforcement resources are extremely scarce in all jurisdictions, the probability of a workplace being inspected in any given year is low. The current approach to enforcement is one of persuasion; more stringent measures such as the power to issue compliance orders or stop-work orders or initiate prosecutions for violations are rarely used, yet they can be much more effective than persuasion. Stop-work orders put an immediate end to potentially dangerous situations because it is usually less expensive for employers to comply with the requested change than to shut down production. At present very few regulations are in place to control exposure to reproductive hazards in the workplace. However, we believe that stop-work orders and prosecution should be used more often by governments as a means to improve compliance with existing health and safety regulations.

The workers' compensation system can also play a role in encouraging compliance by creating financial incentives for employers to protect employees' health. Workers' compensation is funded through employer contributions; some workers' compensation boards have developed funding schemes that encourage employers to maintain safe working environments and penalize those who violate health and safety regulations. In some jurisdictions, these boards have the legal authority to impose penalties on employers whose claims costs are significantly higher than average among employers in similar industries. An approach that places greater emphasis on prevention would involve imposing penalties on the basis of observed hazards, before harm has occurred. At present, however, penalties are imposed only when conditions are detected that are unusually hazardous or that involve a serious violation of health and safety laws, and penalties may not be assessed until the employer has been cited for repeated non-compliance.

In our view, appropriately designed financial incentives administered through workers' compensation boards can play an important preventive role in protecting workers' health. An approach based on using penalty assessments related to observation means employers are less likely to adopt discriminatory employment practices encouraged by other types of approaches. For instance, penalty assessments based on claims cost experience may deter an employer from employing fertile women. Such discriminatory employment practices are, of course, against the law, but violations are difficult to detect. Implementing the other observation-based approach, however, will require that adequate resources be devoted to enforcement.

> **36. The Commission endorses the approach of workers' compensation boards that have established their employer contribution rates using penalty assessments based on observed hazards or health and safety audits. This approach should be adapted to include specific provisions for reproductive hazards.**

The workers' compensation system in each jurisdiction provides compensation for work-induced injuries or diseases, regardless of fault on the part of the worker or employer. To assess the merit of compensation claims, most boards have developed guidelines on what qualifies for compensation, identifying a list of diseases and conditions and a series of criteria, and often identifying the workplace processes in which exposure to a particular substance may have occurred. If the exposure and duration of exposure criteria specified in the guidelines are met, it is assumed that the disease or condition was work-induced, and the worker is therefore entitled to compensation. Claims that do not meet the criteria must be considered on their individual merits.

To date, no guidelines have been issued with respect to reproductive impairment. In theory, the principal reproductive impairments and injuries that might result in a claim for compensation include sexual dysfunction, such as impotence in men; infertility; sterility; miscarriage; medically recommended abortion because of a workplace exposure that could have harmed the fetus; stillbirth; and birth of a child with physical disabilities or intellectual impairment or who is at increased risk of cancer or other health problems. However, good evidence about which exposures are harmful is lacking at present; there are literally thousands of low-level exposures for which there is no reliable information concerning reproductive effects. This lack of knowledge makes it difficult not only to set policy but also for workers' compensation boards to adjudicate claims.

We recognize that the use of guidelines is controversial. In our view, however, guidelines that are developed carefully and implemented appropriately can improve the ability of workers' compensation boards to make decisions with respect to disease claims in general and reproductive impairment more specifically. We believe that workers' compensation boards should review data on the reproductive effects of workplace exposures and, where knowledge exists, consider using the information to develop guidelines regarding compensation for reproductive harm.

> That which is dangerous to a pregnant woman can also be dangerous to women and men prior to conception (affecting the ovaries and sperm). The [Confédération des syndicats nationaux] believes that eliminating the danger at the source and enforcing specific reproductive safeguards is the only way to guarantee that jobs are accessible to everyone and that our places of work are healthy. We would like to broach the problem of fertility and the workplace from this angle. [Translation]
>
> *Brief to the Commission from Confédération des syndicats nationaux, November 22, 1990.*

Information for Workers

In addition to regulatory and control measures, exposure to suspected workplace hazards can be reduced through education of workers. Occupational health and safety legislation in each jurisdiction sets out workers' rights in three key areas: the right to know about hazardous workplace agents, the right to participate in workplace health and safety decisions, and the right to refuse unsafe work.

The Workplace Hazardous Materials Information System (WHMIS), which became part of federal and provincial health and safety laws in 1988, is the legal mechanism that regulates workers' right to know about workplace hazards. WHMIS applies only to hazardous substances, not to hazardous physical agents such as radiation, heat, and noise, and requires that hazardous products be labelled and that they be accompanied by a material safety data sheet. Employers are also required to train workers in the safe use of controlled products and to instruct them on the significance of the information provided on labels and material safety data sheets. If a product is controlled because it is a reproductive hazard, then exposed workers must receive instructions on its safe use.

The federally funded Canadian Centre for Occupational Health and Safety (CCOHS) has also been an important source of information for workers and employers. It operates an international data bank and makes information on hazards, including potential reproductive hazards, available to employers and workers.

Different standards exist in different provinces regarding occupational health and safety. Companies with operations in more than one province must often function, therefore, under a variety of standards. Labour unions with employees in more than one jurisdiction face the same problem. It is important the federal government, in partnership with provincial governments, initiate a process that would allow for the standardizing and harmonizing of standards within Canada. This would eliminate the current expensive duplication of effort that occurs when each province reviews data and develops legislation or regulations to deal with various workplace agents. The Commission therefore recommends that

> **37. The federal government initiate and promote federal/provincial/territorial consultation and information sharing and, in cooperation with other governments, attempt to establish uniform standards in occupational health and safety across the country, in particular in relation to reproductive hazards.**

Worker Participation

The principal way for workers to participate in decisions regarding workplace health and safety standards and policies is through health and safety committees made up of employer and employee representatives. In some provinces, these committees are mandatory for all workplaces over a certain size; in other jurisdictions, committees are established at the employer's discretion. Where they exist, these committees identify situations thought to be hazardous, conduct investigations, and make recommendations to the employer about health and safety issues. In all provinces except Quebec, health and safety committees lack decision-making power. In Quebec, the committees have designated powers, including the right to choose the physician in charge of health services, approve health programs developed by the physician, make decisions about worker training and information, and select personal protective devices.

In no province, however, is there a mechanism for resolving disagreements between workers and employers. This gap should be remedied, because employers and employees may not always have the same view on health and safety issues, and, in most situations, the balance of power lies with the employer. This is a concern, particularly in the case of workers in non-unionized workplaces (mostly women), because if harms occur, they are suffered first by workers. The Commission therefore recommends that

38. Provinces/territories consider how their occupational health and safety legislation could be amended to provide more equal participation by employers and workers, with a view to reducing reproductive workplace hazards. This could include

(a) vesting health and safety committees with the same decision-making powers guaranteed by Quebec's occupational health and safety legislation;

(b) requiring that employers obtain the approval of the workplace health and safety committee for significant workplace changes; and

(c) identifying and appointing external resource persons with health and safety expertise for non-union or small unionized workplaces to provide information on health and safety.

Refusal of Unsafe Work

Although health and safety statutes vary by province, most give workers the right to refuse work when they have reason to believe that the equipment they are using, the physical condition of the workplace, or a breach of the act or regulations is likely to endanger them or another worker. Employers are prohibited from retaliating against workers who exercise their right to refuse unsafe work. In most provinces, the statutes do not give workers the right to be paid during all or part of the work refusal; Quebec and Ontario are the two exceptions. Workers in most provinces therefore face the difficult choice between performing unsafe work and not working and losing pay. The right to refuse unsafe work is exercised overwhelmingly by unionized employees. Non-unionized workers, who are disproportionately women, enjoy less employment security. Because they have fewer resources to support disputes with employers, they are much less likely to exercise their statutory rights (see research volume, *Legal and Ethical Issues in New Reproductive Technologies: Pregnancy and Parenthood*).

Quebec is the only jurisdiction whose health and safety laws currently provide for protective reassignment or compensation. Protective reassignment allows workers to remove themselves from situations considered to be unsafe and to be reassigned or compensated if alternative work is not available. The decision about whether the work is in fact unsafe is made by the Quebec Occupational Health and Safety Commission after a complaint is submitted by the worker's doctor and investigated by the local community health department.

In June 1993, amendments to the *Canada Labour Code* were proclaimed giving a pregnant employee or employee nursing a child the right to request reassignment or job modification should she perceive that continuing any of her job functions might pose a risk to her health or that of her fetus or child. Under the revisions, the employee can submit a request for reassignment or modification accompanied by a medical certificate indicating the expected duration of the potential risk and the activities or conditions to avoid in order to eliminate the risk. In consultation with the employee, the employer then makes a decision to modify the job or reassign the employee if it is "reasonably practicable." Should the employee's job be modified or she be reassigned, she continues to receive the same benefits and wages. If the employer decides that reassignment or job modification is not feasible, or if the employee cannot perform any work, she has the right to maternity-related leave without salary. The employee receives the amount available through unemployment insurance rather than full compensation through the workers' compensation system, as she would in Quebec.

Workers who have suffered some form of occupational injury are covered by workers' compensation and so are not usually permitted to launch tort actions against the employer. It is possible, however, for the spouse or child of a worker to be exposed to reproductive harm as a result of the worker's exposure. For example, workers may bring home toxic substances on their clothes or, through their own exposure, may transmit substances to a developing fetus. Spouses and children are ineligible to claim for workers' compensation, but they can sue the employer. They may also have a cause of action against manufacturers of the substance or product alleged to have caused the harm. In the Commission's view, however, tort liability is not a suitable instrument for encouraging employers to adopt measures to protect pregnant workers.

> In our view, the best way to reduce reproductive harm in the workplace is by developing a knowledge base that provides a solid foundation for definitive preventive action.

In our view, the best way to reduce reproductive harm in the workplace is by developing a knowledge base that provides a solid foundation for definitive preventive action. The fundamental problem is the lack of information on reproductive health in general and on the specific occupational factors that might cause reproductive harm. This information can be generated through research that seeks to produce new data, through analysis and linkage of existing data bases, and through expansion of the scope of existing occupational health and safety research to include reproductive health. At the end of this chapter, we outline recommendations for a research plan that involves these elements.

The Environment and Reproductive Health

Some of the discoveries and conveniences we take for granted in our daily lives (modern transportation, central heating, materials such as plastics) have come at a price. Many industrial products and processes and their resulting wastes have damaged the environment. There are also questions about the effects on human health of many substances used in consumer products and industrial processes that subsequently find their way into the environment.

Contaminants known to be harmful to human beings when they occur in sufficient concentration are generally found in the environment in concentrations lower than those considered to pose a health risk. Although environmental exposure to most harmful substances is low for most people, this is no reason to be complacent about the possible dangers. There is growing concern and some evidence linking exposure to agents in the environment to various diseases, including cancers, respiratory illnesses, neurological problems, and skin disorders.

We are particularly concerned about the classes of substances in the environment that are mutagens and teratogens. "Mutagens" are contaminants that may alter genetic material. "Teratogens" are substances or exposures that may affect the developing embryo or fetus and cause congenital anomalies. Our concern arises because many substances that could be mutagens or teratogens are used for industrial purposes and as a result occur in the environment. We do not have good information, however, about whether many of these substances have health effects, and we have much less information on their reproductive health effects, if any. A major challenge is to show causation of harm when studying environmental agents, since levels of exposure to hazards in the environment are lower than in the workplace, and it is difficult to find "control" populations that have not been exposed. Nevertheless, this issue is of critical importance to our future as a species. Data such as those showing a decline in sperm quality worldwide over the last 50 years sound a warning that must be taken seriously.[3]

Current Knowledge

Exposure

Human beings are exposed daily to both natural and artificial substances that could be harmful if they occurred in sufficiently high concentration. These substances are found in the home, in schools and workplaces, and in the outdoor environment — we come into contact with these materials through the air, water, and soil, as well as the food we eat. Low concentrations of contaminants are transported by air from various sources in the form of gas, fibres, dust, or other bits of matter. Human beings are also exposed to chemical substances in water; for example, more than 300 chemical compounds have been detected in the Great Lakes, and many of these are present in minute quantities in the drinking water of cities located on the lakes. In high concentrations, some of these are known to be carcinogens (cancer-causing agents), mutagens, or teratogens in animals.

Contaminants and chemicals can also enter the body through food and drink. They can be ingested directly or indirectly through the food chain. In the latter case, microscopic amounts of contaminants are absorbed by plants and concentrated there. They then become more concentrated in the organs of small fish and animals that eat the plants. Concentration levels rise as each organism stores the substance before it can be broken down and expelled by the body. This is referred to as "bioaccumulation." Through bioaccumulation, concentrations of substances can reach toxic levels by the time the chemicals are ingested by animals and human beings higher in the food chain. For example, DDT, a pesticide that bioaccumulates, has reached sufficient concentrations in certain geographic areas to have had a severe impact on birds' reproductive systems.

Polychlorinated biphenyls (PCBs) are substances that bioaccumulate; they are insulating oils used until the 1970s, when they were banned. Trace amounts of PCBs are still found everywhere in the environment. Studies have identified a relationship between the amount of local fish eaten by inhabitants of the Great Lakes Basin and levels of PCBs in their blood. One study found that the exposure of pregnant women to PCBs was associated with lower birth weight and smaller head size,[4] although another study did not confirm these findings.[5] Whether or not the long-term development and growth of children exposed to PCBs *in utero* are affected is not known; research findings have been contradictory in this area.

Human beings also absorb some chemicals and other substances through the skin. Although the actual amounts entering the body in this way may be small, absorption contributes to the total load — that is, to the total amount taken in through breathing, ingestion, and absorption. It is difficult to monitor how much of a particular substance has been ingested after exposure to toxic substances in soil and dust, however, and this problem has not been studied in depth.

Substances with Harmful Effects on Human Reproduction

The following discussion on substances found in the environment that in sufficient concentration may have a harmful effect on reproductive health is by no means exhaustive. There is a voluminous literature on suspected harmful agents, although in many cases we lack data on human beings and can only extrapolate from animal studies.[6] Because of the vast nature of the subject, our discussion is intended to be illustrative. It focusses on three factors — metals, pesticides and other chemicals, and radiation — that have been linked clearly to reproductive harm when individuals are exposed to sufficient doses.

Metals can be released into the air through industrial activities, the use of consumer products, and the burning of fossil fuels. Three metals stand out as seriously toxic to the reproductive process: lead, mercury, and cadmium. In 1982 alone, the use of these metals in the United States included 1.3 million pounds of lead, 3.4 million pounds of mercury, and 8.2 million pounds of cadmium. Pesticides, other chemicals, and ionizing radiation have also been associated with serious reproductive harm when they occur in sufficient concentrations. At least 50 chemicals currently in widespread use in U.S. industry have been shown to impair reproductive function in animals. These chemicals include the heavy metals mentioned, glycol ethers, organohalide pesticides, and organic solvents. If these substances occurred in the environment above recommended levels, it would be of grave concern.

Lead: Because lead is prevalent in the environment, it can contaminate food through direct deposit on crops or absorption by plants. Food is the greatest source of exposure to lead for most people. Chronic exposure may produce generalized but serious symptoms, including anaemia, impairment of nervous system function, fatigue, headaches, and kidney problems. Lead and its compounds have been shown to cause adverse effects in both the male and female reproductive systems. Studies have shown increased rates of spontaneous abortion in the wives of workers exposed to lead. The effects of lead exposure on female reproduction include menstrual disorders, infertility, spontaneous abortion, stillbirths, and neonatal deaths. Moreover, lead is now recognized to cause toxic effects on the health of workers at levels of exposure that only recently were thought to be safe. These effects have been shown to occur in workers at levels of exposure to airborne lead that are below the permissible exposure limit of 50 micrograms per decilitre set by the U.S. Occupational Safety and Health Administration. The current action level in Canada — that is, the level at which some action is necessary if lead is in the blood — is 25 micrograms per decilitre. This level is being reviewed by the Federal/Provincial Advisory Committee on Environmental and Occupational Health.

Children and developing fetuses experience much more serious health effects than the general population from given levels of exposure to lead because they absorb 50 percent of the lead they ingest, while adults absorb only 10 percent. Recent research has found that exposure to relatively low levels of lead before birth or during infancy and early childhood may impair intellectual development or hearing, cause behavioural problems, and result in smaller body size.

Mercury: Human beings are exposed to mercury largely through the food chain (primarily through fish), although workers in certain industries may inhale air containing mercury vapour. In the United States, an estimated 40 000 workers are exposed to this form of mercury in manufacturing and mining. At high concentrations, mercury vapour can cause lung irritation and destruction of lung tissue and may eventually cause central nervous system disorders. Certain organs, particularly the liver and kidneys, accumulate mercury more than other organs. The metal also accumulates (although more slowly) in the brain.

Exposure to mercury is known to affect fertility. Research shows that mercury affects sperm production and reduces fertility in male animals. Men who have been accidentally exposed to mercury have been found to have altered libido. Women with occupational exposure to mercury have been observed to have menstrual disturbances. In sufficient concentration mercury affects a developing fetus so that physical growth is retarded and the nervous system is impaired, resulting in motor coordination difficulties or cerebral palsy. The impact of low doses of methyl mercury (organic mercury) in particular may be subtle, including reduced intellectual development and problems with coordination and behaviour.

The risk of damage to the central nervous system in fetuses and children (whose brains are still developing) is especially high for Aboriginal Canadians living in areas affected by mercury used in industrial processes. This is because they may eat large amounts of fish or animals exposed to high concentrations of contaminants such as mercury. During the 1970s, Health and Welfare Canada set up programs to monitor their exposure to mercury by conducting blood and hair tests. High-risk levels were found in 2.5 percent of residents from 43 Aboriginal communities.[7]

Research has been conducted in Canada into prenatal exposure to mercury. Between 1971 and 1978, scientists analyzed a total of 520 blood samples from pregnant women and 739 blood samples from infant umbilical cords. All levels in the women were below 100 parts per billion, the maximum level at which no adverse effects are expected. Infant levels were higher, however, and included four results over 100 parts per billion. No abnormalities were detected in these infants, although the researchers did not rule out the possibility of longer-term development effects.

The federal, provincial, and territorial governments set guidelines for the consumption of fish that are more likely to be contaminated with mercury, and identify where these species are located. They recommend that pregnant women in areas of concern not consume large quantities of fish.

Cadmium: Cadmium is a relatively rare element that occurs naturally in the earth's crust. It is used primarily in electroplating metals or alloys to protect them from corrosion. Industrial and municipal wastes are the major sources of cadmium pollution. Heavily industrialized areas — especially those with nickel or copper smelters — have the highest concentrations of cadmium. Once in the body, cadmium accumulates and is concentrated in the kidneys and liver. Cadmium can cross the placental barrier between the pregnant woman and the developing fetus. Animal studies have found that high levels of cadmium cause congenital anomalies, changes in the testes, and reduced fertility.

Pesticides and Other Chemicals: Chlorine-containing insecticides belong to a family of chemicals known as organochlorines; the pesticide DDT is in this group. At high levels of exposure, pesticides can cause serious harm to human health. For example, dibromochloropropane (DBCP) has been shown to cause testicular atrophy and male sterility. The pesticides DDT and EDB are believed to cause adverse reproductive outcomes in male animals. Because of their chemical structure, pesticides do not break down easily, and they remain in the environment for a long time. As a result, they accumulate in the food chain and may result in toxic concentrations in higher animals and human beings. Organochlorines have been found to interrupt normal breeding cycles and cause congenital anomalies in sea birds and laboratory animals. Because organochlorines bioaccumulate in the food chain, they may have a significant impact on other species, but this effect has not been explored.

Laboratory tests on animals have raised concerns about the impact of two particular families of related chemicals: dioxins and furans. Animals exposed to more than a certain level of the most toxic dioxins and furans experience adverse health effects such as impaired liver function, cancer, and impaired reproduction, including congenital anomalies. The federal government has implemented a wide range of controls to minimize human exposure to dioxins, furans, and PCBs.

Chemicals known as PAHs (polycyclic aromatic hydrocarbons) at high levels can cause cancer in human beings. They have also been implicated in genetic change and problems in development.

Radiation: Radiation from both natural and human-made sources is present everywhere in the environment. "Background radiation" is emitted from natural sources, such as the sun's rays and various elements in the earth, and is impossible to avoid. Other exposures to radiation arise from technologies such as X-rays for medical diagnostic purposes, television sets, and video display terminals. There are three major types of radiation: ionizing radiation, non-ionizing radiation, and electromagnetic fields.

Ionizing radiation is high-energy radiation. It is commonly used in X-rays, in baggage check-in equipment at airports, and as tracers in nuclear medicine. Ionizing radiation can be dangerous to human beings in that it can dislodge electrons from molecules in the body, thereby creating ions that, in turn, can damage cells. High doses of radiation harm the body's mechanisms for defending against infection and may also affect the central nervous system. High doses of ionizing radiation are known to be carcinogenic, mutagenic, and teratogenic.

Non-ionizing radiation refers to low-energy radiation. It is emitted from a variety of sources, including the sun's rays, sun lamps, and microwave ovens. Non-ionizing radiation does not have the capacity to dislodge electrons and damage cells in the same way as ionizing radiation. Nonetheless, at sufficient doses it can penetrate and produce heat in human tissue and cause subsequent damage. Chronic direct exposure to sunlight, for example, harms skin and eyes.

Electrical power creates electric and magnetic fields. Electric fields result from the strength of the electric charge, while magnetic fields result from the motion of the charge. Together, these fields are referred to as electromagnetic fields. Virtually all electrical appliances emit EMFs. EMFs have been found to produce various physiological effects such as changes in the functioning of individual nerve cells as well as the nervous system as a whole. These findings have raised questions about the possible impact of EMFs on reproductive health. Exposures to EMFs may occur at work as we have mentioned with VDTs. They may also occur near power transmission lines, electric blankets, and many other devices. Reports available to date on adverse effects are quite speculative, and present indications from the scientific literature are that low-frequency fields hundreds of times stronger than those usually observed near VDTs, for example, do not produce harmful effects.[8]

Current Legislative Framework

The identification and regulation of environmental hazards fall within the purview of the *Canadian Environmental Protection Act*, which took effect in 1988. CEPA gives the federal government broad powers to define national standards for any given toxic substance in the environment. The act is intended to control toxic substances at all stages of production, including development, manufacture, transportation, distribution, use, storage, and disposal.

CEPA is administered jointly by Environment Canada and Health Canada. The regulations under the act are designed to control toxic substances in the following categories: existing, new, priority, and toxic. "Existing" chemicals are defined by the Domestic Substances List. The list, consisting of about 20 000 substances, serves as an inventory of existing substances.

"New" chemicals or substances are those that do not appear on the current Domestic Substances List. No new substance can be introduced commercially unless it is first assessed for safety. Companies wishing to introduce a substance not on the Domestic Substances List must notify the federal government under the New Substances Notification Regulations and provide enough data for its assessment. If, after assessment, a substance is suspected as harmful, the federal government has several options under the new law: to prohibit manufacture or import, to permit manufacture or import subject to specified conditions, or to request additional information.

"Priority" substances are chemicals that must be assessed before February 1994. A priority list has been developed that identifies 44 substances with the potential to harm the environment or endanger human health. Information on toxicity is obtained from animal testing as well as from studies of disease patterns in populations correlated with levels of exposure.

If a substance is defined as "toxic" under the priority review process, it is moved from the Priority Substances List to the toxic category and becomes subject to controls. These usually take the form of regulations, although guidelines or codes of practice may be used. The government may ban the substance, improve the safety requirements for its use, or limit how much of the substance can lawfully be discharged into the environment. Regulations have already been implemented for substances defined as toxic, and other regulations dealing with the remaining substances will be implemented on a continuing basis.

In addition to federal law, provinces and territories have their own environmental controls. The Ontario Ministry of the Environment, for example, recently released a list of hazardous substances that are candidates for possible ban or phase-out in that province.[9] The list includes contaminants that are present in or discharged into the Ontario environment. They are considered to be hazardous on the basis of their persistence, bioaccumulation, and toxicity. Most of these are carcinogens as well as mutagens and teratogens. A list of candidate substances for ban or phase-out helps identify chemicals that pose the greatest hazard based on their potential to cause damage to the environment or to human health. Where a ban or phase-out is not technically feasible, the province will seek to reduce the use or release of the substance.

Proposed Action on Environmental Exposures

The presence of a regulatory framework at both the federal and the provincial/territorial level provides a basis upon which to take action to protect reproductive health. We believe that two types of action are required. First, steps must be taken to improve our knowledge base. Research is required to identify the impact of designated substances and particular families of chemicals on reproductive health. Studies must consider a broad range of reproductive effects, not only pregnancy losses and congenital anomalies.

We believe that specific consideration of the impact of environmental exposures on reproductive health should be incorporated in the regulations promulgated under the *Canadian Environmental Protection Act*, as well as in the general thinking and approach of federal and provincial/ territorial departments of the environment and departments of health.

Second, action must be taken to ensure that concerns about reproductive health assume a higher profile in all aspects of environmental action. We believe that specific consideration of the impact of environmental exposures on reproductive health should be incorporated in the regulations promulgated under the *Canadian Environmental Protection Act*, as well as in the general thinking and approach of federal and provincial/territorial departments of the environment and departments of health. The Commission therefore recommends that

> **39. Reproductive health experts be asked to examine existing and proposed regulations under the *Canadian Environmental Protection Act* and make appropriate recommendations to ensure that they take into account reproductive health risks.**

and that

> **40. Environment Canada and Health Canada specifically include consideration of the issue of reproductive health in all actions undertaken to protect the environment.**

A Comprehensive Research Strategy

A major conclusion of this Commission, after reviewing the existing data on the effect of exposures in the workplace and the environment on reproductive health, is the vital need for more knowledge in this area. Until we have better information about what agents and substances, at what levels of exposure, pose risks to human fertility, and about who is affected, it will be difficult to develop rational or effective preventive strategies.

Canada is not alone in facing this problem. Indeed, the scope of the issue is too enormous for any single country to take on all the necessary research and analysis. We therefore propose an international cooperative effort to address the problem. There would be significant economies of scale and other benefits in joining forces with occupational and environmental health authorities in other countries to establish the range of tasks to be completed and the priorities for action and then to divide up the responsibilities according to where the necessary expertise and resources are located or can be assigned. This approach could apply to assessing existing data, conducting new research, and developing and evaluating preventive measures, with all countries participating in the effort benefiting from the results.

If this cooperative international approach were adopted, there would be no need, for example, for Canada to review the evidence on each agent or chemical independently; it would be more effective and efficient for groups of experts from different countries collectively to appraise the existing data on various substances. Several data bases that collect literature on occupational and environmental hazards already exist — they include TOXLINE and MEDLINE. What is missing, however, is any critical appraisal of the quality of the studies listed in these data bases or any overall conclusions about substances that should be considered general and/or reproductive health hazards. For example, the U.S. National Institute for Occupational Safety and Health has 79 000 chemicals in its *Registry of Toxic Effects of Chemical Substances*, as well as data on the reproductive effects of almost 20 percent (more than 15 000) of these, but the accuracy, quality, and reliability of these data have not been assessed.

> Commissioners believe that Canada should take the lead in initiating a comprehensive international effort to critically assess the existing data and studies worldwide and identify the chemical, biological, and physical agents that have been associated with reproductive disorders in animals or human beings. Such an effort could be important to the future of our species.

Commissioners believe that Canada should take the lead in initiating a comprehensive international effort to critically assess the existing data and studies worldwide and identify the chemical, biological, and physical agents that have been associated with reproductive disorders in animals or human beings. Such an effort could be important to the future of our species. This research analysis should be conducted to identify substances or agents for which data are (1) sufficient to classify them as reproductive hazards for human beings; (2) inadequate to classify them as reproductive hazards for human beings; or (3) sufficient to indicate that the substance or agent is not a hazard to reproductive health. This important initiative cannot take place without the leadership and commitment of the federal government. The Commission therefore recommends that

> **41.   The federal government organize and provide funding to a working group of Canadian experts in the field of reproductive health and workplace and environmental exposures, to work with the World Health Organization to initiate a cooperative international effort to critically assess the existing data on occupational and environmental substances that may represent risks to reproductive health.**

Where there is sufficient evidence to suggest that a substance or agent does pose a risk to reproductive health, programs must be put in place to monitor the number and locations of individuals exposed and the extent of their exposure. Occupations or industry groups that are shown to be at risk of exposure to a known reproductive hazard should then be targeted for preventive programs. Research should also be undertaken to determine current exposure levels to these hazards among various occupational groups, and, where problems are identified, prevention programs should be put in place to protect the reproductive health of exposed individuals. Accordingly, the Commission recommends that

> **42. The federal government, in conjunction with provincial/territorial governments, develop programs to monitor the exposure of workers in various occupations to known reproductive hazards, with the aim of developing appropriate control and prevention measures.**

Where the evidence is insufficient to categorize the reproductive health risk associated with a substance or agent, additional research will be required. However, given the vast number of substances that will fall within this category, priorities will have to be established. Assessment by an international working group, such as we have recommended, would be the most effective way to address this issue. Consensus on the potential reproductive hazards that should be priorities for further research would help to focus international research efforts in the most important areas of concern. Canada could play an important role by accepting responsibility for conducting the necessary research on some of the priority substances identified through this process. The Commission therefore recommends that

> **43. The federal government and its research funding bodies support research studies on the impact of designated substances and families of chemicals that are suspected of causing adverse reproductive health effects.**

A range of research approaches could be taken to evaluate substances identified as potential reproductive hazards. One approach, discussed throughout this report, is to make better use of data that have already been collected. For instance, existing computerized data bases containing information about workplace exposures, and about health outcomes or medical treatment, could be linked and compared to detect evidence of reproductive impairment, pregnancy complications, congenital anomalies, and so on. Record linkage studies using existing data bases could be done at relatively low cost, since the most expensive part — the data collection — has already been done. Studies have already been carried out that demonstrate the feasibility of this approach for specific purposes. Ensuring this approach is successful on a wide scale will require the cooperation of unions, employers, and governments and their willingness to allow such linkage studies, provided appropriate confidentiality guidelines are in place.

For data bases to be useful in record linkage studies, they need to contain specific items of information. For example, if researchers wanted to look for an association between people's occupations and the risk of specific reproductive outcomes (for example, low birth weight,

Consensus on the potential reproductive hazards that should be priorities for further research would help to focus international research efforts in the most important areas of concern.

congenital anomalies, spontaneous abortion), a data base would have to be available that provided reliable information on men's and women's occupations that could be linked to records, for example, on children with congenital anomalies. Efforts are therefore needed to promote the development of provincial health and vital statistics data collection systems that incorporate these types of information, and, also important, that have standard identifying information across provinces and data bases. As we have discussed elsewhere, Canada needs a system of administrative data collection that is structured in such a way as to allow record linkage. Only then will it be possible to do the necessary analysis of outcomes and consequences (whether after work exposures to particular hazards or suspected hazards or after treatment for infertility) that allow public policy to be based on reliable evidence. Statistics Canada has already done a good deal of work to identify what is needed in the area of health information statistics. For example, the 1991 report of the National Task Force on Health Information addressed this issue in detail. The Commission endorses its work and recommendations.

To be successful, research programs to identify and assess reproductive hazards must be undertaken by researchers who are knowledgeable about complex epidemiological issues. New methodologies that address the complexities of human reproduction will also need to be developed. No effort to evaluate the huge array of data about reproductive health hazards or to conduct new research on suspected hazards can happen overnight — the process will take decades and will require that new researchers be trained in this complex area. Research bodies such as the Medical Research Council of Canada, as well as Health Canada, could play an important role in this respect, for example, with regard to funding training positions and career scientists. The Commission recommends that

> **44. Research funding bodies, such as the Medical Research Council of Canada and Health Canada (National Health Research and Development Program), consider how to increase the pool of trained researchers qualified to conduct research in the area of occupational and environmental reproductive health effects.**

Thus, progress in developing knowledge and prevention strategies regarding risks to reproductive health arising from workplace and environmental exposures will require the involvement and commitment of a significant number of key partners both domestically and internationally. The Commission looks to the federal government in particular to demonstrate leadership and commitment, given its responsibilities with respect to international cooperation, its spending power to influence research and training priorities, and its capacity to promote interprovincial collaboration and harmonization. The Infertility Prevention Sub-Committee of the National Reproductive Technologies Commission could further explore needs in this area and define more precisely what steps need to be taken by the federal government. Its establishment will provide a stimulus to put in place federal initiatives in this field; it will also create a source of continuing public policy advice and public education in this important area.

General Sources

Canada. Environment Canada. *Canadian Environmental Protection Act. Report for the Period Ending March 1990.* Ottawa: Minister of Supply and Services Canada, 1990.

Canada. Health and Welfare Canada. *Health Risk Determination: The Challenge of Health Protection.* Ottawa: Minister of Supply and Services Canada, 1990.

Canada. National Health Information Council. *Health Information for Canada 1991: Report of the National Task Force on Health Information.* Ottawa: National Health Information Council, 1991.

Canada. National Task Force on Health Information. "Report of Project Team on Health Information Analysis: Potentials and Impediments" (Draft). Ottawa: National Health Information Council, 1991.

Fudge, J., and E. Tucker. "Reproductive Hazards in the Workplace: Legal Issues of Regulation, Enforcement, and Redress." In Research Volumes of the Royal Commission on New Reproductive Technologies, 1993.

Hubbard, R. *The Politics of Women's Biology.* New Brunswick: Rutgers University Press, 1990.

Jarrell, J.F., J. Seidel, and P. Bigelow. "Evaluation of an Environmental Contaminant: Development of a Method for Chemical Review and a Case Study of Hexachlorobenzene (HCB) as a Reproductive Toxicant." In Research Volumes of the Royal Commission on New Reproductive Technologies, 1993.

Landrigan, P.J. "Lead in the Modern Workplace." *American Journal of Public Health* 80 (8)(August 1990): 907-908.

Lindbohm, M.J., et al. "Magnetic Fields of Video Display Terminals and Spontaneous Abortion." *American Journal of Epidemiology* 138 (9)(November 1, 1992): 1041-51.

Schrecker, T. *The Pitfalls of Standards.* Hamilton: Canadian Centre for Occupational Health and Safety, 1986.

Sentes, R. *Canadian Occupational Health Standards: A Discussion Paper.* Hamilton: Canadian Centre for Occupational Health and Safety, 1988.

United States. Congress. *Reproductive Health Hazards in the Workplace.* Washington: Office of Technology Assessment, 1985.

United States. Department of Health and Human Services. *Disease Prevention/Health Promotion: The Facts.* Palo Alto: Bull Publishing Company, 1988.

Yassi, A. "Issues in Evaluating Programs to Prevent Infertility Related to Occupational Hazards." In Research Volumes of the Royal Commission on New Reproductive Technologies, 1993.

Specific References

1. United States. Department of Health and Human Services. "Leading Work-Related Diseases and Injuries — United States." *Morbidity and Mortality Weekly Report* 34 (35)(September 6, 1985): 537-44.

2. Preston, F.S., et al. "Effects of Flying and of Time Changes on Menstrual Cycle Length and on Performance in Airline Stewardesses." *Aerospace Medicine* 44 (1973): 438-43; and Cameron, R.G. "Effect of Flying on the Menstrual Function of Air Hostesses." *Aerospace Medicine* 40 (1969): 1020-23.

3. Carlsen, E., et al. "Evidence for Decreasing Quality of Semen During Past 50 Years." *British Medical Journal* 305 (September 12, 1992): 609-13.

4. Fein, G.G., et al. "Prenatal Exposure to Polychlorinated Biphenyls: Effects on Birth Size and Gestational Age." *Journal of Pediatrics* 105 (2)(August 1984): 315-20.

5. Rogan, S.W.J., et al. "Neonatal Effects of Transplacental Exposure to PCBs and DDE." *Journal of Pediatrics* 109 (2)(August 1986): 335-41.

6. See, for example, Roychowdhury, M. "Reproductive Hazards in the Work Environment." *Professional Safety* (May 1990): 17-22.

7. Canada. Health and Welfare Canada. *A Vital Link: Health and the Environment in Canada.* Ottawa: Minister of Supply and Services Canada, 1992, p. 40.

8. Muc, A.M. *Video Display Terminals — Do They Emit Dangerous Levels of Radiation?* Ottawa: National Research Council of Canada, 1987, p. 10.

9. Ontario. Ministry of the Environment. *Candidate Substances List for Bans or Phase-Outs.* Toronto: Queen's Printer for Ontario, 1992.

Other Risk Factors and Infertility

♦

We know that several other risk factors in addition to those already reviewed play a role in infertility, but the limited information available on these factors makes it difficult or impossible to assess how serious the risk is. As we have discussed, a lack of needed information characterizes the entire field of risk factors for infertility, but it is particularly evident for the factors examined in this section. In some cases, this is because their role in infertility has begun to be recognized only recently; in other cases, it is because we have evidence of their role in infertility and adverse reproductive outcomes when exposure is severe, but not in the milder exposures that more commonly occur.

Some of these risks are medical in origin, including diseases such as endometriosis and the unintended effects of medical intervention. Many of these risk factors, however, have to do with personal habits and choices: how the individual eats, exercises, controls fertility, uses substances such as alcohol or drugs, or deals with stress. Exactly what proportion of infertility these risk factors account for is not clear, but they are in the ambit of individuals to control. For instance, women who are trying to conceive or who are pregnant should aim to have moderate amounts of exercise, abstain from alcohol or drug use, and achieve or maintain a normal body weight. Preventing infertility by avoiding these risks is therefore both achievable and cost effective for the individual and for society.

Given the Commission's goal of consolidating the broadest possible understanding of all known risk factors for infertility, we surveyed the extensive literature on all these risk factors, selected the most scientifically rigorous studies, synthesized the findings to establish what is reliably known about these risk factors, and came to conclusions. This is the first time such a comprehensive review has been conducted. The review consisted of a thorough analysis of the extensive international literature and a synthesis of the reliable information that could be obtained from well-designed studies. In all, Commission researchers reviewed more than 500 studies. The conclusions and findings from this review, presented here, in themselves represent a substantial contribution to this field. They also point to the clear need for further research, as these risk factors are relevant to the choices of many women and men who would like to have children. We begin with what is known about the relationship between eating disorders and infertility.

Eating Disorders, Weight, and Exercise

Researchers have identified very low and very high body weight and body fat as factors that may influence reproductive functioning. In particular, an inadequate ratio of body fat to body weight has been linked to infertility in women who exercise excessively, diet to achieve a below-average weight for their height, or have an eating disorder such as bulimia or anorexia nervosa. Excessive weight has also been associated with infertility in women. There has been very little research, however, on how these factors affect male fertility.

Researchers are not yet certain of how these risk factors affect female fertility, but it is suspected that they may disturb the functioning of the hypothalamus and the pituitary gland, which in turn may affect such body functions as hormone production. Even though it is not known exactly how it occurs, there is substantial evidence that infertility may be a consequence of abnormal eating behaviours, excessive exercise, and under- and overnutrition. These effects can be reversed, however, by achieving and maintaining healthy weight and exercise levels and through improved nutrition.

Undernutrition and Eating Disorders

In the Western world, although undernutrition is associated with poverty, drug use, and chronic alcoholism, a substantial amount is also related to self-imposed dietary restrictions, poor eating habits, and eating disorders. Undernutrition and eating disorders may affect women's fertility in terms of both their ability to conceive and their ability to have a healthy pregnancy and birth. Severe nutritional deprivation before and during pregnancy places the fetus at risk; growth retardation, low birth weight, and death or illness among newborns are more common in infants of poorly nourished mothers. As well, the risk of a particular type of congenital anomaly (neural tube defects) is greater in the children of malnourished women who have diets deficient in folic acid.

Eating disorders such as anorexia and bulimia may result in difficulty conceiving, or in pregnancy and birth complications. Anorexia is a psychological disorder that involves extreme dieting to achieve weight reduction. Bulimia is a psychological disorder characterized by induced vomiting or other forms of "purging" such as excessive laxative use. One estimate is that 1 percent of young adult and adolescent women in the general population suffer from anorexia nervosa and that 1.7 percent suffer from bulimia.[1] The prevalence of eating disorders has been reported to be higher than this among infertile women: a Canadian study of 66 infertility patients showed that 7.6 percent had anorexia nervosa or bulimia nervosa, but further studies are needed to ascertain the frequency of eating disorders in women seeking treatment for infertility. The following discussion outlines some possible mechanisms for the association between infertility and eating disorders.

Women with anorexia nervosa often have primary or secondary amenorrhea (cessation of menstrual periods). Anorexic amenorrhea is not attributable solely to weight loss; rather, a combination of physical, psychological, and nutritional stress factors is involved. As well, it has been argued that the loss of body fat rather than body weight per se is a crucial factor. Women who suffer from bulimia have also been reported to experience menstrual disorders that could affect their ability to conceive. The combination of weight loss (although this is generally not as severe as that experienced by anorexic women), inadequate nutrition, chaotic eating behaviours, and psychological distress in bulimic women have been associated with reproductive problems (see research volume, *Understanding Infertility: Risk Factors Affecting Fertility*).

> A complex interplay of biopsychosocial factors appeared to influence the fertility of women who presented with eating disorders, who exercised, or who used dietary restriction as a method of weight control. Weight and percentage of body fat appeared to be critical factors that influenced reproductive functioning. A precise understanding of the physiological links was still unclear, though the majority of evidence suggested a disturbance in the hypothalamic-pituitary axis.
>
> S. Maddocks, "A Literature Review of the Physiological Manifestations Related to Infertility Linked to Weight, Eating Behaviours, and Exercise," in Research Volumes of the Commission, 1993.

Both anorexia and bulimia have been associated with problems in fetal development and pregnancy outcome. Adverse effects such as low infant birth weight, complications of labour and delivery, and increases in perinatal mortality and morbidity have been reported. A recent Canadian study reported on 74 women who had been treated for anorexia nervosa or bulimia, 15 of whom later became pregnant. The researchers observed lower maternal weight gains and infants with lower birth weights for the seven women who were ill with anorexia nervosa or bulimia at the time of conception. The eight women in remission from the disease at the time of conception were found to have healthier infants.[2]   Few studies have been conducted on the effects of anorexia and bulimia on fertility; information from this small Canadian study should therefore be extended and the findings confirmed.

Although eating disorders are much less common in men, it is theoretically possible that undernutrition may affect their fertility.   Although based on small numbers, two studies of 76 men with celiac disease and Crohn's disease (two diseases that affect the body's ability to absorb nutrients from food) found an association between nutritional deficiency and impaired semen quality and infertility.[3]   However, the drugs used to treat the symptoms of Crohn's disease (such as sulphasalazine) may have contributed to the results, and further research is required.

> Young people need to be aware that severe dietary restriction or eating disorders can affect their health, including their fertility ... Young women should be encouraged to identify and evaluate the images of women projected by the media and accepted by many in our society.

Serious eating disorders are tied closely to lack of self-esteem and negative self-image in women.   Unfortunately, women get many messages that they are valued for their appearance and that perpetuate unrealistic expectations about women's body size and shape.   A consequence of this focus on "ideal" body weight is that many young women feel that they could be more attractive or more popular if they could change their appearance to fit with what they perceive to be the ideal.   This same preoccupation leads many young women to smoke as a means of "controlling" their weight.   While severe forms of dieting are clearly linked to infertility, again we lack data on whether the dieting that many young women engage in has any impact on fertility.

Young people need to be aware that severe dietary restriction or eating disorders can affect their health, including their fertility.   As is the case with sexuality education, this information is best presented in the context of developing individual self-confidence and self-esteem.   Young women should be encouraged to identify and evaluate the images of women projected by the media and accepted by many in our society.   The Commission recommends that

> **45.   Health Canada initiate and promote consultation and information sharing with provincial/territorial ministries of health and education to ensure that goals and objectives for health education incorporate information about the effects of severe dietary restrictions and severe weight**

> control on health and fertility. This information
> should be conveyed in a context that
> encourages young people to question popular
> myths about female beauty and to develop a
> healthy sense of self-acceptance.

Most obese women are fertile, but obesity has also been reported to be associated with anovulation and menstrual cycle disturbances. There is some evidence that obesity is more common among infertile women. One study of 312 sterile women found that 8.7 percent were obese.[4] Negative effects on pregnancy development occur among obese women (mainly the risk of high blood pressure), and such women may also give birth to infants that are large for their gestational age, although this is generally considered a less serious problem than low birth weight.

Mild reproductive disturbances in obese men have also been reported by researchers; for example, testosterone levels have been reported to decline, which might affect sperm production or sperm function. More research is required on the relationship between male obesity and fertility.

We have already noted that a proportion of women undergoing infertility treatment have an eating disorder that could have affected their fertility. These women need to be informed of the importance of eating a healthy diet and achieving a normal weight to their wish to conceive and have a healthy pregnancy. Physicians and other health care workers should include weight and diet assessment as a part of the preliminary investigation preceding infertility treatment. The Commission recommends that

> 46. **Physicians and health care workers ask women
>   who are seeking infertility treatment about their
>   eating habits to determine whether their diet and
>   weight may be factors contributing to their
>   infertility. Women who are severely underweight
>   or overweight should be encouraged to restore
>   their weight to a normal level for a reasonable
>   time to see if they still do not become pregnant
>   before embarking on any form of fertility
>   treatment; counselling and support to help them
>   accomplish this goal should be made available.**

Excessive Exercise

There is no association between moderate exercise (for example, up to 60 minutes per day) and ovulatory dysfunction. However, excessive exercise may cause delayed onset of menstrual periods, the absence of menstrual periods, and other problems that would make establishing a pregnancy difficult or impossible. Studies have consistently reported an association between infertility and vigorous extended daily exercise (for example, more than 60 minutes per day of running, aerobics, tennis, or downhill skiing). Infertility resulting from this level of exercise is reversible, however.

Researchers have not established an accurate estimate of the prevalence of exercise-induced infertility among women. Surveys show that the incidence of menstrual irregularities among competitive athletes ranges from 1 to 50 percent, compared to the estimated 2 to 5 percent in the general population. These widely varying results are attributable to differences in the way researchers define menstrual dysfunction and are influenced by whether the training intensity of the athletes is taken into consideration.

Some have hypothesized that certain risks to fetal development and pregnancy outcome may be associated with prolonged excessive exercise during pregnancy. These include hyperthermia leading to teratogenesis, miscarriage, premature rupture of membranes, placental abruption (premature separation of placenta), premature labour, and long-term low oxygen supply to the fetus (hypoxia).[5] Normal levels of activity during pregnancy do not carry these risks.

In summary, excessive strenuous exercise can have negative effects on fertility and pregnancy, but infertility associated with this factor is reversible. Pregnant women or women who are trying to conceive should be encouraged to undertake *moderate* exercise, as this is beneficial, but prolonged intensive daily exercise should be avoided. The Commission recommends that

47. (a) **Physicians and other health care workers inform women of reproductive age of the possible effects of excessive exercise on their fertility; if they are trying to conceive or are pregnant, they should exercise in moderation.**

    (b) **Physicians and health care workers routinely evaluate the exercise history of women seeking infertility treatment to determine whether excessive exercise (more than 60 minutes of vigorous activity per day) might be a contributing factor in their infertility. Women who are exercising to this extent, including high-performance**

athletes, should be encouraged to reduce their level of activity to a moderate level to restore their fertility. This should be a first step before any form of fertility treatment is attempted.

Endometriosis

Endometriosis is a chronic condition in which endometrium (the tissue lining the uterus) is found in other parts of the body, including the fallopian tubes, the ovaries, the ligaments that suspend the uterus, the outside of the uterus itself, and, in severe cases, the intestines, bowel, and bladder. The endometrial tissue in these locations can bleed during menstruation, but the tissue and blood remain trapped in the body, and this may cause inflammation, the formation of cysts and scar tissue, and consequent medical problems.   While many women with endometriosis have no symptoms, in others the symptoms include chronic pelvic pain, pain during sexual intercourse, and painful menstrual periods, bowel movements, and urination. Physicians classify endometriosis according to stages: Stage I (minimal disease), Stage II (mild disease), Stage III (moderate disease), and Stage IV (severe disease). The disease is generally thought to be progressive if left untreated, but whether in fact this is the case is not clear. Endometriosis has also been identified as a risk factor for infertility, but again the exact relationship is not clear. There is clear evidence that it can cause infertility when anatomical distortion or obstruction of the fallopian tubes occurs. Whether the presence of endometrial implants alone, without distortion or disruption of the fallopian tubes, can cause infertility is not known definitively, but it appears much less likely. Some women with mild endometriosis have difficulty conceiving, but others with mild or even moderate endometriosis do not experience any difficulty becoming pregnant.

In the past endometriosis was considered a "career woman's disease" because it was diagnosed most often in childless women between the ages of 30 and 40. It is now known that this is false; endometriosis can affect any woman and is relatively common among adolescents.   Estimating the prevalence of endometriosis among women of reproductive age is difficult because many experience symptoms long before they seek help

> Some women with mild endometriosis have difficulty conceiving, but others with mild or even moderate endometriosis do not experience any difficulty becoming pregnant.

from a doctor, while others experience no symptoms at all. Despite these limitations, researchers estimate that 10 to 20 percent of all women of reproductive age have endometriosis.[6] It is therefore not surprising that endometriosis is often identified during preliminary infertility investigations: between 10 and 40 percent of infertile women are found to have endometriosis (see research volume, *Understanding Infertility: Risk Factors Affecting Fertility*); one study puts the incidence rate at 14 percent.[7] The answer to the key question of whether the condition is more common among infertile women than among fertile women has not been established, however. Women experiencing difficulty conceiving are usually investigated using procedures such as laparoscopy, so that if endometriosis is present it will be identified; it would not be justifiable to investigate healthy women in the same way, however, simply to establish whether they are more or less likely to have endometriosis.

Some clinicians consider endometriosis (even mild endometriosis, which causes no visible obstructions) that is found to co-exist with infertility to be its cause. The available evidence does not show a causal relationship, however, and a comprehensive investigation of potential factors in a large group of infertile women showed that endometriosis without adhesions did not alter the cumulative conception rate.[8] Nor does medical treatment of endometriosis enhance the chances of conception in infertile women. However, additional research is required to confirm this conclusion further.

In contrast to milder forms of the condition, it is quite clear that endometriosis that produces visible anatomic distortions and scarring to the reproductive organs and surrounding areas within the pelvic cavity does cause infertility. Bands of scar tissue can impair the function of the ovaries and fallopian tubes by binding them together. Scar tissue can also interfere with the release of eggs from the ovaries or the pick-up of the eggs by the finger-like fimbria at the end of the fallopian tubes. A further barrier to pregnancy is that severe endometriosis can make sexual intercourse very painful.

> Medical investigators have developed a general understanding of basic cellular activities within peritoneal fluid during the menstrual cycle, and they have ascertained that both the peritoneal fluid environment and the reproductive cycles of infertile women with endometriosis are dysfunctional in comparison to those of healthy women. However, as yet, investigators offer only suggestions for the cause of the defects, and for the specific relationship or relationships between minimal or mild endometriosis and infertility, projecting that future research will confirm or modify their theories.
>
> *A. Ponchuk, "The Physiological Links Between Endometriosis and Infertility: Review of the Medical Literature and Annotated Bibliography (1985-1990)," in Research Volumes of the Commission, 1993.*

There is no "cure" for endometriosis; physicians can only reduce the symptoms of the disease, by surgically removing endometrial tissue that has implanted outside the uterus, or by using drug therapy.   Drugs commonly prescribed for endometriosis suppress ovulation, preventing the monthly build-up and shedding of endometrial tissue, and are effective in reducing pain. Drug treatment is thought to help cause the implants to shrink and disappear, but there is no evidence that this is effective in treating infertility.

Researchers have considered how endometriosis might affect reproduction. Both the peritoneal fluid environment and the reproductive cycles of infertile women with endometriosis have been shown to vary from what is considered normal. Researchers have reported abnormalities in some of the phases in the menstrual cycle in women with endometriosis; this in turn may affect their fertility. As well, variations in the volume and content of peritoneal fluid in the cavity surrounding the internal organs have been observed that might help explain the occurrence of endometriosis and a relationship between endometriosis and infertility. A link between the altered peritoneal environment of women with endometriosis and the survival and motility of sperm within their bodies has also been suggested. This alteration might cause problems with sperm-egg interaction, embryo implantation, or early embryonic development, or it may cause spontaneous abortion.

So many mechanisms have been proposed to explain the occurrence of minimal or mild endometriosis that this, in itself, is evidence that we do not yet understand what leads to this condition. It is clear that further research is needed in such areas as the possible contribution of abnormalities in peritoneal fluid in the development of endometriosis. It may also be that multiple co-existing factors are responsible for both endometriosis and infertility. It is evident that we know little in a definitive way about this condition and that it needs to be studied further.

Since the causes of endometriosis are not well understood, it is impossible to know how to prevent women from developing endometriosis and thus reduce the prevalence of infertility resulting from severe forms of this disease.   However, educational efforts could help to inform women of the possible impact of endometriosis on their fertility and encourage them to consider this in making their childbearing plans.   For example, one 1990 survey found that only about half the 618 Canadian women interviewed

Since the causes of endometriosis are not well understood, it is impossible to know how to prevent women from developing endometriosis and thus reduce the prevalence of infertility resulting from severe forms of this disease. However, educational efforts could help to inform women of the possible impact of endometriosis on their fertility and encourage them to consider this in making their childbearing plans.

knew about endometriosis. Another quarter of the women recognized the term, but knew little or nothing about the condition.[9] Such a finding suggests a need for efforts to inform women of the symptoms of endometriosis, and the need to provide information about the possible impact on their fertility to those with the condition. The Commission recommends that

> **48. Health professionals such as physicians, gynaecologists, and nurses ensure that women who have endometriosis know about the possible implications of the condition for their fertility so that they can take this information into account when making their childbearing plans.**

Substance Use and Abuse

Alcohol

Many studies have confirmed the existence of an association between chronic alcohol abuse and negative effects on male reproductive function, such as impotence, testicular atrophy (shrinking of the testes), sperm abnormalities, and reduced sperm production. Chronic alcohol use by men has also been associated with a reduction in testosterone levels, even after only a few months of daily alcohol consumption. Exactly what level of alcohol consumption produces these problems is not known, however. It is therefore clear that people who abuse alcohol are more likely to experience reproductive problems. Whether the amounts of alcohol that Canadians commonly consume have an effect on their reproductive health is not known.

The situation is similar with regard to women — chronic alcoholism has been associated with menstrual irregularities — but researchers have not found any statistically significant associations between low or moderate levels of alcohol intake and a woman's ability to conceive.

However, the risks associated with heavy alcohol consumption (defined as more than six drinks, glasses of wine, or bottles of beer per day)[10] during pregnancy are well documented; they include spontaneous abortion and fetal anomalies. The evidence is also clear that heavy drinking has a high risk of causing alcohol-related birth anomalies, ranging from full fetal alcohol syndrome (growth retardation, central nervous system dysfunction, characteristic facial anomalies, and often congenital heart disease) to one or more of such problems. Fetal alcohol syndrome is reported to be the third most common known cause of congenital anomalies and mental retardation in newborns.[11] It is also the most preventable cause of these conditions. At any given level of alcohol intake during pregnancy, far more children will have alcohol-related birth anomalies than will have full fetal alcohol syndrome. As a result, many more children in the population will have intellectual deficits and minor physical problems than will have the full syndrome. The proportion of children affected decreases with reduced levels of alcohol intake, so that at less than two drinks per day the risk of these problems is minimal. At the same time, results of animal studies suggest that even a single episode of heavy drinking at a critical time in pregnancy may cause fetal damage.

Alcohol Consumption in Canada

The prevalence of alcohol consumption has declined slightly over the last 10 years in Canada. This has occurred largely among the younger and older segments of the population: between 1985 and 1989 the proportion of young people between the ages of 15 and 19 who were current drinkers dropped from 81 percent to 74 percent. Regardless of age, a higher percentage of men than women consume alcohol; men also consume alcohol more frequently and in greater quantities.

On average, Canadians consume 3.7 drinks per week. The Addiction Research Foundation estimates that approximately 477 000 Canadian adults (3 percent of the adult population) are alcoholics; 70 percent of these are men.

Efforts to prevent alcohol abuse, and thus to reduce the impact of alcohol as a risk factor for infertility and adverse birth effects such as fetal alcohol syndrome, must begin with young people. The earlier people start drinking regularly, the more likely they are to develop alcohol problems. *Opportunities for Health: A Report on Youth,* from the Chief Medical Officer of Health, published by the Ontario Ministry of Health, suggests that although the number of young people who drink has declined over the past few years, binge and problem drinking have increased.

To reduce alcohol consumption among young people, a comprehensive strategy is required that involves programs to influence both the environment and the individual. The social conditions and personal circumstances that lead individuals to abuse alcohol need to be recognized and addressed. Easy access to alcohol and the glamorization of drinking through advertising and the media promote consumption. Preventive efforts designed to influence the environment can include, for example, limiting access to alcohol by strictly enforcing drinking age regulations. School policies and programs can also help shape young people's attitudes toward alcohol consumption; providing leisure and recreation activities as an alternative to adolescent drinking and teaching young people in health education programs how and why to avoid alcohol use are necessary components of a strategy to prevent alcohol abuse. The Commission recommends that

> **49. Health Canada, in cooperation with provincial/territorial ministries of health and education, review and evaluate existing programs to reduce alcohol consumption among young people and, where necessary, develop new or improved initiatives to accomplish this objective.**

Educational efforts are also necessary to inform women of the adverse effects of alcohol consumption during pregnancy. Women who are hoping to conceive or for whom pregnancy is a possibility should be aware that much of fetal development occurs before they are even aware or certain they are pregnant. Strongly worded labels on alcoholic beverages, advising pregnant women of the risks of consuming alcohol during pregnancy, may reduce the likelihood that those who wish to conceive or who are pregnant will drink alcoholic beverages. A 1987 report by the U.S. Department of Health and Human Services concluded that health warning labels can have an impact on consumers if the labels are designed effectively. In the United States, manufacturers of alcoholic beverages are now required by law to include warnings about the risks of alcohol consumption to pregnant women and fetuses.

In Canada, no such law exists, although a pilot project is under way to evaluate whether labelling influences drinking behaviours. Alcohol consumption represents more than a risk to fertility; the dangers associated with drinking and driving are also cause for concern, and chronic alcohol consumption is associated with a host of other adverse health risks. It would therefore make sense to have warnings regarding all these risks on alcohol labels, similar to the approach that has been taken with health warnings on cigarette packages. Warnings about the effects of alcohol on fertility should not be directed solely to women — men too have fertility risks from chronic alcohol consumption, and both sexes are at risk from the range of other adverse health effects. If the results of the pilot project show they have an effect, the Commission recommends that

> **50. Health Canada make it mandatory for manufacturers to include on all containers of alcoholic beverages health warnings about the risks of alcohol consumption, including risks to the fetus.**

and that

> 51. **Physicians and health care workers provide**
>   **information about the reproductive health effects**
>   **of alcohol consumption to women who plan to**
>   **become pregnant and to couples trying to**
>   **conceive.**

Couples who are experiencing infertility need to be made aware that although moderate consumption of alcohol by either partner has not been shown to affect fertility, chronic consumption of alcohol has been linked to fertility problems in men. Men are less likely to consult a physician when a couple wants to become pregnant, and providing information to their partners about the effects of alcohol use on male fertility may be a way of helping this information get to them.

Because of the association between heavy alcohol consumption and harm to the fetus, as well as the fact that a safe level of alcohol consumption for pregnant women has not been established, it is common sense for women who are trying to conceive to avoid consuming alcohol. Unless there is no possibility they will become pregnant, women of childbearing age should avoid heavy alcohol consumption or binge drinking, not only for their own health but because of the possible risks to the fetus in an unplanned or undetected pregnancy. The Commission recommends that

> 52. **Physicians and health care workers provide**
>   **information to couples seeking infertility**
>   **treatment on the effects of alcohol consumption**
>   **on fertility and on pregnancy outcomes and**
>   **make sure couples trying to conceive**
>   **understand the importance of minimizing**
>   **alcohol use.**

and that

> 53. **Physicians and health care workers routinely**
>   **evaluate the drinking history of both partners in**
>   **couples who are infertile. If a problem is**
>   **identified, counselling and support should be**
>   **offered to change alcohol consumption before**
>   **they undergo infertility treatment.**

Illicit Drugs

Some drugs used illicitly may inhibit the activity of the central nervous system (anaesthetics, analgesics, sedatives, and tranquilizers). Others stimulate the activity of the central nervous system (anti-depressants, stimulants, and hallucinogens). Drugs in both categories have the potential to affect reproductive function by influencing various body processes and nervous system functioning associated with the production of sex hormones by the pituitary. Changes in hormone production could in turn affect ovulation or sperm production. Psychoactive drugs might also influence reproductive function by affecting the autonomic nervous system, which controls erection and ejaculation in men and sexual arousal in women.

Illicit Drug Use in Canada

Cannabis (marijuana/hashish) is the most commonly used illicit drug in Canada. In 1989, approximately 6.5 percent of Canadian adults had used it in the past year, and approximately one in five of these used it at least once a week. More than twice as many men as women were users, with the highest rate of use in the 20 to 34 year age group.

In 1989, approximately 1.4 percent of Canadian adults had used cocaine or crack at least once in the past year. The highest rate of use was among adults 25 to 34 years of age: approximately 4.9 percent of men and 1.8 percent of women in this age group had used cocaine in the past year.

Use of LSD, speed, and heroin in the year preceding the survey was reported by 0.4 percent of Canadian adults.

Source: Canada. Health Promotion Directorate. Health and Welfare Canada. *National Alcohol and Other Drugs Survey: Highlights Report.* Ottawa: Minister of Supply and Services Canada, 1990.

One problem with assessing the effects of illicit use of such drugs is that regular users often engage in other unhealthy practices, making it difficult to separate the effects of drug use from these other factors. It is estimated, for example, that 67 percent of women who are addicted to heroin support their habit by prostitution, which puts them at higher risk of contracting sexually transmitted diseases. As a result, there is a high incidence of pelvic inflammatory disease, and consequently tubal infertility, among heroin users. Malnutrition and the concurrent use of other drugs are also confounding factors. Despite these research complexities, there is strong evidence to suggest that certain illicit drugs have an adverse effect on the fertility of men and women.

Cocaine

Cocaine use in men has been associated with problems with sperm motility, density, and morphology. One group of researchers found that cocaine consumption over a period of two years was strongly associated with low sperm concentration (compared to men who had never taken cocaine). Cocaine use over a five-year period was associated with low sperm counts, low sperm motility, and a greater incidence of abnormally shaped sperm. These researchers also found that the frequency of cocaine use was less strongly related to infertility than was the duration of use or how recently it had been used. They concluded that, given the number of men who use cocaine (particularly men between the ages of 20 and 35), it could play a significant role in infertility. Other researchers have found that cocaine directly affects the first stages of sperm production and can cause constriction of the blood vessels, which in turn may have harmful effects on testicular function.

Cocaine use during pregnancy is potentially harmful to both the woman and the fetus. Some studies suggest that the risks are severe, including maternal heart attack and higher rates of spontaneous abortion and fetal death, as well as congenital anomalies, growth retardation, and stillbirth. Cocaine has a well-documented constrictive effect on blood vessels. An increased frequency of neurological problems and brain damage in fetuses (resulting from the death of areas of brain tissue when their blood supply is cut off) has been reported by several groups of researchers. However, the many reports on adverse effects must be interpreted with some caution, as it is difficult to isolate the effects of cocaine use itself from the impact of poor diet, poor social circumstances, and other problems that are common among chronic cocaine users. Evidence of an increased likelihood of placental abruption due to cocaine use is fairly clear, however.

Heroin

In men, frequent use of heroin has been reported to reduce sex drive and affect sexual performance. The effect of heroin consumption on male sex hormone levels is not clear, as both increases and decreases have been reported. In women, heroin abuse has been associated with menstrual irregularities, including lack of ovulation. (Morphine use has also been found to have similar consequences.)

Marijuana

Some researchers have reported an association between marijuana use and declining levels of the hormones that control ovulation. It is not possible to say definitively whether marijuana or one of its components causes infertility, but some researchers believe that it may delay conception. Overall, however, relatively little is known about the effects of marijuana use on human reproduction.

It is not clear how heroin, morphine, and marijuana affect pregnancy outcome. All three drugs pass easily through the placenta, and heroin use during pregnancy has been associated with negative effects such as withdrawal symptoms, which have been observed in 40 to 80 percent of infants born to heroin-addicted women.[12] The symptoms can last as long as three weeks after birth.

Low birth weight in infants born to women who used heroin during pregnancy has also been reported. It is difficult in most cases, however, to dissociate the effects of heroin use from other factors contributing to the poor health of the pregnant woman. Finally, no consistent associations have been drawn between heroin use during pregnancy and the risk of congenital anomalies in infants.

In view of the risks to general health associated with the use of illicit drugs, it is obviously common sense for all individuals to avoid their use. Women and men also need to be aware of the potential effects of illicit drugs on their reproductive

> Most of the studies surveyed ... indicate that licit and illicit drugs can affect the physiological parameters linked to male and female fertility to varying degrees. However, none of them clearly demonstrates that any one of these drugs causes infertility. Consequently, considerable care should be taken in interpreting research into the effects of these drugs on fertility.
>
> At the same time, it is impossible to overemphasize the need for experimental methods that lend themselves to multifactorial analysis. Human beings do not live in antiseptic laboratories. Attempts must therefore be made to assess the impact of multiple variables that cannot be submitted to very strict experimental control. Furthermore, the majority of people dependent on licit and illicit drugs do not limit their consumption to only one of those drugs. For example, smokers are more likely to consume alcohol than non-smokers ... Multiple drug use may have harmful effects that a simplistic statistical analysis cannot reveal.
>
> H. Boyer, "Effects of Licit and Illicit Drugs, Alcohol, Caffeine, and Nicotine on Infertility," in Research Volumes of the Commission, 1993.

health. The evidence suggests that we should be particularly concerned about use of these drugs by young people, especially those between the ages of 20 and 34. These individuals may experience a reduced ability to conceive; they may also have an increased risk of problems in pregnancy or birth complications if they have a pregnancy while using drugs.

Health education in schools can help to reduce illicit drug use among young people by imparting information about the risks and by teaching skills to help them resist social pressures to use drugs. Public education programs can also help to convey messages about the risks of using drugs, and both federal and provincial/territorial governments have been involved in this area. Specific efforts targeted at high-risk groups such as drug users, prostitutes, and youth who have dropped out of school are also required, as these individuals are less likely to be reached through such traditional channels as school programs. Heavy consumers of drugs within these groups must be reached with messages that encourage them to seek help, and counselling and treatment services must be made available to them. In particular, special programs are required to help young women who become pregnant while abusing drugs to stop using them.

In view of the number of known or suspected risks to reproductive health and fertility associated with the use of illicit drugs, people who are trying to conceive should avoid their use. Physicians should routinely ask couples seeking infertility treatment about their drug history, to ensure that use of drugs is not a factor contributing to their infertility. The Commission recommends that

54. **Health Canada and provincial/territorial ministries of health coordinate their efforts to develop school-based and public education programs for young people concerning drug use.**

55. **Federal, provincial, and territorial governments ensure that funding for school health and public education programs related to drugs also include funding for the evaluation of program effectiveness.**

56. **Health Canada and provincial/territorial ministries of health develop specific programs targeted at high-risk individuals such as drug users, prostitutes, and street youth regarding drug use and, in particular, ensure that counselling and treatment programs be made available to help women who become pregnant while abusing drugs to stop using them.**

57. **Physicians routinely take a drug history from couples seeking infertility treatment to ensure that illicit drug use is not a possible contributing factor to their infertility.**

Caffeine

Caffeine, widely consumed in coffee, tea, and soft drinks, enters the bloodstream very easily and is distributed throughout various body tissues. Its presence can be detected in the brain, testicles, secretions of the uterus, early embryonic cells, fetal tissue, amniotic fluid, and breast milk. Very few specific studies have been conducted on the effects of caffeine consumption on male and female fertility.   Some studies have indicated a delay in conception as a result of caffeine consumption by women, but the methodology of these studies has been strongly criticized.[13]

Many studies have looked at the risk of congenital anomalies or spontaneous abortion as a result of caffeine intake (moderate drinking of coffee, tea, or colas) during pregnancy.   The data on which to base judgements about moderate caffeine intake are fairly sound; in general, they show that the risks are minimal. Although some studies have shown a higher incidence of spontaneous abortion, premature labour, fetuses that were small for their gestational age, and congenital anomalies in these studies, it is difficult to isolate the effects of caffeine from other factors such as cigarette smoking. In summary, most well-designed studies have shown no link between caffeine and fetal anomalies.   Data on which to base judgements about higher levels of caffeine intake are not available.

Although no clear link has been established between caffeine consumption and reduced fertility or pregnancy complications, it would nevertheless seem prudent for women who want to become pregnant to consume caffeine in moderation, particularly because research shows that caffeine does pass through the placenta to the fetus. The existence of a few studies suggesting an association between caffeine consumption and a delay in conception, notwithstanding their methodological shortcomings, suggests that women should err on the side of caution.

Less is known about the effect of caffeine consumption on male fertility.   A few studies have associated caffeine consumption with potentially beneficial effects on male fertility, including increased sperm density and motility. Further research is required to determine whether there is an association between caffeine consumption and increased (or decreased) male fertility.

Stress and Psychological Factors

There is a very large literature on the effect of stress and psychological factors on infertility; it is a field in which there are many hypotheses but relatively few studies with data meeting a good standard of evidence. It is a difficult and complex area to study and in which to show cause and effect. Several psychological factors are suspected as potential risks to fertility. Some researchers believe that psychological problems associated with psychosexual maladjustment, stress, lack of self-esteem, anxiety, mood disorders, depression, and psychosocial distress can have adverse effects on fertility in both men and women. The extensive literature devoted to these questions is often speculative, anecdotal, and contradictory. Psychological stress can result in decreases in testosterone levels and sperm counts in men and amenorrhea in women. Whether such stress-induced changes in hormone levels or reproductive functioning account for infertility is unknown. Definitive associations or cause-effect relationships between stress or other psychological factors and infertility have yet to be well documented in either men or women. A major difficulty in designing studies is how to measure stress and other psychological problems, as they are common in both fertile and infertile people.

Recently, researchers have begun to hypothesize about how stress might affect sperm production and ovulation. Stress stimulates several hormonal responses that help the body adapt to real or perceived threats by affecting the cardiovascular, energy-producing, and immune systems. Proper reproductive function depends heavily on the healthy functioning of these three major body systems, but it remains unclear how the body's reaction to stress might specifically affect or compromise reproductive ability.

> There is a very large literature on the effect of stress and psychological factors on infertility; it is a field in which there are many hypotheses but relatively few studies with data meeting a good standard of evidence. It is a difficult and complex area to study and in which to show cause and effect.

Stress may also play a role in infertility by interfering with sexual desire or performance. Problems cited in this area include impotence, retarded ejaculation, ejaculation prior to intromission, infrequent intercourse, and vaginismus. However, no firm conclusions about the impact of stress on sexual desire or performance in men or women can be drawn on the basis of existing research in this area.

Psychosocial distress has been reported to be more common in couples who are infertile than in other couples. Researchers recently reviewed 30 existing studies to determine whether (1) stress causes infertility; (2) the experience of infertility (and/or associated treatment) brings about a certain level of stress; or (3) the two are interdependent, each having a causal effect on the other.[14] They found some evidence for all three hypotheses, particularly for the latter two. They concluded that in a small but consistent percentage of patients who are infertile, stress is likely to precede infertility and could play an important causal role in infertility among members of this group.

Recent studies have examined whether being treated for infertility places additional stress on couples who are infertile and sometimes exacerbates an infertility problem. A decrease in semen quality has been reported in men whose female partners were undergoing *in vitro* fertilization.[15] A recent study of women undergoing infertility treatment, conducted at Concordia University in Montreal, found that, contrary to popular belief, it is not the treatment itself that creates the most stress for women, but rather finding out that the treatment has been unsuccessful. The authors suggest that women who are infertile need to be informed about and helped to cope with treatment failure — they need to develop strategies to help them deal with the stress occasioned by this.[16]

Medical Intervention and Infertility

Infertility can be an intended or unintended consequence of medical intervention or treatment. The infertility may be desired — for example, as a result of contraceptive use or after a tubal ligation or vasectomy. In some cases, medical intervention may be necessary and the resulting infertility anticipated — for example, after a hysterectomy. Much less frequently infertility may be an unintended side effect of a diagnostic or treatment procedure. In this section we discuss infertility associated with each of these categories.

Method of Contraception

Although the use of contraception indicates a desire to control fertility, certain methods of birth control carry a risk of unintended infertility or delay in the return to fertility when the method is discontinued. Other methods of contraception do not present such risks, but nor do they protect fertility. Methods that provide no protection against the transmission of STDs and thus no protection against this cause of infertility include the rhythm method, natural family planning, periodic abstinence, coitus interruptus/withdrawal, IUDs, oral contraceptives, post-coital contraceptives, hormonal implants, and injectable progesterone. Contraceptive methods that provide protection against STDs include condoms and, to a lesser extent, diaphragms, cer-

> Professionals and the public should be educated that the concomitant use of two contraceptive systems (dual protection) is necessary for both pregnancy control and the prevention of infection-based infertility. There is a need for public and professional education regarding the expert use of contraceptives with a view to protecting against unwanted pregnancy and an equal concern for future reproductive health.
>
> N. Barwin and W. Fisher, "Contraception: An Evaluation of Its Role in Relation to Infertility — Can It Protect?" in Research Volumes of the Commission, 1993.

vical caps, and spermicides. These categories are particularly important for individuals who are likely to have more than one sexual partner, or whose partner has had other sexual partners.

Commission research, reported in Chapter 9, shows that, excluding those who are surgically sterilized, about 4 out of 10 Canadian women between the ages of 18 and 49, who are married or cohabiting with a male partner, use some form of contraception. The 1984 Canadian Fertility Survey shows that if those who are surgically sterilized are included, 7 out of 10 Canadians between the ages of 18 and 49 are using contraception.

Sterilization

Voluntary sterilization is the most widely used form of contraception in Canada. As shown in Table 14.1, in 1984 approximately 35 percent of those women 18 to 49 years of age who used some form of birth control had undergone a tubal ligation; and 12.7 percent of the women surveyed indicated that their male partner had undergone a vasectomy. (Tubal ligation involves surgery to block or sever the fallopian tubes so that the egg and sperm cannot meet. Male sterilization by vasectomy involves cutting and sealing the vas deferens, the tube that carries sperm from the testes.)

As shown in Table 14.2, in 1991-92, 22.9 percent of cohabiting women aged 18 to 44 years had a tubal ligation, and 18 percent of their male partners had a vasectomy. Overall, in 41 percent of couples, one or both members were sterilized. Not surprisingly, the proportion who have had surgical sterilization rises with age, and in 61 percent of couples in the 40 to 44 age group one or both members were sterilized. Data gathered by the Commission in 1991-92 suggest that the difference in the proportion of women who have undergone a tubal ligation and the proportion of men who have undergone a vasectomy is narrowing.

Voluntary sterilization is most likely to be chosen by men and women who are over the age of 35 and have had all the children they want. Uncertainty remains, however, about the percentage of those who have been surgically sterilized who come to regret this decision and seek to regain their fertility. One study of couples in Quebec found that about 15 percent of all sterilized couples felt "some regret" about their choice, and 10 percent would have tried to have another child were it not for the sterilization. A Scandinavian researcher who conducted a literature review estimated that between 1.3 and 12.7 percent of women who had undergone sterilization regretted their decision to some extent.[17] Research shows that women who regret having had a tubal ligation and who seek reversal are more likely to have been sterilized at an early age and to have had complex marital histories.[18]

Regret about sterilization may occur when a partnership has ended, for example by divorce or death, and the man or woman would like to have children with a new partner. Some couples may regret their earlier decision

Table 14.1. Percent Distribution of Women 18 to 49 Years of Age Using Contraceptives, by Method of Contraception and Age Group, Canada, 1984

Age group	Number of respondents	Percentage using contraception	Percent distribution of women using contraception, by method						
			Total	Female sterilization	Male sterilization	Pill	IUD	Condom	Other*
18-24 years	1 323	56.9	100.0	2.1	1.6	76.6	6.5	8.1	5.0
25-29 years	986	67.7	100.0	16.5	7.9	39.2	11.7	14.5	10.2
30-34 years	925	74.8	100.0	35.7	16.8	17.3	13.4	10.0	6.8
35-39 years	846	78.5	100.0	54.1	17.8	6.5	8.6	7.4	5.7
40-44 years	644	76.2	100.0	61.3	21.6	2.9	3.9	4.7	5.7
45-49 years	591	63.6	100.0	67.6	15.4	0.3	1.6	8.8	6.4
Total (18-49 years)	5 315	68.4	100.0	35.3	12.7	28.0	8.3	9.1	6.6

* Including diaphragm, spermicides, rhythm, withdrawal, and others.

Source: Balakrishnan, T.R., K. Krotki, and E. Lapierre-Adamcyk. "Contraceptive Use in Canada, 1984." *Family Planning Perspectives* 17 (5)(September-October 1985), Table 3.

Table 14.2. Percentage of Cohabiting Couples Who Were Contraceptively Sterilized (Either Tubal Ligation or Vasectomy) in 1991-92

Age group	Tubal ligation and vasectomy combined		Tubal ligation (%)	Vasectomy (%)
	Number	Sterilized (%)		
18-24 years	119	—	—	—
25-29 years	291	15.8	7.6	8.2
30-34 years	429	40.0	21.0	19.1
35-39 years	387	58.7	31.0	27.6
40-44 years	272	60.9	40.1	20.9
Total (18-44 years)	**1 501**	**40.8**	**22.9**	**18.0**

Note: Percentages may not sum to overall rates due to rounding.

Source: Commission analysis of data from Dulberg, C.S., and T. Stephens. "The Prevalence of Infertility in Canada, 1991-1992: Analysis of Three National Surveys," in Research Volumes of the Royal Commission on New Reproductive Technologies, 1993.

to be sterilized when one partner or both decide they would like to have additional children. Couples in this situation can attempt to have the sterilization surgically reversed — although the surgery can be complicated and success is not guaranteed in reversing tubal ligation or vasectomy. An alternative to reversal for a vasectomy is for the woman to attempt to conceive using donor sperm, although in this case the man will not have a child who is genetically related to him. In the case of tubal ligation, a woman can attempt *in vitro* fertilization, which bypasses the fallopian tubes.

Health Canada data on the number of individuals who undergo a rejoining of the vas deferens or fallopian tubes provide an upper estimate of the number of sterilization reversals being performed in Canada, although some of this surgery is done for reasons other than the desire to regain fertility after sterilization. For example, tubal surgery may be done for tubal blockage as a result of sexually transmitted diseases. In 1980-81, 1 711 procedures on the fallopian tubes or vas deferens were performed; in 1989-90, 4 433 were performed.[19] Estimated success rate for reversal of tubal ligation is 60 percent, and for vasectomy 39 to 78 percent.

Based on a survey of fertility clinics conducted for the Commission, it was estimated that between 5 and 15 percent of patients requesting *in vitro* fertilization had had tubal ligation. A similar percentage of people seeking assisted insemination were reported to have requested that procedure because of a vasectomy. In total for 1991, therefore, an estimated 10 percent (630 of 6 300) of couples having one of these treatments (3 400 assisted insemination, 2 900 *in vitro* fertilization; see research volume, *Treatment of Infertility: Current Practices and Psychosocial Implications*) would have previously had surgical sterilization. Given that there are approximately 1.5 million Canadian couples, in which the female partner is between the ages of 18 and 44, who have been surgically sterilized, this figure represents an extremely small proportion of all sterilized couples. It does, however, represent a significant minority of couples seeking infertility treatments in a given year. Moreover, more women are being sterilized at a younger age, and this may affect the number of couples seeking reversal of sterilization (see research volume, *The Prevalence of Infertility in Canada*).

Surgical sterilization must be viewed as permanent; it is essential that the decision and all its implications be considered carefully to minimize the likelihood that it will be performed on people whose desire to have children is likely to resurface or where change in life circumstances is likely to lead to regret about sterilization. The Commission recommends that

> 58. **Physicians counsel couples considering surgical sterilization to ensure that they view the decision as permanent and to inform them what the likelihood of pregnancy is after reversal of tubal ligation or vasectomy.**

Oral Contraceptives

As shown in Table 14.1, oral contraceptives (the pill) are the next most common form of contraception after surgical sterilization. Twenty-eight percent of Canadian women between the ages of 18 and 49 use the pill, the majority of them under the age of 34. In Chapter 10, we emphasized that women who use the pill for pregnancy prevention need to be aware that it provides no protection against sexually transmitted diseases. Women who are not in long-term monogamous relationships should therefore be encouraged, particularly by physicians prescribing oral contraceptives, to ensure that their partners use condoms for protection against STDs. Some data show that use of the pill may reduce the likelihood that an infection will move into the upper genital tract and may thereby lessen the risk of STD-induced pelvic inflammatory disease; it is not known how or why this is the case. However, use of the pill has also been reported to increase the risk of cervical infection caused by chlamydia; it is therefore important for physicians to recognize that oral contraceptives on their own are not appropriate for women who are not in long-term monogamous relationships. The Commission recommends that

> **59. Physicians and health care workers counsel young women and men who are not in long-term monogamous relationships about the need for dual forms of protection against pregnancy and sexually transmitted diseases. In particular, oral contraceptives should be used in conjunction with a barrier form of contraception to protect against not only pregnancy but also sexually transmitted diseases.**

As discussed in Chapter 10, there is also a need for school and community sex education programs to convey to young women (and men) that oral contraceptives, while offering an effective means to avoid pregnancy, do not protect them against sexually transmitted diseases. Pharmaceutical companies can also promote awareness of this important message by including package inserts in oral contraceptives to communicate the importance of using condoms for protection against sexually transmitted diseases by individuals who may be at risk.

Some women who stop using oral contraceptives may experience a delay before they become fertile again. One study of 5 580 fertile women who had stopped using contraception to conceive found that the proportion of previous pill users who conceived in the first month was 30 percent less than users of other contraceptive methods, but this difference disappeared by the third month.[20] A similar study confirmed that conception delays were temporary among oral contraceptive users, but found the delay to be longer. While most of the difference disappeared by 24 months, very small differences were detectable up to three years later.

Women who are using oral contraceptives and plan to become pregnant in the future should be informed of the possibility of a delay before they are fertile again, so they can take this into account in their childbearing plans.

Intrauterine Devices

The IUD, which prevents pregnancy by stopping a fertilized egg from implanting in the wall of the uterus, is used by 8.3 percent of women who use some form of contraception. Women aged 25 to 34 are the group most likely to use an IUD. In the late 1970s and early '80s case control studies showed an association between the use of IUDs and several health risks, including pelvic inflammatory disease, ectopic pregnancy, and spontaneous abortion. Following this information, as well as the controversy surrounding the Dalkon Shield® and its removal from the North American market, there was a dramatic decline in the use of IUDs. The Dalkon Shield® is associated with a higher risk of pelvic inflammatory disease, and data on women who used it had been included in these earlier studies.

A recent international study by the World Health Organization used the largest data base of any IUD study, including 22 908 IUD insertions and more than 50 000 woman-years of follow-up, to evaluate the possible relationship between pelvic inflammatory disease and IUD use.[21] The study found a higher risk of PID during the first 20 days after IUD insertion. After that time, there was little difference between the incidences of PID among IUD users and other contraceptive users; the risk was low and constant during follow-up. The short-term risk of PID during the first days after insertion is likely related to the insertion procedure rather than the IUD itself. If bacteria are present in the woman's vagina at the time of insertion, or if they are introduced during the procedure, there is an increased risk of infection. This means IUDs should not be replaced routinely, but should be left in place for their maximum lifespan if the woman wishes to continue use.

Other studies have shown that in women who have had only one sexual partner, there is no increased risk of tubal infertility (which may result from PID) associated with IUD use.[22] However, the risk of pelvic inflammatory disease is greater in IUD users who were more likely to have been exposed to sexually transmitted diseases than among IUD users who were at low risk of exposure. This is to be expected, because the IUD does not provide protection against sexually transmitted diseases. Women who have had multiple partners, or whose partner has had multiple partners, are at greater risk of contracting a STD and subsequent pelvic inflammatory disease. This points to the need for physicians to ensure that a woman does not have a sexually transmitted disease, and is not at risk of exposure to STDs, before inserting an IUD. Women should be advised to seek prompt medical attention if they experience symptoms of an infection after IUD insertion. They should also be warned that an IUD does not provide protection against sexually transmitted diseases. It also suggests the need for a trial to evaluate whether antibiotic use prior to an IUD insertion reduces the risk of subsequent infection.

The estimated incidence of ectopic pregnancy among IUD users is approximately 102 per 1 000 woman-years (a unit used to measure use — for example, 500 women using an IUD for two years would account for 1 000 woman-years of IUD use).[23] This is 2.5 times less than the chances of ectopic pregnancy in women who are sexually active and who use no contraception, but 200 times greater than the chances of ectopic pregnancy in women who use oral contraceptives (because they are very unlikely to become pregnant at all) and 10 times greater than for women whose partners use condoms. It would appear that the IUD does not cause ectopic pregnancies, but, unlike the oral forms of contraception, which prevent fertilization and thus also ectopic pregnancy, IUD use does not prevent ectopic pregnancy in predisposed women. Women who have a history of pelvic inflammatory disease (which increases their risk of ectopic pregnancy) or a previous ectopic pregnancy should therefore choose other forms of contraception.

In rare cases, women conceive despite using an IUD. The pregnancy rate is estimated to be 20 in 1 000 woman-years.[24] In these situations, there is an increased risk of pregnancy complications such as premature delivery if the device cannot be removed, which sometimes occurs because the thread attached to the IUD has retracted into the uterus. If the device is removed early in pregnancy, however, the risk of pregnancy complications is very low.

Research shows that the majority of women who stop using the IUD return to fertility in 12 months or less. One study found that 89 percent of women under the age of 30, and 78 percent of women 30 years of age and over, became pregnant within 12 months of having an IUD removed.[25]

Condoms

Condoms are the method selected by 9.1 percent of women using contraception (see Table 14.1). Condom use lessens the risk of transmission of STDs and subsequent infertility. In Chapter 10, we described the clear and urgent need for prevention programs to encourage condom use by sexually active young people. However, the values and mores that contribute to the inequality of women also make it difficult for some women to persuade their partners to use or to insist they use a condom. This points to the need for contraception methods to be developed that are much more directly under the control of women (as may become the case with vaginal condoms) as well as for education of both men and women to change attitudes toward condom use.

Other Forms of Contraception

Other forms of contraception (rhythm methods, natural family planning, periodic abstinence, coitus interruptus/withdrawal, spermicides, diaphragms, cervical caps, post-coital contraceptives, hormonal implants, and injectable progesterone) are used by 6.6 percent of women using contraception in Canada (see Table 14.1). Spermicides, diaphragms, and cervical caps provide some protection against STDs and subsequent infertility, but the rest do not. Injectables and implants have also been linked with delays in the return of fertility after their use is discontinued (see research volume, *Understanding Infertility: Risk Factors Affecting Fertility*): these types of contraceptives either are not available, however, or are used rarely in Canada. This is also the case for post-coital contraceptives (the morning-after pill).

Based on our review of what is known about the various methods of contraception, the Commission recommends that

> **60. Physicians inform women about the protection against sexually transmitted diseases provided by various forms of contraception and whether their use may be associated with a delayed return to fertility after contraceptive use is discontinued. Women who have had more than one sexual partner (or whose partner has had other partners) should be counselled to use protection against both pregnancy and STDs. Oral contraceptives should not be prescribed for those individuals without counselling about the need to protect against STDs as well as pregnancy.**

Surgical Procedures in Women

Some surgical procedures for women may make it difficult or impossible for them to conceive. Hysterectomy always leads to infertility, as it involves removal of the uterus and usually the fallopian tubes and may also include removal of the ovaries. Certain other surgical procedures are associated with a low risk of complications that may lead to infertility.

Cervical surgery can affect fertility, as it may lead to incompetent cervix, a condition that results in the inability to carry a pregnancy to term. Cervical traumas associated with surgeries, such as conization of the cervix, dilation and curettage, and induced abortion, or with childbirth (either in natural delivery or with instrument use) are reported to be responsible for 30 to 50 percent of cases of incompetent cervix. However, in most cases women who are infertile because of an incompetent cervix can be treated successfully with a procedure that involves circling the cervix with a suture. This improves the fetal survival rate in women with the condition from between 20 and 50 percent to between 70 and 90 percent (see research volume, *Understanding Infertility: Risk Factors Affecting Fertility*).

Many studies have been undertaken to determine whether induced abortions affect subsequent fertility and pregnancy outcomes since they are a frequently performed surgical procedure; in 1990, more than 92 600 abortions were performed in Canada, with the highest rates among women between the ages of 18 and 24.[26] The risk of infertility associated with induced abortion is complex to assess because factors such as the abortion technique used, the conditions under which the abortion is performed, whether the abortion is a first or subsequent abortion, and the age and other characteristics of the woman involved may influence the outcome, as well as the surgery itself. Despite these complexities, the most recent and rigorous studies do not demonstrate an increased risk of infertility or complications in a subsequent pregnancy after induced abortion. Statistics Canada data show that the rate of complications following abortion is low, at 1.1 percent in 1991. This is consistent with existing research studies, which show that between 1 and 2 percent of women have a significant post-abortion complication.

Complications that could lead to infertility include pelvic inflammatory disease, endometrial lesions, or haemorrhaging leading to the need for a hysterectomy. However, secondary hysterectomies (removal of the uterus) as a complication following an abortion are very rare: in Canada, the rate is less than one in 10 000 procedures. Estimates of the incidence of pelvic inflammatory disease following an induced abortion range from 0.1 percent to 5.0 percent, depending on the study.[27] The risk of developing pelvic inflammatory disease following an abortion is strongly influenced by whether the woman had a history of sexually transmitted diseases and PID and whether she was infected at the time of the abortion. We believe that research should be conducted to determine the benefit of screening women in high-risk groups who wish to undergo an induced abortion to ensure they do not have a sexually transmitted disease before the procedure is performed. The preventive use of antibiotics for such women should also be assessed and the results taken into account when the *Canadian Guidelines for the Prevention, Diagnosis, Management and Treatment of Sexually Transmitted Diseases in Neonates, Children, Adolescents and Adults* are updated.

Research has also examined whether there is an increased risk of ectopic pregnancy, spontaneous abortion, or premature delivery associated with subsequent pregnancies among women who have undergone an induced abortion. The risk of ectopic pregnancy following an abortion, if it exists, is too low to be detected in large-scale studies. Studies concerning the possible association between abortion and future spontaneous abortion or premature delivery suggest that the risk is minimal. Whether repeated abortions over time are a risk factor for infertility is not yet known — some studies have reported an association, while others have found no association.

Caesarian sections do not appear to be a risk factor for infertility, although there is a slightly higher risk of spontaneous abortion in subsequent pregnancies than following a vaginal delivery.

Surgical Procedures in Men

Some forms of surgery on the male genital organs and accessory organs may have a subsequent effect on fertility. For example, urological procedures involving resection of the bladder neck or the prostate have been reported to lead to infertility through retrograde ejaculation. Following removal of the prostate glands to treat cancer, impotence has been reported in 60 to 90 percent of cases. The great majority of these procedures are performed at an age when it is likely that no further children are desired, so their impact is of importance not for fertility but for sexual functioning.

Testicular cancer may occur in younger men and has been reported to cause lowered fertility. Surgical removal of both testes, which might have to be done to remove a cancerous growth, will obviously result in infertility. Ways to modify treatment procedures to prevent subsequent infertility are being explored, and sperm samples can be frozen and stored before surgery if the man wants to retain the capacity to father a child later.

Radiation Therapy

The levels of radiation exposure that have a documentable effect on fertility are usually approached only when radiation is used in the treatment of cancer. The average man or woman will not be exposed to levels of radiation that could impair their fertility. Women and men who are to undergo radiation therapy should of course be informed of the possible effects on their fertility, and men who foresee wanting to have children should be made aware of the option to freeze their sperm in the event that they become infertile following a surgical procedure or radiation treatment; it is not possible to freeze eggs at present, but a couple could consider the possibility of freezing zygotes.

Diagnostic Testing Procedures for Infertility

Like other invasive medical procedures, testing procedures used to diagnose infertility in women and men have risks, including a slight risk that the procedure itself will lead to complications that may affect fertility.

Laparoscopy is the most commonly performed diagnostic procedure to assess fertility in women. It involves the introduction of an instrument through the abdominal wall, or into a hollow organ, to visualize the tissues. It is used to observe the ovaries, fallopian tubes, and external walls of the uterus, and it is also used in egg retrieval for *in vitro* fertilization. In rare cases, the instrument used to elevate and manipulate the uterus during the procedure may perforate the uterus, resulting in internal bleeding. The risk of this occurring has not been documented for laparoscopies used in infertility diagnosis, but a 3 percent chance of this occurring has been reported during sterilization procedures via laparoscopy.[28] This is not usually a serious complication, and we found no data concerning the impact of it on fertility.

Hysteroscopy involves the insertion of a small scope through the cervix to visualize the interior of the uterus, to identify the existence of tumours, adhesions, and/or congenital anomalies. The test has a small risk of exacerbating an undiagnosed pelvic infection. Physicians should therefore ensure that women undergoing this procedure have been screened to eliminate the risk of a pelvic infection.

Hysterosalpingography is a test to determine whether a woman's fallopian tubes are structurally intact and her uterus is shaped normally. It involves the injection of a radiopaque dye directly into the uterine cavity. Normally the dye fills the uterine cavity and then flows through the fallopian tubes into the peritoneal cavity. If the dye does not pass through the tubes, then a blockage may be identified, either through X-ray or by observation during a laparoscopy. The incidence of infection following a hysterosalpingography has been reported to be between 0.3 and 3.1 percent in various studies. Our review did not reveal any studies of the impact of this test on fertility.

Endometrial biopsy is used to determine whether certain hormone levels, and the body's response to them, are normal. It involves the removal of a small sample of the endometrium for analysis. We found no data on the risk of infection or infertility following this test. If the woman is pregnant at the time of testing, there is a risk of removal of a conceptus during biopsy (0.6 to 6.3 percent).[29]

Vasography is a test used to detect the location of blockages or leaks in the duct leading from the testicles to the prostate (the vas deferens). Radiopaque dye is injected into the vas deferens to trace the path of the semen.   One study found that 3 percent of 509 azoospermic men experienced obstruction of the vas deferens *after* undergoing a vasography.[30] Reducing the risk of complications is possible by performing a vasography on one vas deferens initially, instead of both. Only if an obstruction is found will a vasography be required for the other vas deferens as well, because one open vas deferens is sufficient to allow sperm to be transported out of the body during ejaculation.

Testicular biopsy is recommended only when a man has an extremely low sperm count that cannot be explained. It involves making a very small incision in the scrotum to remove a small quantity of testicular tissue for examination under the microscope.   Some studies have reported that testicular biopsies may lead to a temporary decrease in sperm production. Infection has been reported in only a few cases as a result of this procedure, and infertility as a result of undergoing a testicular biopsy is likely to be very rare.

Prescription Drugs

The use of certain prescription drugs is associated with fertility problems as a side effect. Infertility caused by chemotherapy treatment for cancer is common in both men and women, but it is not considered to be a permanent effect of this treatment. As well, pregnancy loss and some teratogenic effects in the fetus have been reported from chemotherapy treatment for cancer during pregnancy (the effects varying with the dose and length of the treatment period).

Use of barbiturates has been associated with menstrual abnormalities in women and with hormonal changes in both men and women, although neither of these conditions necessarily implies fertility problems. Barbiturates have also been reported to pass quite easily through the placenta to the fetus.

It is suspected that anti-depressants may have side effects on erection and ejaculation ability in men and menstruation in women. As well, neuroleptic drugs may cause a decline in the volume of sperm produced. To date, however, no studies have directly examined the reproductive effects of these two types of drugs. Very few epidemiological data are available on the effects of these drugs when taken during pregnancy, but the risk of teratogenic effects as a result of *in utero* exposure is thought to be very small.

Studies have documented that drugs to control high blood pressure have the side effect of loss of sexual desire in some patients, difficulty in achieving or maintaining erection, and difficulty in achieving orgasm. These drugs have also been associated with menstrual disorders. Researchers note that it is difficult to determine with certainty whether these effects are a direct result of drug use, or whether they are related to the condition for which the drugs are taken. Some anti-hypertensive drugs have been associated with a substantial risk of oligohydramnios (too little fluid around the developing fetus) and fetal distress or death when taken in the latter part of pregnancy. But no studies of congenital anomalies in infants born to women who have been treated for hypertension have been reported.

Certain drugs used to treat gastrointestinal illnesses have been associated with sexual dysfunction and limited sperm production. However, gastrointestinal illnesses themselves can affect the reproductive system by altering concentrations of certain hormones. Our review did not identify any good data on the effects of these drugs on fetal development.

It is clearly important that physicians inform their patients about the risks associated with any drug they prescribe, including its possible effects on their fertility. These risks must be weighed against the potential benefits of taking the drugs and the need to treat the illness. There are, however, obstacles to informing about the risks — good data may simply not be available, or such data as do exist may not have been widely disseminated in an arm's-length and objective way. Currently, many doctors receive much of their information on drugs from pharmaceutical companies or from the *Compendium of Pharmaceuticals and Specialties.* No body or mechanism exists at present to assemble good data regarding drugs and to make this information accessible to physicians (see Chapter 18).

General Sources

Audebert, A., et al. "Endometriosis: A Discussion Document." *Human Reproduction* 7 (3)(1992): 432-35.

Bai, J., et al. "Drug-Related Menstrual Aberrations." *Obstetrics and Gynecology* 44 (5)(November 1974): 713-19.

Balakrishnan, T.R., and R. Fernando. "Infertility Among Canadians: An Analysis of Data from the Canadian Fertility Survey (1984) and General Social Survey (1990)." In Research Volumes of the Royal Commission on New Reproductive Technologies, 1993.

Balakrishnan, T.R., K. Krotki, and E. Lapierre-Adamcyk. "Contraceptive Use in Canada, 1984." *Family Planning Perspectives* 17 (5)(September-October 1985): 209-15.

Barwin, B.N., and W. Fisher. "Contraception: An Evaluation of Its Role in Relation to Infertility — Can It Protect?" In Research Volumes of the Royal Commission on New Reproductive Technologies, 1993.

Bracken, M.B., et al. "Association of Cocaine Use with Sperm Concentration, Motility, and Morphology." *Fertility and Sterility* 53 (2)(February 1990): 315-22.

Frisch, R.E. "The Right Weight: Body Fat, Menarche and Ovulation." *Baillière's Clinical Obstetrics and Gynaecology* 4 (3)(September 1990): 419-39.

Green, B.B., et al. "Exercise as a Risk Factor for Infertility with Ovulatory Dysfunction." *American Journal of Public Health* 76 (12)(December 1986): 1432-36.

Highet, R. "Athletic Amenorrhoea: An Update on Aetiology, Complications and Management." *Sports Medicine* 7 (1989): 82-108.

Millson, P., and K. Maznyk. "Pilot Study on Determining the Relative Importance of Risk Factors for Infertility in Canada." In Research Volumes of the Royal Commission on New Reproductive Technologies, 1993.

Smith, C.G. "Drug Effects on Male Sexual Function." *Clinical Obstetrics and Gynecology* 25 (3)(September 1982): 525-31.

Smith, C.G., and R.H. Asch. "Drug Abuse and Reproduction." *Fertility and Sterility* 48 (3)(September 1987): 355-73.

Sobel, R.J., et al. "Medical Conditions Leading to Infertility." In *Infertility: Male and Female*, ed. V. Insler and B. Lunenfeld. Edinburgh: Churchill Livingstone, 1986.

Stanton, A.L., and C. Dunkel-Schetter. *Infertility: Perspectives from Stress and Coping Management*. New York: Plenum Press, 1991.

United States. Congress. *Reproductive Health Hazards in the Workplace*. Washington: Office of Technology Assessment, 1985.

Specific References

1. Stewart, D.E., et al. "Infertility and Eating Disorders." *American Journal of Obstetrics and Gynecology* 163 (4)(Part 1)(October 1990): 1196-99.

2. Stewart, D.E., et al. "Anorexia Nervosa, Bulimia, and Pregnancy." *American Journal of Obstetrics and Gynecology* 157 (5)(November 1987): 1194-98.

3. Farthing, M.J.G., et al. "Male Gonadal Function in Coeliac Disease: 1: Sexual Dysfunction, Infertility, and Semen Quality." *Gut* 23 (1982): 608-14; Farthing, M.J.G., and A.M. Dawson. "Impaired Semen Quality in Crohn's Disease — Drugs, Ill Health, or Undernutrition?" *Scandinavian Journal of Gastroenterology* 18 (1983): 57-60.

4. Kusakari, M., et al. "Relationship Between the Delayed-Reaction Type of LH-RH Test and Obesity in Sterile Women with Ovulatory Disturbances: A Preliminary Report." *International Journal of Fertility* 35 (1)(1990): 14-18.

5. Maddocks, S.E. "A Literature Review of the Physiological Manifestations Related to Infertility Linked to Weight, Eating Behaviours, and Exercise." In Research Volumes of the Royal Commission on New Reproductive Technologies, 1993.

6. Olive, D.L., and L.B. Schwartz. "Endometriosis." *New England Journal of Medicine* 328 (24)(June 17, 1993): 1759-69; Ponchuk, A. "The Physiological Links Between Endometriosis and Infertility: Review of the Medical Literature and Annotated Bibliography (1985-1990)." In Research Volumes of the Royal Commission on New Reproductive Technologies, 1993.

7. Olive and Schwartz, "Endometriosis."

8. Dunphy, B.C., et al. "Female Age, and the Length of Involuntary Infertility Prior to Investigation and Fertility Outcome." *Human Reproduction* 4 (5)(1989): 527-30.

9. Ponchuk, "The Physiological Links Between Endometriosis and Infertility."

10. TERIS Advisory Board. Summaries for Alcohol, Caffeine, Heroin, Cocaine, and Marijuana. Seattle: University of Washington, 1990.

11. Boyer, H. "Effects of Licit and Illicit Drugs, Alcohol, Caffeine, and Nicotine on Infertility." In Research Volumes of the Royal Commission on New Reproductive Technologies, 1993.

12. TERIS Advisory Board, Summaries for Alcohol, Caffeine, Heroin, Cocaine, and Marijuana.

13. Wilcox, A., C. Weinberg, and D. Baird. "Caffeinated Beverages and Decreased Fertility." *Lancet* (December 24-31, 1988): 1453-55; Olsen, J. "Cigarette Smoking, Tea and Coffee Drinking, and Subfecundity." *American Journal of Epidemiology* 133 (7)(1990): 734-39.

14. Wright, J., et al. "Psychosocial Distress and Infertility: A Review of Controlled Research." *International Journal of Fertility* 34 (2)(1989): 126-42.

15. Harrison, K.L., V.J. Callan, and J.F. Hennessey. "Stress and Semen Quality in an In Vitro Fertilization Program." *Fertility and Sterility* 48 (4)(October 1987): 633-36.

16. Boivin, J. "Comparison of Prospective and Retrospective Measures Evaluating Psychological Reactions to Infertility Treatment." Paper presented to the Annual Meeting of the American Fertility Society, New Orleans, November 1992. Montreal: Concordia University, 1992.

17. Kjer, J.J. "Regret of Laparoscopic Sterilization." *European Journal of Obstetrics and Gynaecology and Reproductive Biology* 35 (2-3)(May-June 1990): 205-10.

18. Marcil-Gratton, N., et al. "Profile of Women Who Request Reversal of Tubal Sterilization: Comparison with a Randomly Selected Control Group." *Canadian Medical Association Journal* 138 (April 15, 1988): 711-13.

19. There are two caveats to interpreting these data: 1) These figures may overestimate the number of reversals because they do not distinguish between procedures to reverse a previous sterilization and those to treat damage caused by disease. However, they set an upper limit on the number of reversals done in those provinces reporting. 2) The 1989-90 figure may underestimate the number of reversals done in Canada in this period because it does not include procedures performed in Nova Scotia or Alberta (which no longer pay for reversals), or British Columbia.

20. Harlap, S., and M. Baras. "Conception-Waits in Fertile Women After Stopping Oral Contraceptives." *International Journal of Fertility* 29 (2)(1984): 73-80.

21. Farley, T.M.M., et al. "Intrauterine Devices and Pelvic Inflammatory Disease: An International Perspective." *Lancet* 339 (March 28, 1992): 785-88.

22. Cramer, D., et al. "Tubal Infertility and IUD's." *New England Journal of Medicine* 312 (1985): 941-47; Daling, J.R., et al. "Primary Tubal Infertility in Relation to IUD Use." *New England Journal of Medicine* 312 (1985): 937-41.

23. Franks, A.L., et al. "Contraception and Ectopic Pregnancy Risk." *American Journal of Obstetrics and Gynecology* 163 (4)(Part 1)(October 1990): 1120-23.

24. Ibid.

25. Struthers, B.J. "Sexually Transmitted Disease, Infertility, IUDs and Epidemiology." *Advances in Contraception* 3 (1987): 82-96.

26. Canada. Statistics Canada. "Therapeutic Abortions 1990." *Health Reports* (Suppl. 9) 3 (4)(1991).

27. Dumas, S., E. Guilbert, and J-É. Rioux. "The Impact of Medical Procedures on Fertility." In Research Volumes of the Royal Commission on New Reproductive Technologies, 1993.

28. White, M.K., H.W. Ory, and L.A. Goldenberg. "A Cost-Control Study of Uterine Perforations Documented at Laparoscopy." *American Journal of Obstetrics and Gynecology* 129 (6)(November 15, 1977): 623-25.

29. Dumas et al., "The Impact of Medical Procedures on Fertility."

30. Wagenknecht, L., et al. "Vasography — Clinical and Experimental Investigations." *Andrologia* 14 (2)(March-April 1982): 182-89.

Preventing Infertility

♦

As we have seen, our knowledge about the contribution of various risk factors to the overall prevalence of infertility is incomplete. Nevertheless, what remains compellingly clear is the urgent need for national leadership and cooperation among the key partners — the federal government, the provinces and territories, health professionals, educators, volunteer groups, and others — so that as many people as possible can be spared the pain of wanting but not being able to have a child.

We have made specific recommendations to reduce the prevalence of infertility by preventing exposure to risk factors in the sections dealing with each of those factors. In some areas, such as sexually transmitted diseases and smoking, the risk is sufficiently clear and the route to prevention sufficiently known that it is possible to make fairly detailed recommendations; in other areas, such as environmental and workplace hazards, the need for more information limits the ability to develop effective prevention measures, but we have outlined some steps that can be taken. What is clearly evident, however, is that we lack any comprehensive or coordinated approach to promoting the reproductive health of Canadians generally or preventing infertility in particular. What is also evident from the Commission's work in this field is that prevention is a feasible and desirable approach. We have the ability to design programs to address specific known risk factors, and methods of evaluating those programs for effectiveness are being developed.

Prevention of infertility is a subject that naturally prompts questions about prevention in general and infertility prevention in particular. Does prevention work, and can it be effective enough to make a discernible impact on the prevalence of infertility and the demand for infertility treatment? How do we know when an infertility prevention program is effective or successful? What types of prevention approaches work for what kinds of risk factors? Posing questions of this type is consistent with the Commission's evidence-based approach to new reproductive technologies.

The Commission has concluded that there are indeed risk factors for infertility, such as sexually transmitted diseases and smoking, that can be addressed through prevention programs; that some risk factors, especially environmental and workplace exposures, can be identified, studied, and contained with appropriate countermeasures; that other risk factors, including those related to weight, eating disorders, and exercise, may be amenable to counselling and related responses; and that the potential effects of the less reversible risk factors, such as endometriosis and biological aging, can be addressed through timely and accurate information about their implications for individual decisions about childbearing.

As many Canadians recognized in their testimony before the Commission, the current emphasis on treating infertility after it has occurred must be rebalanced to include more attention and resources to preventing infertility in the first place. Although this perspective is tempered with the recognition that some infertility will not be amenable to prevention — even if we had unlimited resources to devote to this effort — there remains a strong sense among Canadians that many women and men who seek infertility treatment would not have needed such services if timely and appropriate prevention programs had been in place.

> There is a need to increase public awareness of the risk factors that lead to infertility. Nurses are in a key position to disseminate information about the causes of infertility through educational programs aimed at reaching those involved in at-risk activities ... The need for health promotion and disease prevention strategies related to the infertility is extremely important for adolescents.
>
> *Brief to the Commission from the Association of Registered Nurses of Newfoundland, April 28, 1992.*

In this chapter, therefore, we set out our strategy for a national action plan to reduce the prevalence of infertility and, in general, to improve the reproductive health of Canadians. We developed this plan in keeping with our commitment to our guiding principles and an evidence-based approach to health care provision. We believe that one entity must be given formal responsibility for developing policy and identifying broad strategies. We therefore propose the establishment of a permanent sub-committee of the National Reproductive Technologies Commission, the Infertility Prevention Sub-Committee, and our recommendations to this effect are presented at the end of this chapter.

In calling for a greater emphasis on infertility prevention, the Commission is among the many and growing voices advocating a new approach to health, some of which are detailed later in this section. While medical care can be vital in restoring health when specific problems occur, there is increasing recognition that acute care is actually quite limited in its ability to influence overall health. We discuss this shift in emphasis from acute care to prevention in this section. This shift implies that adequate resources should be devoted to prevention. To date, however, that has not been the case; this has presented further obstacles to an effective and comprehensive approach.

Commissioners believe that the best strategy for preventing infertility in men and women involves a coordinated and integrated approach within a larger context; to be successful, a national prevention effort must place prevention in the larger context of social and health policy in Canada. For instance, as we note in the chapter on aging and infertility, workplace policies and the

Commissioners believe that the best strategy for preventing infertility in men and women involves a coordinated and integrated approach within a larger context; to be successful, a national prevention effort must place prevention in the larger context of social and health policy in Canada.

availability of accessible and affordable child care could have a significant impact on the decision to delay childbearing. Similarly, broadening definitions of occupational health and safety to include reproductive health could result in the more timely identification of hazards to reproductive health and the development of measures to reduce exposure to them. Prevention thus requires a multifaceted approach, with coordinated action on many fronts simultaneously and the involvement of a diverse range of partners in these efforts. This will help to overcome some of the barriers we described — the lack of definitive knowledge of the links between various risks and infertility, the inter-relationships among the various risk factors, and the complexity of the contexts and systems within which risk factors arise and prevention responses must take place.

The most important priorities for a national reproductive health strategy that emerged from our review of the evidence on risk factors for infertility are as follows:

- reducing the incidence of sexually transmitted diseases, particularly among young women;

- reducing smoking among women and men and preventing smoking among young people; and

- increasing public awareness of the effect of delaying childbearing on fertility.

Also important are the expansion of scientific and medical knowledge about workplace and environmental risks to infertility, and encouraging women and couples who want to have a child not to drink alcohol, use drugs, or exercise excessively and to maintain sound eating habits and a healthy body weight.

The Commission has identified several key areas for action in reproductive health, where priorities need to be identified and strategic plans for action established, including the following:

- Research into risk factors for infertility, so that we have the information needed to guide prevention policy — evaluation of prevention programs is an essential part of this research effort, as is stable and continuing funding of research, program development, and evaluation.

- Education of the public and practitioners to promote awareness and understanding of risk factors and how to protect reproductive health. Public education programs should be non-judgemental, reflect the pluralistic nature of Canadian society, and address the complex issues surrounding sexuality in our society. They should also be evaluated periodically to determine whether they are having the desired effect.

- Working with provincial/territorial education ministries and school boards to incorporate information on fertility protection into school-based health promotion programs. In addition, special programs will be needed to reach young people at high risk who are not in school.

- Developing and providing relevant and clear information to assist women, men, and couples in making decisions related to their reproductive health, to prevent specific problems, and to seek appropriate assistance when necessary. This information must be culturally relevant to different target groups, including adolescents, Aboriginal people, and those who speak neither English nor French.

- Persuading all levels of government to fund and support reproductive health promotion and infertility prevention programs and their evaluation.

- Identifying and encouraging needed legislative change, such as changes in occupational health and safety and environmental legislation, to make it more effective in protecting reproductive health.

- Facilitating the involvement of key partners, such as the education, legal, and social service sectors, in prevention and promotion efforts. Pharmaceutical companies have a role to play with respect to including information inserts regarding condom use in packages of contraceptive hormones.

- Identifying and promoting professional and support services such as counselling and outreach that are not in place but are needed to make prevention possible. This should be within the context of larger prevention and health promotion efforts, building, for instance, on campaigns to reduce smoking so that they include risks to fertility, or on existing contraceptive counselling so that it includes STD prevention and targets specific populations, particularly adolescent women.

- Encouraging relevant changes in the training of health care providers in reproductive health promotion and infertility prevention at both the undergraduate and postgraduate levels. Curricula should address the factors that affect fertility, as well as the general reproductive health and well-being of both women and men. Continuing medical education in these areas is vital not only for physicians, but for all health care providers, whether they are working in the institutional or community health sector or in private practice.

We believe the National Reproductive Technologies Commission has a key role to play in these efforts, and we discuss the various initiatives we propose at the end of this chapter.

The Role of Prevention

There appears to be strong support in many parts of the country for initiatives that redirect resources toward disease prevention and health promotion. The federal government has been involved in formulating new conceptual frameworks for health and health care services. As early as 1974, the Department of National Health and Welfare in its document *A New Perspective on the Health of Canadians: A Working Document* took a strong position showing that factors other than health care services — such as human biology, environment, lifestyle, and health care organization — are key determinants of health. In 1986, the Department of National Health and Welfare issued a paper entitled *Achieving Health for All: A Framework for Health Promotion*, which set out three major strategies for promoting health: fostering public participation, strengthening community health services, and coordinating healthy public policy. In the same year, an international conference on health promotion sponsored by the World Health Organization, the Department of National Health and Welfare, and the Canadian Public Health Association produced the *Ottawa Charter for*

> We have been disturbed by the media coverage of these hearings pitting women who are cautious about new reproductive technologies against women who feel they may benefit from them. We believe an approach including public education, research, and funding that emphasizes prevention benefits all women.
>
> *R. Kilpatrick, Association of Ontario Midwives, Public Hearings Transcripts, Toronto, Ontario, November 20, 1990.*

Health Promotion, setting out a blueprint to help the international community develop strategies for promoting health.

The federal government has not been alone in trying to encourage a shift of effort and resources toward prevention and health promotion. Over the past few years, many provincial governments have appointed commissions and task forces. A common theme in their recommendations has been the need for initiatives that shift resources from curative treatments toward prevention.

In 1983, the Quebec government commissioned a provincial study on health promotion (*Objective: A Health Concept in Quebec: A Report of the Task Force on Health Promotion*). The task force set out 10 measurable health objectives and what was needed to achieve these objectives. Following this review, a 1986-87 commission of inquiry (Commission d'enquête sur les services de santé et les services sociaux — commonly known as the Rochon Commission) assessed the operation and financing of the health and social service systems in the province. Among its 27 recommendations for improving these systems was a proposal to reorganize infertility health services along a continuum — starting with health promotion, followed by treatment of infertility and, finally, recourse to reproductive technologies. In response to these and other reports of the task forces that it had struck throughout the 1980s, the Quebec Ministry of Health and Social Services released a document in April 1989 entitled *Improving Health and Well-Being in Quebec: Orientations*. The ministry proposed four major strategies for future action — one

> What reason is there for resorting on a wide scale to the use of technologies which counter infertility without first carrying out some in depth research into the causes and treatment of infertility? No serious, ongoing effort has been made to inform teenagers about sexually transmitted diseases which are one of the leading causes of sterility and involuntary infertility. While education and training may not be sensational or newsworthy approaches, from a social standpoint, they are extremely effective. Once more, prevention is being overshadowed by the rush to find a cure. [Translation]
>
> *Brief to the Commission from Confédération des organismes familiaux du Québec, February 2, 1991.*

> We also urge the Commission to recognize that the real problem is not how to "cure infertility" but rather how to lay the framework for a series of strategies that will prevent infertility and enhance the reproductive wellbeing of all Canadian women.
>
> *S. Ballangall, YWCA of Canada, Public Hearings Transcripts, Toronto, Ontario, November 20, 1990.*

of which was the prevention of health problems and the promotion of health and well-being.

Ontario has also been active: the Ontario Premier's Council on Health Strategy was established in 1987 in response to the recommendations of three major provincial inquiries into health and health care. The Council's mandate was to provide leadership and guidance in achieving health for all citizens of Ontario. It developed guiding principles that included greater emphasis on promoting and maintaining health and access to a balanced system of treatment. Based on these principles, the Council outlined a vision of health that took account of the importance of economic and social determinants of health, as well as the importance of equitable access to affordable and appropriate health care.

Increased emphasis on prevention and health promotion was also one of the key directions for change identified by the Premier's Commission on Future Health Care for Albertans in 1989. The Premier's Commission recommended that, by April 1995, a minimum of at least an additional 1 percent of the total Alberta health budget be allocated to health promotion and illness prevention programs.[1]

In 1989, the Nova Scotia Royal Commission on Health Care identified several principles to guide change in the provincial health care system, including the need to attain a better balance between the curative and preventive components of health care. Health promotion and disease prevention accounted for 2 percent of the budget of the Nova Scotia Department of Health in 1990-91. In response to that commission's recommendations, the department plans to increase its spending on community health to 4 percent of total departmental spending. These funds will be channelled to the development, implementation, and evaluation of comprehensive health promotion and disease prevention programs.

The 1990 Saskatchewan Commission on Directions in Health Care also called for greater emphasis on health promotion. It recommended that the mandate of traditional public health programs be expanded to place

> In terms of public policy priorities, we recommend that research funding be redirected to the following areas:
>
> Firstly, to research into the causes of infertility linked to the environment, to sexually transmitted diseases, and to the use of certain methods of contraception.
>
> Secondly, to research into the long-term effects of all reproductive technologies, including so-called "routine" prenatal exams and hormonal drugs.
>
> Thirdly, to research into no-risk contraceptive methods. [Translation]
>
> *M. Bégin, Canadian Research Institute for the Advancement of Women, Public Hearings Transcripts, Ottawa, Ontario, September 20, 1990.*

more emphasis on health promotion and maintenance of good health through programs of disease prevention, public education, personal and group counselling, and monitoring of environmental and community factors that affect the health of individuals.[2]

Similarly, the 1991 report of the British Columbia Royal Commission on Health Care and Costs noted that almost all health care funds are devoted to treatment; less than 1.5 percent of funds are spent on trying to prevent illness or injury. This report, too, makes a strong and clear call for a shift in priorities: "More money should be spent on the prevention of illness or injury and on protecting health. The least amount of money possible should be spent on providing the necessary high quality curative services."[3]

> For the sake of the public's health, your Commission should formulate social policies aimed at modifying lifestyles or behaviours that cause infertility, much in the same way as there are social policies aimed at eliminating certain lifestyles or behaviours associated with the use of toxic substances (alcohol, tobacco, drugs). There is no logic in increasing the number of infertility treatment clinics without addressing the lifestyles that cause infertility. Similarly, it would make no sense to increase the number of lung cancer treatment centres without also stepping up our efforts to eliminate smoking. [Translation]
>
> *L. Simard, Action Famille, Public Hearings Transcripts, Montreal, Quebec, November 22, 1990.*

In short, prevention is an idea whose time has come. The approach we are advocating, based on our guiding principles, the ethic of care, and evidence-based medicine, is part of a broader trend evident not only in the reports of provincial royal commissions and inquiries and documents issued by provincial/territorial and federal health departments, but also in the work of community health organizations, health policy advocates, and consumers across the country. It is clear, then, that prevention is going to assume a more prominent role in the future of public policy, resource allocation, and individual decision making in this country.

Obstacles to Shifting Resources to Prevention Programs

Despite clear recognition by governments of the need for greater emphasis on prevention, substantial change in provincial budget allocations has not occurred. The greatest proportion of health dollars continues to be spent on acute care. At present and for the foreseeable future, new dollars are not likely to be made available to be allocated to prevention and health promotion. This means that shifts *within* existing provincial budgets will be necessary to make a new emphasis on prevention and health promotion anything more than words. Deciding where these shifts should occur is very difficult, however, because the evidence on which to make such decisions is incomplete — few data have been collected, for example, on what medical treatments work, which are ineffective (or even harmful), and what approaches to prevention are successful. Such decisions are also very difficult politically, given the strong public perception that more medical care means better health. Canadians need to understand that not all medical care is of equal value, and that it may often be wiser to allocate funding to effective prevention than to ineffective treatment.

Resistance to reallocating funds to prevention also stems from the fact that it is much easier to advocate the allocation of resources to meet the needs of identifiable individuals than to devote them to serving unidentified individuals. Preventive programs also help individuals, but it is difficult to identify who they are, whereas medical programs relate to particular individuals in a direct, immediate, and documentable

Establishing the relative frequency and severity of various risk factors for infertility in the Canadian population is an important initial step in any priority-setting exercise aimed at deciding what resources are needed to tackle the prevention of infertility. Since resources are inevitably limited, such a study could help to direct the most effective resource allocation. Without a systematic effort to establish the relative importance of various identified causes of infertility, there is a risk that important preventable causes of infertility will not receive the attention they deserve. This could lead to resources being focussed on treatment of problems deemed treatable. In turn, this tends to displace attention from the relative costs of this approach versus a prevention-oriented approach, or from attempts to introduce prevention where it could be potentially beneficial.

P. Millson and K. Maznyk, "Pilot Study on Determining the Relative Importance of Risk Factors for Infertility in Canada," in Research Volumes of the Commission, 1993.

way. It is easier to justify public expenditures when moving media stories and articulate advocates of identifiable individuals are involved. People sympathize with someone anxiously awaiting medical treatment they perceive to be needed, even if it has not been proven to be of benefit. It is less easy to generate public sympathy for the unidentifiable people helped by promotion and prevention programs, even if the suffering avoided is equally real and even, in collective terms, greater. It is difficult to stop providing expensive treatments that deal with identifiable individuals, even if the treatment is of questionable value to many of those who receive it.

Reallocating funds from medical treatments to prevention does not require, however, that effective programs be closed down. There is room within many therapeutic programs to save money by allocating resources appropriately within them — through early discharge programs, for example, or establishing criteria for receiving a given treatment based on evidence of what works for what indications. Rigorous application of these and other approaches would make it largely unnecessary to withdraw funding from efficacious treatment programs in order to generate funds for prevention.

In categories of cases where no proof of effectiveness exists, or where treatments have been demonstrated ineffective, we believe funding should be withdrawn and reallocated to effective prevention programs. We recognize, however, that many groups (health care workers, physicians, hospital employees, pharmacists, and others employed in the health care industry) have a strong interest in maintaining or increasing funding for treatment; these groups, together with the public, can exert significant pressure against resource reallocation, giving politicians little room to manoeuvre when they try to shift resources to fund prevention programs.

> At present and for the foreseeable future, new dollars are not likely to be made available to be allocated to prevention and health promotion. This means that shifts *within* existing provincial budgets will be necessary to make a new emphasis on prevention and health promotion anything more than words.

Another impediment to resource reallocation is that prevention programs seem to have required a greater burden of proof before being funded than medical treatments. Even though many medical and drug treatments have not been proven effective through appropriate testing and evaluation, they are widely used and funded by provincial health care systems. Yet funding requests for prevention programs are often turned down because their impact has not been established with certainty. Even where prevention programs have been shown to be effective, funds may not be provided to maintain or extend a program.

> Prevention programs are hard to evaluate. Not all infertility is preventable, and it would be difficult to count the number of cases of infertility averted. However, common sense dictates that prevention programs are the most obvious and the least expensive step in reducing infertility, and that these programs must be available to all potential parents.
>
> *M. McGovern, Women's Issues Group, Canadian Federation of University Women, North York, Public Hearings Transcripts, Toronto, Ontario, October 31, 1990.*

A further difficulty inherent in using assessments of prevention programs is that it is not always possible to generalize from the results of one effective program. For example, sexuality education and support services designed to alter the sexual attitudes or behaviours of high school students cannot be applied to youth who have dropped out of school, even if they have been demonstrated effective in a high school setting.

Prevention programs must be designed with the identified needs, knowledge base, and motivations of specific target groups in mind.

One reason cited for the shortage of data evaluating the results of prevention programs is the difficulty of measuring these results. For example, many prevention programs are intended to elicit behaviour changes in individuals, and both the change and whether the change produced the intended results are difficult phenomena to measure. Similarly, people are exposed to many factors, including peer pressure, media images, and the home environment, that make it difficult to assess whether it was the prevention program itself or other factors that actually influenced behaviour. However, many preventive programs are just as easy to measure as many treatment programs. Many medical treatments (for example, coronary bypass surgery in patients over 65 years of age) are equally problematic to assess because other factors (such as social support, socioeconomic status, diet, exercise, tobacco use) influence the health of patients who have undergone the procedure. However, even in a short time, it is possible to measure reduced incidence of disease (for example, sexually transmitted diseases, reduction in incidence of low birth weight) in a population that has received a prevention program, so that prevention programs are not necessarily more difficult to evaluate than medical treatments.

In the view of the Commissioners, it is generally inappropriate to subject preventive efforts to more stringent effectiveness criteria than medical treatments before funding them. The effectiveness of the great majority of treatments — like the effectiveness of most prevention programs — remains unproven. Society's approach to resource allocation for medical treatments and prevention programs should be the same — both need to be evaluated rigorously before they are disseminated widely and then regularly after that to determine their continuing effectiveness. Funding for prevention programs should include funding designated for measuring outcomes. This is analogous to the evidence-based approach we recommend for treatment programs.

We recognize that this is not a simple task. Prevention is a complex undertaking in its own right, and one that cannot be taken for granted in terms of the need for information to support program evaluation and provide guidance of resource allocation and policy decisions.

Moreover, we also recognize that the standards of evidence for treatment and prevention may vary, even though an evidence-based approach should apply to both. There is an additional onus, for example, on those responsible for disease prevention and health promotion programs aimed at those who consider themselves healthy to ensure that they do no harm. This is not always the case with treatment; for instance, even in the absence of definitive evidence, a risk of causing harm by trying an untested procedure may on occasion be justified to help someone with a very serious illness if there is no alternative treatment available. Such a risk would not be justifiable in the context of prevention, which might require a higher standard of evidence of the effectiveness of a new program before its use could be justified if the potential for harm is great.

Building on Success

Despite the difficulties associated with evaluating prevention programs, there is enough evidence to show that some programs are effective in preventing exposure to some of the risk factors for infertility. For example, a comprehensive approach to reducing smoking among Canadians, including legislation, public education, school programs, and high taxation, has significantly reduced the prevalence of this risk factor.[4] Building on this successful approach to include a specific infertility prevention component could add significantly to these successes.

Similarly, AIDS education that combines information and skills building and motivates individuals to use these skills has been shown to reduce high-risk behaviour significantly. Such an approach has also proven successful in reducing pregnancies among adolescents and college students.[5] As discussed in this Part, an approach that combines these three elements could also reduce rates of sexually transmitted diseases among young people by "piggybacking" infertility prevention onto existing efforts.

It is clear, then, that the real issue in prevention is not feasibility but political will. Given that prevention programs can be evaluated, there is nothing in principle preventing governments from making informed decisions about prevention program development and resource allocation in general and infertility prevention and reproductive health promotion in particular. This Commission has concluded that preventing infertility and promoting reproductive health have at least as much to contribute in terms of rationalizing the use of scarce resources as treating fertility problems after they have occurred. Other inquiries have reached similar conclusions;

> This Commission has concluded that preventing infertility and promoting reproductive health have at least as much to contribute in terms of rationalizing the use of scarce resources as treating fertility problems after they have occurred.

what is missing is the will to make policy in light of this information. In our view, the onus is no longer on advocates of prevention to make their case but rather on policy makers to show why they have not acted to make prevention a more important part of government priorities and agendas for action.

Cost Effectiveness

Some advocates of prevention cite cost effectiveness (saving money) as the reason why resources should be shifted from medical treatments to prevention, assuming that prevention will cost less than treatment. There are two problems with this argument. For prevention programs to be more "cost effective," they must yield more health benefits than use of the same funds in treatment. In other words, the cost of the prevention program must be less than the cost of providing medical treatment to people affected by the health problem in question — prevention must result in better health status for a larger number of people. Some prevention programs, such as fluoridation of drinking water and childhood immunizations, clearly meet these standards and save substantial health care dollars. However, many other prevention programs are less cost effective than acute care would be, because they are aimed at preventing diseases that affect only a relatively small proportion of the population. Programs that aim to reduce individual exposure to risk factors associated with infertility may well be cost effective in the long term when compared to medical treatments for infertility, as many of these have substantial direct and indirect costs associated with them, but the data that would make it possible to determine this do not exist.

This brings us to the second problem with the cost-effectiveness argument and to the discussion that began this section. Evaluating programs solely on the basis of cost effectiveness ignores the ethical basis for preventing the harms associated with injury, disability, and disease. There are compelling reasons for a compassionate society to protect the fertility of individuals that go well beyond economic arguments. Infertility treatments are invasive and not always successful; like any medical treatment they entail risks, and there are also emotional and financial costs associated with them. The most humane approach is to help people protect their fertility, rather than providing treatment to help them conceive after they have already become infertile — to avoid harm rather than try to ameliorate its effects after the fact.

> When so many determinants of reproductive health are outside the medical care system, viewing change in that system alone as the way to produce reproductive health is using the wrong tool to do the job.

The cost-effectiveness argument paints too limited a picture, because it tends to frame the issues in terms of resource reallocation within the health care system. It is important to be clear that prevention is not simply — or even mainly — the concern of the health care system. In fact, effective prevention will be possible only if there is change outside the medical system — in the educational, legal, and social sectors as well. Prevention is a shared responsibility of a broad range of sectors in society and has important implications for individual Canadians as well. When so many determinants of reproductive health are outside the medical care system, viewing change in that system alone as the way to produce reproductive health is using the wrong tool to do the job. What is needed is a coordinated and multifaceted response — no individual sector has all the tools or resources to do what is needed. The Commission is therefore urging strong national leadership to begin the job of mounting a concerted effort to encourage all relevant sectors to work together to prevent infertility and promote the reproductive health of Canadians.

We recognize that provincial budgets are under tremendous pressure and that policy makers are hard pressed to find funds to maintain existing services. In this environment, reallocating resources to prevention will be difficult. Moving toward an evidence-based approach to medicine, however, with new funding provided only for treatments that have been demonstrated to be beneficial for specific medical conditions, together with evaluation of unproven treatments now in use, would permit reallocation for prevention. Prevention programs that are funded in this way should also be evaluated to determine their effectiveness. In other words, the same approach that we are advocating for assessing and funding medical treatments should also be used with prevention initiatives.

It is critical that we use our common resources effectively to achieve optimal health for all Canadians. If policy makers continue to pay only lip service to this concept, prevention will not be given the necessary emphasis, and we will continue to see an increasing proportion of our tax dollars being consumed by medical care; eventually, the health care system will collapse under the strain. This does not have to be the result if we make the decision now to move in a new direction.

> Moving toward an evidence-based approach to medicine, however, with new funding provided only for treatments that have been demonstrated to be beneficial for specific medical conditions, together with evaluation of unproven treatments now in use, would permit reallocation for prevention.

It is clear that most prevention efforts, however, will have to take place outside the health care system if they are to be effective. The education, social services, and legal systems are essential partners in effective prevention strategies and programs. Tackling the issue of infertility at its source means adopting a comprehensive, coordinated strategy for protecting the reproductive health of Canadians; reallocation of some resources within the health care system is not enough and should be only part of Canada's response.

A Comprehensive Response

In earlier chapters of this Part, we recommended programs, guidelines, and legislation that could help to reduce the exposure of individuals to the various factors that pose a risk to fertility. They ranged from improving sex education programs in schools to evaluating substances in the workplace and the environment for their reproductive health effects. In this final section, we review the role we propose for the Infertility Prevention Sub-Committee of the National Reproductive Technologies Commission in leading, supporting, and supplementing existing efforts by governments, health professionals, educators, volunteer groups, and others to reduce the prevalence of infertility in Canada and to improve the overall reproductive health of Canadians.

We have noted that there is no infertility prevention policy or strategy in Canada at present that is national in scope. Existing programs address aspects of reproductive health in a fragmented way, with little coordination between federal and provincial/territorial governments, health organizations, health care professionals, and those involved in public education. This is in contrast to what has been achieved, for example, in the field of reducing tobacco consumption, where a national committee, with representatives from federal and provincial/territorial governments and non-governmental health organizations, has successfully developed a national strategy involving a full range of actions by many sectors and groups to reduce tobacco use in Canada.

Infertility in particular, and sexual and reproductive health in general, clearly merit a similar comprehensive and coordinated response, because they are issues that affect all Canadians. It is essential that efforts to prevent known reproductive health hazards, such as sexually transmitted diseases, be integrated and coordinated to maximize their efficiency. At the same time, it is necessary to intensify and coordinate public and private research efforts directed at improving the existing pool of knowledge about the incidence, impact, and prevalence of reproductive health risks, whether caused by environmental, workplace, medical, or other factors. It is important that programs directed to infertility prevention and reproductive health be evaluated for effectiveness. Finally, it is imperative to raise public awareness about reproductive health hazards and to increase public accountability in decision making related to the development and implementation of programs and initiatives aimed at infertility prevention. The Commission therefore recommends

> **61. The establishment of a permanent sub-committee of the National Reproductive Technologies Commission, with primary responsibility in the field of infertility prevention and reproductive health promotion.**

The Infertility Prevention Sub-Committee would play an important role in all the areas just enumerated. As we explained in Chapter 5, the Infertility Prevention Sub-Committee would be one of six permanent sub-committees of the National Commission, along with those dealing with assisted insemination services, assisted conception services, prenatal diagnosis, embryo research, and the provision of fetal tissue for research and other designated purposes. Like National Commission members themselves, we recommend that at least half the Infertility Prevention Sub-Committee members be women, and that all members be chosen with a view to ensuring that they have a background and demonstrated experience in dealing with a multidisciplinary approach to issues, as well as an ability to work together to find solutions and recommend policies to address the complex challenges of infertility prevention and reproductive health promotion in a way that meets the concerns of Canadian society as a whole.

The Infertility Prevention Sub-Committee would have several functions. In addition to the priorities identified at the beginning of this section, the Sub-Committee could decide to establish ad hoc working groups to deal with one of more of these functions, if appropriate:

- Promoting and supporting consultation and cooperation among federal and provincial/territorial departments of health, labour, and the environment, among agencies such as the Canadian Centre for Occupational Health and Safety and the Canadian Centre on Substance Abuse, provincial workers' compensation boards, and other governmental bodies with responsibilities related to the field of reproductive health.

- Consulting with the provinces/territories, directly or through the Conference of Deputy Ministers of Health, on matters related to infertility prevention and reproductive health.

- Advising the federal and provincial/territorial governments on legislative and regulatory issues related to infertility prevention and reproductive health promotion, including in the areas of environmental protection and occupational health and safety.

- Consulting with health care professionals, community and public health personnel, educators, family planning organizations, and others involved in public education efforts in the field of reproductive health.

- Initiating, evaluating, disseminating, and contributing to the exchange of existing and new data and research on suspected reproductive risks, their incidence, and their reproductive effects.

- Assessing available information on existing and new infertility prevention and reproductive health promotion programs and initiatives and advising on how these can be designed and delivered more effectively.

- Working with other National Commission Sub-Committees on issues related to infertility prevention and reproductive health promotion, including training, ethical, legal, and related matters.

- Encouraging the federal government and federal research funding organizations to place greater priority on the funding of infertility-related research, including research related to program evaluation, in the public, quasi-public, and private sectors.

- Encouraging the federal and provincial/territorial governments to enhance support for infertility prevention initiatives and activities by health, labour, community, and other organizations with an interest and expertise in the field of reproductive health promotion.

- Promoting, on behalf of the federal government, international cooperation in research, information gathering, and public health initiatives related to infertility prevention. (See, for example, our recommendations in Chapter 13 with respect to a cooperative international effort to assess existing data on workplace and environmental exposures that may pose risks to reproductive health.)

- Promoting public awareness and discussion about the causes, incidence, and preventability of infertility in Canada, in part through the National Commission's annual report.

As suggested earlier, heightening public awareness about reproductive health hazards and increasing accountability in decisions about infertility prevention priorities and strategies are integral aspects of the mandate we propose for the Infertility Prevention Sub-Committee. Public awareness about reproductive health hazards will be increased as a result of the Infertility Prevention Sub-Committee's activities in promoting and disseminating further research into the causes and preventability of infertility in Canada. In addition to the National Commission's annual report, we anticipate that the Sub-Committee will make use of a variety of public consultation mechanisms to inform Canadians of new research findings in this area and to promote informed debate on their regulatory and policy implications.

Public debate and accountability will also be promoted by the composition of the Infertility Prevention Sub-Committee, which should include a balance of National Commission and outside membership, designed to ensure multidisciplinary perspectives and broad representation of the various interests involved. In particular, we recommend that this Sub-Committee include membership with a particular interest and expertise in the area of reproductive health and infertility prevention, including, for example, members from federal and provincial/territorial governments, health care professionals, community and public health personnel, educators, non-governmental health organizations, and other community organizations such as women's groups and family planning groups.

We are confident that with such a range of input, the Infertility Prevention Sub-Committee will be in a better position to identify and monitor research priorities, to evaluate existing initiatives, and to plan and coordinate future programs in a way that responds to widespread public demands for greater emphasis on infertility prevention and reproductive health promotion in any public policy response to the challenges posed by new reproductive technologies.

Conclusion

It should be clear from the discussion in this chapter that preventing infertility and promoting reproductive health are extremely complex. The old adage about medicine being as much an art as a science applies with equal force to prevention in general and infertility prevention in particular. A great deal obviously remains to be learned about all aspects of prevention as a dimension of health care, social policy, and other public policy fields. This assessment should not, however, be interpreted as meaning that prevention is not a viable response to infertility. Instead, the Commission's research has shown that there is both an opportunity for creativity in program design and a concomitant need for the disciplined and evidence-based development of initiatives that are effective in preventing infertility and promoting reproductive health.

Our research has shown further that the cost to individual Canadians and to society of failing to pursue these issues through further research and program development, together with the cost of failing to act on what we know already, will be great. There is a growing body of research and practical knowledge about what works and what does not work with respect to prevention as a policy response to public health issues. There is every reason to believe that this momentum will increase, leading to the development of more targeted, more sophisticated, and ultimately more effective efforts to prevent infertility.

Finally, our review of this field has shown that preventing infertility and promoting reproductive health are, for the most part, not the preserve or the responsibility of the health care system. Indeed, when the social determinants of behaviour

> There is a growing body of research and practical knowledge about what works and what does not work with respect to prevention as a policy response to public health issues.

that puts fertility at risk are considered, and when workplace and environmental risk factors are taken into account, it becomes clear that the health care system is not the main custodian of prevention efforts. Thus, whatever the outcome of the current debate about the appropriate proportion of health care resources that should be devoted to prevention and acute care, it must always be remembered that this debate also needs to be initiated and action taken in other sectors as well, including those dealing with schools, the workplace, and the community. This is why the approach we recommend is premised on coordination and collaboration among all key partners with the tools and resources to make the reproductive health of Canadians and the prevention of infertility a priority, with the Infertility Prevention Sub-Committee to provide focus and impetus for these efforts.

The Commission's research shows that infertility affects at least a quarter of a million Canadian couples at any given time. Unfortunately, our current knowledge does not allow us to make accurate predictions of the proportion of infertility that could be prevented. We believe, nevertheless, that a substantial proportion of infertility could be prevented if the range of measures we suggest were implemented to prevent individual exposure to the factors that pose a risk to fertility; there would be additional, more general benefits to the health of Canadians from these measures as well. We have outlined in this chapter the most urgent priorities for action and how we think they should be addressed.

Clearly, however, even if we had unlimited financial resources to devote to these efforts, and even with the most effective prevention programs in place, many people will still find themselves unable to have the children they want. In the next few chapters, therefore, we examine practices and procedures that can assist infertile couples to conceive and have healthy children.

General Sources

Quebec. Commission d'enquête sur les services de santé et les services sociaux. *Rapport de la Commission d'enquête sur les services de santé et les services sociaux.* Quebec: Government of Quebec, 1988.

Quebec. Conseil des affaires sociales et de la famille. *Objective: A Health Concept in Quebec: A Report of the Task Force on Health Promotion.* Translated by M.S. Gayk. Ottawa: Canadian Hospital Association, 1986.

Quebec. Ministry of Health and Social Services. *Improving Health and Well-Being in Quebec: Orientations.* Quebec: Government of Quebec, 1989.

Specific References

1. Alberta. Premier's Commission on Future Health Care for Albertans. *The Rainbow Report: Our Vision for Health. Vol. II. Final Report.* Edmonton: The Commission, 1989, p. 36.

2. Saskatchewan. Commission on Directions in Health Care. *Future Directions for Health Care in Saskatchewan.* Regina: The Commission, 1990.

3. British Columbia. Royal Commission on Health Care and Costs. *Closer to Home.* Victoria: The Commission, 1991, p. B3.

4. Canada. Statistics Canada. *Production and Disposition of Tobacco Products* 18 (12)(Cat. No. 32-022). Ottawa: Minister of Supply and Services Canada, 1989.

5. Canada. Health and Welfare Canada. *Guidelines for Sexual Health Education* [Draft]. Ottawa: Health Canada, 1993.

Adoption

During our public hearings and other consultations, adoption was the most frequently mentioned non-technological alternative for couples who are not able to have a child together. Couples in this situation may contemplate adoption as a solution, as an alternative to infertility treatment, or as an option if treatment proves unsuccessful. For example, in a study done for the Commission, 30 percent of IVF patients surveyed had applied for adoption by the time their treatment was under way or completed.

The attitudes expressed by intervenors reflect Canadians' views generally: fully 90 percent of people responding to a national survey conducted for the Commission considered adoption an acceptable option for couples who cannot conceive a child together. Indeed, more than half the respondents in another national survey said they would adopt a child if they were in this situation. Fewer respondents indicated they would choose other options, such as assisted insemination and *in vitro* fertilization, or choose to live without children.

However, the Commission's review of the adoption situation in Canada revealed that, in practice, adoption is not an easy alternative for most couples and is even less likely to provide a means for single people or people in non-traditional relationships to form a family. Although hard data are difficult to come by — in part because adoption systems and record-keeping methods vary between provinces and even within provinces — it is clear that trends over the past two decades are making domestic adoption a less accessible option and a more complex and difficult choice than ever before. Far more people are applying to adopt than there

> Far more people are applying to adopt than there are infants available for adoption in Canada.

are infants available for adoption in Canada. These findings place options such as donor insemination and *in vitro* fertilization in another light as we consider how societal resources should be apportioned to help people have children.

Analogous to what we heard about many of the technological options, people who conveyed their experiences to the Commission talked about their frustration with the long and complex adoption process. As explained later in this chapter, this results in part from the disparity in number of available infants and numbers wishing to adopt in Canada. Indeed, Commissioners were struck by the similarities between the experiences of couples awaiting adoption and those undergoing infertility treatment. Both processes involve intense emotions and considerable stress, which are heightened, couples

> Our daughter ... is the joy of our lives. Adopting her was no less of a miracle than our subsequent GIFT children. And this cannot be emphasized enough ... It is not really talked about as a therapy or anything, but adoption is one complete answer for infertility. It is a wonderful answer, with no physical risks, other than the birth mother's pre-existing pregnancy.
>
> [We] are greatly distressed that adoption is as difficult as it is today, because it is very difficult.
>
> *In Camera Sessions, Personal Experiences, Toronto, Ontario, May 1, 1991.*

reported, by the uncertainty of the outcome and the feeling that they have no control over the process or its result. Many who embark on infertility treatment will not have a child, just as many who apply for adoption will not be successful. For older couples in particular, these strains are intensified by the sense that they are racing against time, with the chances of a successful outcome declining as they approach the age of 40.

When Commissioners reviewed the current state of adoption in Canada, some of the reasons for these frustrations became clear. Just under 1 700 infants were placed for adoption in Canada in 1991, the latest year for which figures are available. Indeed, research

> Indeed, research conducted for the Commission shows that for every infant placed for adoption by public adoption agencies across Canada, eight applicants are waiting to adopt.

conducted for the Commission shows that for every infant placed for adoption by public adoption agencies across Canada, eight applicants are waiting to adopt. Given this, the availability of IVF and AI as options take on added importance. We estimate that between 2 000 and 4 000 children were born as a result of assisted insemination, *in vitro* fertilization, and related reproductive technologies in 1991. Thus, while the number of Canadian infants available for adoption has been declining, the number of infants born in Canada through assisted conception has been rising and now exceeds the number of infants adopted in Canada.

Although adoption was not mentioned in the Commission's mandate, Commissioners considered it important to review the current situation, given the assumption apparent in testimony before the Commission that adoption is a viable non-technological alternative for infertile couples. We therefore discuss current trends in adoption and the implications for people who are involuntarily childless in this chapter.

Methods of Adoption in Canada

Public adoption: facilitated by a public child welfare agency or provincial ministry facility; no fees

Private adoption: facilitated by non-government agency or private practitioner; prospective parents pay a fee for the service; services may be provided on a for-profit or non-profit basis

International adoption: coordinated by a public child welfare agency, a private practitioner, or, in some instances, the adopters themselves

---

Trends in Adoption in Canada

Records on adoptions from 1981 to 1990* were examined in research conducted for the Commission. As shown in Figure 16.1, the data revealed several important trends, reflecting dramatic changes in adoption over the past 10 years. The number of infants available for adoption in Canada has declined by more than half in the past decade, despite overall growth in the population. In 1981, 3 521 infants were placed

> The number of infants available for adoption in Canada has declined by more than half in the past decade, despite overall growth in the population.

---

* Statistics were gathered from the provinces, and a national survey of approximately 350 adoption service providers was conducted (202 public service agencies, 130 private practitioners, and 16 private adoption agencies). The data come with some caveats. For example, it is rare to find complete and comparable adoption records in provincial ministries over a substantial period of time. Nor has there been a sustained effort to collect specific categories of adoption information across the country, making it difficult to combine or compare information from various provinces. The fact that the Commission had to rely on estimates in some cases underscores the need for data collection in support of public policy in this area.

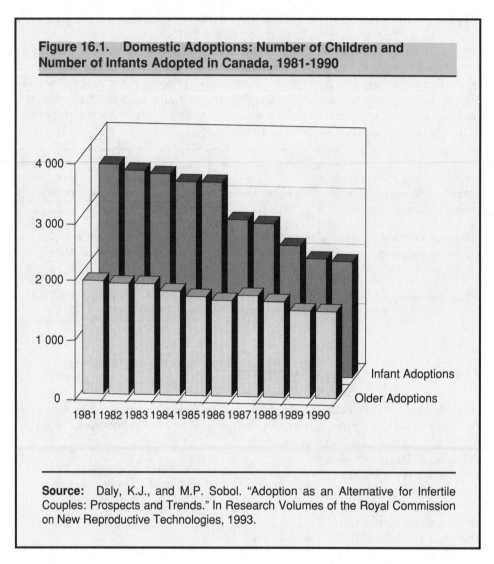

Figure 16.1.   Domestic Adoptions: Number of Children and Number of Infants Adopted in Canada, 1981-1990

Source: Daly, K.J., and M.P. Sobol. "Adoption as an Alternative for Infertile Couples: Prospects and Trends." In Research Volumes of the Royal Commission on New Reproductive Technologies, 1993.

for adoption, compared to 1 698 in 1990. Given that Canada's population increased by 9.3 percent over the same period, the decline appears even more dramatic.

This trend is attributable largely to two factors: the general availability of contraception, which has reduced the overall number of pregnancies that might result in a child becoming available for adoption, and the fact that many more young women are choosing to keep their children in circumstances where, in the past, they might have chosen to place them for

The assumption that the availability of abortion has reduced the number of infants available for adoption appears to be unfounded.

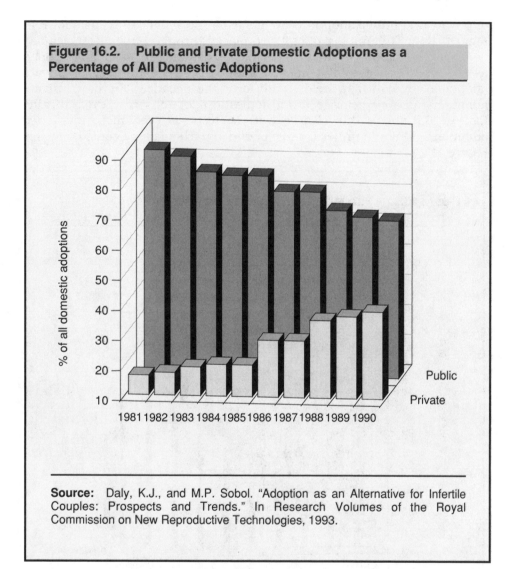

Figure 16.2.   Public and Private Domestic Adoptions as a Percentage of All Domestic Adoptions

Source: Daly, K.J., and M.P. Sobol. "Adoption as an Alternative for Infertile Couples: Prospects and Trends." In Research Volumes of the Royal Commission on New Reproductive Technologies, 1993.

adoption. Of all births to unmarried mothers, data for 1959 suggest that 64 percent ended in adoption, whereas recent data available for unmarried women under 25 years of age suggest less than 4 percent gave them up for adoption. The assumption that the availability of abortion has reduced the number of infants available for adoption appears to be unfounded. Among women under the age of 25, who make up the vast majority of those who place infants for adoption, the number of abortions declined steadily over the past decade, yet the number of infants available for adoption also declined.

Adoptions can be facilitated by public or private agencies (see earlier box). Within the shrinking number of domestic adoptions, the proportions of private and public adoptions are also shifting significantly, as shown in Figure 16.2. The number of children placed through public agencies has declined significantly in the past decade, as has the rate of such adoptions as a proportion of total domestic adoptions. The number of private adoptions, by contrast, held steady over the decade. However, private adoptions as a percentage of all domestic adoptions rose dramatically. Figure 16.2 shows this clearly, but the trend is even more marked if adoptions of infants under the age of one in particular are considered (see Figure 16.3).

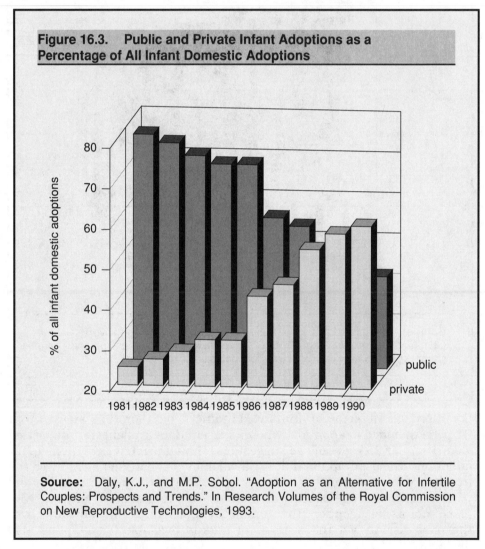

Figure 16.3. Public and Private Infant Adoptions as a Percentage of All Infant Domestic Adoptions

Source: Daly, K.J., and M.P. Sobol. "Adoption as an Alternative for Infertile Couples: Prospects and Trends." In Research Volumes of the Royal Commission on New Reproductive Technologies, 1993.

Figure 16.3 also illustrates the current reality of adoption in Canada: infants are available for adoption primarily through private rather than public adoption agencies. In 1990, for example, the number of applicants for public adoption exceeded the number of infants actually placed for adoption by a factor of almost eight to one. Overall, the ratio of applicants to children of all ages placed for adoption is about three to one.

> Infants are available for adoption primarily through private rather than public adoption agencies ... Overall, the ratio of applicants to children of all ages placed for adoption is about three to one.

As a result of these trends, the number of people who want to adopt far exceeds the number of children available for adoption in Canada. This is no doubt one reason for the rising number of international adoptions, along with the desire of couples to avoid the long wait for domestic adoption of an infant. International adoptions are now thought to outnumber domestic adoptions (public and private combined); best estimates (extrapolated from the figures for Quebec, which is the only province that keeps complete records) are that for every two domestic adoptions of infants, three international infant adoptions take place.

Canada's Adoption System

Those who want to adopt a child in Canada can choose one of three methods: public, private, or international adoption. All provinces and territories except Quebec and Newfoundland permit both public and private adoption. Quebec prohibited private adoptions in 1980; since then, all adoptions, including international adoptions, have been coordinated through a public system. Since 1972, all adoptions in Newfoundland have been coordinated through a public system as well. No independent agencies or practitioners provide adoption services for a fee; only government social workers are permitted to act as service providers. Ontario requires all private practitioners to be licensed. In Alberta, agencies operate on a non-profit basis and a licence is required only if the agency is charging a fee to adoptive parents. No other province or territory requires private agencies or practitioners to be licensed, and none places an upper limit on the fees private agencies can charge.

> We desperately need more educated professionals in the issues of adoption to help us and our children cope with all the feelings in, around and about adoption. Perhaps, in time, there will be a Parent's Aid Society that works together with Children's Aid Societies to help the whole family.
>
> *Brief to the Commission from the Adoptive Parents Association of Halton, November 8, 1991.*

Public Adoption

Public adoptions are financially the most accessible type of adoption, as no fee is involved. Applicants must pass a screening process, however, and waiting lists for public adoption are long — six years on average to adopt a healthy infant, compared to three years for privately arranged adoptions where no fee is involved and just under two years through private agencies or practitioners that charge a fee. In fact, some 16 percent of the public agencies contacted for the National Adoption Study have closed their waiting lists — they are not accepting any new applications from people wishing to adopt.

In testimony and submissions to the Commission, many people described the various public adoption systems as difficult and frustrating, citing long waiting lists, the small number of children available for adoption, and application and screening procedures that prospective parents see as complex and intrusive, contributing to their feeling of powerlessness and lack of control over the adoption process.

On the other hand, public systems offer several advantages, primarily in the services offered to birth and adoptive parents. Thirty-two percent of public adoption agencies, for instance, offer support groups for new adoptive parents, compared to 21 percent in the private sector. Two-thirds (66 percent) of public providers offer short-term support to the birth parents, compared to 47 percent of private providers. The availability of this structured support, including professional staff, can be important for both the biological and the adoptive parents.

A benefit of public adoption for the children is the large pool of adoptive families from among whom agency personnel can select prospective parents. Other features of public adoption include more complete records of children's medical and social history (and storage of these records for an indefinite period); alternative resources in the event of a disruption in the adoption; more equitable access, regardless of socioeconomic status; and continuing availability of counselling services for all parties involved. This helps to ensure, through the structure and operation of the adoption process, that the best interests of the child are promoted.

Private Adoption

Private adoption is an appealing alternative for those who can afford it. Prospective parents face shorter waiting lists and a greater chance of adopting an infant, and they have more control over how the adoption is handled. These factors are reflected in the rise of private adoptions as a proportion of all domestic adoptions during the 1980s. The number of private adoptions remained relatively steady over this period, but they rose from 17.4 percent of domestic adoptions in 1981 to 39 percent by 1990, while the number of public adoptions declined.

Prospective parents using a private agency can expect to pay fees of up to $6 000, with the average being about $3 600. For adoptions facilitated by a private practitioner (a lawyer or social worker), the average fee is about $3 100 according to data provided to the Commission, although some practitioners involved in private arrangements charge no fee. The higher fees usually mean that the adoptive parents have agreed to pay for additional services, such as pre- and post-adoption counselling for the birth parents, other expenses of the birth mother, and home study updates.

One of the perceived advantages of private adoption is that it offers both the birth mother and the adoptive parents more opportunities to control the adoption process and have more personal influence in decisions about it. Research conducted for the Commission shows, for example, that private adoptions are more likely than public adoptions to be "open" — with birth and adoptive parents knowing about and even meeting each other. Some have argued that it is in the best interests of the child to know about his or her birth parents and for adoption arrangements to be open. The research showed that twice as many private practitioners as public service providers (41 percent compared to 20 percent) have facilitated a fully open adoption, where birth parents and adoptive parents meet before the placement and exchange identifying information. Similarly, 62 percent of private practitioners have facilitated an adoption where the birth and adoptive parents exchanged information anonymously through the practitioner; 55 percent of the public agencies surveyed had done this.

> We came through the [private] adoption route ...
>
> IVF was a piece of cake compared to everything else.
>
> We were treated by the Children's Aid workers and case workers and social workers as less than human, and it cost us a fair amount of money in trying the adoption route ...
>
> And we came up with nothing.
>
> *In Camera Sessions, Personal Experiences, Ottawa, Ontario, May 14, 1991.*

At the same time, private adoption raises questions about whether and how the best interests of children are being served. Private adoption is available only to those who can afford the fees, giving rise to apprehension about commercialization of this activity. Nor is private adoption closely regulated in 10 of the 12 provinces and territories that permit it. This raises concerns about standards in adoption services — for example, the training and qualifications of personnel involved in placing children for adoption, follow-up and support services for adoptive families, and the content, completeness, and availability of adoption records. It could also be argued, however, that if a private system encourages openness in adoptions, adopted children could benefit.

International Adoption

International adoption has become the most common method of infant adoption for Canadians, reflecting the small number of infants available for adoption within the country. Canadians made an estimated 2 448 international adoptions in 1991.

One adoptive parent who testified before the Commission placed the cost of adopting a child from outside Canada at between $12 000 and $15 000. In addition to the financial cost, international adoptions may pose challenges to the adoptive family. For example, as in some domestic adoptions, poor pre- and post-natal conditions may result in future physical or mental disabilities in the child, while missing or incomplete medical records may compound the difficulties associated with caring for and raising the child.

International adoptions also raise complex issues for families — such as the challenge of raising a child of a different racial or ethnic background — and for Canadian society, including such issues as how to ensure that international adoptions conform to Canadian standards with respect to ethics, law, and the protection of the child's best interests. Among the ethical issues involved are the possible pressures on parents in difficult financial or social circumstances to allow their children to be adopted by families in wealthier countries and the potential for international adoptions to encourage the view that children can be "bought" or "sold."

Custom Adoption

The Commission also learned during its public hearings that adoption in Aboriginal communities can take place without the formal involvement of public agencies or officials. People in these communities follow their traditional rules or customs in a practice known as custom adoption. Whether permitted by provincial or territorial law or practised without this authority, custom adoption is among the means for Aboriginal people to ensure that their children remain in Aboriginal communities and in contact with their family and cultural origins.

As the Commission was told in Whitehorse and Yellowknife, custom adoptions involve a fertile couple or woman "giving" a child to a childless cou-

> Some women who are indeed infertile ... in talking with their own family members and elders [have been told] ... children are a gift and if you haven't received that gift, then maybe your love should be shared in some other way with the extended family. And that's why it's ... so much more common for them to take in the child of a sister or a cousin because there isn't quite the same pressure, I feel, on them having their own natural child ... access to custom adoption is probably a little more free than down south.
>
> *L. Hudson, Tawow Society, Fort Smith, Public Hearings Transcripts, Yellowknife, Northwest Territories, September 12, 1990.*

ple, sometimes but not necessarily because one or both birth parents are unable to care for the child. The adoptee knows who the birth parents are, and some relationship between the birth parents and the child continues. This is an accepted part of many Aboriginal cultures and does not devalue the child — on the contrary, the cultural perception may be that the child "belongs" to the community more than to the individual who gave birth to or raises the child. In the Northwest Territories, such adoptions are recorded to ensure that the adoptive family is entitled to family and educational benefits for the child.

Given current efforts by many Aboriginal communities to gain control of child welfare services, as well as the work of the Royal Commission on Aboriginal Peoples, which has a comprehensive mandate in relation to Aboriginal child welfare and many other issues, we believe it would be inappropriate for this Commission to comment on this practice.

Access to Adoption

In private sessions with Commissioners, Canadians said that they had considered adoption, but some had not pursued it actively because of the low number of infants available for adoption, the complex and lengthy public adoption process, the length of waiting lists, or the prohibitive cost of private and international adoptions. Others had pursued adoption despite these difficulties.

Thus, the statistics discussed earlier in the chapter were given a human face in the Commission's private sessions; many people who had explored adoption after discovering their infertility saw adoption as a relatively undesirable or inaccessible option for them. Some rejected adoption because they wanted a genetically linked child or wanted to experience pregnancy and birth. For others, however, access to adoption was the more important issue. In addition to long waiting lists for public adoption and high costs

> If we prohibit pregnancy contracts and limit access to other technologies, then couples who wish to have children must have greater access to other courses of action. Adoption appears to be one solution that does not of course settle all the problems but which might be more feasible. At present, there are very great limitations to international adoption and adoption within Canada, and these need to be resolved. Those who cannot sort out the issues involved in international adoption should be given access to the psychosocial methods and resources to help them reconcile themselves to not having children. [Translation]
>
> *C. Coderre, Fédération des femmes du Québec, Public Hearings Transcripts, Montreal, Quebec, November 21, 1990.*

for private or international adoption, some thought they had been denied access to adoption because of personal characteristics such as their age, marital status, religion, or sexual orientation.

The Commission's research showed that some of these perceptions accurately reflect adoption agency policies. The criteria used by both private and public agencies to screen prospective parents generally reflect the traditional concept of the family — a relatively young married couple. Our research also showed that some adoption agencies have reservations about placing a child with single people, people of a different race or religion from the child, and couples over the age of 40. Gay and lesbian couples encounter the greatest difficulty when trying to adopt.

The age criterion is particularly relevant to people undergoing infertility treatment. By the time they discover their infertility and seek treatment for it, couples are usually in their early 30s. There may be a substantial waiting period before the couple is able to receive treatment. If treatment is unsuccessful (again requiring a year or more to find out), the couple may wish to adopt. They will discover, however, that the waiting period for a public adoption averages six years, bringing one or both of them perilously close to the age cut-off used by many adoption agencies to screen prospective parents.

> What you have been hearing about the dramatic efforts of some to bear children should incline your Commission to come out as an ardent promoter of social policies to facilitate adoptions.
>
> In today's world, for every Canadian couple striving to have a child there are hundreds, even thousands, of children in need of parents. Many of them are not adopted because they are perceived to be imperfect. You can urge that it be a priority for all levels of government in this country to adopt measures to reduce the difficulties and delays that now frustrate many who want to adopt children. These measures should include educational efforts to help people overcome fears and prejudices about adoptions.
>
> They should also include international accords, to establish procedures that are respectful of the needs of children and would-be parents. It is inhumane not to have better programmes than today's to promote and facilitate adoptions.
>
> *Brief to the Commission from Action Famille, February 5, 1991.*

This is among the reasons we have recommended elsewhere in this report that infertility treatment clinics improve their information and counselling services with respect to options and alternatives when a couple first seeks treatment (see Chapters 19 and 20). We believe that infertility treatment centres should not exclude people who are on an adoption waiting list. In addition, adoption agencies should not screen out people waiting for or undergoing infertility treatment. Canadians told us that these practices are occurring, but our surveys of *in vitro* fertilization clinics and adoption agencies did not reveal the existence of such policies. Nevertheless, since people may withdraw from either waiting list for reasons such as spontaneous pregnancy, there is no good reason for such policies.

An Adoption System in the Best Interests of Children

The principle of the best interests of the child guided the development of adoption policies in Canada. The evolution of the adoption field over the last decade led us to question, however, whether this principle continues to be the basis of such policies or, in some cases, the lack of policy.

Children are important as individuals and as members of society; this should be reflected in all arrangements society makes for their care, including adoption systems. We question whether the current mix of private and public adoption systems is the best means of protecting children's interests and of supporting people's ability to form families through adoption. Many issues can arise — emotional, psychological, developmental, and social — in the period leading up to an adoption and as the parents raise the child, and we question whether current adoption policies and practices provide the necessary support for parents and children alike.

> Individual and cultural values play key roles in determining the acceptability of adoption as a viable alternative. Historical changes in the meaning of adoptive relationships have had an impact on the interpersonal experiences of adoption, the delivery of adoption services, and adoption legislation and policy. Recent social-psychological research has provided insight into some of the unique and predictable tasks that are encountered when becoming adoptive parents. Identity has emerged as a central focus in the adoption literature, with the accessibility of information about biological heritage being a key to healthy adoption adjustment.
>
> *K. Daly and M. Sobol. "Adoption as an Alternative for Infertile Couples: Prospects and Trends," in Research Volumes of the Commission, 1993.*

In addition to protecting the interests of children and meeting the needs of adoptive families, we also believe that adoption systems, including Canadian policies with respect to international adoption, should reflect concern for other principles that are part of our ethical prism, such as the non-commercialization of reproduction, equality or non-discrimination in access, and scope for autonomy in decisions on the part of both birth parents and adoptive parents.

In the Commission's view, a comprehensive review of Canadian adoption systems is warranted at this time. The recently completed National Adoption Study, sponsored by Health Canada, was a step in this direction. The study gathered information on demographic trends (much of the information available for the first time in Canada), adoption law and policies in various jurisdictions across the country, and the policies and practices of public and private adoption providers. Although the study appeared too late in this Commission's mandate for us to address the issues it raises or evaluate its recommendations in detail, it is clear that its subject matter warrants continuing public policy attention from both federal and provincial/territorial governments. The Commission therefore recommends that

> **62. Federal and provincial/territorial governments undertake a joint review of adoption in Canada, with a view to addressing such issues as the relative merits of public and private adoption systems in promoting the best interests of the child and in meeting the needs of the other parties involved (including birth parents, adoptive parents, and siblings of the adopted child); access to adoption and barriers to access; cost; record keeping and disclosure; counselling and consent; the advantages and drawbacks of interprovincial harmonization of policies, services, and practices; and issues in relation to international adoptions.**

Commissioners are of the view that the ethical and other issues raised by the existence of a private adoption system, as well as by the practice of international adoption, necessitate a thorough review and coordinated action in this regard. This could occur in the context of the continuing consultations suggested by the National Adoption Study or as a separate exercise.

In summary, the Commission found that adoption is not a feasible alternative for many Canadians who are involuntarily childless, mainly because the number of children, particularly infants, available for adoption has declined so markedly. As we have noted, fewer infants are adopted in Canada each year now than are born as a result of assisted conception techniques. In the next few chapters we examine these techniques, their role in treating infertility, and their place in Canada's response to the problem of involuntary childlessness.

General Sources

Daly, K.J., and M.P. Sobol. "Adoption as an Alternative for Infertile Couples: Prospects and Trends." In Research Volumes of the Royal Commission on New Reproductive Technologies, 1993.

Daly, K.J., and M.P. Sobol. *Adoption in Canada: Final Report.* Study funded by National Welfare Grants, Health Canada. Guelph: University of Guelph, National Adoption Study, 1993.

Hepworth, H.P. *Foster Care and Adoption in Canada.* Ottawa: Canadian Council on Social Development, 1980.

Infertility Treatments: Introduction and Social Context

♦

There is no easy way for couples to discover they are infertile. Trying to have a child but not being able to conceive means hopes and plans for the future are dashed. Often, this happens after a couple has spent several years controlling their assumed fertility through contraception, which may make the discovery even more difficult. Also, it is quite common that by the time infertility is diagnosed, the couple may already be well into their reproductive years and have spent a significant amount of time trying to conceive naturally; they want to know what they can do before it is too late.

The three reproductive technologies covered in this section are separate but linked types of infertility treatment: fertility drugs; assisted insemination; and *in vitro* fertilization and its related techniques. These treatments can be seen as existing along a continuum. At one end there are fertility drugs, the most frequent and least invasive fertility treatment, often prescribed by family physicians or obstetricians and gynaecologists. For many couples, this is the only infertility treatment used. Others move on to increasingly invasive and complex treatments. Assisted insemination, the next treatment we consider in this section, used primarily for male infertility, is used less commonly than fertility drugs and is practised not only by family doctors and obstetricians but also in clinic-based fertility programs. The most invasive and most expensive technique is also the one most people associate with new reproductive technologies: *in vitro* fertilization. This is performed only in clinic-based fertility programs. A final chapter in this section looks at egg and embryo donation, rarely used in this country, examining the issues that arise because of the availability of IVF and the capacity to retrieve eggs, fertilize them for use in assisted conception, then preserve the remaining zygotes outside the human body.

Many individuals — the single largest group of those treated for infertility — are treated with fertility drugs prescribed by family physicians.

These are women who may never go any further with infertility treatment, never see specialists or enrol in a fertility program. For other patients, however, the initial treatment with fertility drugs is the start of a long and demanding journey of referrals to specialists and increasingly invasive treatments. The Commission examined all three areas — fertility drugs, assisted insemination, and *in vitro* fertilization — with equal rigour, using the principles of evidence-based medicine, discussed in Part One, as well as our ethical framework. One of our goals was to right the balance of attention, which has previously been weighted toward IVF. The research we carried out with respect to clinical effectiveness and safety, as well as practices and procedures, has not been done as comprehensively in Canada before. Our approach was innovative, and our findings, which will be presented in detail over the next three chapters, were unsettling. Commissioners were disturbed by the state of practice in this area.

We found, for instance, that little research has been done into the effectiveness or adverse outcomes of fertility drug use, with many practitioners accepting that they all work well, without necessarily having the evidence to support this view. We also found that IVF has been shown to be effective only for the one condition it was developed to treat — fallopian tube blockage — but that its use proliferated over the 1980s, so that it is now being used to treat a wider and wider range of conditions without evidence that it is effective for them. There is also marked variation in practices and procedures in fertility programs across the country, including some practices that are simply unsafe. Of particular concern was the fact that our 1991 survey of fertility programs across the country found that some programs were not quarantining donated sperm and retesting sperm donors for HIV six months after the donation before using the sperm for assisted insemination. At least three private practitioners surveyed were using fresh sperm for donor insemination, despite the existence of professional guidelines since 1988 requiring sperm to be frozen and quarantined to allow for testing of donors. We considered these findings so serious that we brought them to the attention of Canadians and the relevant professional bodies in releasing the survey findings in April 1993.

A treatment cannot be assumed to be effective unless it has been demonstrated to be so through well-designed clinical research. Second, data must be collected to track long-term health outcomes to ensure that effective treatments are also safe treatments.

In the Commission's view, the joining of an egg and sperm *in vitro*, and transfer of the resulting zygote to a woman's body, are not unethical or inappropriate in and of themselves, provided they are carried out in circumstances that ensure ethical and responsible use of the technologies. However, our research in the field of infertility treatments led to one inescapable conclusion: Commissioners believe it is time to get back to basics. First, a treatment cannot be assumed to be effective unless it has been demonstrated to be so through well-designed clinical research. Second, data must be collected to track long-term health outcomes to ensure that effective treatments are also safe treatments.

The question of whether there are safe and effective IVF treatments must be addressed by evaluating evidence. In our view, medical procedures should move from the realm of research to that of treatment only if they can be demonstrated to be effective and beneficial and if information on their risks and effects is available. With respect to IVF, information from this type of assessment facilitates decisions on two levels: societal decisions about the allocation of health care resources to provide IVF and related procedures; and specific decisions about treatment of individuals. We believe it is important, however, that this same evidence-based approach apply just as rigorously to the less invasive and less "high-tech" treatments (fertility drugs and assisted insemination) as it does to IVF. These treatments are provided to thousands of Canadian women each year, with potential implications for their health and that of their children and partners; these treatments should not be spared assessment simply because the technology they involve is not "high" technology. Decisive national leadership is needed to put the mechanisms in place to facilitate this more balanced approach, which would be spearheaded by the National Reproductive Technologies Commission we propose be established. Our specific recommendations for how this should be done are set out in the next four chapters.

We did not arrive at our conclusions lightly. We came to them, rather, as a logical outgrowth of our ethical foundation and guiding principles and our commitment to evidence-based medicine. Commissioners believe that demanding safe and effective treatment is not patronizing of individuals who are infertile; rather, it is the prudent approach based on society's responsibility to defend vulnerable interests — both those of individuals and those of the wider community. Adherence to the ethic of care makes it imperative to reduce risk to minimum acceptable levels, but this is not invariably the situation with infertility treatment in Canada today. We recognize that adoption of our proposals may mean that some couples will not have access to treatments they, and indeed some physicians, may have come to consider necessary. The statement of one woman who is infertile appearing before the Commission exemplifies what others also told us; she said that infertile people want treatment, but they do not want unsafe or ineffective treatment.

> Infertile people want treatment, but they do not want unsafe or ineffective treatment.

We also recognize that the standards we propose place greater demands for evidence on this area of medical care than is currently the case in other areas of medicine. But we believe that setting high standards of quality here is appropriate because we are dealing with human reproduction, an area that must be approached with caution and an eye to future generations, and because such standards are within our reach as a society and within the reach of the health care system through which infertility treatments are provided.   Infertility treatment involves both individual and collective aspects, combining complex diagnosis and treatment procedures with socially significant and far-reaching implications for others as well.   This combination of factors means it is even more important to approach infertility treatment responsibly.   There is the potential to provide a model of how evidence-based medicine should work, an example that may be valuable for other areas of medical care.   The approach we propose will also provide the needed evidence upon which governments will be able to base rational and accountable resource allocation decisions about providing coverage under provincial/territorial health insurance plans for infertility treatments that have been demonstrated effective and safe.

Although infertility treatments are provided in a medical context, they have profound social significance as well.   The remainder of this introductory section examines the social context for infertility treatment.

The Social Context for Infertility Treatments: What We Heard

Decisions about infertility treatment take place at two levels. At the personal level, individuals and couples who are infertile must decide whether they want to undergo treatment to attempt to have a child, basing the decision on their individual circumstances, values, and knowledge. These decisions are not made in a vacuum, however, but in a context of societal values and attitudes and previous societal decisions. Issues such as how society views technology and the medicalization of women's health, particularly their reproductive health, and decisions about which procedures qualify as medical treatments, what kinds of resources to allocate to them, and who has access to them, form the social context for understanding infertility treatments. Some of these issues were discussed in a more general sense in Part One of this report but will be touched upon again because of their immediate relevance to infertility treatment.

The values, opinions, and behaviours of Canadians, and their attitudes toward reproduction and IVF in particular, also form part of the social context for IVF and the background to our discussion of how society should address the issues raised by use of the technology at the collective level. *In vitro* fertilization was one of the most extensively debated technologies in the Commission's mandate; this is reflected in the amount of attention it received from the media and from individuals and groups that participated in the Commission's work, through public hearings, private sessions, roundtables, panel discussions, letters, and submissions. In addition, the Commission sought further understanding through national surveys and a survey of people enrolled in fertility programs across the country. The findings of these surveys will be discussed throughout the next few chapters. These consultation activities were complemented by extensive research projects examining not only the medical, but also the psychological and social aspects of infertility treatment.

> Thus, although we support the use of *in vitro* fertilization techniques for childless couples, the use of donor sperm and ova and surrogacy breaks, or, at least, severely strains the bond of mutuality between partners as well as between parents and children. The issue, in other words, is about the use of technology in relationships, not just about setting the limits to technology.
>
> *J. Olthuis, Citizens for Public Justice, Public Hearings Transcripts, Toronto, Ontario, October 29, 1990.*

The national dialogue on infertility treatment that resulted from the Commission's work in this area gave Commissioners a rich and multifaceted basis from which to consider the issues. This multidimensional perspective was necessary because no single vantage point can provide a comprehensive overview of the personal, medical, social, ethical, economic, and legal dimensions of the issues surrounding infertility treatment.

Despite the issues and concerns they raise, most Canadians see infertility treatments as valuable reproductive options. For example, we found from our survey that the majority (58 percent) support donor insemination for couples in which the male partner has a sperm problem that affects his fertility, whereas almost 80 percent approve of IVF, a much more complex and high-tech procedure, when it involves the use of the couple's own eggs and sperm. Many women and couples impressed upon the Commission that these treatments have given them the chance to experience parenthood and have children and urged the Commission to ensure that they remain a reproductive option. The Commission also heard concerns, however, about how the treatments are provided and how records about the treatments and their results are kept. These concerns, many of which were borne out by the Commission's research, are discussed in greater detail in the following sections.

How Society Views Technology

The ambivalence with which many in society view technology is clearly illustrated by attitudes toward *in vitro* fertilization. A cursory examination of media coverage demonstrates the contradictory images of, on one hand, bouncing babies and their overjoyed parents and, on the other hand, complex technology, gleaming laboratories, and the power of medical scientists who can manipulate human zygotes.

In fact, society's attitudes toward the whole field of infertility treatment reflects such an ambivalence. Heartfelt calls for solutions to infertility co-exist with a sense of suspicion and scepticism about the solutions now being offered. For instance, experiences with some drugs (such as thalidomide and DES) have made many people wary of the effects of fertility drugs on the women taking them and on their children.

Women's Reproductive Health and Well-Being

While understanding people's desire to have children and to have access to treatment that may make this possible, many Canadians have strong reservations about infertility treatment as it is now provided.

> Like all other medical techniques, NRTs are used in a growing number of pregnancies, and are evolving from their original foundations of therapy and prevention to involve the rationalized management of human reproduction.
>
> This has major consequences, such as women's relinquishment of the maternity experience, and increased dependence of individuals on the priorities set by the medical staff and NRT accessibility criteria. What will become of couples' freedom to make their own decisions about fecundity if NRTs continue to develop at the current rate? [Translation]
>
> *Brief to the Commission from Confédération des organismes familiaux du Québec, February 2, 1991.*

Many of these reservations focus on IVF because of its highly technological nature, but the concerns the Commission heard reflect the hesitancy with which many people view other infertility treatments as well.

Individuals and groups, among them the major women's groups in Canada, are concerned that, just as the movement to de-medicalize women's reproductive health, through services such as midwifery, is making strides, infertility treatment may encourage a return to a medicalized model of women's reproductive health. They are concerned that women are socialized to believe they must be mothers, and that they are being pressured to seek medical solutions to social dilemmas. Further, the Commission heard, this re-medicalization has been carried out irresponsibly, endangering women's health in the process, and experimental procedures, primarily IVF, are being used as treatment without any evidence of effectiveness or safety. Intervenors were also concerned that women are treated as the patients in assisted insemination programs, with any risks that entails, when, in fact, assisted insemination is a treatment for the male partner's infertility.

There is also a wider public perception that infertility treatments, because they take place in clinics or doctors' offices, are "safe." This belief explains in part the sense of betrayal experienced when the perception is shown to be unfounded, as was the case with the Commission's survey of fertility programs, which found that some physicians and programs were not taking the necessary precautions to prevent the transmission of HIV, the virus thought to cause AIDS.

Concerns about safety were why some groups and individuals called for a moratorium on infertility treatments. Some groups would like to see a halt to the expansion of all services until the necessary evidence on effectiveness and safety can be gathered. In particular, they think more information is needed on whether infertility drugs work and whether they have long-term health effects for women and children.

Other groups focussed on IVF, opposing any provision of this procedure, regardless of evidence of its effectiveness, because of the ethical issues surrounding the creation and storage of zygotes outside the human body. The fact that zygotes created but not needed for IVF treatment are sometimes discarded or used for research offends their beliefs about the status of the embryo/zygote.

These views were juxtaposed to those of individuals and couples who are infertile and who told the Commission that having a child is very important to them and who saw infertility treatment as their only chance to achieve this. They felt strongly that they were capable of making their own decisions about their use of the technologies, provided information was available to them.

> I ... want to express my views to you today as a wife, an infertile woman, a feminist and a recipient of in vitro fertilization.
>
> My concern is that too many others, mainly parents and those who are childless by choice, portray people with infertility problems as mindless guinea pigs, obsessed by [an] unnatural desire to procreate at any cost regardless of any risk to the health of the child which we might have or risk to our own health. Infertile women especially seem to be pictured as victims of a male-dominated medical profession and/or dominated by a husband's need to produce progeny to secure his immortality, or some such version ... others speak for us assuming that somehow we are not capable of rational decision-making when managing our infertility ... This stereotypical view of infertile people is false.
>
> *J. McDonald, Kingston Infertility Network, Public Hearings Transcripts, Ottawa, Ontario, September 20, 1990.*

Contrary to what some observers have said about external pressure, our survey of 1 395 women who participated in infertility programs across the country showed that women's own desire for children was the strongest motive for seeking help at an infertility clinic. We discussed in Chapter 2 how social construction has a part to play in shaping people's attitudes about having children, but the women we surveyed felt their own desire was much more important than any other motivating factor, including a spouse's desire for children, and very few reported pressure.

Many intervenors in the Commission's public consultations were also disturbed by the links between the use of new reproductive technologies in animals and in human beings. For instance, IVF is used to help people have children, but it is used in animals to improve genetic traits, and there were fears expressed that this use could be transferred to human beings. These issues are discussed in greater detail in Chapter 22.

Decision Making About Infertility Treatments

Canadians told the Commission that they want more opportunities to influence decisions about the use of technologies and the allocation of public resources to them; they do not want to leave decisions about how the technologies are practised and who has access to them solely in the hands of medical practitioners and researchers. Although we heard the view that society should look to the medical profession as both the repository of knowledge about new reproductive technologies and the best source of decisions regarding their use, more often we heard the view that practitioners and researchers should not be making moral and ethical judgements for individual patients or for the community at large. In fact, many physicians told the Commission that they do not want to be placed in that position, yet they have been placed there unwillingly because of the absence of other forms of societal ethical decision making.

> I have worked with several couples who are infertile and have gone through the use of new reproductive technologies and some of the anguish they have gone through in trying to get pregnant and not succeeding ... I have also worked at the other end of [the] spectrum for many years ... with very poor women who have had extremely premature births because they don't get adequate nutrition throughout their pregnancy, and their babies don't survive ... And the discrepancy of those two things ... in one culture like ours, just continues to flabbergast me ... this is money that we have to choose how we are going to spend in the society.
>
> D. Marshall, Citizens for Public Justice, Public Hearings Transcripts, Toronto, Ontario, October 29, 1990.

Need for Informed Choice

The controversy about whether infertility treatments, especially IVF, amount to experiments on women or valid treatments was often presented as a polarized debate, but in reality the Commission found that there was more common ground than confrontation. One of the key areas of agreement was on the need for more information about all technologies, not just IVF, and about their effectiveness and safety, so that individuals and couples considering using the technologies can exercise informed choice.

There was also agreement that this information must be accessible to a wide range of prospective patients, reflecting the pluralistic nature of Canadian society.

Women and couples felt that they did not have enough information about the short- and long-term effects of undergoing treatment. The Commission's survey of patients in fertility programs across Canada found that the issues about which they wanted most information were those on which the material provided by programs placed least emphasis and was least helpful. These included the psychosocial aspects of treatment, their chances of having a child, the short- and long-term effects of treatment, and treatment alternatives.

Individual attitudes and choices about infertility treatments are often conditioned by underlying assumptions or beliefs about the role of technology, the determinants of women's reproductive health and well-being, and the need for informed choice. Several other more explicit issues can also affect an individual's or couple's decisions about whether to accept infertility treatment and, if so, which one.

Funding for Infertility Treatments

Public funding for infertility treatments is a major determinant of how much they are used. The Commission's study of fertility programs found that 70 percent of IVF treatments are carried out in Ontario, which has 37 percent of Canada's population. Ontario is the only province that covers the procedure under its health insurance plan.

Canadians communicated a range of views on whether infertility treatments should be part of the publicly financed medical care system. Some people believed that infertility is a physical condition that should be treated through the health care system, and others believed that the health care system is already too overburdened to provide high-tech solutions to infertility, regardless of whether they are effective and safe. We also heard testimony that safe and effective procedures that could help those who are infertile should be included in the health care system on the grounds that infertility is just as important in the lives of those affected as

> Canada's health care system does not take infertility seriously. Nowhere has the prevention, diagnosis or treatment of infertility been acknowledged as a priority ... infertility is marginalized as a health care issue through excessive waiting lists, restrictions on access to treatment, and a constant threat of funding cutbacks. Those who seek access to treatment are demoralized by their exclusion from a health care system which claims to be universal but repeatedly tells them that infertility is an insignificant health care issue.
>
> *Brief to the Commission from the Infertility Awareness Association of Canada, April 30, 1992.*

many other conditions now treated in the health care system. We heard many people talk about the importance of children in the lives of individuals, couples, and society in general. Because of this importance, many people believe that if safe, ethical, and effective medical procedures are available to assist people who are infertile to have children, a caring society should provide them through the health care system. Others, however, have no objection to funding some treatments, such as assisted insemination, if they are effective, but believe that extending funding to expensive and high-tech procedures such as IVF diverts attention and resources from other reproductive health services, including preventing infertility in the first place.

Access

For many Canadians, the decision about whether to use one of these technologies has been removed from them, because of lack of access. These include people who live in isolated or rural areas and who do not have the resources to travel to fertility programs; those who are not part of stable, heterosexual relationships; and those who cannot afford the procedures if they are not covered by their provincial/territorial medical insurance plan. In addition, those who do not speak English or French may be less likely to have access to information on programs or procedures, and so have less access to them.

Some intervenors stated that physicians control access to fertility clinics and that access to treatment is easier for highly educated, high-income, married, heterosexual couples. We heard that the route to the use of reproductive technologies is currently unclear and complex, and people with less education are less likely to find access to it. It is expensive, and, in many provinces, the cost has to be borne directly by the users. This means level of income may determine access.

> The gap between women's access to the knowledge about NRT's and the rapid advancements in the field is increasingly adding to the power of the professionals over the consumers ... The lack of communication between immigrant women and health professionals increases immigrant women's vulnerability to be exploited ... thus further reducing this group of women's power. The NRT's have enormous potential to further add to sexism and racism.
>
> *Brief to the Commission from the Immigrant Women of Saskatchewan, October 25, 1990.*

Some of these people give up their hopes of having a child. Others seek alternative routes to conception, such as single women or lesbians who use self-insemination using donor sperm. This process, which is discussed in the section on assisted insemination, redresses part of the problem of access (by removing the necessity for medical involvement), but it also raises issues about safety.

Commissioners heard specifically from single women and lesbians who described how they had been discriminated against in the traditional medical setting. Some witnesses told the Commission that the over-medicalization of assisted insemination using donor sperm has created a situation in which medical practitioners have become gatekeepers, enforcing what they perceive to be community standards about family formation by establishing access criteria that exclude single or lesbian women.

Impact on the Family and Its Biological Relationships

Infertility treatments have direct effects on familial relationships, because they can be carried out using donated gametes (donated sperm for assisted insemination, or donated eggs, sperm, or both for IVF). Our surveys showed that Canadians hold strong opinions about breaking the ties between biological and social parenthood. For instance, when asked about assisted insemination using the partner's sperm, almost all survey respondents found this acceptable; fewer approved of using donor sperm. When asked questions about using donated sperm, 58 percent of Canadians approved of DI in general. Forty-seven percent said they would use DI personally, but 22 percent were opposed to the use of DI (see research volume, *Social Values and Attitudes Surrounding New Reproductive Technologies*).

Views about the acceptability of separating the biological and the social aspects of parenthood differ among individual Canadians and among specific groups that make up Canadian society. We deliberately reached out to solicit the views of Aboriginal people and Canadians who are members of racial or ethnic minorities in roundtable discussions and focus groups. From these we gained insights into cultural values that affect how people see donor insemination — we learned, for example, that many Aboriginal cultures emphasize passing on one's spirit to the next generation through one's children. We also heard from people in these groups who spoke about the importance of continuing their "family line." Groups representing ethnic minorities told the Commission that children are a priority in part because they enable a community to pass on its cultural and ethnic heritage.

This social context of infertility treatments provides a backdrop for our more detailed discussion of these aspects with regard to each treatment. The remaining chapters in this section on infertility treatments present our findings on fertility drugs, assisted insemination, *in vitro* fertilization, and egg and embryo donation. It is important to remember, however, that the treatments are not discrete, but intertwined: fertility drugs are often used in both assisted insemination and *in vitro* fertilization; IVF is sometimes used as a diagnostic test of male fertility before making the decision to use donor sperm rather than the sperm of the male partner; and patients often progress from one treatment to another.

General Sources

Decima Research. "Social Values and Attitudes of Canadians Toward New Reproductive Technologies." In Research Volumes of the Royal Commission on New Reproductive Technologies, 1993.

Decima Research. "Social Values and Attitudes of Canadians Toward New Reproductive Technologies: Focus Group Findings." In Research Volumes of the Royal Commission on New Reproductive Technologies, 1993.

Dutt, S. "Survey of Ethnocultural Communities on New Reproductive Technologies." In Research Volumes of the Royal Commission on New Reproductive Technologies, 1993.

Infertility Treatments: Fertility Drugs

◆

Fertility drugs are hormones that affect the reproductive system. They are the most common treatment for infertility — general practitioners and gynaecologists often prescribe them alone, and some are also used at infertility clinics in support of more complex treatments, such as *in vitro* fertilization. A review of current fertility drug treatment practices must take account of the two quite distinct contexts in which fertility drugs are prescribed: in the offices of family practitioners and obstetricians/gynaecologists consulted by women or couples having difficulties conceiving, and in specialized clinics where drugs are used to promote the maturation of multiple eggs for *in vitro* fertilization procedures. The number of women treated in each sector is difficult to estimate accurately on the basis of available data. Nevertheless, a rough comparison of annual Canadian sales of fertility drugs (excluding those for endometriosis) to the use of such drugs by IVF clinics would suggest that about three-quarters of the fertility drugs prescribed each year in Canada are prescribed by family practitioners and obstetricians/gynaecologists practising outside the specialized clinics. The existence of these two practice areas, as well as the different concerns brought before the Commission with respect to them, necessitates a two-pronged approach. The issues and the options for dealing with them (mechanisms available for ensuring appropriate use of the drugs) are different in each sector.

Of particular concern are variations in the expertise and facilities available in the two sectors to deal with any adverse consequences of

> About three-quarters of the fertility drugs prescribed each year in Canada are prescribed by family practitioners and obstetricians/gynaecologists practising outside the specialized clinics.

fertility drug use. Ovulation induction drugs and other drugs used to treat infertility can have powerful effects on the body, especially if used in high doses. As a result, complications can occur, making it necessary for women taking the drugs to be monitored closely for side effects. This can be difficult to do without the specialized knowledge and laboratory facilities (needed to detect side effects biochemically even before other symptoms appear) that are available at specialized clinics.

Because these drugs play such an important role in the treatment of infertility, Commissioners needed information on several aspects of them. This chapter therefore begins with a description of the concerns we heard from Canadians. We go on to review briefly the development of fertility drugs and the purposes for which they are used in treating infertility. Then we present our analysis of the effectiveness and risks of the fertility drugs prescribed most commonly, based on our review of the limited available evidence, and we examine the current regulatory environment for the development and introduction of new drugs; we then review current practices in the prescription and use of these drugs in the two sectors just identified — infertility treatment clinics and the broader practitioner community. Finally, we present our conclusions and recommendations for ensuring that fertility drugs are used only in ethically responsible ways that take into account protection of the health of women and their children, respect for women's autonomy in making decisions about their reproductive health, and the need to generate the information necessary to ensure that policies and practices with respect to fertility drug use evolve in appropriate and beneficial ways.

The Views of Canadians

During our public hearings and through our surveys of fertility clinics and patients, the Commission heard many concerns about the way fertility drugs are currently used in practice. Many groups and individuals made representations relevant to the use of fertility drugs; the Commission heard from infertility patients and practitioners and those involved with the women's health movement; and we obtained information from pharmaceutical

> Most of what I know today I wish I had known 10 years ago, and it comes about directly as a result of my having read everything I could get my hands on ... the doctors never volunteered that information ... but, you know, I came into this process reasonably well educated, middle class, knowing how to ... go about finding things out. What happens to people who don't have those advantages?
>
> *D. Allen, private citizen, Public Hearings Transcripts, Toronto, Ontario, October 29, 1990.*

manufacturers and regulators, and many others. One category of concerns brought before the Commission related to the development and regulation of fertility drugs in Canada today. Commissioners agreed that a full understanding of the issues surrounding fertility drugs required an examination of both the commercial context for the development and marketing of these products and the regulatory environment governing their introduction and use. The conclusions arising from our review of the commercial context for the development and marketing of drugs are presented in Chapter 24, while the regulatory environment is examined later in this chapter.

Many groups and individuals who appeared at the public hearings or made submissions to the Commission expressed concern that commercial motives may be inappropriately driving the development of reproductive technologies (including fertility drugs), that these motives may promote high-tech approaches to the treatment of infertility to the detriment of other alternatives, and that industry research funding policies are emphasizing drugs and other infertility treatments at the expense of prevention. Many intervenors expressed concern about the activities of the pharmaceutical industry in developing and marketing fertility drugs and raised issues regarding drug safety, efficacy, and regulation. The Commission also heard views that pharmaceutical companies do not consider ethical aspects sufficiently when developing drugs. It was suggested to the Commission that some pharmaceutical companies avoid Canadian safety standards by testing drugs on women in developing countries, where standards of safety and informed consent are less stringent than in the developed world. This, they say, amounts to exploitation, with negative consequences for the lives and health of women and their families in the developing world.

Pharmaceutical companies told the Commission that the drugs they market were tested and monitored extensively according to Canadian regulations before being introduced into practice. Many Canadians expressed a belief, however, that manufacturers are insufficiently concerned with safety and that the government does not demand rigorous enough testing of fertility drugs before they are made available for general use. Not all individuals feel this way: some couples who were undergoing infertility treatment told the Commission they feared that too stringent

> Medical questions that need to be researched include, are there any effects of taking fertility drugs that do not become apparent until later life? ...
>
> And for the women who have taken fertility drugs, I would think they would have to be watched for perhaps 20 years afterwards to see if they differ statistically from any other group.
>
> *D. Ellis, The Canadian Federation of Business and Professional Women's Clubs, Public Hearings Transcripts, Toronto, Ontario, October 29, 1990.*

testing of fertility drugs in Canada is driving up prices and delaying development of new techniques.

A second category of concerns brought before us related to treatment and prescription practices. Commissioners learned through public consultations that many Canadians believe that fertility drugs are being overused or used too routinely, sometimes without the benefit of complete diagnoses of the infertility problems they are intended to treat. Women who had been treated for infertility told the Commission that doctors prescribing drugs for unapproved indications or at excessive dosages had put their health at risk, yet they felt they had not been adequately informed about the nature,

> Also we are concerned about the health risks posed to women, medication which is given to women as fertility drugs ... The emotional cost and then translated into physical health cost do become phenomenal.
>
> *N. Javed, Immigrant Women of Saskatchewan, Public Hearings Transcripts, Saskatoon, Saskatchewan, October 25, 1990.*

effectiveness, and risks of the drugs they had been prescribed.[1] Medical professionals and many women's groups were concerned that there is little follow-up to identify the health effects of drug use, so that if there are short- or long-term harmful consequences, these may not be identified. Intervenors were also concerned that women were not being adequately informed about the known side effects.

For example, some women who had taken clomiphene citrate (a drug used to induce ovulation) told the Commission they had experienced side effects such as hot flushes, bloating, abdominal pain, dizziness, and insomnia. Some said they had not been told enough about what to expect; others said that their doctors had downplayed the seriousness of some of the symptoms (blurred vision, for example, though not life-threatening, could be alarming or create serious situations). Some women reported increased anxiety, depression, and mood swings — psychological effects that are considered mild and are not usually recorded by medical professionals. We

> When I asked the specialist about the side effects of Pergonal®, her attitude was distinctly unfriendly, like there was something wrong with me that I chose to ask a question about whether or not multiple births would happen as a result of taking Pergonal®, and she looked at me like I was being totally ungrateful and that I should just be very grateful that they were doing anything for me. And when I said that I want to know more about Pergonal®, she dismissed my concerns by giving me a leaflet on Clomid®, which I already had read.
>
> *D. Flanagan, private citizen, Public Hearings Transcripts, Toronto, Ontario, November 19, 1990.*

also heard testimony that insufficient attention is paid to a side effect that can have lifelong consequences for couples and their children — the higher incidence of multiple births following fertility drug use.

Commissioners also heard testimony from Canadians who fear that those who develop, approve, and prescribe fertility drugs have forgotten the lessons of the past. The harmful consequences of drugs such as DES and thalidomide have led Canadians to question whether fertility drugs on the market today are truly safe. Many believe that the possibility of unanticipated harm means there is a clear need for more information about the long-term effects of drugs used to treat infertility. Again, we heard concerns that women considering fertility drug use are not being adequately informed of the fact that little is known about the long-term effects of fertility drug use on women and their children.

> The experimental nature of procedures, drugs used, and risks involved must be clearly explained to potential users of new reproductive technologies. Informed consent must be stringently enforced. The use of the drugs Clomid® and Pergonal® to stimulate women's ovaries in *in vitro* fertilization comes with a number of disturbing side effects and little long-term follow-up studies. The use of DES in the '50s and '60s had long-range consequences that were not anticipated at that time and that children of that generation are dealing with now.
>
> *J. Hutchinson, Social Issues Committee, YWCA, Calgary, Public Hearings Transcripts, Calgary, Alberta, September 14, 1990.*

The Development of Fertility Drugs

Estrogen, a naturally occurring hormone that is responsible in part for regulating the female reproductive system, was first synthesized in the 1930s. This made possible many treatments that are now an accepted part of medical care. Hormones are used to treat menstrual disorders, to prevent pregnancy, and to prevent miscarriage when hormone insufficiency has been diagnosed. They are also used to alleviate the discomforts of menopause and prevent consequent complications. Progesterone, another hormone of the reproductive cycle, was also discovered and extracted during the same decade. Also, discovery of these two key hormones enabled researchers to influence menstruation and ovulation in mammals and thus to understand the reproductive process more fully.

These discoveries led to synthesis of the first fertility drugs — those that induce ovulation. The first of these was clomiphene citrate, which was developed and tested initially for its potential as a contraceptive in the 1950s. In 1961 it was shown to stimulate the ovaries when ovulation was not occurring, and by 1967 it was being used to treat this condition. The development and use of clomiphene were followed closely by the introduction of human menopausal gonadotropin or hMG, a purified preparation of naturally occurring hormones produced by the pituitary gland. It induces ovulation by stimulating the development and maturation of the follicle and corpus luteum, the structures in the ovaries in which eggs develop and mature, leading to ovulation (see Chapter 7). Human menopausal gonadotropin was first used in 1958, but because it was expensive and difficult to extract (from human urine), it was not marketed widely until the 1960s, when a less expensive and easier method of extraction was discovered.

Once drugs were developed that could affect the various phases of ovulation, it became feasible to develop other techniques of assisted reproduction. The control over ovulation and the production of multiple eggs made possible by these drugs thus supported the development of assisted reproduction procedures during the last two decades. For example, *in vitro* fertilization is feasible largely because fertility drugs can be used to induce the ovaries to produce more than one egg — without these additional eggs the chances of fertilization, implantation, and development

> We have met women who have been given a trial of drugs like Clomid® or Pergonal® "just to see if it would help," before they have even learned the rudimentaries of charting their own cycles. In fact a recent article in the *Medical Post* suggests clomiphene citrate is the first step to solving the frustration of treating unexplained infertility. I'm sure there will be other intervenors who will address the risks of such medication or the concerns.
>
> *M. MacDonald, Fertility Management Services, Public Hearings Transcripts, Toronto, Ontario, October 31, 1990.*

would be lower. At the same time, as discussed in Chapter 20, the use of these drugs in the context of assisted reproduction raises its own concerns.

There are about a dozen fertility drugs on the market in Canada; clomiphene and hMG are the most commonly used fertility drugs at present. Neither was ever fully evaluated before it was introduced — in fact, the exact metabolic pathway by which clomiphene acts is still not known. When these drugs were introduced into clinical practice in the 1960s, the need for rigorous standards in assessing the safety and effectiveness of drugs was not as clear as it is now. Today this need is evident, as is the need to follow up on drug use and to gather information on adverse effects that, if infrequent, can be gained only from studies of their use by large numbers of people over many years.

Effectiveness and Risks of Fertility Drugs

In keeping with our evidence-based approach, the Commission reviewed the available evidence on the drugs now used to treat infertility, looking for information that could be used as the basis for judgements about their effectiveness, side effects, and risks. This field is not static, however, and the many different clinical situations involved make it difficult to establish and apply general rules; in this evolving field, it would not be appropriate to make detailed recommendations about every drug that currently is used or may be used. It is nevertheless useful to outline our findings with respect to some of the most commonly used drugs. An initial assessment does not, however, preclude the need for continuing follow-up to monitor the effects of drug use and to adjust policies and guidelines in light of the knowledge gained.

A formal meta-analysis of the effectiveness of most fertility drugs is not possible because of the deficiency of data from a sufficient number of well-designed, large-scale studies. The Commission therefore used two criteria to determine whether a drug could be categorized as a treatment that is of benefit. First, the drug had to have been tested and been shown to be of benefit in appropriately designed randomized control trials with at least 200 subjects in each of the control and treatment groups. Alternatively, the drug had to be shown clearly to affect a specific pathway or factor known to cause infertility — there had to be a clear and plausible biological reason for the drug to "work."

> In fact, we know that incredible amounts of money go into trying to ensure that the drugs on the market are innocuous, and for all that, mistakes are made, such as thalidomide, something that everyone remembers. I am not referring to the malformations that still occur today due to the ingestion during pregnancy of drugs that are damaging to the fetus. These days, however, we no longer see such malformations, as they are eliminated as soon as they are detected in the mother using another new medical breakthrough — ultrasound. [Translation]
>
> *C. Bouchard, Campagne Québec-Vie, Public Hearings Transcripts, Quebec City, Quebec, September 26, 1990.*

Unless the evidence showed that the drug fell into one of these two categories, we judged it unproven — that is, we found that the evidence is insufficient to say whether use of the drug is either better or worse than receiving no treatment.

The fertility drugs available today, when used alone, attempt to restore fertility by acting on various biological mechanisms in reproduction. They do not bypass any of the vital steps in the process that culminates in fertilization of an egg; instead, they attempt to correct disorders in women and men that can cause hormonal imbalance, or to reverse the effects of an illness that blocks fertility. Most fertility drugs on the market today fall into one of three broad categories: ovulation induction drugs, ovulation suppression drugs, and those used to treat male infertility. We begin by describing their present use and our assessment of their effectiveness for these uses, given the limited data available, then go on to examine the risks identified to date.

Ovulation Induction Drugs

The most common use of fertility drugs is to correct ovulatory defects. If a woman is not ovulating, she cannot conceive — no egg is released to be fertilized. Disturbances in the hypothalamus — leading to either high or low hormone levels in the blood — or problems in the ovary, such as polycystic ovary disease, may be associated with irregular or absent ovulation. In these conditions the delicate balance of hormones has been upset, with the result that ovulation, if it occurs at all, does not occur regularly. As well, a small proportion of women (estimated at between 1 and 5 percent) who stop taking birth control pills after using them for a number of years do not resume normal cycles with ovulation for six months or longer,[2] and these drugs may be used by such women.

Ovulation Induction Drugs

Ovulation induction drugs are used for women who are anovulatory and also to promote regular menstrual cycles for women who have never had periods or who subsequently stop having them. They may also be used for women with oligomenorrhea, irregular cycles, ovarian failure (due to abnormal development, premature menopause, or damage to the ovaries by chemicals or radiation), or other hormonal dysfunctions that may cause a problem in ovulation, including those caused by polycystic ovary disease.

The drugs are also used in association with other infertility treatments, such as IVF, GIFT, and some assisted inseminations to maximize their effectiveness. They do this by stimulating production of multiple eggs per cycle — even if the woman was ovulating normally. Having more eggs to fertilize in a cycle increases the likelihood of a live birth.

The three main fertility drugs used to induce ovulation are clomiphene citrate, human menopausal gonadotropin, and bromocriptine. A fourth — gonadotropin-releasing hormone — is used in treatment of a specific syndrome.

Clomiphene Citrate

Clomiphene citrate (brand names Clomid®, Serophene®) is usually the first choice for treatment of women with irregular or absent ovulation. If used in appropriate doses, it is considered by practitioners and experts in the field to be a relatively mild, safe drug with only a few adverse health effects. Although it carries a small risk of some potentially life-threatening side effects, these are much less frequent with clomiphene than with other ovulation induction drugs (see section on Risks of Ovulation Induction).

Clomiphene is generally accepted to be an effective treatment for all ovulation disorders and has become a standard treatment for them (see research volume, *Treatment of Infertility: Current Practices and Psychosocial Implications*). Even though there have been few randomized clinical trials on clomiphene citrate for ovulation disorders, several studies have demonstrated that clomiphene is effective in inducing ovulation in women who are anovulatory, and the biological mechanism makes sense. In addition, physicians who have had extensive experience with the drug have observed that women who have not been having periods are likely to resume normal cycles when they use this drug.

It is estimated in the literature that when used to treat infertility resulting from anovulation, clomiphene use results in pregnancy in 30 to 40 percent of cases, although a Commission study found that practitioners often overestimate clomiphene success rates (see research volume, *New Reproductive Technologies and the Health Care System: The Case for Evidence-Based Medicine*). In the Commission's assessment, then, clomiphene citrate has been proven effective and is of low risk when used at the proper dosage to treat lack of ovulation resulting from primary amenorrhea, secondary amenorrhea, and oligomenorrhea. When prescribed at approved doses when these disorders have been diagnosed, clomiphene citrate should be considered an accepted treatment. Because of the lack of definitive data from large-scale studies, however, continuing data collection on the results of clomiphene use is essential. In addition, women contemplating the use of clomiphene for an ovulation problem should be informed about the limited availability of reliable data on its use, and the effects of the dosages used should be monitored closely.

> When prescribed at approved doses when these disorders have been diagnosed, clomiphene citrate should be considered an accepted treatment.

Clomiphene has also been used in the treatment of unexplained infertility, which is the diagnosis for about one-quarter of couples seeking treatment at Canadian infertility clinics. When no reason or condition can be found in either partner to explain their infertility, it is the judgement of practitioners and experts in the field that clomiphene is a low-risk, fairly simple treatment that could help rectify a hormone imbalance not detected by current methods.

Couples who have been trying to conceive for some time (particularly if they are at the age when they feel their reproductive time is running out) often feel a sense of urgency about treatment, especially the need to feel that they are "doing something" to increase their chances of becoming pregnant. Physicians may conclude in these situations that prescribing clomiphene represents a compassionate response to a couple whose infertility cannot be explained, and there is always the hope that the drug might increase their chance of pregnancy, perhaps by correcting an undetected hormonal imbalance that may be affecting the couple's fertility. In fact, our survey of infertility clinics showed that 29 percent of women in couples with unexplained infertility are treated first with clomiphene, and there is some evidence to suggest that clomiphene citrate is effective when used in this way, although the mechanism is not understood.

Based on our assessment of the current data, clomiphene citrate may be an effective treatment for couples who have had unexplained infertility for a minimum of three years.[3] We therefore see a need to evaluate short-term treatment with clomiphene for this purpose in the context of a clinical trial, with stringent requirements for informed participation. Our review of the available evidence also showed, however, that the use of clomiphene citrate by women in couples with unexplained infertility of *less* than three years' duration is not justified. There is a greater probability that such couples will be able to conceive without treatment, and physicians should counsel these couples accordingly. The possible risks associated with clomiphene citrate, together with the likelihood of conception occurring naturally, mean it is not justified to prescribe clomiphene in these cases. However, if a woman's older age indicates that she has little chance of conceiving naturally before the three-year time period, she should be considered for inclusion in a clinical trial investigating clomiphene as treatment for unexplained infertility in older women.

Clomiphene citrate is also a common form of first treatment for infertile women with minimal or mild endometriosis. The evidence to date, however, is insufficient to draw any conclusions. This question should also be addressed through well-designed clinical trials.

Human Menopausal Gonadotropin

The second most common fertility drug prescribed to induce ovulation is hMG (brand names Pergonal®, Humegon®). Human menopausal gonadotropin is a much stronger drug than clomiphene citrate and it may induce ovulation in some women who do not respond to clomiphene. Its most common use is therefore to induce ovulation in women with amenorrhea, oligomenorrhea, or irregular cycles when clomiphene has not worked. It has more risks, however, and its side effects are quite severe (see section on Risks of

hMG can be an appropriate treatment for women who are anovulatory and who have not responded to clomiphene citrate.

Ovulation Induction). To help avoid more serious side effects, hMG is often prescribed in conjunction with gonadotropin-releasing hormone (Gn-RH).[4]

There is a clear and plausible biological mechanism by which hMG works, and physicians have observed that the drug is effective in producing ovulation in many women with amenorrhea. Although side effects are more common than with clomiphene and may be severe, the Commission believes that fully informed women may wish to take this risk. In the Commission's assessment, then, hMG can be an appropriate treatment for women who are anovulatory and who have not responded to clomiphene citrate.

We did not find enough evidence, however, to state that treatment with hMG is effective for cases of oligomenorrhea and irregular cycles or for unexplained infertility. Women with these conditions still ovulate, albeit irregularly, so in theory they still have a chance of becoming pregnant. There is no convincing evidence that hMG corrects a specific biological pathway in this situation, and as the side effects are considerably more serious than those of clomiphene citrate, Commissioners believe that hMG is not an appropriate treatment for these conditions. There is not enough evidence to categorize hMG as effective, there is no pathway that would logically be corrected by hMG in this situation, and there is risk to the patient. Human menopausal gonadotropin is of unproven value for these diagnoses and should not be offered as treatment, nor should this use of hMG be a priority for research.

Bromocriptine

The effectiveness of bromocriptine (brand name Parlodel®) has not been proven in randomized control trials, but its mechanism of action is specific, and it has been shown to correct the high blood prolactin occurring in some women experiencing infertility. Based on what we currently know about how it works, its use is justified only to treat women who have documented high levels of prolactin, and it should not be used without this documentation.

Gonadotropin-Releasing Hormone

Gn-RH is prescribed for women in whom Kallman syndrome has lowered the level of Gn-RH to abnormal levels, causing amenorrhea. It is an effective treatment for this specific condition, and it works through a precise and convincing biological mechanism by restoring Gn-RH to normal levels. The Commission therefore concludes that the use of Gn-RH to treat amenorrhea caused by Kallman syndrome is effective and should be considered medically necessary.

Risks of Ovulation Induction

To determine what is known about the adverse effects of ovulation induction drugs, Commission researchers searched 15 computerized data bases, looking at more than 500 journals from 1955 to the present. They found 4 840 references to research studies in this area. By the time they eliminated duplicates and studies that were unobtainable, they were down to 1 651 studies, 937 of which met the criteria for meta-analysis, allowing their results to be compared with each other. The complete results of this review are available in the research volumes accompanying this report (see research volume, *New Reproductive Technologies and the Health Care System: The Case for Evidence-Based Medicine*).

To determine what is known about the adverse effects of ovulation induction drugs, Commission researchers searched 15 computerized data bases, looking at more than 500 journals from 1955 to the present. They found 4 840 references to research studies in this area.

This comprehensive review showed that there has been a lack of systematic research on adverse side effects of ovulation induction drugs. Perhaps the most striking fact about the review is that it was the first comprehensive attempt ever in Canada to compile evidence on the adverse effects of ovulation induction drugs. The review showed that although these are immensely powerful drugs, there has been a relative vacuum in research attention directed to examining the results of their use; by contrast, drugs used for chemotherapy and cardiac arrhythmias are extensively reviewed. A commitment to the tenets of evidence-based medicine requires that this deficiency be remedied.

As with any medication, side effects occur in some women treated with ovulation induction drugs; in a small proportion of cases, serious health problems occur. The most serious side effect is a condition called ovarian hyperstimulation syndrome, which can be mild, moderate, or severe. Depending on the drug used, some women experience hot flushes, ovarian enlargement resulting in abdominal discomfort or pain, breast tenderness, dizziness, headache, nervousness, nausea or vomiting, fatigue, and visual disturbances. Women experiencing mild or moderate symptoms can be treated with rest, medication, and monitoring. However, the complications associated with severe cases (which occur in between 0.4 and 4 percent of cycles), though rare, can be life-threatening.[5] The highest risk of severe ovarian hyperstimulation syndrome is with the use of hMG. Women receiving ovulation induction drugs must therefore be monitored closely for signs of the syndrome, with careful attention paid to dosages, and steps must be taken to counteract the syndrome if it occurs.

Women receiving ovulation induction drugs must therefore be monitored closely.

Another of the adverse effects that has been shown clearly to result from ovulation induction drug use is an increased rate of multiple birth.

The use of hMG carries the greatest risk, with multiple pregnancies reported in as many as 32 percent of women in some studies. The rate of multiple births in Canada has increased dramatically since the advent of fertility drug use. The statistics show a dramatic increase in the multiple-birth set rate in the 1980s and early 1990s as fertility drug and IVF use became more common. Recently published data for Canada between 1974 and 1990 show that the multiple-birth set rate rose from 912.8 in 1974 to 1 058.9 per 100 000 confinements in 1990. During this same period, the birth rate for triplets, quadruplets, and quintuplets rose from 8.3 to 21.7 per 100 000 confinements.[6]

Canada is not alone in showing such an increase in multiple births. For example, in 1985 in Wales and England, there were 14 sets of triplets per 100 000 births; by 1989, it had risen to 27 sets per 100 000, and, since then, it has increased even more dramatically. An American study, too, has shown similar recent marked increases in the frequency of high-order multiple births. Interestingly, the increases there have occurred primarily among white women in their late 20s and early 30s who are of higher socioeconomic status. The explanation for all these rises is almost certainly the use of fertility drugs and techniques such as *in vitro* fertilization. In fact, the Statistics Canada study found that the increase in rate of multiple births of three or more children was highest in Ontario, which also has the greatest number of fertility clinics and is the only province where IVF is covered under the provincial health care plan.

Further evidence that infertility treatment is the cause of the increase in multiple births is found in a study in Britain in the early to mid-1980s, which found that 70 percent of mothers of quadruplets and 36 percent of mothers

> Another of the adverse effects that has been shown clearly to result from ovulation induction drug use is an increased rate of multiple birth.

of triplets had been prescribed ovulation-stimulating drugs. A decade later, with increasing use of these drugs and other techniques, it is likely that an even greater proportion is attributable to this.

It is logical to assume that fertility drug use is largely responsible for the increase in the multiple birth rate. Although a substantial percentage (38 percent) of all individuals born following *in vitro* fertilization in Canada are from a multiple pregnancy, the absolute number of IVF births for the Canadian population is still small; thus, fertility drug use, particularly ovulation induction drugs, must have made a greater contribution to the marked rise. As discussed in Chapter 20, multiple pregnancies pose significant risks for pregnant women, for the fetuses, and for the eventual children, as well as costs for the health care system and society generally as these children grow up.

The possibility has also been raised that fertility drug use could be associated with subsequent ovarian cancer. A large recent study for the

National Institute of Child Health and Human Development found that the data available at that time (January 1993) were inadequate to estimate whether there is an increased risk and, if so, its magnitude. However, this possibility is a cause for concern, pointing to the need for further research.

In general terms, further research is needed to provide full information on the long-term health effects of fertility drug use on women and their children. Although clomiphene has been in use since the late 1960s, for example, only recently have any data been available on its longer-term health effects. There has been considerable conjecture about the effects of clomiphene on the health of children; in particular, an Australian study raised the possibility of an increase in the occurrence of neural tube defects, but this has not been confirmed in other studies or in a large recent case-control study on this topic.[7] Overall, studies of children at birth have shown that the incidence of congenital anomalies among the children of women who took fertility drugs has been similar to that in the general population.[8]

> Studies of children at birth have shown that the incidence of congenital anomalies among the children of women who took fertility drugs has been similar to that in the general population.

Ovulation Suppression Drugs

The second group of drugs used to treat infertility, ovulation suppression drugs, are used primarily to treat women with endometriosis, one of the risk factors associated with infertility. Ovulation suppression is a highly invasive step, yet it is used, with no evidence that it is effective, to treat a condition whose cause and pathogenesis are not even understood, simply in the hope that treatment will have an effect on the woman's fertility. The drugs are used to suppress her menstrual cycle for at least six months, in the hope that the symptoms affecting fertility will subside and conception will be more likely to occur once drug use is discontinued and menstrual cycles resume.

The Commission analyzed the data available in the worldwide literature on three types of common ovulation suppression drugs — danazol, norethindrone, and Gn-RH analogues — and their effect on endometriosis-related infertility. Based on this analysis, it is the Commission's assessment that the use of danazol, norethindrone, Gn-RH analogues, or any ovulation suppression drug is ineffective in treating infertility thought to result from endometriosis or unexplained infertility. Their use should be discontinued, as they have moderate to severe side effects; moreover, they eliminate the possibility of conceiving naturally for the duration of treatment. Such risks should not be undertaken when there is evidence that the use of these drugs is ineffective.

Drugs to Treat Male Infertility

The Commission evaluated data on the drugs used most often to treat male infertility; they include clomiphene citrate, gonadotropin-releasing hormone, oral kallikrein, bromocriptine, and androgens (male hormones).

Seminal Defects

Since it is usual for a man's sperm count to vary, an accurate diagnosis of a seminal defect can be made only if several sperm samples are collected over a period of time. Data collected from Canadian academic infertility clinics show that in couples where the man had a seminal defect, 74 percent had oligospermia (reduced sperm count) and 26 percent had azoospermia (no sperm).

Azoospermia clearly results in infertility, but the relationship between low sperm count and male infertility is less clear. The partners of men with oligospermia have a live birth rate of 2 percent per month of unprotected intercourse, compared to about 20 to 25 percent for the population at large. Although 20 million sperm per millilitre is regarded as the dividing line between oligospermia and a normal sperm count, men with lower sperm counts (less than 5 million) have been known to conceive. Many physicians believe that as-yet-undetectable subfertility in the female partner adds to the problem in cases where a couple in which the man has oligospermia cannot conceive. This would help to explain why the partners of some men with low sperm counts are able to conceive while the partners of others cannot.

Clomiphene Citrate

The Commission found that there is not enough evidence to determine whether clomiphene citrate is an effective treatment for men with oligospermia. It is inappropriate to continue to expose men to the risks of clomiphene use without collecting the data that would allow evidence-based decisions about whether its use constitutes appropriate medical practice; this drug should therefore be a priority for investigation in the context of a well-designed clinical trial, but it should not be used as an accepted treatment.

Gonadotropin-Releasing Hormone

Gn-RH is prescribed for men in whom Kallman syndrome has lowered the level of Gn-RH to abnormal levels, causing azoospermia. It is an effective treatment for this specific condition, and it works through a precise and convincing biological mechanism by restoring Gn-RH to normal levels. The Commission therefore concludes that the use of Gn-RH to treat azoospermia caused by Kallman syndrome is effective and should be considered medically necessary.

Oral Kallikrein

The Commission found no evidence that oral kallikrein is an effective treatment for oligospermia, and as there is no biologically plausible way it would work we conclude that it should not be used for this treatment purpose. Nor should it be a research priority.

Bromocriptine

Bromocriptine is prescribed for oligospermia with the aim of reducing estrogen levels. The Commission's analysis of international data revealed insufficient evidence to categorize bromocriptine as effective or ineffective.[9] However, there is a potential mechanism by which it could work, so we conclude that its effectiveness should be investigated in a clinical trial.

Androgens

The male hormones (androgens) mesterolone and testosterone are sometimes prescribed for men with oligospermia in the hope that sperm production will be stimulated. As a group, androgens have been shown to be ineffective in treating oligospermia. They should therefore not be offered as treatment and should be considered a low priority for research.

Need for Research

Male infertility has been a neglected area in research, despite the fact that 24 percent of couples seen at Canadian infertility clinics are infertile because of a diagnosed problem in the male partner (see research volume, *Treatment of Infertility: Current Practices and Psychosocial Implications*). Medical science is unable to identify a specific cause for 30 to 40 percent of cases of male infertility, and researchers have estimated that only 11 percent of infertile men are potentially treatable at present. As we pointed out earlier, the area of male infertility warrants much greater research emphasis. Assigning a higher research priority to investigating male infertility would promote greater understanding of the causes, diagnoses, and treatments of seminal disorders and might enable a reduced use of treatments in female partners who are fertile because of male infertility.

Ensuring Safe and Effective Fertility Drug Treatment in the Future

In summary, the Commission concludes that ensuring the effectiveness of fertility drug treatment requires that clinical trials on the uses of drugs we identified as requiring more research be carried out in licensed clinics and approved by the National Reproductive Technologies Commission. While it is not current practice for provincial/territorial ministries to be involved in funding clinical trials, provincial departments do have a responsibility to ensure efficient management of the health care system. Therefore, as discussed in Chapter 4, funding should be provided in part by provincial/territorial health ministries, in part by arm's-length contributions from the pharmaceutical manufacturers of the fertility drugs used, and in part by federal research funding bodies. The Commission therefore recommends that

> **63. Randomized controlled trials of fertility drugs already on the Canadian market be designed and carried out by licensed clinics providing assisted conception services, in conjunction with the National Reproductive Technologies Commission and the Health Protection Branch, Health Canada. Participation of women and men in these trials should involve their fully informed consent, and research proposals should obtain prior approval of both the Assisted Conception Sub-Committee of the National Commission and local research ethics boards.**

and that

> **64. Funding for well-designed clinical trials of fertility drugs be made available by pharmaceutical companies (with arm's-length administration of the funding), medical research funding bodies such as the Medical Research Council, provincial/territorial ministries of health, and Health Canada through the National Health Research and Development Program.**

The Drug Regulatory System

The legacy of harm caused by two drugs formerly prescribed during pregnancy, thalidomide and DES, raises questions for many Canadians about whether the drug regulatory system is as well designed as it could be to screen drugs for safety and effectiveness before they reach the market. No scheme can offer absolute assurances of safety; it is only when a drug is used by thousands of people over a significant period of time that uncommon or longer-term effects on health can be identified and assessed. It is possible, nevertheless, to design the initial screening process and post-marketing surveillance procedures in such a way as to ensure that any unforeseen harmful consequences are identified, assessed, and dealt with quickly and appropriately.

The Current System

We reviewed the process by which drugs are approved in Canada before they go on the market and the mechanisms in place to monitor the safety of drugs following their approval. The production and marketing of drugs used to treat infertility, like all other human prescription drugs, are heavily regulated in Canada. Canada's drug laws were changed in 1963 after the harmful effects of thalidomide were identified, to require that companies submit evidence of effectiveness of a new drug before they can be licensed. From their initial development to the approval for sale to consumers, drugs are subject to a lengthy process of testing and evaluation. The research leading to the marketing of a safe, effective drug can take decades and cost a pharmaceutical company millions of dollars.

The process begins with the manufacturer conducting animal and laboratory studies (pre-clinical trials) to identify the therapeutic uses and risks of a new compound, to determine new uses of an existing compound, or to test the use of an existing compound produced in a new way. This research may take place in Canada or another country where the pharmaceutical company has research facilities. If the laboratory and animal research demonstrates that the drug has the desired therapeutic effect and has an acceptable level of safety, the next step is to conduct research using human subjects. If the research is to be conducted in Canada, the company must first obtain permission from the Drugs Directorate, Health Protection Branch, Health Canada, to begin clinical trials with human subjects. Companies must then submit data from three phases of clinical research to gain approval to market a new drug. In phase I clinical trials, designed to assess safety, a small number of healthy volunteers receive the drug. In phase II trials, small numbers of selected patients receive the drug to see whether it affects the condition it is intended to treat. If both phases show appropriate results, several hundred or even thousands of patients participate in formal, randomized double-

> Improvements are needed to the existing process of regulating the use of pharmaceutical products. IVF involves the use of a number of substances and technologies the long-term effects of which on the health of women and children are not yet known. D.E.S. Action proposes that the regulations governing the use of pharmaceutical products and medical procedures include a criterion which takes into consideration the current "social need" for any new product and procedure. [Translation]
>
> *Brief to the Commission from D.E.S. Action Canada, June 1991.*

blind trials (phase III). (Neither patients nor researchers know what drug is being administered or whether it is a placebo.) The purpose of phase III trials is to assess the therapeutic and adverse effects of the drug at the recommended dosage and also to identify other medications with which the new drug may interact.

If the three phases of clinical trials demonstrate that the drug is effective and safe, the pharmaceutical company files a New Drug Submission (NDS) with the Drugs Directorate, indicating trial results, dosage strengths and the form in which the drug will be marketed, and details about known side effects and efficacy. The Drugs Directorate conducts a detailed review of the NDS to assess whether the drug should be approved for the Canadian market. Foreign research results are accepted if the research is judged to be of sufficient quality. If the drug is approved, it receives a Notice of Compliance, and the recommended dosage ("approved dosage") and uses for the drug ("approved indications") are set. If a company subsequently wants to promote the drug for additional uses or at different dosages, it must submit additional evidence that the drug is proven effective and low-risk at those dosages and for those uses.

Drugs are also subject to post-marketing surveillance for seven years following their introduction, but as we discuss later in this chapter, this system, known as the Adverse Drug Reaction Reporting Program, has several shortcomings.

Changes in the Drug Approval System

Although our country is considered to have one of the most stringent and rigorous drug regulatory systems in the world, concerns have arisen regarding its capacity to ensure that drugs used in Canada are effective and safe over the longer term. We heard criticisms that Canada's system is too isolated from drug regulatory systems in place in other industrialized countries and that, once drugs are approved for sale in Canada, there is negligible follow-up and limited monitoring to identify harmful side effects. Many critics of the current system also argue that Canada's slow approval process prevents Canadians from obtaining access to new or improved drugs in a timely fashion.

Several reports have evaluated the current regulatory system and made recommendations to address various of these concerns. The most recent of these include *Working in Partnerships: Drug Review for the Future,* by Denis Gagnon (1992); *Developing a National Postmarketing Pharmaceutical Surveillance Program,* by J.N. Hlynka (1991); *Towards an Improved Drug Regulatory System: Progress Since Stein,* by the Drugs Directorate, Health and Welfare Canada (1992); and *Benefit, Risk and Cost Management of Drugs,* report of the Canadian Public Health Association National Advisory Panel on Risk/Benefit Management of Drugs (1993). Other reports, such as *Breast Cancer: Unanswered Questions,* by the

Parliamentary Sub-Committee on the Status of Women, have also addressed issues related to drug regulation.

A common theme of these reports, and a recurring one heard from the Health Protection Branch, industry, health care professionals, and consumer groups, is the need to change the drug regulatory system. The proposed reforms include streamlining the approval process, making the regulatory system more accountable to decision makers outside the system, and in particular strengthening follow-up on monitoring procedures for drugs already on the market.

Among the reforms being considered to speed up the drug approval process is aligning it with internationally accepted standards such as those of the European Community or the U.S. National Institutes of Health.[10] This would involve, for example, taking foreign reviews of drugs into account during the review process; becoming more involved in cooperative drug reviews with comparable countries such as Australia and Sweden; and adopting the European Community criteria for drug evaluation, which have become the standards in many industrialized countries.

In the Commissioners' view, however, different countries could well have varying views on what constitutes an acceptable level of drug safety. In some cases, Canadians may be unwilling to accept a level of risk or a side effect associated with a drug that another country finds acceptable, and vice versa. International data and studies will continue to be useful to Canadian regulators, but we believe that fertility drugs in particular should be approved or rejected according to standards of safety and efficacy that are acceptable to Canadians. We conclude that Canada should maintain sovereignty over the review process leading to approval or disapproval of fertility drugs, as the drugs used are powerful and have the potential to do harm. The Commission therefore recommends that

> We conclude that Canada should maintain sovereignty over the review process leading to approval or disapproval of fertility drugs, as the drugs used are powerful and have the potential to do harm.

> **65. The evaluation of drugs used in assisted conception be considered an area where Canadian specifications for evaluation are required, in recognition of the potential long-term health effects of these drugs on women, men, and children.**

A second way to streamline the system would be to make greater use of external reviewers (outside the Drugs Directorate) to evaluate drug submissions and provide expert advice in specific areas. We agree that this is appropriate, provided the external reviewers are objective (their objectivity would be compromised, for example, if they performed contract work for both the Drugs Directorate and pharmaceutical companies) and they have the appropriate training and expertise in regulatory matters if asked to conduct complete drug reviews. Drug evaluations require two distinct types of expertise: clinical assessment of a drug and regulatory analysis. External reviewers may be well qualified to give a medical analysis of a drug, but they may lack the knowledge about regulation necessary to conduct a complete drug review.

In investigating the effectiveness and safety of existing fertility drugs, the Commission found that there is a small network of physicians in Canada who have both practical experience prescribing fertility drugs and extensive experience conducting clinical trials and evaluating existing research on effects of the drugs. We believe that these individuals would be highly qualified to assist the Drugs Directorate in clinical assessments of new fertility drugs and in addressing issues that arise with respect to the safety or effectiveness of existing drugs. The Commission recommends that

66. **When assessing new fertility drugs for approval, the Drugs Directorate consult with experts who have clinical and research experience with fertility drugs, to ensure that the benefits and risks have been evaluated comprehensively. Consideration should be given to forming permanent advisory committees of individuals qualified to assess specific categories of drugs, such as those used in treating infertility.**

Recombinant Fertility Drugs

The active ingredients of many fertility drugs are natural hormones; for example, in the past, gonadotropins were extracted from the urine of women who were post-menopausal — a complex, time-consuming, and inefficient process. In the future, genetic engineering will enable production of large quantities of gonadotropins using human genes spliced into microbial or other non-human cells. Because recombinant drugs will be produced by genetically altered organisms, they must be assessed to determine whether the organism used in the production process has also left behind significant impurities.

The Drugs Directorate has developed broad guidelines for the safety and testing of biotechnology products. Some observers believe, however, that the guidelines should be more comprehensive and specific and should have the capacity to evolve as the science develops. While assessing the appropriateness of the guidelines for safety testing of recombinant drugs is beyond the mandate of this report, we believe that this issue should be addressed by the federal government. The Commission therefore recommends that

> 67. **The federal government develop up-to-date criteria, to be used in the approval process, appropriate for screening the safety and efficacy of new biotechnology products, including recombinant fertility drugs.**

Ethical Review of Trials

Finally, the Commission notes that some fertility drug research trials are not conducted in hospitals and universities, where they are subject to review by institutional ethics review boards, but in the offices of individual physicians under the auspices of pharmaceutical companies. Because of the potential for serious effects on the health of users and their children, we believe that all such trials should be reviewed by research ethics boards, regardless of the setting in which they are conducted. This would ensure that the research is conducted in accordance with existing guidelines for medical research involving human subjects, including the requirement that participants be fully informed before consenting to participate, and that they are not charged for any drugs used in the trial. There may be costs involved in this ethical review, and these costs should be recoverable from the pharmaceutical company by the institution conducting the review. We recommend that

> 68. **The federal drug approval process include a requirement that any proposed trial of a fertility drug be reviewed by the research ethics board of a major hospital or university.**

Current Treatment and Prescription Practices

The Commission identified three issues of particular relevance here: the practices surrounding how drugs are prescribed and used; the information available to women and couples about the drugs they are considering taking; and the information available on short- and long-term health effects of drug use.

Prescription Practices

Drugs are tested and government-approved for certain uses and at certain doses, but once they reach the market doctors can prescribe them as they see fit. Doctors often hear of alternative unapproved uses of drugs from medical journals, at conferences, and from colleagues in other countries where drugs may be approved for different indications. Many fertility drugs are therefore commonly used for unapproved indications, and they are also used at unapproved dosages. In this context "unapproved" does not mean the drugs have been assessed and refused approval: it means that this particular use or dosage has not been assessed and approved in Canada. Some of the unapproved uses are in conjunction with new and emerging technologies that themselves have yet to be evaluated adequately.

There are often good reasons why physicians prescribe drugs for unapproved uses; certain drugs that are valuable in treating rare medical conditions could not be used if physicians were limited only to approved uses in their prescription decisions (see research volume, *New Reproductive Technologies and the Science, Industry, Education, and Social Welfare Systems in Canada*). This is because pharmaceutical companies do not wish to absorb the cost of the additional testing that would be required to gain government approval for uncommon indications where the market return would be small.

Nevertheless, the Commission sees no benefit in allowing fertility drugs to be prescribed at unproven doses and for new indications outside the context of clinical trials. The risks of prescribing fertility drugs for unproven uses and at unproven doses should not be taken unless the drugs are administered in such a way that the information gained can be used to decide whether they work and are of acceptable risk. A woman taking high doses of an unproven fertility drug may be putting her health at risk without good evidence that she is any more likely to have a child.

Without the comparisons made possible by well-designed trials — in which results can be compared between those who did and those who did not take the drug — risk is undertaken without even resulting in an increase in knowledge in the field, knowledge that is needed to minimize the number of women exposed to potential harm. Doctors should be cognizant of the fact that prescribing drugs in this manner is experimentation and should therefore be governed by the checks and balances of any research involving human subjects. The Commission therefore concludes that clear protocols and guidelines for the use of fertility drugs by practitioners, both in licensed clinics and practising outside them, are needed. In particular, the Commission recommends that

> **69. The Assisted Conception Sub-Committee of the National Reproductive Technologies Commission develop, with input from the relevant professional bodies, standards and guidelines for use by practitioners prescribing fertility drugs in licensed clinics providing assisted conception services.**

and that

> **70. The College of Family Practitioners of Canada and the Society of Obstetricians and Gynaecologists of Canada develop and disseminate similar guidelines for use by practitioners prescribing fertility drugs outside the context of licensed clinics. In particular, these guidelines should recommend against the prescribing of drugs where safe use requires specialized expertise and hormonal monitoring of women taking the drugs.**

In addition, physicians need an objective source of information on these drugs. At present, the most widely used source is the *Compendium of Pharmaceuticals and Specialties* (CPS). The CPS is published and distributed by the Canadian Pharmaceutical Association and lists the names, uses, and side effects of drugs on the Canadian market. The information in the CPS is supplied by drug manufacturers, who also subsidize the Canadian Pharmaceutical Association. Thus, the CPS is not an objective source of drug information. One study found that 46.9 percent of drugs listed in the 1977 edition of CPS could be classified as "probably useless," "obsolete," or "irrational mixtures," and that more than 60 percent did not list well-known risks, dangers, or adverse effects.[11] The Commission was troubled to find research showing that many doctors rely solely on CPS information for their drug data. If this is a doctor's only source of information about prescription drugs, the health of patients could be jeopardized. The Commission therefore believes that

> Government, as the guardian of the public interest, should take a role in facilitating the provision of objective sources of drug information independent of pharmaceutical manufacturers so that doctors have a practical alternative to the CPS.

government, as the guardian of the public interest, should take a role in facilitating the provision of objective sources of drug information independent of pharmaceutical manufacturers so that doctors have a practical alternative to the CPS. This is not an issue that is going to be resolved in the short term; it is one faced by all developed countries and will need the ongoing cooperation of several sectors. If the interests of Canadians are to be protected, however, physicians must have better access to practical, useful, and objective information on drugs.

We therefore conclude that the federal government should identify mechanisms to meet the need for development and dissemination of comparative, objective assessments of drugs, including fertility drugs. In the meantime, our recommendations with regard to fertility drug use in clinics and in the broader medical community, together with our recommendations regarding collection and dissemination of information on drugs, will help meet this need with regard to fertility drugs in particular.

Monitoring is already done by several bodies, but the Commission is of the view that the promotional activities of companies marketing fertility drugs in particular in Canada should be monitored on a continuing basis and therefore recommends that

> **71. The promotional activities of companies marketing fertility drugs in Canada be monitored on a continuing basis by the Assisted Conception Sub-Committee of the National Reproductive Technologies Commission and that any inappropriate activity be publicly identified.**

Informed Consent

As we have noted, most women who take fertility drugs obtain them from their general practitioner or gynaecologist. The Commission was contacted by some patients who were prescribed fertility drugs by physicians practising outside clinics. Their information, though valuable, is not likely to be representative, and in fact there is no practical way at present to identify or obtain representative information concerning use of fertility drugs prescribed by general practitioners or gynaecologists.

The Commission did, however, survey 1 395 clinic patients, and their views can be used to draw conclusions about patient perceptions of fertility drug treatment as practised at clinics. About half the women had already had some kind of fertility drug treatment before coming to the clinic. At the clinics, a majority of patients were prescribed fertility drugs, either alone or in conjunction with other treatments. Patients receiving only fertility drugs reported receiving much less information or counselling than those undergoing other treatments — fewer than half those taking fertility drugs said they received counselling or took part in discussions about their treatment, compared to 89 percent of patients who had IVF (see research volume, *Treatment of Infertility: Current Practices and Psychosocial Implications*).

The data collected for the Commission on the practices of fertility clinics and attitudes of patients showed that counselling, information provision, and support for informed decision making do not measure up to patients' expectations with respect to informed choice or indeed to the standards set by physicians' professional organizations. The Commission also found that this information deficit seriously limits patients' ability to make decisions about their health. Without sufficient information about fertility drug treatment and its attendant risks, benefits, costs, and possible outcomes, patients must cope with added physical and psychological stresses. The Commission therefore recommends that

> **72. Fertility drug treatment provided in licensed clinics offering assisted conception services be administered in a context of informed choice for patients. Standard protocols should include the availability of professional, non-directive counselling, and full, unbiased information on what is known about the side effects and long-term outcomes of the drug(s) to be used.**

and that

> **73. The Assisted Conception Sub-Committee of the National Commission develop, with input from relevant professional bodies, unbiased and readily understandable information materials on fertility drugs for distribution to patients by physicians and clinics providing assisted conception services.**

Identifying Short-Term Effects

Neither the government nor pharmaceutical companies have effective systems in place to monitor the results of fertility drug use after a drug has been approved for sale. There is a need for more data on both the short-term risks associated with their use and, especially, any long-term health effects on women or their children.

As we have discussed, no drug approval process, no matter how rigorous, can guarantee that a drug is safe when it is approved for market.

Only after a large number of people have used a drug over a long enough period of time does it become possible to predict all the potential adverse effects of a drug with any accuracy. Clinical trials generally involve 2 000 to 3 000 patients who have used the drug. With a sample of this size, rare adverse effects, or effects that occur many years after the end of the trial, cannot be identified. For these reasons, monitoring drugs after they come on the market (called post-market surveillance) is essential for physicians, consumers, and regulators alike.

The current system for collecting and analyzing data on the adverse effects of drugs has several important shortcomings. Under the Adverse Drug Reaction Reporting Program, doctors submit a report of observed adverse drug reactions (ADRs) to the pharmaceutical company that manufactures the drug or directly to the Drugs Directorate's Bureau of Pharmaceutical Surveillance. But the ADR Reporting Program is little used. There are two basic problems. There is no meaningful system by which ADR report events are gathered, collated, analyzed, and published. Also, physician compliance with reporting is low. The reporting system is inadequate. It lacks criteria telling physicians what the Drugs Directorate wants them to report. Health care professionals are not well informed about ADR reporting procedures. Moreover, there is lack of feedback to health care professionals when an ADR report is filed.

The rate of reporting ADRs by physicians is low. One industry representative told the Commission that only 10 percent of all adverse reactions are reported by doctors. Two factors contribute to the low reporting rate. Without a clearly defined system, there is little incentive for physicians to participate. As one expert told the Commission, "Physicians are very pragmatic people. They won't report adverse drug reactions unless they can see results." At the same time, the reporting system is strictly voluntary, and physicians are offered no compensation, despite the time required to complete the necessary paperwork, to follow up on patients, and to participate in any further investigation.

Regulatory requirements for adverse drug reactions do not cover all drugs; after a drug has been on the market for seven years, for example, it is no longer considered necessary to monitor for adverse reactions. Another weakness is poor analysis and follow-up on adverse drug reactions. As a result, reports of adverse drug reactions constitute anecdotal and unstandardized evidence that has not been collected following a rigorous scientific approach; as such, they are valuable only in indicating a potential problem and the need for appropriately rigorous study of it.

A recent proposal by the Drugs Directorate would require health care practitioners to report adverse drug reactions to five regional ADR reporting centres or to the manufacturer. The regional centres would transmit the reports to the national ADR reporting centre, which would compile the reports and distribute them to manufacturers, the regional centres, and the WHO Collaborating Centre in Sweden. The national centre would then evaluate the data to identify drugs requiring further study. The federal government has committed funding to a regional pilot project using this approach but has not committed funds to implement the national program.

We strongly agree that the post-market surveillance system should be improved, but we believe that further steps are needed as well. The financial burden of follow-up on prelimi-nary indications of adverse side effects or outcomes should not fall solely on the federal govern-ment. We believe that drug companies should be required to help fund investigations into problems identified through analysis of ADR data. Pharmaceutical companies have a lot to gain or lose, depending on the findings of researchers: profits increase if a drug is found to be safe, and costly legal action can be avoided if findings show at an early stage that a drug is dangerous. Therefore, the Commission believes companies should not do the investigations themselves but should be required to provide arm's-length financial support for investigations on the adverse effects of their products emerging from ADR data. We also believe that pharmaceutical companies that market fertility drugs should be required to help fund studies on fertility drugs done by the National Reproductive Technologies Commission using its data base to link with other health data bases to assess long-term outcomes of drug use, as discussed below. This funding should have no conditions attached other than it is to be used to study outcomes of fertility drug use. To minimize the possibility of influencing the Commission in any way, an intermediary body should receive the funding and administer it. The Commission therefore recommends that

> Companies should not do the investigations themselves but should be required to provide arm's-length financial support for investigations on the adverse effects of their products emerging from ADR data.

> **74. The federal government require pharmaceutical companies marketing fertility drugs to contribute funding for studies found by Health Canada to be required based on incoming adverse drug reaction data. This funding should be administered by national research funding agencies, but the studies should be facilitated and overseen by the National Reproductive Technologies Commission.**

Appropriate data collection and recording are necessary to permit assessments of the effects and outcomes of fertility drug use. The Commission believes that the data base established within the National Reproductive Technologies Commission must be structured and maintained so as to make possible evaluation of the short- and long-term health effects of fertility drugs. Submission of data to enable this would be required from every licensed fertility clinic.

Analysis of outcome information on fertility drugs, facilitated by the collection of standardized data by the National Reproductive Technologies Commission, will make possible the establishment of appropriate clinical standards; will inform policy decisions about drug treatment and its place in reproductive medicine; and will encourage priority setting for research in this field. Harmful drug effects identified by the NRTC through this data collection and analysis could also be made available to the ADR regional centres for distribution to practitioners, as well as to the public generally. The Commission recommends that

> **75. Categories of data established by the National Reproductive Technologies Commission on the use of fertility drugs, information on individuals receiving them, and data on adverse effects and outcomes be reported annually by infertility clinics to the National Reproductive Technologies Commission as a condition of licensing. Data collected in this manner should be analyzed and evaluated regularly by the National Reproductive Technologies Commission.**

> **76. The National Reproductive Technologies Commission issue an annual report giving significant findings resulting from data collection and analysis, and that aggregate data be used in the development of written information materials on the drugs used most commonly to treat infertility, to be distributed to clinics, regulators, and people contemplating the use of fertility drugs.**

and that

> **77. General practitioners and obstetricians/ gynaecologists prescribing fertility drugs should continue to report adverse effects from the use of fertility drugs through the Adverse Drug Reaction Reporting Program or the proposed regional system if it is implemented.**

Tracking Long-Term Outcomes

A major problem in assessing the long-term health effects of ovulation induction drugs (and many other drugs) is that no mechanism is in place to track long-term consequences. Provincial and federal bodies that have studied the current situation with regard to the long-term effects of prescription drugs have found it lacking. Concerns about long-term tracking of outcomes of fertility drug use are particularly important, and the Commission took this issue very seriously.

The Commission found no Canadian data available on these drugs because of the absence of a mechanism to gather and assess data on long-term outcomes. There are, however, innovative ways of using data already being collected by the health care system (such as hospital admission and discharge records), to determine whether women who took fertility drugs subsequently had health problems requiring treatment.

> Rational decision making in health care — whether by patients, practitioners, or policy makers — must be based on sound evidence, which can be provided only by collecting appropriate follow-up information over time ... Monitoring mechanisms are necessary to evaluate data in an ongoing way to inform decisions at many levels.

Computerized record linkage using existing data bases could drastically reduce costs and widen the scope of study by using health and vital statistics data already being collected by governments or institutions for other reasons and linking it to data — for example, on drug use — collected by other facilities.[12] This kind of data linkage is possible without violating people's privacy and would allow evaluation of any long-term effects of taking medications, including ovulation induction drugs. What is required is a uniform method of collecting information on people who have taken the drugs, so that record linkage studies of this type can be carried out.

Rational decision making in health care — whether by patients, practitioners, or policy makers — must be based on sound evidence, which can be provided only by collecting appropriate follow-up information over time. The Commission finds it disturbing that no mechanism is in place to allow the long-term health effects of fertility drugs (or, indeed, other drugs) to be assessed, particularly because those effects could have implications for women and men taking the drugs today as well as for their children. Current systems set up to store health and hospital records often do not provide for a mechanism to pull those data together into groupings that would permit analysts to assess the effects of past treatments. Moreover, after drugs are approved for use, little is done to ensure they are used appropriately or to track their use and effects. Monitoring mechanisms are necessary to evaluate data in an ongoing way to inform decisions at many levels. In the field of fertility drugs, this information would allow assessment of new and existing drug treatments, would make possible the establishment of clinical standards, and would inform policy decisions about drug treatment and its place in reproductive medicine. It would allow decisions to be made more quickly about the appropriateness of treatments and would encourage priority setting for research in this field.

Health-related data are accumulated across the country in a variety of forms: in hospital records, physician billing data for health insurance plans, death and birth records, and a host of other data bases. Using the example of the province of Saskatchewan (which has data available on hospital, medical, and prescription drug use — see research volume, *New Reproductive Technologies and the Health Care System: The Case for Evidence-Based Medicine*), researchers for the Commission investigated the feasibility of linking information from different data bases through time and across health sectors, to see whether outcomes of treatments could be assessed. This is a specific example of the kind of valuable study that could be carried out in the field of human reproduction, and we conclude on the basis of our investigation that such approaches would be feasible.

For example, clomiphene citrate use would be a good subject for a pilot record linkage study in Saskatchewan, where appropriately structured data bases exist. Health care data amassed since 1967 (the period during which clomiphene has been in use) could be accessed to answer outstanding questions and contribute useful information and analysis to the field of infertility research without involving the added major expense of primary data collection. Such a study could link data on clomiphene use with data from health and vital statistics data bases to assess its effectiveness, the factors associated with successful and unsuccessful outcomes, and any later negative impacts of the drug during the study period. Such studies could also provide data on the direct costs to the health care system. Not only could such studies link ovulation induction using clomiphene with outcomes, it could also compare outcomes in the children of women who took the drugs with outcomes in the children of similar women who conceived without them. Women could be matched by age, socioeconomic status, and place of residence, as such data are contained in the existing data bases. For example, it would be possible theoretically to assess whether prematurity, low birth weight, neonatal death, or hospitalizations were more common in the children of women who took clomiphene citrate.

One of the aspects essential to address in any record linkage study is stringent protection of any personally identifying data. If coded identifiers are assigned to each individual covered by a province's health programs and these identifiers are used when information about individuals is recorded in various data bases, it is possible to link the use of services over time by a given individual without researchers knowing the identity of the individuals involved. Fortunately, then, there are proven ways to meet the critical need to protect privacy while also allowing the evaluation of health consequences that is needed for appropriate policy and decision making.

Record linkage studies would also overcome the problems associated with following up individually in direct studies of patients who have used fertility drugs. Research has shown that the majority of infertility patients do not wish to participate directly in follow-up studies; they express a desire to put the experience behind them, regardless of whether the outcome was positive or negative. This too is a reason for developing alternative means of obtaining data on outcomes without intruding on patients' privacy. Using record linkage and data that are already collected for other purposes removes the necessity to contact patients.

Other useful "piggybacking" approaches on existing data bases may also be feasible. For example, it may be possible to structure pharmacists' data bases to make them amenable to linkage and to collect information when certain kinds of prescriptions are being filled, or to incorporate a data collection method into the system physicians use to bill provincial health insurance

> There are proven ways to meet the critical need to protect privacy while also allowing the evaluation of health consequences that is needed for appropriate policy and decision making ... Using record linkage and data that are already collected for other purposes removes the necessity to contact patients.

plans. The feasibility and practicality of these approaches would naturally vary from province to province and the territories given their different systems, but the benefits would be considerable in terms of gathering sufficient country-wide data — within a relatively short period of several years and at much less cost than primary data collection — to draw reliable conclusions about outcomes. In the Commission's view, provincial/territorial ministries of health could collaborate with each other to apply such approaches not only in reproductive health care but also in other areas to support rational decision making and appropriate use of public resources.

The Commission's research indicates that, with appropriate development of data bases on patients undergoing infertility treatment, it would be feasible to evaluate the long-term health effects of drug treatments on patients and their children. We believe that federal research funding agencies and provincial/territorial ministries of health should fund appropriate research proposals in this area. The Commission therefore recommends that

> **78. The licensing requirements for facilities providing assisted conception services ensure that data collected on use of infertility treatments (including fertility drugs) contain sufficient standardized information on individuals to permit linkage with other data**

bases on health outcomes, so that approved research can be conducted into possible long-term health effects of new reproductive technologies and into the effect of treatments on fertility.

and that

79. Pharmaceutical companies marketing fertility drugs be required by the federal government to contribute funding to be used for studies sponsored by the National Reproductive Technologies Commission linking data in its data base to data on longer-term health outcomes of individuals who have taken fertility drugs.

To safeguard the interests of patients in this process, the Commission recommends that

80. Patients be informed that non-identifying data on them will be used for studies on long-term outcomes; that this will not involve any contact with them; that only coded data will be used; that no named identifying information on any individual will be released to researchers; and that any published data will be in sufficient aggregation that individuals could not be identified.

and that

81. Access to data collected by the National Reproductive Technologies Commission be restricted to use of coded data by researchers conducting research projects that have been evaluated and approved by the National Reproductive Technologies Commission.

Conclusion

Fertility drugs occupy a unique place in the infertility treatment spectrum. Many do not consider fertility drugs to be a "new reproductive technology," yet fertility drugs are developed and used to act on the same biological processes as new reproductive technologies, with the aim of correcting some of the same disorders, and they have the same far-reaching implications — they could potentially affect not only the women who use them but also their children.

Fertility drugs are the most prevalent infertility treatment and are used in most other assisted conception techniques. The prevalence of fertility drug use makes it important to collect information on their short- and long-term outcomes. The side effects and long-term outcomes of fertility drug use have implications for society that are just as great as those of drugs used to treat heart disease or cancer. The evaluation of long-term outcomes is not easy, however, in part because the use of some drugs (especially clomiphene citrate) occurs most frequently outside the context of specialized treatment facilities, and in part because information on both the individuals receiving treatment and their children is relevant to this assessment.

It is not in society's interests that the use of these drugs continue without thorough and ongoing evaluation of their risks and effectiveness. Present federal regulatory bodies are not equipped to be solely responsible for appropriate and adequate evaluation of the safety and effectiveness of fertility drugs. The Commission's findings in this area suggest that data collected by the National Reproductive Technologies Commission are needed to allow evaluation of fertility drugs. The evidence gathered through analysis must be fed back continuously into shaping appropriate and safe practice.

The Commission's research and consultations with patients and clinics indicate that some of the concerns about fertility drugs raised at the Commission's hearings and private meetings are valid. We have identified the problems we found with existing systems and mechanisms, as well as the gaps in the research and evaluation of these drugs. The current process for approving and regulating drugs that come onto the market and for monitoring the side effects and long-term health effects of fertility drugs is inadequate. Although the Canadian drug evaluation and approval system is now being overhauled, the Commission believes that further steps are necessary. The existing system of post-marketing surveillance of drugs in Canada is seriously deficient in providing good data on the short- and long-term effects of fertility drugs on women and their children. The involvement and interaction of the proposed National Reproductive Technologies Commission with the emerging drug approval system would be beneficial in this area. Additional post-marketing mechanisms are called for; data on treatments provided at infertility clinics should be

> Adopting the approach we propose will provide Canadians with the assurance they seek that governments and professional bodies are fulfilling their responsibilities to protect citizens from unethical, unproven, or unsafe practices and treatments.

collected in a standardized way, as a condition of licensing, to facilitate post-marketing surveillance. In addition, research using record linkage to assess long-term health outcomes should be pursued and facilitated by the NRTC.

The Commission also found that some treatment practices with regard to fertility drugs are putting the health of patients at risk without the prospect of benefit. It is clear from the evidence before the Commission that there is a need to protect patients from unproven or experimental drug therapies and that guidelines for appropriate use of these drugs should be developed and disseminated widely. The Commission believes that our proposed system for licensing assisted conception clinics, including compliance with professional guidelines on drug use as a condition of licensing, will be a major step in the right direction. Moreover, it is essential — and the Commission has recommended — that the College of Family Physicians of Canada and the Society of Obstetricians and Gynaecologists of Canada develop the guidelines for the use of such drugs by practitioners outside clinics and that these be disseminated by the two organizations to their membership.

The Commission recommends that, apart from clomiphene citrate (which should be used only according to guidelines developed by the College of Family Physicians of Canada and the Society of Obstetricians and Gynaecologists of Canada), all other drugs should be used only if the patient can be closely monitored with appropriate specialized clinical and laboratory expertise. Thus, it will usually be inappropriate to use them outside infertility treatment clinics. Furthermore, only drugs that meet the standards of effectiveness we have established should be included in guidelines for practice used by licensed clinics. Use of fertility drugs in clinics other than in this way would be conditional on participation in clinical research trials designed to evaluate outcomes, so that the interests of patients can be protected while still allowing progress in knowledge and improvement of practice.

Many patients are receiving inadequate information about drug treatment. Full, understandable, and unbiased information should be available to patients before they take fertility drugs; this is why we have recommended that such information be developed by the Assisted Conception Sub-Committee of the NRTC and be

> Only the drug treatments that have been demonstrated effective at acceptable levels of risk should be offered. Others should be offered only in the context of multicentre clinical trials, in which standards of ethical research are adhered to. Yet others should be discontinued altogether.

made available for distribution by physicians and clinics. Data collected by the NRTC should be made available in a timely fashion to practitioners through annual aggregate reports and should be passed on to patients in accessible and useful form. Appropriate information and counselling to facilitate informed choice should be available to patients in licensed clinics as a condition of licensing. All experimental treatments should be identified as such to the patients participating in them in the context of clinical trials.

In summary, the Commission believes that only the drug treatments that have been demonstrated effective at acceptable levels of risk should be offered. Others should be offered only in the context of multicentre clinical trials, in which standards of ethical research are adhered to. Yet others should be discontinued altogether. Adopting the approach we propose will provide Canadians with the assurance they seek that governments and professional bodies are fulfilling their responsibilities to protect citizens from unethical, unproven, or unsafe practices and treatments.

General Sources

Collins, J., E. Burrows, and A. Willan. "Infertile Couples and Their Treatment in Canadian Academic Infertility Clinics." In Research Volumes of the Royal Commission on New Reproductive Technologies, 1993.

Hughes, E.G., D.M. Fedorkow, and J.A. Collins. "Meta-Analysis of Controlled Trials in Infertility." In Research Volumes of the Royal Commission on New Reproductive Technologies, 1993.

Jarrell, J.F., J. Seidel, and P. Bigelow. "Adverse Health Effects of Drugs Used for Ovulation Induction." In Research Volumes of the Royal Commission on New Reproductive Technologies, 1993.

Rochon Ford, A. "A Socio-Historical Examination of the Development of *In Vitro* Fertilization and Related Assisted Reproductive Techniques." In Research Volumes of the Royal Commission on New Reproductive Technologies, 1993.

Rowlands, J., N. Saby, and J. Smith. "Commercial Involvement in New Reproductive Technologies: An Overview." In Research Volumes of the Royal Commission on New Reproductive Technologies, 1993.

SPR Associates Inc. "An Evaluation of Canadian Fertility Clinics: The Patient's Perspective." In Research Volumes of the Royal Commission on New Reproductive Technologies, 1993.

Vandekerckhove, P., et al. "Treatment of Male Infertility: Is It Effective? A Review and Meta-Analyses of Published Randomized Controlled Trials." In Research Volumes of the Royal Commission on New Reproductive Technologies, 1993.

Specific References

1. A concern expressed frequently by participants at the Commission's public hearings and in numerous written submissions centres on the use of fertility drugs in dosages that exceed recommended levels and for purposes not envisioned at the time they were approved for sale in Canada. There is ample evidence that this occurs, even though the long-term effects of such usage are unknown. For example, the drug Lupron® (leuprolide acetate) is approved in Canada only for the treatment of prostate cancer but is being prescribed for the treatment of endometriosis, and in conjunction with IVF.

2. Mullens, A. *Missed Conceptions: Overcoming Infertility.* Toronto: McGraw-Hill Ryerson, 1990, p. 115.

3. Glazener, C.M.A., et al. "Clomiphene Treatment for Women with Unexplained Infertility: Placebo-Controlled Study of Hormonal Responses and Conception Rates." *Gynecological Endocrinology* 4 (2)(June 1990): 75-83.

4. Gonadotropin-releasing hormone (Gn-RH or LH-RH): controls excessive release of FSH and LH by the pituitary gland, thus preventing ovarian hyperstimulation; prevents spontaneous LH surge that may result in ovulation, which may hinder egg retrieval. Brand names Lupron®, Buserelin®, Decapeptyl®.

5. Medical Research International. "Adverse Effects of Ovulatory Stimulants." Report submitted to the National Institute of Child Health and Human Development. Burlington: MRI, 1993.

6. Millar, W.J., S. Wadhera, and C. Nimrod. "Multiple Births: Trends and Patterns in Canada, 1974-1990." *Health Reports* 4 (3)(1992): 223-29.

7. Mills, J.L., et al. "Risk of Neural Tube Defects in Relation to Maternal Fertility and Fertility Drug Use." *Lancet* 336 (July 14, 1990): 103-104.

8. TERIS data base summary for clomiphene. Seattle: University of Washington, September 1992. The frequency of congenital anomalies was no greater than expected among infants of women who had been treated with clomiphene to induce ovulation in three cohort studies involving respectively 225, 340, and 935 children (Harlap, S. "Ovulation Induction and Congenital Malformations." *Lancet* (October 30, 1976): 961; Barrat, J., and D. Leger. "Avenir des grossesses obtenues après stimulation de l'ovulation." *Journal de Gynecologie, Obstetrique et Biologie de la Reproduction* 8 (1979): 333-42; Kurachi, K., et al. "Congenital Malformations of Newborn Infants After Clomiphene-Induced Ovulation." *Fertility and Sterility* 40 (2)(August 1983): 187-89) or in a case-control study of 4 904 infants with major congenital anomalies (Mili, F., M.J. Khoury, and X. Lu. "Clomiphene Citrate Use and the Risk of Birth Defects: A Population-Based Case-Control Study." *Geratology* 43 (5)(May 1991): 422-23).

9. Vandekerckhove, P., et al. "Treatment of Male Infertility: Is It Effective? A Review and Meta-Analyses of Published Randomized Controlled Trials." In Research Volumes of the Royal Commission on New Reproductive Technologies, 1993.

10. Gagnon, D. *Working in Partnerships: Drug Review for the Future: Review of the Canadian Drug Approval System.* Quebec: Université Laval, 1992, p. 107. Recommendation 101.

11. Lexchin, J. *The Real Pushers: A Critical Analysis of the Canadian Drug Industry.* Vancouver: New Star Books, 1984, p. 148; Bell, R., and J.W. Osterman. "The Compendium of Pharmaceuticals and Specialties: A Critical Analysis." *International Journal of Health Services* 13 (1)(1983): 107-18.

12. Tugwell, P. Volume review comments, research volumes of the Royal Commission on New Reproductive Technologies, August 24, 1992.

Infertility Treatments: Assisted Insemination

Assisted insemination is the oldest known remedy for women who do not have a male partner who is fertile. Although in its commonest form it is a relatively simple procedure, the social and ethical implications of AI* are potentially as significant as those of other more technically complex assisted conception methods. AI can be used in quite different situations — the sperm can come from the woman's husband or partner, or it can come from a donor; the woman can be married, single, or a lesbian; the procedure can be performed by a doctor in a medical setting or by the woman herself or with the assistance of her partner.

The Commission's investigation of AI found that the practice is worthy of much more scrutiny, assessment, and policy attention than our society has afforded it in the past. We found that researchers and commentators have often neglected AI in favour of more technologically complex infertility treatments, perhaps perceiving AI as a simple practice that is adequately monitored and controlled. The Commission's examination of AI and the issues it raises showed that this is not the case.

We discovered that the lack of enforceable regulation and inadequate monitoring of the practice of AI have the potential to endanger the health of AI recipients, their partners, and their children; that inadequate record keeping is making it impossible to meet the current and future needs of AI children and their families for information; and that families formed through assisted insemination exist in a legal vacuum in most provinces, with the potential for conflict and distress if disputes over a child's parentage, custody, or inheritance arise. Our examination of the current

---

* In this text, "AI" is used to indicate all forms of assisted insemination (insemination using donor sperm, assisted insemination using the partner's sperm, intrauterine insemination using donor or partner sperm, and self-insemination using donor sperm). The specific terms are used when only one form of AI is referred to.   .

situation with respect to assisted insemination thus led us to conclude that the issues and concerns it raises for Canadians individually and as a society make it imperative to include the practice within the comprehensive licensing, monitoring, and record-keeping framework we propose for reproductive technologies, under the oversight of the National Reproductive Technologies Commission.

We begin this chapter with an examination of the social context in which AI is practised, then assess its past development and current practice. Next we examine issues that arise from the three stages in the process — sperm donation and banking; the clinical practice of insemination itself; and concerns about families formed through assisted insemination. (For details on the Commission's research in this area, see research volume, *Treatment of Infertility: Assisted Reproductive Technologies.*) We go on to lay out a comprehensive framework for the safe and effective delivery and monitoring of assisted insemination in Canada in a way that protects the current and future health and well-being of AI recipients and their families.

The Views of Canadians

AI involves personal decisions for the participants, but it also has broader implications for society. To reach a better understanding of the social context for AI in Canada, the Commission conducted two national surveys, each involving a representative sample of Canadians. In total, the views, attitudes, and opinions of more than 3 500 Canadians were gauged in personal interviews, telephone surveys, focus groups, or written questionnaires. The social context for donor insemination was also illustrated by the views and opinions conveyed in public hearings, private sessions, and written submissions, which gave the Commission the opportunity to hear from DI recipients, their partners, and their families, as well as from donors, AI practitioners, and others involved in the delivery of AI in Canada. We also heard a wide range of views from groups representing the interests of women, medical professionals, lesbians, churches and religious groups, legal professionals, and others interested in this field.

> It is very important that gamete banks be established in accordance with federal regulations ... to overcome problems related to the quality of donor gametes, the selection of donors, and accessibility generally.
>
> J. Dillon, Canadian Bar Association, Public Hearings Transcripts, Vancouver, British Columbia, November 27, 1990.

Many of the issues identified through these activities are echoed throughout this chapter: concern about the use of donor sperm and its implications for offspring and families; differing opinions about whether single women and lesbians who want to have children should have access to AI; and questions of how to maintain safety while ensuring broad access. AI has been performed for much longer than newer techniques such as IVF. It is only as it has moved from being a socially hidden to a more socially acceptable practice, however, that these issues have surfaced in public discussion. The public debate was also further focussed by Commission findings that some physicians and fertility programs are not adhering to existing professional guidelines intended to prevent the transmission of HIV, the virus thought to cause AIDS, through donor sperm. These findings were made public in April 1993 before our final report was released. The Commission also wrote at that time to provincial colleges of physicians and surgeons, whose mandate is to protect the public interest, to urge them to act in the interim before our report and its recommendations became public, so that women's health would not be put at risk by use of unsafe sperm.

> With the increasing incidence of AIDS in our society ... we have to recognize that [AI] ... can pose a risk to the health of the prospective mother and her baby.
>
> *K. Arnup, private citizen, Public Hearings Transcripts, Toronto, Ontario, November 20, 1990.*

Our surveys showed that Canadians generally support the use of AI to help a couple having difficulty conceiving, although opinions varied when the use of donor sperm was mentioned. Almost all survey respondents found AI using the male partner's sperm acceptable, but when asked about using donated sperm to help a couple who have difficulty having children, 58 percent of Canadians approved of DI use, and 22 percent were opposed. When asked if they would be likely to use sperm from a sperm bank if they were in this situation themselves, 47 percent said they would.

As mentioned in the introduction to this section, we also made deliberate efforts to solicit the views of Aboriginal people and Canadians who are members of racial or ethnic minorities in roundtable discussions and focus groups. From these we gained insights into the cultural values that affect how people see DI — we learned, for example, that many Aboriginal cultures emphasize passing on one's spirit to the next generation through one's children. We also heard from people in these communities who spoke about the importance of continuing their "family line" (see research volume, *Social Values and Attitudes Surrounding New Reproductive Technologies*).

As part of our national survey, the Commission also asked men whether they would consider donating sperm. We found that 26 percent would be very or somewhat likely to donate sperm to a sperm bank, while

73 percent would not be likely to donate. Twenty-five percent said they would consider donation if their identity was kept confidential.

Despite the issues and concerns it raises, we found general support among Canadians for AI as a reproductive option. Many women and couples impressed upon the Commission that DI had given them the chance to experience parenthood and have children, and they urged the Commission to ensure that DI remained a reproductive option. Some spoke about DI as a way to avoid passing on genetic disease and to make parenthood possible for couples who would otherwise feel they could not have children.

> Sperm donation and alternative insemination are non-invasive, low-risk procedures ... The technology is easy to use, cheap, and versatile, making decentralized and non-specialist use easily available.
>
> *S. McDonald, Ontario Advisory Council on Women's Issues, Public Hearings Transcripts, Toronto, Ontario, October 29, 1990.*

Single women and lesbians told the Commission about how DI helped them form families. Many witnesses also pointed out that DI is non-invasive, inexpensive, and relatively low-tech when compared to other methods of assisted conception.

The Commission also heard concerns about how DI is practised and about its implications. The increasing incidence of HIV and other sexually transmitted diseases prompted concerns about the safety of the sperm being used, leading to calls for regulation and monitoring of DI while maintaining the accessibility of the procedure. Numerous groups had suggestions for regulating sperm banks and establishing mechanisms to ensure safe and ethical use of the procedure by AI practitioners. It was clear that most did not endorse a system based on commercial sperm banks but were looking to the government to control DI and sperm banking in Canada.

Canadians were concerned about record keeping and the needs of DI recipients and their children with respect to genetic, medical, and other information about donors. Issues such as the anonymity of donors and the lack or unavailability of records were raised, and the need for complete confidentiality of donor informa-

> Abuses may be centred around the ... commercialization of sperm banks ...
>
> *R. Murray, Prairie Prolife of Portage la Prairie, Public Hearings Transcripts, Winnipeg, Manitoba, October 24, 1990.*

tion was questioned. It was clear that many of those involved in DI, whether as donors, recipients, DI children, or practitioners, felt that the process of DI should become more open. Many saw a need to protect donor anonymity and familial privacy but were also cognizant of the expressed needs of DI families, especially of some children for information about their genetic origins. There were clear indications that Canadians see a need for record-keeping mechanisms adequate to accommodate the lifelong implications of DI. Many Canadians urged the Commission to look to the adoption experience for lessons about how to deal with the needs of children born as a result of DI.

Canadians were also concerned about the broad ethical, social, and legal issues raised by the use of donor sperm and the formation of families through DI. For example, the issue of access to DI was an important one for Canadians. Some saw insemination as a health service, with access to it falling within the scope of *Canadian Charter of Rights and Freedoms* and human rights legislation. Others saw it as analogous to adoption, so that the principle of the best interests of the child should determine access.

Perhaps the most controversial aspect of the practice evident in testimony before the Commission was the use of DI by single women and lesbians. This mirrors attitudes found in the Commission's national surveys. Many respondents were of the view that because DI gives women without a male partner

[AI] using the sperm of an outside donor is considered by a majority of our members to be immoral and would conflict with their view of the sanctity of marriage and procreation.

H. Hilsden, Pentecostal Assemblies of Canada, Public Hearings Transcripts, Toronto, Ontario, November 20, 1990.

AI is acceptable between husband and wife; insemination where the sperm is brought from outside is not acceptable.

Brief to the Commission from the Muslim Women's Auxiliary, July 29, 1990.

The vitality and stability of society require that children come into the world within a family and that the family be firmly based on marriage.

Brief to the Commission from the Canadian Conference of Catholic Bishops, January 28, 1991.

the chance to have children, it devalues the role of males in relation to their children and deprives children of a father. Some respondents said that assisted conception should be limited to heterosexual couples because they felt the resulting child would be disadvantaged in other types of family settings.

At the same time, some Canadians pointed to constitutional and legal prohibitions on discrimination on the basis of single status or sexual orientation. Some witnesses stated that physicians control access to fertility clinics and that, given their attitudes, it is easier for married, heterosexual couples to obtain treatment. Commissioners heard specifically from single women and lesbians who described how they had been denied access and thus discriminated against in the traditional medical setting.

The issue of medicalization of AI was raised, particularly when more invasive techniques of insemination with partner sperm were used. Some intervenors warned that doing this gives rise to other, more serious problems. We heard the view that it is inappropriate to treat women as the patients in AI programs, with the risks that entails, when in fact AI is a treatment for their male partner's infertility. On this point, we also heard that AI involving treatment of the partner's sperm and placement of it higher in the woman's reproductive tract may be the only way for such couples to have a child together; this is important to both partners and is the reason why women decide to undergo the more invasive treatment. Indeed, women who had had AI told the Commission that their main motivation was their own desire for children; pressure from a spouse or partner was a distant second, they said, and support or pressure from family and friends was of very little importance (see research volume, *Treatment of Infertility: Current Practices and Psychosocial Implications*).

> We are concerned that persons conceived of donor sperm ... may be cut off from any knowledge of [their] genetic parents by policies of confidentiality. We feel this may be harmful to them as it has been for many adoptees.
>
> *H. Kramer, Canadian Adoption Reunion Register, Public Hearings Transcripts, Toronto, Ontario, November 20, 1990.*

As alluded to earlier, the medicalization of AI has also created a situation in which medical practitioners are the gatekeepers of DI in particular, enforcing what they perceive to be community standards about family formation by establishing access criteria to it. There were also concerns that despite being viewed as within the medical sphere, some aspects of DI are in fact under-controlled and not monitored, so that the procedure is not as safe as it should be.

Finally, many Canadians pointed out that the law ignores the interests, roles, and responsibilities of DI participants, making such families vulnerable. Many linked this legal void to the secrecy surrounding DI, arguing

> Most Canadians see DI as an option that should be available, provided it is offered in a safe manner.

that if the interests of donors, recipients, and children were better protected, the process could become more open (see the section on Secrecy in DI Families).

Emerging from this range of views and concerns was a distinct sense that most Canadians see DI as an option that should be available, provided it is offered in a safe manner. These views and the issues identified helped form the basis for the Commission's research into assisted insemination.

Our decisions on these questions were not easily made. There were a few occasions, for instance, when our moral reasoning led us to conclusions that were not strongly supported by the responses to some specific questions in our surveys of Canadians. This kind of situation usually arose when a value that Canadians strongly endorsed and said was important to them, such as equality, was not upheld in answer to a question on a specific situation, such as whether single women should have access to donor insemination or whether people who are disabled should have access to IVF.

We gave great thought to this dilemma. We were guided by and took into consideration what Canadians said about both their fundamental values and their attitudes toward specific issues, but they were not the only determinant of decision making in this complex area. Where there was a divergence on specific policy questions, we decided that our moral reasoning should have greater weight if it was in line with fundamental values endorsed by Canadians, because we had spent much time weighing the evidence and thinking through the implications of different policies on such specific questions.

> Increasingly the use of all of the new reproductive technology is being limited to married or at least co-habiting heterosexual couples. Single women, whether they are heterosexual or lesbian, find themselves denied access to fertility treatment and to artificial insemination. And I am here today to suggest that it is critical that these technologies not be limited to a select population. I believe that access to AI should not be influenced by race, class, physical disability, marital status or sexual orientation.
>
> *K. Arnup, private citizen, Public Hearings Transcripts, Toronto, Ontario, November 20, 1990.*
>
> I urge you not to consider [AI] for lesbians and unmarried women ... Our Canadian society does not need more confused, emotionally deprived children.
>
> *Brief to the Commission from E. Kelly, December 17, 1990.*

History and Development of Assisted Insemination

Although AI has been known to human beings since early civilization, the first recorded insemination in women took place in Britain in 1793. American scientific literature indicates six women were inseminated with donor sperm in 1866, while the earliest recorded DI in Canada was in 1950 (although it was probably practised, unrecorded, before that time).

Techniques of Assisted Insemination

Assisted Insemination (AI): Includes all forms of insemination without intercourse using donor or partner's sperm.

Assisted Insemination Homologous (AIH): Term for AI when sperm from the woman's husband or partner is used. Also known as *Assisted Insemination by Husband*. AIH is used most frequently for oligospermia or when the woman has an immune response to the husband's sperm, since it allows the sperm to be treated to make it more likely to fertilize an egg. The sperm of the woman's partner is placed in the vagina, near the cervix, or in the uterus.

Intrauterine Insemination (IUI): Term for AIH when the sperm is placed in the uterus; it is the most common form of insemination in a site other than the vagina. Others include *peritoneal insemination (PI)*, in the peritoneal cavity, and *synchronized hysteroscopic insemination of the fallopian tubes (SHIFT)*, in the fallopian tubes. IUI is used for oligospermia thought to be caused by poor sperm mobility, or unexplained factors, or when there is a cervical mucus problem. The sperm of the woman's partner is placed in the uterus or fallopian tubes with a catheter inserted through the cervix. IUI is thought to increase the chance of conception by allowing the sperm and egg a better chance of contact.

Donor Insemination (DI): Term for AI when the sperm comes from a man other than the woman's husband or partner. Also known as *artificial insemination* and *assisted insemination by donor (AID)*. DI is the only known way to circumvent azoospermia that is not caused by a male tubal blockage or ejaculatory defect. It is also used by couples in which the male is oligospermic and AIH is ineffective, or to prevent the transmission of a genetic disease carried by the male partner. DI is also used by women who wish to have a child but do not have a male partner. Sperm from a donor is placed in the vagina near the cervix.

Self-Insemination (SI): Term for DI when it is performed without medical assistance by the woman, her partner, or other non-medical support. Also known as *alternative insemination*. SI is used by women who cannot or choose not to take part in clinical AI programs. SI takes place outside a medical setting with no medical intervention. Donor sperm is placed in the vagina by the woman or her partner.

Today AI is used in several situations: when a woman's partner is infertile or subfertile; when both partners are subfertile; and when a woman without a male partner wishes to have a child. The procedure itself is simple: a fertile man's semen is placed in the woman's body using a syringe or other instrument, with fertilization, pregnancy, and birth following naturally if the procedure succeeds. AI can also be used to increase the chances of fertilization where male factor infertility (for example, low sperm count) has been diagnosed. Although it may not be possible to achieve pregnancy through sexual intercourse in these cases, the chances of fertilization may be greater if the sperm is concentrated and enhanced, if it is placed in the woman's body at sites other than the vagina (such as the uterus or the fallopian tubes), if the woman is prescribed fertility drugs, or if a combination of these techniques is used. The term assisted insemination homologous (AIH) includes all these methods where the sperm is that of the woman's partner.

AIH is not an option if a woman does not have a male partner, if her partner is at risk of passing on a genetic disease, or if his infertility cannot be treated through sperm enhancement techniques. Women and couples in these situations may choose to bypass these problems by using donor sperm.

In addition to women whose partners are infertile, single women or lesbian couples who want to have children have also looked to DI. They have found that marital status or sexual orientation is sometimes a barrier to services. As a result, single women and lesbians in some cities have set up alternative DI systems. The women obtain sperm from friends or other donors and do the insemination themselves; known as self-insemination (SI), this practice carries its own risks and societal concerns.

An important development in the history of AI was the discovery that sperm can survive freezing. Fresh sperm can live only a few hours outside the body, and then only if kept at a moderate temperature,[1] but semen frozen in liquid nitrogen (cryopreservation) can be kept indefinitely. The first successful insemination using thawed human sperm occurred in the 1940s.

Cryopreservation opened the door to sperm banking; sperm samples are frozen at a central location, then shipped to practitioners and thawed for use when required. Two types of sperm banks emerged — those affiliated with medical schools and hospital fertility clinics (which usually collected and stored sperm solely for their own use), and private banks operating at a profit by selling sperm to AI practitioners. The first large sperm banks appeared in the United States in the 1970s. Because donors to these banks are recruited from a wide geographic area, couples may be able to use sperm from a donor whose physical features are similar to those of the husband or partner, or from a donor with the same racial or ethnic characteristics. Some sperm banks also offer recipients a choice of donors with above-average intelligence, certain levels of schooling, or professional status, reviving the debate about selective breeding.

While the U.S. experience with DI was defined by private enterprise in the 1970s, the same decade saw the emergence of government-sponsored programs in some other countries, for example a sophisticated government-regulated system in France. The Centre d'étude et de conservation des oeufs et du sperme humains (CECOS), a self-regulating group of clinics, was established in 1973 to license sperm clinics according to rigorous standards of practice, recently incorporated into national legislation. Costs of AI when performed by licensed clinics have been covered by France's state-funded social security since 1978.

The current practice of AI in Canada has emerged as a combination of publicly supported and private, for-profit services. Donor sperm is collected by hospitals, by doctors in private practice, and by commercial sperm banks. Inseminations are performed in hospital-based fertility programs, by private practitioners, and in private fertility clinics, as well as through the alternative networks mentioned earlier. The insemination procedure is covered by provincial health insurance in half of Canadian provinces, although costs for donor sperm and cryopreservation may be charged directly to the recipient. Many hospital-based DI programs collect and store donor sperm in-house, but the majority of private fertility programs buy donor sperm from commercial sources. There are four major commercial sperm banks in Canada — Repromed (Toronto), Gamete Services (Toronto), the University of Calgary, and L'Institut de Médecine de la Reproduction de Montréal Inc. — and several U.S. banks will ship sperm to Canada. A Commission survey of Canadian fertility clinics found that Repromed is the most frequently used commercial source of sperm.

> The current practice of AI in Canada has emerged as a combination of publicly supported and private, for-profit services.

In the past 15 years, professional medical associations in Canada and the United States have become concerned about the safety of AI practice. In 1980, the American Fertility Society published the first guidelines for insemination. The first Canadian guidelines, *Storage and Utilization of Human Sperm*, were published in 1981 by Health and Welfare Canada. Today, many professional associations outline specific safety guidelines for every step of the process, and both the American and Canadian fertility societies (representing practitioners involved in fertility treatments) updated their guidelines for DI practice in 1993. However, these guidelines remain voluntary; as the evidence will show, they are not uniformly adhered to, and some practitioners are not even aware of them.

AI in Canada: Current Practice

Of the 24 assisted insemination programs across Canada, 19 are offered at teaching hospitals, while five are located in other hospitals and private clinics. The Commission found that about 3 400 women used these services in 1991, more than any other infertility treatment procedure offered in Canada. AI is also offered by family practitioners and obstetricians; data on the number of women treated in these settings are not available, in some

> AI is a solution in practice for many more couples who are infertile than IVF is and affects far more children and families.

cases because no records are kept, and because no mechanism exists to identify individual AI practitioners and collect information from them.

Although the Commission conducted a survey of all these clinics and of a small sample of AI practitioners in the community, it was not possible to obtain a good estimate of the number of children born as a result of AI in this country. Our 1991 survey found, for example, that 778 DI pregnancies were recorded by Canadian AI services, but this is an underestimate because many clinics do not record pregnancies or births — some do not even keep an exact count of the number of women treated, instead counting only the number of treatment cycles. While medicare billings give some information on how often AI is used in the provinces where it is an insured service, that system generally does not differentiate between DI and AIH and does not link AI to pregnancy care and birth. If both inseminations at clinics and those occurring in informal networks using self-insemination are included, estimates are that between 1 500 and 6 000 DI children are born each year — that is, between 0.4 and 1.5 percent of all children born in Canada. This is many more children than are born through *in vitro* fertilization (about 400 in 1991) — in fact between 4 and 15 times more. Thus, AI is a solution in practice for many more couples who are infertile than IVF is and affects far more children and families.

The details of insemination practices vary, but sperm banks, clinics, and solo practitioners (doctors who offer DI in their own offices) must go through the same three basic stages. The process begins with the collection of donor

> **Azoospermia:** Absence of living sperm in the semen.
>
> **Oligospermia:** Scarcity of sperm in the semen.

sperm. Canadian sperm banks usually recruit donors through university newspapers or physicians' personal contacts. The currently recommended standard screening process for donors begins with a personal medical history, family history, and social history, including collection and recording of both identifying and non-identifying information. Non-identifying physical information includes such aspects as height, weight, age, build, eye and hair colour, complexion, and ethnic background. Potential donors are given a physical examination, blood samples are taken, and candidates are asked to provide a semen sample.[2] Only about 15 percent of potential donors are accepted; the most common reason for non-acceptance is that their sperm does not survive freezing and thawing well, but some donors are rejected because they are at risk of passing on an infectious or genetic disease.

Blood and semen samples are sent to a laboratory for analysis, including sperm count, analysis of sperm shape and motility, and testing for sexually transmitted infectious diseases. The rest of the semen is cryopreserved in "straws" (small glass tubes each holding about one-tenth

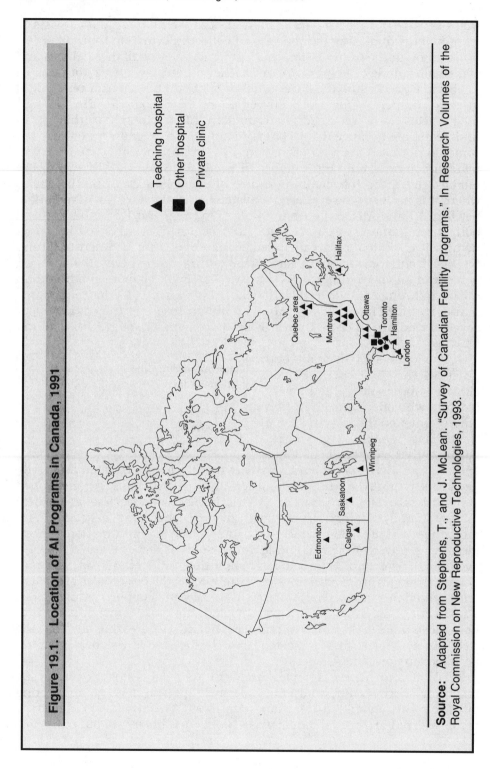

Figure 19.1.   Location of AI Programs in Canada, 1991

Teaching hospital
Other hospital
Private clinic

Source: Adapted from Stephens, T., and J. McLean. "Survey of Canadian Fertility Programs." In Research Volumes of the Royal Commission on New Reproductive Technologies, 1993.

of the sperm from an average ejaculation) and held in reserve. If the initial test results do not identify a problem, the frozen samples are kept aside until the donor can be tested again a few months later. If antibodies to HIV[3] are not found in the donor's blood at this time (they can take six months or longer to develop), the frozen semen is then considered acceptable for insemination. Professional guidelines recommend that donors continue to undergo blood and semen tests every three months for as long as they continue donating, with the semen being kept aside until results are available. Sperm considered acceptable for insemination is labelled and kept frozen until a practitioner requests a sample; currently, only physicians can obtain donor sperm from Canadian sperm banks.

> There should be no restrictions on access to [AI] apart from medical reasons, that is, no criteria or requirement that married women have permission of spouses and no exclusion of women for sociological reasons.
>
> *C. Micklewright, British Columbia Federation of Labour, Public Hearings Transcripts, Vancouver, British Columbia, November 27, 1990.*

The donor sperm used in fertility clinics is obtained either from in-house sperm banks or from commercial banks. Two AI programs (2 of 33) told the Commission they allow relatives or friends of the patient to act as donor. If the donor sperm is provided by the clinic, recipients can exercise some choice based on non-identifying information — usually, the donor's physical characteristics are matched as closely as possible with those of the woman's partner. Patients pay a fee for each straw of donor sperm, and there are additional charges if the type of sperm is in short supply (such as sperm from an ethnic minority donor) or is shipped from the United States.

At most clinics (12 of 18) the recipient is asked to sign forms giving her consent for the practitioner to perform AI. At half (9 of 18), her spouse must also give consent. In cases of DI, the woman's spouse is usually (14 of 18) asked to provide written acknowledgement of the insemination. Without this consent it would be possible for him to contest his paternity after the child is born. As we discuss later, this is among the legal issues raised by DI.

Women undergoing AI may have an infertility work-up to verify their fertility, and they may also be prescribed fertility drugs to ensure that they ovulate and to make the time of ovulation easy to pinpoint. The woman is then asked to chart her ovulation cycles. When a woman determines that she is ovulating, she alerts the clinic or her practitioner. If her partner's sperm is being used, a sample is collected and may be treated or enhanced to increase the chances of fertilization. If donor sperm is being used, a sample is thawed and prepared for use; it is allowed to liquify (this takes about 10 minutes) and must then be used within the next two hours. The semen is usually placed in the woman's vaginal canal with a sterile syringe or in a small cup that covers the cervix and is left in place for about four hours. The woman may lie with her pelvis elevated for 30 to 40 minutes. The procedure is usually done the day the woman ovulates and repeated one or two times in the few days that follow. This process is referred to as one "treatment cycle." If pregnancy is achieved, the clinic or practitioner usually has no more involvement with the woman or couple.

Effectiveness of AI

In some treatment programs, about 60 to 70 percent of women inseminated with donor sperm become pregnant within six treatment cycles — this is about the same as the natural pregnancy rate (see Figure 9.1). Other clinics say that 30 to 40 percent of inseminations result in pregnancy within six cycles. Obviously, the success rate at any given clinic will depend on the

> The likelihood of having a live birth after donor insemination is much greater than for IVF.

ages of the women treated and on what proportion of them are subfertile (in addition to their partners being oligospermic). Nevertheless, the likelihood of having a live birth after donor insemination is much greater than for IVF. By contrast, the pregnancy rate after AIH depends on the male partner's diagnosis and the method used to treat the sperm or inseminate the woman; some studies have shown that AIH is of little benefit in achieving pregnancy.[4]   Currently, it is not standard practice to follow up once pregnancy is achieved or to record the number of children born after DI. Our survey showed that many clinics left it up to the sperm bank to keep records about donors and recipients and that each sperm bank has different standards of record keeping. The Commission found that the number of inseminations allowed from one donor varies widely, and the number of inseminations may not be recorded or tracked. No central records are kept about the number of inseminations or children born per donor, pregnancy outcomes, or the health of children born after AI.

The Commission assessed each form of assisted insemination (AIH, IUI, and DI) for both risks and effectiveness.

Effectiveness of AIH

AIH is the most medically complex form of AI, although it raises fewer social and ethical concerns, as only the couple's gametes are involved. If a semen analysis identifies a problem with the male partner's sperm,[5] the sperm can be treated by various methods aimed at enhancing its ability to fertilize the egg. The treatments include

- sperm washing, the most common procedure, which is used to separate viable sperm from other elements of the semen, such as prostaglandins, antibodies, and micro-organisms, and concentrate viable sperm into a smaller volume;

- sperm swim-up, also known as sperm rise, which is used to concentrate the most highly motile sperm; and

- drug treatments, such as the addition of caffeine or other stimulants to the semen sample, in the hope of improving sperm motility. Antibiotics may also be used to eliminate bacterial infection.

Treated sperm are usually placed directly in the uterus rather than in the vagina or near the cervix because the volume is very small and, it is reasoned, closer access to the fallopian tubes may help to compensate for this. However, it is not clear whether these treatments in fact increase the likelihood of having a child, and there is no evidence from suitably controlled observations that it is effective. AIH has a clear role in cases where the male partner has a spinal cord injury and intercourse cannot occur, but, apart from this, there is not sufficient evidence to conclude that sperm treatments are effective either in increasing sperm motility and function or in increasing the probability of conception.

In addition to treatments aimed at enhancing the viability of the sperm, insemination can be performed in such a way as to increase the chances of fertilization by mixing the partner's sperm with donor sperm, allowing the possibility that any child born could be genetically linked to the male partner. This is no longer considered good practice as it creates ambiguity about the child's parentage. Other adjuncts to AIH may include the treatment of the woman, either with fertility drugs or with different methods of insemination, because in some couples both partners may be subfertile.

Risks and Effectiveness of Intrauterine Insemination and Related Techniques

Insemination in the uterine cavity may be used in some cases of poor sperm motility or low sperm count, for a cervical mucus problem,[6] or where the sperm may be prevented from ascending to the fallopian tube. As outlined above, the sperm is usually treated first. The Commission found that 20 percent of couples with unexplained infertility undergo IUI as their first treatment in fertility clinics (see research volume, *Treatment of Infertility: Current Practices and Psychosocial Implications*). IUI may be done using natural (unstimulated) cycles or may be used in conjunction with fertility drugs, the rationale being that if more than one egg is released from the ovaries, this may increase the chance of pregnancy. IUI carries a small risk of complications such as cramping, allergic reaction, fever, shock, or infection.

Research comparing the effectiveness of IUI for couples with unexplained fertility with that of sexual intercourse timed to coincide with ovulation has failed to demonstrate any benefit to using IUI, although weaknesses in study design limit the reliability of these results (see research volume, *New Reproductive Technologies and the Health Care System: The Case for Evidence-Based Medicine*). When intrauterine insemination is conducted in conjunction with drug therapy using hMG (see Chapter 18), there is some evidence that it is more likely to be effective, but, again, methodology problems with the studies render the evidence inconclusive. This is an important area for further study; at present there is simply not enough evidence to categorize intrauterine insemination as effective or ineffective, either with or without fertility drugs.

> At present there is simply not enough evidence to categorize intrauterine insemination as effective or ineffective, either with or without fertility drugs.

Cervical Mucus Incompatibility

The cervix, at the entrance to the uterus, secretes mucus throughout the menstrual cycle according to hormone levels in the woman's body. During most of the cycle, the mucus creates an acidic barrier preventing bacteria, sperm, or other foreign substances from entering the uterus. Sperm that encounter the mucus die within a few hours. In response to increased estrogen produced around the time of ovulation, however, the mucus changes to "mid-cycle mucus," becoming much thinner and more hospitable to sperm. For up to three days, this type of mucus is produced and facilitates sperm movement into the uterus and toward the egg. After ovulation, the mucus goes back to its acidic state.

In some cases, inadequate mid-cycle mucus can impair fertility, especially in cases where the sperm is of low motility, and sperm die before entering the uterus. IUI is meant to circumvent this problem by bypassing the cervix and depositing the sperm directly inside the uterus.

Evidence is also lacking about the effectiveness and risks of two related techniques — peritoneal insemination (PI), in which semen is injected into the peritoneal cavity, and synchronized hysteroscopic insemination of the fallopian tubes (SHIFT), in which semen is injected into a fallopian tube. These are therefore unproven treatments.

Risks and Effectiveness of Donor Insemination

Statistics show that DI with frozen sperm, quarantined until the donor has been tested for infectious diseases, is the safest and most effective method of circumventing the lack of a male partner who is fertile. This is not surprising, as both the woman and the donor are presumably fertile, and no drug therapy, surgery, or other invasive procedures are required. In the past, frozen sperm was less viable than fresh sperm, but cryopreservation and insemination procedures have improved, and some recent studies show little difference in success rates between frozen and fresh sperm.

DI properly performed after appropriate testing of the donor poses no physical risks, but there may be psychological effects on the recipient, her partner, or both. DI pregnancies can be accompanied by feelings of ambivalence, fear, or nightmares for some women. Some women report being depressed after a DI birth, while their partners report feelings of guilt, impotence, and resentment (see research volume, *Treatment of Infertility: Assisted Reproductive Technologies*). Many of the psychological effects of DI can be minimized or avoided with proper counselling and informed consent before a woman or couple agrees to undergo the procedure; these and other related issues are discussed later in this chapter.

Issues in Sperm Donation, Collection, and Storage

The DI process begins with the donor. Studies show that men donate sperm for different reasons: altruism, for example, or a wish to "test" their fertility. Donors have been neglected in the study of DI, however, perhaps because they are wary of jeopardizing their anonymity and because current record-keeping practices make most of them impossible to contact. The donor's interests and responsibilities should not be ignored, however. Issues such as anonymity and informed consent, as well as the standards and practices of facilities that collect and use sperm, have implications for the donor's health and psychological well-being, as well as that of the recipient and her child.

Donor Anonymity

One of the most controversial issues in DI is whether the donor should remain anonymous; the issue is also related to secrecy about the procedure (see section on Secrecy in DI Families). For decades, practitioners believed that anonymity made DI easier for everyone involved and have protected the identity of both the donor and the recipient. In interviews, many donors have said that they value the guarantee of anonymity because they want to ensure that they are not forced to assume the legal responsibilities of parenthood; they trust

> I think it is clearly a necessity for the [children] to know the genetic heritage they are carrying and not run into a roadblock when they go searching for that genetic heritage.
>
> *J. Harrington, Thomas More Centre for the Family, Public Hearings Transcripts, Toronto, Ontario, November 19, 1990.*

clinicians and sperm banks not to reveal their identity, and they have no interest in meeting recipients or their children. It has been argued that eliminating donor anonymity would make it more difficult to find men willing to donate sperm; in a national survey done for the Commission, men identified confidentiality as the number one condition for donating sperm. Most women and couples contemplating DI also prefer an anonymous donor, usually to avoid unwanted involvement by the donor in the life of the family and the child. Although two (2 of 33) AI programs surveyed by the Commission allow patients to designate a donor, few patients request this.

Donor anonymity may, however, work against the interests of DI children, for example if they want to know about their origins. Some DI children and parents told the Commission that without information about the donor, the children could feel cut off from their genetic origins, might be unaware of potential health problems, or might marry a blood relative unknowingly (see section on Lessons from the Adoption Context).

The Commission considered three options for making donor information available to DI families:

1.   full disclosure of all information — donations would be made on the understanding that recipients and their children would have full access at some time to both identifying and non-identifying information about the donor;

2.   a dual system — donors could choose to have their identity known or to remain anonymous, and recipients could choose whether they wanted an anonymous donor or a named donor; and

3.   a system giving DI recipients and children full social, medical, and genetic information about the donor, but concealing his identity unless there was a pressing medical need to reveal further information.

These options are discussed below.

Full Disclosure

Access to the donor's name and identity would put DI children in the same situation as most other children with respect to knowing who their parents are. Proponents of this approach told the Commission that the social and psychological need to know about their origins is no different for DI children (or indeed for adoptees) than it is for other children. This is not a straightforward issue, however. Full disclosure of identifying information about donors also raises ethical and practical issues that may work against the best interests of the DI child. Disclosing the identity of the donor invades the privacy and security of the newly formed DI family, it may go against their wishes, and it may threaten parent/child bonds. The recipient has contributed genetically to the child, has carried the child to term, and has shared the experience of pregnancy and birth with her partner, and her partner is usually the child's social and legal father — it is in their child's best interests that a strong, mutually supportive, and nurturing family unit be established without the unwanted intrusion of a known donor.

A sperm donor cannot in any way be compared to a parent or family member — he has not entered into any personal relationship with the recipient, and he has undertaken none of the duties or responsibilities of fatherhood. The social parents, no matter what the child's origins, must be able to define how the family will live and interact — they may find any role for the donor in their lives intrusive and disruptive. Knowing the identity of the donor may be seen by them to belittle their shared experience, as well as actual parenthood. If revelation of the donor's identity is unwanted but is mandatory, it may well be at the expense of the well-being of the child and the social parents and their ability to form family bonds as they see fit. Indeed, it may contribute to or encourage secrecy about the method of conception.

> It will be important for children who are conceived through alternative insemination to know later what their genetic history is, particularly ... health risks, but also probably ethnic and racial background ... [perhaps with] a code attached to it which states the genetic [and] medical [background].
>
> *B. Beagan, Halifax Lesbian Committee on New Reproductive Technologies, Public Hearings Transcripts, Halifax, Nova Scotia, October 17, 1990.*

DI children are not the only ones who may not know the name of their father — for example, adoptees have access to birth records only if their birth mother agrees — and children in other families may not know either. It has been estimated that the birth certificates of between 6 and 10 percent of children born in Canada do not contain an entry for the father. Even in cases where paternity is presumed, children born as a result of extra-marital affairs or relationships that broke up before the current union are often raised thinking they are biologically linked to both their parents — society does not demand disclosure in these instances. In fact, in North America, the likelihood of non-paternity in the children of couples in the general population is in the range of 1 to 5 percent and may be as high as 10 percent.[7] A man's name

> This issue is related to donor anonymity, and I would also like to bring another element to the attention of the Commission — an element that may be peculiar to Quebec, but I think that the same principle holds true for all other Canadian provinces: the equality of all children regardless of the circumstances of their birth. [Translation]
>
> *E. Deleury, Faculté de droit, Université Laval, Public Hearings Transcripts, Quebec City, Quebec, September 26, 1990.*

on a child's birth certificate is one indication of his willingness to be identified as the father, but it is not a guarantee that he is in fact genetically linked to the child.

Paradoxically, a system of full disclosure might well encourage secrecy about the DI process. Parents who want no contact with the donor could arrange insemination privately and simply conceal the circumstances of conception from the child, so that he or she would never have reason to request information about a donor. Moreover, evidence before the Commission shows that secrecy in families can be very harmful (see section on Lessons from the Adoption Context). If parents were secure in the knowledge that a donor would not be identified and intrude on their lives, they might be more likely to feel free to raise their children in an open and honest environment, revealing the circumstances of a child's conception but not the particular individual involved.

As with adoptees, disclosure of a donor's identity could be postponed until the child reached the age of majority. As we discuss further in the next section, however, this presumes that a donor can anticipate how he will feel 18 or more years later.

Finally, full disclosure is likely to affect the supply of donor sperm. When Sweden changed its law in 1985 to require that identifying information be made available to the child upon request to the social services authority, the number of clinics was reduced by half (from 10 to 5), and Swedish couples began travelling to other countries for DI.

Dual System

Another system proposed to the Commission would allow men, at the time of donation, to choose one of two options: (a) not to have identifying information released, or (b) to be willing to be identified by name when the child reached the age of majority. DI recipients and their partners could choose either an anonymous donor or one willing to be identified, based on their values and perceptions of the role of the donor. The system has analogies to current adoption law in some jurisdictions, where adoption records are revealed to the child if the birth mother wishes to be contacted.

As explained previously, however, the Commission believes DI families *are* different from those formed through adoption. When a couple raises an adopted child, neither is biologically related to that child; when a couple raises a DI child, only one of them is the biological parent. In adoption, the child already exists and is placed for adoption because the mother is unable to raise the child; in DI situations, the child is conceived

> DI families *are* different from those formed through adoption ... Adoption deals with finding a family for an existing child, while DI deals with the deliberate formation of a family by having a child.

deliberately with the intent of nurturing and raising it. Adoption deals with finding a family for an existing child, while DI deals with the deliberate formation of a family by having a child.

Moreover, a dual system would create two classes of DI children — those who may have named information on their genetic father, and those who may not. This seems intrinsically unfair since if it is beneficial for one group, it must be for the other as well. Whatever system is chosen should treat all DI children equally.

Finally, a dual system in which the donor's identity is revealed when the child reaches the age of majority assumes that, at the time of donation, a donor can anticipate how he will feel at least 18 years later. By that time most donors will have entered into marriages or relationships, perhaps with children, with the result that their families would be affected by such a revelation. Now, with the advent of cryopreservation, a child born from donor sperm could be born years after a donation, pushing the date of disclosure even further into the future. It is unrealistic to believe that a donor's feelings and beliefs about his role are unchanging — as discussed later in this chapter, some donors told the Commission that they regretted their donation. As a result, a donor might wish to withdraw his consent to be contacted by his biological child, perhaps years after he or she is born. Unless revocation were disallowed, DI parents could choose a donor based on his willingness to be identified, only to have that option revoked by the donor at a later date, making their choice meaningless.

Non-Identifying Information Disclosure

The reasoning just outlined led Commissioners to endorse the concept of non-identifying information disclosure; identifying information would be collected and maintained, however, and could be made available in extraordinary circumstances of medical need under strictly controlled conditions. The Commission believes that this is the best way to balance the needs of children and families. It is a system that acknowledges the need of individuals for social, genetic, and medical information about their biological parent, but it also acknowledges the need for DI families to flourish and form a strong unit if the best interests of the child are to be served. It is an option that does not impose specific roles on participants and that respects marital and familial privacy. Moreover, this system accords greater importance to family relationships and actual parenting than to the source of genetic material.

> The Commission proposes a system whereby information (standard non-identifying genetic, social, and medical information) about a donor would be available at any time to DI parents and children. Such information would be stored by the National Reproductive Technologies Commission for 100 years after the birth of the last child from the donor's sperm.

The Commission therefore proposes a system whereby information (standard non-identifying genetic, social, and medical information) about a donor would be available at any time to DI parents and children. Such information would be stored by the National Reproductive Technologies Commission for 100 years after the birth of the last child from the donor's sperm. Identifying information on donors (name, date of birth, city of residence) would also be stored for the same length of time, under conditions of strict security. Only in very rare cases would this information be revealed if the physical or psychological health needs of the child warranted. In these cases, and only if a situation were deemed to be a medical necessity by a court of law, identifying information should be available to parents or children. This should be very rare, as, even in the case of an inheritable medical disorder, for example, it would not usually be necessary to release named information.

Informed Consent to Sperm Donation

Researchers conducting interviews for the Commission were told that sperm donation is not necessarily a simple isolated act; some donors said they had not considered the full implications of DI until years after donating. Some said they strongly regretted donating; some felt frustrated by the lack of access to basic information about the children born as a result of their donation. Many reported that they had regarded

> Sperm donation is not necessarily a simple isolated act; some donors said they had not considered the full implications of DI until years after donating.

donation very casually until they were married or had children of their own, when they began considering the implications of having a genetically linked child growing up elsewhere. Some donors also reported that their wives or partners were upset by their past donations — and said they worried that their children could marry a half-sibling unknowingly. One donor told the Commission that his wife's concerns about his donation were a major factor in the break-up of their marriage.

Gamete donation is a decision that should not be taken lightly. Donors should have access to professional counselling and should be aware of the implications of their actions. They should also be aware of the policies that govern sperm donation, including the requirement for full disclosure of genetic or health information. Donors should be advised that although their identity will not normally be disclosed to recipients, their identity could be released in the event that a court deemed it necessary. Donors should also be made fully aware that decisions about how donations are used in inseminations, and whether they are used at all, will be made by the collection/storage facility and recipients and their doctors — the donor should realize that he will not be able to control who receives his gametes or influence the storage or practice policies of facilities or physicians.

Men considering sperm donation need access to standardized written information about the implications of sperm donation and should be required to sign a statement that they have read the information and understand the short- and long-term implications of donation. Given that donated sperm can be used not only in assisted insemination, but in other ways as well, the donor should be informed about and give consent for the possible uses of his donation if he consents to be a donor. The other two purposes for which donor sperm could be used are fertilization of eggs *in vitro*, to create zygotes for donation to infertile couples, and fertilization of eggs to create zygotes for research purposes under controlled conditions. Counselling should be available if requested, and men considering sperm donation should also be informed and counselled about the tests they will be required to undergo if they donate. This is particularly important with regard to testing for HIV — potential donors should know that their blood will be tested for HIV antibodies, as they may not wish to have this testing. Similarly, they should be aware that although the identity of a sperm donor is protected today, the same may not be true in decades to come; this, too, may influence the decision to donate.

> Men considering sperm donation need access to standardized written information about the implications of sperm donation and should be required to sign a statement that they have read the information and understand the short- and long-term implications of donation.

Commercialization

Commissioners are strongly opposed to commercializing human reproduction, as are Canadians generally. We heard clearly from Canadians that they are uncomfortable with any situation involving the development of reproductive technologies or services on the basis of their profit potential, particularly where only those with the means to pay can have access to them. In our view, no profit should be made from the selling of any reproductive material, including eggs, sperm, or zygotes/embryos, because of its ultimately dehumanizing effects. Two aspects are relevant here — payment for donors and sperm banking and distribution.

> No profit should be made from the selling of any reproductive material, including eggs, sperm, or zygotes/embryos, because of its ultimately dehumanizing effects.

Payment for Donation

Because donors must spend considerable time giving a medical history, having a physical examination and coming back for repeated blood tests, and giving sperm samples, the Commission feels it is reasonable to compensate donors for their time and inconvenience. Such compensation should not be high enough, however, to provide a financial incentive to donate. What level of remuneration, if any, is appropriate for sperm "donation"? Most sperm donors in Canada receive money intended to reimburse their out-of-pocket expenses — currently around $75 per donation. This is unlikely to act as a financial inducement, given the inconvenience involved, but we believe this level should not increase except perhaps to maintain its value relative to inflation.

Storage and Distribution

Another aspect of DI that lends itself to commercialization is the storing and distribution of sperm. The principle of non-commercialization means that commercial sperm banks are unacceptable in Canada, as are the purchase and use of sperm from commercial banks in other countries. In the United States, assisted insemination is a $164-million-per-year industry,[8] and data gathered by the Commission show that the potential exists for substantial profit in this country too — each sperm donation (for which the donor receives $75) produces 8 to 10 straws or containers of sperm, which are sold to practitioners for about $125 each. Since many women and couples undergoing DI have to pay in advance for a six-month supply of donor sperm — and are not reimbursed if a pregnancy occurs in an early cycle (see research volume, *Treatment of Infertility: Current Practices and Psychosocial Implications*) — sperm banks can potentially earn far more than it costs them to test, freeze, and transport sperm and maintain adequate records, despite the significant cost of stringent testing and detailed record keeping. Making a profit from sperm banking is unacceptable from the perspective of our guiding principles.

Safety Issues

Because most sexually transmitted diseases can be transmitted in semen, it is essential to ensure that donors do not infect recipients. Precautions to prevent this occurring are now critical because HIV, the virus associated with AIDS, is transmitted in semen. For good practice, professional organizations have identified several tests that should be performed before donated sperm is used for insemination. The American Fertility Society, for example, recommends that sperm be cryopreserved and quarantined for six months to allow testing for HIV, cytomegalovirus, hepatitis B, herpes simplex, chlamydia, gonorrhoea, syphilis, ureaplasma, mycoplasma, streptococcal species, and trichomonas. The Canadian Fertility and Andrology Society guidelines recommend even more stringent testing for other sexually transmitted diseases, such as genital warts, and some genetic diseases. However, these tests are only "recommended" by professional guidelines; they are not compulsory, and there is no way of assessing whether guidelines are being adhered to by the physicians who perform DI, especially outside clinics.

Every Canadian sperm bank contacted by the Commission said they followed the professional guidelines for testing and record keeping. However, fewer than half the programs surveyed in a research project for the Commission in fact performed the full complement of recommended tests. At least two fertility clinics said that sperm donors were tested for tuberculosis, when in fact the bank from which the clinics purchased sperm did not perform such a test. Just 12 of the 33 programs tested for genital warts, while 17 tested for herpes or trichomoniasis (Table 19.1).

> Failure to observe existing professional guidelines constitutes dangerous and unethical practice, which puts the health and well-being of women, their partners, and their children at risk. Implementing the Commission's recommendations would mean safe frozen sperm could be sent to smaller communities through the distribution system we propose. Our recommendations not only would make safe sperm available but also would ensure proper records are kept, thus protecting the best interests of the child.

Commissioners were very disturbed to find from this 1991 survey of clinics and practitioners that, in some parts of Canada, donor sperm was being used without proper testing for HIV and some other STDs. One program did not test donors for HIV at the time of donation, and two sperm banks said they did not test donors for HIV at an appropriate interval after donation (this infection can take up to six months or more to be detectable by blood tests). In addition, at that time a small survey of 11 private practitioners showed that 3 of them used donor sperm that had not been frozen, a process necessary to allow the time to ensure that the sperm donor is not infected with HIV. The physicians in question said they were convinced the sperm was safe because they "trusted the donors."

It is not known how many physicians in Canada are performing DI in their offices or whether there are many others who are also not adhering to guidelines. Some family practitioners and others have argued that the use of fresh sperm is justified, for example, in smaller communities where facilities to test and freeze sperm are not available and women cannot afford the expense of travelling to a larger centre. Commissioners disagree and believe strongly that failure to observe existing professional guidelines constitutes dangerous and unethical practice, which puts the health and well-being of women, their partners, and their children at risk. Implementing the Commission's recommendations would mean safe frozen sperm could be sent to smaller communities through the distribution system we propose. Our recommendations not only would make safe sperm available but also would ensure proper records are kept, thus protecting the best interests of the child.

Table 19.1. Screening of Potential Sperm Donors in 1991			
	All settings (28)*	Teaching hospitals (16)**	Other hospitals and private clinics (12)***
Gonorrhoea	27	15	12
Hepatitis A & B	27	15	12
HIV 1&2	27	15	12
Syphilis	27	15	12
Chlamydia	25	14	11
Genetic history	25	14	11
Sexual activity	25	13	12
Sexual orientation	24	13	11
Cytomegalovirus	19	10	9
Herpes	17	8	9
Trichomoniasis	17	10	7
Ejaculate culture and sensitivity	16	8	8
Chromosomal analysis	13	8	5
Human papillomavirus	12	6	6
Tuberculosis	8	3	5

*   There are 33 settings, but one did not respond; for 4, it was not applicable.
**   There are 18 teaching hospitals, but, for 2 hospitals, it was not applicable.
***   There are 15 other hospitals and private clinics, but one did not respond; for 2, it was not applicable.

Source: Stephens, T., and J. McLean. "Survey of Canadian Fertility Programs." In Research Volumes of the Royal Commission on New Reproductive Technologies, 1993.

Other Uses for Sperm Banking Facilities

Sperm banks can have uses other than the collection and storing of sperm for donation. They can also store sperm for men whose fertility is in jeopardy — for example, men undergoing testicular surgery or radiation therapy for cancer. Samples of their healthy sperm can be frozen for future use according to agreed conditions (for example, that it will be destroyed at their death; released only into their control).

Issues in the Practice of Insemination*

In this section we discuss the medicalization of AI, access to DI, alternatives to the medical setting, patient needs and characteristics, and treatment protocols such as informed consent and counselling.

Medicalization

Couples in which the infertility can be treated simply by self-insemination using partner's sperm are very rare; these would be cases where intercourse cannot take place but normal sperm is produced. AI using the husband's or partner's sperm is almost always performed in a fertility clinic to allow that sperm to be treated with the goal of enhancing the likelihood of conception; this may on occasion involve more invasive placements of the sperm higher in the woman's reproductive tract. However, people who choose to have donor insemination in a medical setting do so not mainly for medical reasons but because this is where the service is most readily available at present and they are most comfortable with the process. Treating the insemination as a medical procedure reduces some of the sexual connotations and maintains anonymity of the donor and secrecy about the process. In addition, many women feel safer when a procedure is performed under a doctor's supervision. It is important, however, to re-examine the consequences and implications of medicalization. Factors such as the invasive nature of diagnosis and treatment, costs of medicalization, and the availability of alternatives must be considered.

AI patients, as well as many groups presenting their views during the Commission's public hearings, expressed concerns about the invasive and impersonal nature of the AI process. Many questioned the necessity of invasive investigative or diagnostic procedures on women when AI is a remedy for male infertility.[9] The Commission's survey of clinics showed that more than half the AI programs (which included both AIH and DI) routinely required that women undergo hysterosalpingograms[10] before treatment, and a third required endometrial biopsy.[11] One clinic required a laparoscopy — a surgical procedure done under general anaesthetic to rule out tubal blockage or scarring — before going ahead with AI.

---

* Other countries have grappled with these issues, and it is instructive to look at their experiences. These are outlined briefly in Appendix 1 to this chapter.

Physicians consider this approach to be medically indicated, because even if sperm tests show some problems, the female partner may also have less than optimal fertility. It is important that invasive diagnostic or insemination procedures be kept to a minimum; at the same time this must be balanced with a recognition of a couple's desire to identify and treat their problem in a timely fashion and to try to conceive a child using their own gametes. Many of the couples in AI programs have unexplained infertility and have been trying to become pregnant for at least a year, so unless male-factor infertility can be clearly identified immediately, it may be appropriate to investigate the female partner more extensively.

However, it is good medical practice to perform the least invasive, risky, or costly diagnostic

> **Hysterosalpingogram**: An X-ray of the uterus and fallopian tubes, which has been the standard screening test for tubal patency since the 1960s. Dye is injected into the uterus through a catheter inserted into the cervix. The X-ray measures how the dye flows through the fallopian tubes (tubal blockage, scarring, or endometrial growths or fibroids can be identified). For some the procedure can be painful, inducing strong uterine cramping, while others report little pain.
>
> **Endometrial biopsy**: This test is the final confirmation of ovulation and confirmation that the endometrium is being properly primed by hormones. A speculum is inserted in the vagina, the cervix is dilated, and a sample of the lining of the front wall of the uterus is scraped with a metal curette and read under a microscope for characteristic changes. The procedure is unpleasant, can be painful, and causes some bleeding.

techniques first, and only if indicated. In AIH programs, male infertility should be diagnosed or ruled out before more invasive diagnostic investigations of the woman are considered. There should also be some prior evidence that there is a female factor blocking fertility — invasive diagnostic procedures should not be performed routinely. Unless a treatable male or female factor is identified, adjuncts to AI that pose risks for women, such as fertility drug therapy or insemination at sites other than the vagina, should not be initiated until after three unsuccessful cycles of AIH with sperm manipulation and vaginal insemination, and then only in the context of clinical trials for insemination at sites other than the vagina. Experts in this area recommend that at least three cycles be attempted before moving to more invasive methods, because the data indicate that virtually all AIH conceptions occur within the first six cycles and the majority of conceptions are achieved within three to six months. If time is short, three unsuccessful cycles would be an indication that AIH is probably not the best option.

In DI programs, unless there is evidence to the contrary, it should be assumed that women are fertile, and they should not undergo invasive diagnostic tests unless repeated inseminations are unsuccessful, indicating the likelihood of infertility in the recipient. The same progression should be followed: vaginal insemination, vaginal insemination with fertility drugs, and insemination at sites other than the vagina (such as the unproven and invasive techniques of intrauterine insemination and peritoneal insemination). However, insemination at other sites should be used only after unsuccessful vaginal insemination and should be offered only in the context of a clinical trial. Physicians and couples should make decisions about treatment without unnecessary delays, but a couple's feelings of urgency should not supersede the ethics of good medical practice.

Medicalization of a procedure naturally leads to higher costs. Patients in clinical AIH programs reported an average cost of about $900 per cycle of treatment, while DI patients reported costs of about $500 per cycle. If travel and accommodation are necessary, clinical AI programs can become too expensive to be an option for many women and couples — clinics are concentrated in urban centres in central Canada (a third of them in southern Ontario), and treatment can span months. The

> [A] problematic ... recommendation is a designation of alternative insemination as the practice of medicine ... This would make self-insemination subject to legal prosecution.
>
> *M. Patrell, Halifax Lesbian Committee on New Reproductive Technologies, Public Hearings Transcripts, Halifax, Nova Scotia, October 17, 1990.*

financial and psychological costs of time off work and of regular travel are unaffordable for many women or couples who are infertile.

Some have avoided high travel costs by seeking out a local private practitioner to perform AI, although the cost of sperm (and the insemination, if not covered by public or private health insurance) is still charged to the patient. We also found that one clinic had out-of-town couples come to the clinic once, where they were shown how to self-inseminate — sperm for subsequent cycles was then sent to them for self-insemination, so that the costs of repeated travel could be avoided.

Although a private practitioner's office may offer a less expensive alternative or a more relaxed setting than fertility clinics, Commission research showed that individual doctors operating outside the confines of a clinic are more likely to report poor clinical practice, such as using fresh sperm or sperm

> It is evident that a mechanism is required to ensure that AI is offered only by practitioners following standard guidelines for good practice, and that all DI is done using safe sperm and appropriate donor testing.

from untested donors, performing procedures that do not conform with professional guidelines, or keeping inadequate records (see research volume, *Treatment of Infertility: Assisted Reproductive Technologies*). The

Commission believes that solo practitioners may be a valuable alternative, but they must meet the same safety and practice standards as fertility clinics. It is evident that a mechanism is required to ensure that AI is offered only by practitioners following standard guidelines for good practice, and that all DI is done using safe sperm and appropriate donor testing. Similarly, if a source of safe sperm were available, women could inseminate themselves alone or with a partner's help (see section on Alternatives to the Medical Setting).

Access to Treatment*

To find out who was having AI in Canada, the Commission surveyed 150 AIH patients and 150 DI patients at 21 of the 33 fertility clinics across the country (see research volume, *Treatment of Infertility: Current Practices and Psychosocial Implications*). The two groups of patients were demographically very similar — predominantly between 30 and 40 years old, English-speaking, and educated to at least the community college level. More than 60 percent of female partners and more than 80 percent of male partners were employed full time. Close to 80 percent of AI patients' households had an annual income of at least $40 000 (compared to close to 60 percent in the general population[12]). Everyone who responded to the Commission's survey was married or cohabiting in a stable relationship with a male partner.

Although our sample of AI patients was not exhaustive, it seemed to bear out the perception that single women and lesbians, as well as unemployed and low- to middle-income couples, are not represented among patients at fertility clinics. In a separate study, researchers asked 33 clinics about their policy and practices. Twenty would exclude single women, and 19 of the 33 AI programs surveyed told the Commission that lesbians would be refused treatment at their clinic. Other factors were also taken into consideration with regard to access: 16 clinics said "below-average intelligence" would be grounds for refusing treatment; 10 clinics said "doubtful parenting ability," including financial factors, would be a factor; and 6 specified low income as grounds for refusal.

Clinic staff said admission policies are usually set by clinic directors and treatment teams, and only about 5 percent of applicants were rejected. They also said that they rarely received applications from single women and lesbians, and other data show that DI programs within the traditional medical milieu receive few inquiries from these women. It is probable that single women and lesbians are not applying to fertility clinics because they know they will be rejected. Many such women told the Commission they did not attempt to gain access on the advice of other patients, or because of what they had heard from their family doctors and gynaecologists. One

---

* See Annex for dissenting opinion.

single woman said her doctor had asked for reference letters concerning her ability to parent before he would refer her to a fertility clinic.   Although clinicians may believe that these women are using alternatives to the medical setting out of choice, interviews with 19 women who helped other women perform DI outside a medical setting showed that half believed that women would use a medical route for DI if it were available — the dominant reasons being well-screened sperm and easier access to donors.

> The sole criterion determining who has access to the NRTs should be medical in nature. The criterion of whether a woman would make a good mother or not is very subjective, and neither the medical staff nor the government nor anyone else besides the woman in question should make such judgments, except in extreme situations.
>
> *Brief to the Commission from New Brunswick Advisory Council on the Status of Women, October 1990.*

The Commission believes that the criteria used to determine access to publicly funded medical services must be fair and applied equally to all. We believe this as one of our fundamental guiding principles, and we believe this because it reflects basic principles of human rights law. Non-discrimination in the provision of public services is a clear requirement under the Canadian Charter and federal and provincial human rights legislation, which prohibit discrimination on the basis of such historically disadvantaging factors as sex, marital status, sexual orientation, and social or economic status.

We do believe that it is within the purview of practitioners to make decisions about medical indications for services. That is their responsibility, and it is what they are trained to do. In the case of DI, however, there are no medical indications for this service, in that, other than in rare cases, it is performed on healthy women who are fertile. Whether heterosexual or homosexual, married or single, all women undergoing DI are in the same situation — they are unable to have a child, either because their partner is infertile or because they do not have a male partner. The Commission believes it is wrong to forbid some people access to medical services on the basis of social factors while others are permitted to use them; using criteria such as a woman's marital status or sexual orientation to determine access to DI, based on historical prejudices and stereotypes, amounts to discrimination as defined under human rights law and contravenes the Commission's guiding principle of equality. There is no intent to force any practitioner or clinic to provide new reproductive technologies if they do not wish to do so — our recommendations are to ensure that services provided and funded by provinces' health budgets are not offered in a discriminatory way contravening the Canadian Charter. Clearly, religious institutions exist and should not be forced to contravene their religious beliefs, but publicly supported health care should be delivered in a universal and non-discriminatory way.

The Commission recognizes that some Canadians are uneasy about family forms that might be facilitated by such access to AI. Our survey of national values and attitudes, for instance, found that the Canadians surveyed are most supportive of AI when it is used by a married, heterosexual couple, and least supportive when it is used by a lesbian couple. Almost half the people surveyed oppose or strongly oppose its use by single women.

Although most Canadians surveyed did not support lesbians having access to DI, to provide a service in a discriminatory way by denying access, without evidence that a resultant child would be harmed, is contrary to the Charter and also contravenes our ethic of care. The available evidence does not show different outcomes in children born to or raised by lesbians when compared to outcomes in children born to heterosexual women and couples.[13] Thus, the "best interests of the child" cannot be used as a reason to deny access simply because a woman is a lesbian. The ethic of care dictates that people should be treated equally unless there is evidence that others will be harmed.

> The available evidence does not show different outcomes in children born to or raised by lesbians when compared to outcomes in children born to heterosexual women and couples. Thus, the "best interests of the child" cannot be used as a reason to deny access simply because a woman is a lesbian.

As we made clear in Part One of this report, the Commission believes that society's approach to new reproductive technologies should be governed by the social values of Canadians. We are also aware, however, of the difference between social values and individual opinions. We believe that the social values held by Canadians are reflected in the *Canadian Charter of Rights and Freedoms*, and the prohibitions on discrimination it contains must be our guide in this matter.

There might be grounds to over-ride this provision, of course, if it could be determined that discriminatory criteria for access to DI were in the best interests of the children who would be born; this would have to be specified in law and be shown to be demonstrably justified in a free and democratic society, as required by section 1 of the Charter. Commission research found no reliable evidence, however, that the environment in families formed by single women or lesbian couples is any better or worse for the children involved than that in families formed by heterosexual couples. It found that other factors such as time invested, nurturing, and emotional commitment to the child are more important than sexual orientation per se. There is therefore no demonstrated basis for restricting the experience of parenting to heterosexual or married couples for the best interests of the child.

> There is therefore no demonstrated basis for restricting the experience of parenting to heterosexual or married couples for the best interests of the child.

Studies show that although a majority of Canadians (54 percent) think others should be able to use DI, fewer, even in a married relationship, would use it themselves. Moreover, it is likely that only a very small minority of women would consider using donor insemination if single or in circumstances where raising a child would be difficult. Women deliberately trying to conceive a child by DI are likely to have thought through the decision carefully; it is not taken in the heat of the moment. As a caring society, we have an obligation to protect from harm all those who would use DI to form their family. Forming a family is of deep importance to the vast majority of Canadians, regardless of their sexual orientation, marital status, or financial situation. If practised with adherence to standards, DI is an effective, safe, and non-invasive way of enabling this.

Excluding single women or lesbians from DI programs not only contravenes their equality rights, it also puts their health at risk, by forcing them to resort to unsafe practices while heterosexual women in traditional marital relationships have access to safe and effective procedures. In both situations there is a strong desire for a child, but no male partner who is fertile; there is in fact no greater medical need in a woman whose partner has no sperm than in a woman who has no partner.

> If a service is to be available, women should be treated equally, unless there is good evidence that the best interests of the child will suffer.

If a service is to be available, women should be treated equally, unless there is good evidence that the best interests of the child will suffer. Current practice is inequitable and reflects discriminatory attitudes. The same standards of access to DI should apply to all women choosing this route to pregnancy and parenthood, to ensure that all can do so safely.

Alternatives to the Medical Setting

Some women who have been rejected by medical DI programs, or fear they would be rejected, choose self-insemination as an alternative. Although SI can be used by any woman who wishes to have control over the process, it is used most often by single women and lesbians. Some heterosexual couples may also choose to use SI because they wish to have a known donor. Establishing how frequently SI is used is difficult, because by definition it takes place in a private setting. Since the early 1970s, alternative insemination networks in Britain, the United States, and Canada have grown in both numbers and sophistication. One U.S. estimate suggests that 1 000 to 3 000 children are conceived by lesbians using SI each year, and it is generally agreed that the practice is increasing. However, given the total number of children born each year, this is still a very uncommon way for children to be conceived.

The Commission learned about self-insemination in Canada through studies based on the experiences of women who have used SI and others who have been involved in its provision. It appears to be practised primarily in larger urban areas, particularly Toronto. Participants say they chose SI to have control over the process, to avoid intercourse, to avoid unnecessary medications, or to avoid having to justify one's wish to be a parent to clinic personnel. The majority of women who chose SI used anonymous donors for fear of legal complications and from a desire to raise the child without the involvement of the donor.[14]

An exploratory study of women involved with SI showed that some communities have sophisticated networks that find donors, provide women with suitable donor sperm, and teach women how to pinpoint ovulation and perform the insemination. Although some said they were able to get safe frozen sperm from "friendly MDs," this was the exception, not the rule.

> Small volunteer networks cannot afford the equipment to cryopreserve sperm ... Only if the sperm can be frozen for later use are test results on the donor's blood at six months after donation relevant to the decision to use the frozen sperm for insemination.

Two small studies of SI networks showed that all used fresh sperm and that little information was available about donors. Donor sperm is so scarce outside a medical setting that most networks were able to accommodate only the request that donors be of the same race as recipients.

Finding donors and ensuring the safety of the sperm are the most difficult aspects of SI. In the past, gay men frequently acted as donors for lesbians, but this option has become riskier because of the prevalence of HIV in the gay community. Screening of donors is also problematic; although donors participating in SI networks were often asked about their medical history, HIV testing and screening for STDs or genetic disorders were less common — in interviews with 19 women involved in SI networks, only 9 reported that donors were tested for HIV, and only 7 used frozen sperm. These small volunteer networks cannot afford the equipment to cryopreserve sperm. This makes testing for infectious diseases, particularly HIV, irrelevant — because only if the sperm can be frozen for later use are test results on the donor's blood at six months after donation relevant to the decision to use the frozen sperm for insemination. The Commission heard of only one group of women in a small Ontario city with their own equipment for freezing sperm.

Few of the networks keep records; access is limited to word-of-mouth. Most of the networks contacted by Commission researchers said they would give any woman access to their services, although one woman told researchers that because donor sperm was so scarce and heterosexual women could gain access to the traditional medical system more easily, the network she was involved in reserved donor sperm for the use of lesbians.

> If society supports the use of donor insemination to have children, it should be provided in a fair and equitable manner.

The Commission believes that if society supports the use of donor insemination to have children, it should be provided in a fair and equitable manner. There is no medical necessity limiting the practice of DI to the medical setting; there is no clear reason to deny single women and lesbians access to safe donor sperm (they essentially have the same diagnosis as married women — lack of a male partner who is fertile and a strong wish to have a child); and there is no reliable evidence that children raised by single women or lesbians are disadvantaged because of their parents' sexual orientation or marital status. Thus, principles of equality dictate that these women should not be prevented from forming a family. Self-insemination is going to go on; making it unavailable in the medical system will not stop it. It is therefore important that safe sperm be available so that women do not have to risk their health and lives. Because many women and indeed many couples would prefer the control, comfort, and affordability of SI, the Commission feels it is important to allow and facilitate the safe practice of SI in Canada.

Commissioners believe that society has a responsibility to ensure that women choosing this alternative are not forced to jeopardize their health by using unsafe donor sperm. In addition, they and their children

> Both heterosexual couples and women without a male partner can avoid the costly and medicalized aspects of clinical DI programs by choosing SI, and that choice should be made available to them without compromising the standards for sperm safety or comprehensive record keeping that are offered to recipients in clinical DI programs.

should not be forced to give up the benefits of proper record keeping on donors and recipients simply because they have chosen a less medicalized procedure. Both heterosexual couples and women without a male partner can avoid the costly and medicalized aspects of clinical DI programs by choosing SI, and that choice should be made available to them without compromising the standards for sperm safety or comprehensive record keeping that are offered to recipients in clinical DI programs.

Information, Counselling, and Consent

Participants in AI programs told the Commission they valued a sense of personal control about their treatment. Close to 90 percent of AI recipients surveyed by the Commission read literature about the procedure, discussed the procedure with doctors and others who had had the procedure, or informed themselves in other ways before deciding to go ahead with AI; 68 percent had counselling before making their decision. Two things are necessary for people to make their own decisions about treatment: full information and appropriate counselling. If these are provided in a way that meets the needs of prospective AI recipients, it can be said with confidence that they are exercising informed choice.

The provision of information enables couples to learn the facts about their diagnosis, their chances of success (both general success rates for the procedure and the success rates at the particular clinic), and the details of their treatment. It can also assist them in making an informed choice about their treatment path — information about non-medical alternatives, treatment costs and benefits, and possible outcomes is an essential basis for informed discussion and decision making. Various professional guidelines have outlined what AI patients should be told about the procedure, but there is evidence that recipients are either not receiving or not absorbing the recommended information.

Professional standards outline the importance of providing information in the following areas: the nature of the fertility problem, alternatives to treatment, chances of success, the physical and emotional demands, and the long- and short-term effects of treatment. Although more than three-quarters of AI recipients identified these as the most important types of information,

> These findings show clearly the need to develop standard, accurate, comprehensible information materials about AI that meet high standards of content and accessibility. Provision of these materials should be mandatory for all AIH and DI programs, and any woman or couple considering DI should receive these.

less than a third were satisfied with the information their clinic provided in these areas — in fact, AI recipients were the least satisfied of all the patient groups in our survey of 1 395 people treated at Canadian fertility clinics.

Furthermore, an analysis of the information materials on AI provided by clinics found them to be too technical and complex for a general audience.[15] Reading levels required ranged from grade 10 to four years of post-secondary education. Those whose mother tongue is neither English nor French had to provide their own translation — none of the clinics had information in any other language. These findings show clearly the need to develop standard, accurate, comprehensible information materials about AI that meet high standards of content and accessibility. Provision of these materials should be mandatory for all AIH and DI programs, and any woman or couple considering DI should receive these.

Commission survey results also showed that women seeking AI were dissatisfied with the counselling they received. Only 13 percent of AIH patients and 23 percent of DI patients said their needs were met (compared to 35 percent of IVF patients), and only 10 percent of AIH patients and 18 percent of DI patients were satisfied with the counselling their male partners received (compared with 31 percent of IVF patients). Given the strong psychosocial implications of DI, people need the opportunity to discuss and weigh their options with a qualified counsellor. Existing studies in this area have found that couples contemplating DI must first work through their infertility (which can include strong feelings of loss, depression, guilt, anger, and ambivalence for both members of the couple, particularly the male). Then they must deal with the implications of DI, its impact on the couple's marriage, the future family, and the complex social dynamics involved.

As was the case with the information materials, the Commission found that the provision of counselling did not live up to the professional standards set in this area. Although guidelines recommend counselling of the woman by a

> It is essential to see the couples as a couple, then each separately, then as a couple again at least once more. They have to be willing to focus on the effect of the imbalance in the relationship — "I'm all right, you're not all right" — and be willing to discuss their feelings about a child that is hers but not his. What of the tendency she may have to look for his rejection? What of his possible jealousy? What of the donor? ... He must have time to grieve over his lost fertility ... She must have time to focus on the grief of not bearing her partner's child and feelings about carrying a "stranger's child." As a couple, would they want the child to know about their donor status? If not, what are their fears? If so, what are their ideas about when and how to tell? ... Is there anything they wish to explore, before going on to DI — AIH, IVF ... etc.? Have they discussed these options?
>
> B. Mostyn, "Counselling the Infertile Patient," in Infertility: Guidelines for Practice, Fertility Committee of the Royal College of Obstetricians and Gynaecologists. London: RCOG Press, 1992.

clinical psychologist, this is often not provided.[16] Only 5 of 33 programs said that all women received counselling on their own; 18 said couples were counselled together. In the Commission survey of patients, 50 percent of those in DI programs and 48 percent in AIH programs said they received no counselling at all, and those that did were more likely to speak to a physician or nurse than to a professional counsellor.

The Commission believes that patients would benefit significantly from counselling before, during, and after treatment, and from discussing their situation and the options before them. Not everyone wants counselling — half the women who underwent DI did not want follow-up counselling after treatment, perhaps to help maintain secrecy about their involvement and appear as close to a "normal" family as possible. The Commission believes nevertheless that the availability of counselling is an essential component of responsible practice, especially in DI programs. On-site counselling services, or referral to appropriate services, should be a standard and mandatory part of AI programs, should be completely confidential, and should be provided by health care and helping professionals with specialized training in this area.

A final component of informed choice for patients is consent to treatment. Medical standards dictate that patients be aware that they can refuse to participate in treatment, and that consent and refusal are both revocable (see research volume, *New Reproductive Technologies: Ethical Aspects*). At present there are no standard methods of obtaining consent from women undergoing AI or from their partners; Commission research found 28 distinct consent procedures in place at various Canadian fertility clinics, and at least two years of post-secondary education were needed to understand many consent forms. Many survey participants told the Commission that they were not given copies of the consent forms they were required to sign, and few were told that they could revoke their consent at any time.

Patients need fact-based information, as well as counselling about feelings and decision making, in order to make informed choices about treatment. AI provides a good setting for the participatory ideal in informed choice: prospective patients are usually able to comprehend information and make well thought out decisions, most are young and healthy, the treatment is elective, and they have the time to digest and discuss their options, so real choice is possible. Decisions about DI in particular involve personal values, which patients are better equipped to factor into their decision than

> The availability of counselling is an essential component of responsible practice, especially in DI programs. On-site counselling services, or referral to appropriate services, should be a standard and mandatory part of AI programs, should be completely confidential, and should be provided by health care and helping professionals with specialized training in this area.

physicians are. Yet our findings indicate that many programs do not seem to facilitate genuine informed choice for patients (see research volume, *Treatment of Infertility: Current Practices and Psychosocial Implications*).

The Commission's findings with respect to information provision, counselling, and consent are a further indication of a discrepancy between published professional guidelines and actual clinical practices and of a gap between patient needs and the services they receive.

Familial and Societal Implications of DI*

Complex issues face families formed using DI, and from them emerge new societal dilemmas. At the individual level, the secrecy surrounding DI can give rise to conflict within the DI family, but at the societal level it has also resulted in significant gaps in relevant research, legal direction, and record keeping. The legal status of DI families, what records should be required and who should have access to them, and how best to balance the needs of DI participants remain unaddressed in law or policy. Many DI participants liken their situation to that of adoptive families, so it is important to consider whether there are lessons to be learned from the evolution of Canada's adoption policies.

> Canadians attach importance to having a genetic link between themselves and their children; we found that most Canadians would seek medical help to conceive before looking into adoption because of the importance of this link.

Surveys and research done for the Commission show that Canadians attach importance to having a genetic link between themselves and their children; we found that most Canadians would seek medical help to conceive before looking into adoption because of the importance of this link. Many aspects of Western and other cultures reflect as well as reinforce the importance of the genetic link between parent and child. As a result, many practitioners suggest that DI be kept secret, even from the child, to preserve the appearance that the family does not differ from most other families. Some clinics even require couples to sign a form stating that they will never tell anyone about their DI procedure. At the same time, our society values honesty and openness in personal relationships. This results in great ambivalence for many individuals involved, as secrecy often implies something to be ashamed of.

Parents deal with these pressures in different ways. There is a marked preference among recipients at the time of insemination to keep the procedure secret (although this may become more difficult as time passes

---

* See Annex for dissenting opinion.

and the child is growing up), and they are encouraged in this by our laws and medical standards. Secrecy is preferred because it seems to solve so many problems: the man's infertility is hidden, an image of normalcy is maintained, children do not grow up feeling different from their peers, and any potential legal tangles are avoided. In addition, keeping it a secret sidesteps the issue of acknowledging a division between social and biological parenthood for these couples.

Secrecy in DI Families

On the surface it would seem that secrecy about DI is fairly easy to maintain. Once conception has occurred, the pregnancy continues like any other. In the long run, however, the Commission found that secrecy places great strains on families. Parents must always remain on guard lest they give away the secret, and differences between father and child must be

> The cultural norm of parenthood assumes that an individual undertakes both biological and social roles. When these roles are severed, deviation from the cultural norm is reflected in additional descriptors to the parental roles. In the case of adoption, biological parents are known as birth parents and social parents are the adoptive parents. A stigma is attached to non-biological parental roles. As Kirk pointed out, "adoptive kinship is not and cannot be the equivalent of blood relationship."
>
> DI severs the relationship between biological and social fatherhood. In this sense, DI participants are social innovators in family forms ... Successful adjustment to DI requires clarification and identification of the distinct roles, including the rights and the responsibilities, of biological and social paternity.
>
> *R. Achilles, "The Social Meanings of Donor Insemination," in Research Volumes of the Commission, 1993.*

minimized or ignored. The father may feel incomplete or inadequate, but he has to suppress those feelings. Some fathers said they felt fraudulent about how they fit into the family narrative.

When Commission researchers interviewed married DI mothers, many expressed relief at finally being able to talk about the facts of their child's conception. They said they avoided talking about the issue at home, out of sensitivity for their husbands' feelings. Some women said they felt they were "living a lie," pretending that their husband was the genetic father of the children. Lesbian DI mothers told the Commission they did not feel the same pressure to keep their child's origins a secret because DI is more accepted in the lesbian community. Some said they paid a price for this openness — some were already estranged from parents and siblings who could not accept their sexual orientation, and undergoing DI added to the strain.

Commission research showed that maintaining secrecy about the means of conception can be contrary to the best interests of the child (see research volume, *The Prevalence of Infertility in Canada*). Adults born through DI reported that the decision to keep DI a secret was very damaging — they felt deceived and said they had always sensed that something was "wrong" in the family. Some told the Commission that they found out about the method of conception at a time of family crisis, such as divorce or death in the family — a time when secrets are difficult to keep. Discovering the truth in this way is doubly traumatic; the shock of discovery during an already stressful period is coupled with the realization that your parents had lied to you all your life.

Adoptive families used to be advised to keep this secret from the community and from the child; studies have since shown, however, that openness and honesty about adoption are healthier for all concerned.[17] Secrets kept within families put added pressure on marriages, and children often sense something is being hidden. Many professionals who have experience with adoption, such as social workers, psychologists, doctors, and sociologists who have seen the damage that secrets can cause, as well as some adoptees themselves, advocate openness about the fact of DI.[18]

Ultimately, the decision about whether and whom to tell should be made by the parents, as it is rooted in personal values and beliefs. However, given the long-term psychological and familial implications of secrecy, particularly for the resulting child, women and couples should make their decision based on full information and discussion about their options. Provision of information to the recipient about the issue should be a required part of the DI process.

Legal Status of DI Families

Family law has not kept pace with the advent of new reproductive technologies. Most current legislation in Canada was enacted before these new familial realities became apparent. Although DI is not new, secrecy about its practice has compounded the legal vacuum for participants. Legal rights and obligations of parents are set out in provincial family law, governing such matters as maternity, paternity, filiation, custody, access, and support. Only three jurisdictions have amended their laws to deal explicitly with donor insemination — Yukon, Newfoundland, and Quebec[19] — with a view to protecting the interests of DI children, recipients, and donors. In the rest of the country, DI participants exist in a virtual legal limbo.

It has been argued that DI recipients, their partners, and their children are adequately protected by existing family law. Commission analyses of the relevant statutes indicate that this is not true (see research volume, *Legal and Ethical Issues in New Reproductive Technologies: Pregnancy and Parenthood*). A basic tenet of family law establishes the "best interests of the child" as the governing principle in the determination of an award of custody between two legal parents. Many situations could arise in which the best interests of DI children are not served by existing family law.

Single DI Recipients

In most Canadian jurisdictions, it is recognized that the woman who gives birth to the child is the legal mother; thus, DI recipients have virtually undisputed maternal rights. At present, if the recipient is single and there is no male partner legally presumed to be the father, a donor could establish paternity and seek parental access to the child. Conversely, recipients and children could have a legal basis to pursue the donor for support or inheritance rights. Only in the three Canadian jurisdictions with DI-specific legislation have these matters been clarified by absolving the donor of parental rights and responsibilities.

Male Partners

In a heterosexual partnership (marriage or common-law), the male partner is legally presumed to be the father of any children born of that union. That presumption of paternity could be contested in jurisdictions with no DI-specific legislation if a donor could establish a genetic link to the child.[20] If a donor successfully contested the paternity of the social father and could prove to a court that the best interests of the child would be served, he could conceivably gain custody of or access to the child.

> A first step would be legislation to give full legal standing to the [DI] child, recognizing the social father as the child's father in law and the donor as having no legal rights or responsibilities for support and maintenance.
>
> *P. Creighton, private citizen,
> Public Hearings Transcripts,
> Toronto, Ontario, November 19, 1990.*

Also, male partners of DI recipients may not be legally compelled to act as a father to a DI child. In jurisdictions with no DI-specific law, the male spouse or partner of a woman undergoing DI, even if he consented at the time of insemination and intended to act as a parent to the child, could possibly disavow paternity when the child was born, leaving the child without a legal father.[21] Conversely, if the relationship broke up before the child was born, the recipient could challenge her partner's paternity and seek to deny him access to the child.

Female Partners

Lesbian couples are the most legally vulnerable after having a child by DI. Even in a stable, long-standing lesbian relationship, the law does not grant the legal status of parenthood to a female partner of a DI recipient (see research volume, *Treatment of Infertility: Assisted Reproductive Technologies*). It is legally impossible for a child to have two parents of the same sex, so if the biological mother died, or in cases of custody, access, or child support, the non-genetically linked lesbian partner would have the status of a "legal stranger."[22] This is the case even when the partner has shared in the parenting of the child all his or her life. The best interests of the child do guide court decisions about custody in these cases, so a lesbian partner who had been in a nurturing relationship with the child would not necessarily be precluded from obtaining custody or access. However, lesbians understandably want to guard against court decisions based on discriminatory attitudes.[23]

DI Children

Given that family law in most provinces contains the gaps just described, the situation of DI children is characterized by uncertainty with respect to inheritance, custody, access, and support. It is clearly not in the best interests of DI children to allow these gaps to persist. In addition to creating unwarranted stress, confusion, and uncertainty in DI families, the lack of legal recognition of DI participants fosters unsafe DI practices and secrecy about the process. Reforms in Canadian family law are needed to define the roles and responsibilities of DI participants and to avoid further confusion in this area. The Commission therefore recommends that

82. **Legislation be adopted, in those provinces where it does not already exist, to ensure that**
     (a) the donor's rights and responsibilities of parenthood are severed by the act of sperm donation;
     (b) the married or cohabiting male partner of a DI recipient, if he has given his written consent at the time of insemination, is considered the legal father of the child;
     (c) the married or cohabiting male partner of a DI mother at the time of birth should be able to initiate a disavowal of paternity only if:
          (i)   he did not consent in writing to the insemination or he did not enter into a parental relationship with the child knowing he was not the genetic father;
          (ii) he consented to the insemination under duress, coercion, or fraud;
          (iii) he had acted as a father to the child only because he believed he was the genetic father;

> **(d)   if the legal mother of the child has no male partner, the child has the legal status of "father unknown";**
>
> **(e)   if the legal mother enters into a relationship with a male partner who acts as a parent toward the DI child, such a relationship be recognized by the courts in determining the best interests of the child for purposes of custody, access, and support, or in the event of the death of the child's mother;**
>
> **(f)   if the female partner of a DI child's mother acts as a parent toward the child, such a relationship be recognized by the courts in determining the best interests of the child for purposes of custody, access, and support, or in the event of the death of the child's mother.**

The Commission believes that such legislation would remedy the ambiguities of current family law as it relates to DI families. It would enable the formation of secure families, free of unwanted contact with or by donors, in the best interests of DI children. In addition, it would assure DI children the benefits of two legal parents or, in the case of single women and lesbians, clear legal authority for the mother to form her family according to her values. Third, such legislation would maintain the privacy of the donor and protect him from any unexpected or unwarranted claim for support or inheritance.

Lessons from the Adoption Context

At present, DI record-keeping practices are unregulated — in fact, there is no requirement for sperm banks, individual physicians, or fertility clinics to maintain any donor records at all. An analysis of the evolution of law and policies relating to adoption may help in developing a framework for DI policies. Although adoptive and DI families are different, the experience of adoptees can suggest what DI children need with regard to access to information about their social and genetic background. Many adoptees who have little or no information about their origins feel as if their life stories "began at chapter two." These adoptees may develop an incomplete sense of identity and may make the search for their biological roots a primary life focus.

All jurisdictions have some means of providing for the release of non-identifying information about birth parents to adoptive families, in recognition of its importance to the emotional well-being of adoptees. In more open arrangements, non-identifying information on the birth mother may be provided to the adoptive parents at the time of placement; an adopted child can request further non-identifying information at any time, although the permission of the adoptive parents is required until the child reaches the age of majority. Disclosure without the birth parent's permission is not allowed unless the health, safety, or welfare of the child requires such disclosure, and such cases would be rare. Where there are no legislative provisions, courts have tended to guard the confidentiality of the birth family when asked by an adopted child to open court records related to the adoption.

The goals of adoption record keeping are based on a concern for the best interests of the adopted child. Full adoption records, kept on file for generations, mean that genetically transmitted health problems can be identified and traced; two family members can be prevented

> As adoptees who have been reunited with birth parents and siblings, we can personally attest to the importance of the genetic link. To us the view that such a link could ever be erased or eradicated is extreme folly.
>
> We believe that the genetic third parent of children born of DI ... procedures will be a fundamental reality in their lives and one which cannot be dismissed or debased without eventually causing harm.
>
> We feel that the very existence of a central registry for information on these births would tend to swing public opinion away from the notion that such procedures are best concealed. This Commission has the opportunity to promote an atmosphere of truthfulness and greater openness in these matters by recommending that the future information rights of these children be acknowledged now.
>
> *H. Kramer, Canadian Adoption Reunion Register, Public Hearings Transcripts, Toronto, Ontario, November 20, 1990.*

from marrying or conceiving a child unknowingly; and adoptive families can have enough information about the child's biological background for their own psychological needs. Record-keeping practices in the field of DI should have similar goals.

Canadian practitioners, particularly solo practitioners, have kept haphazard or even no records on sperm donors, inseminations, and DI births. This effectively closes off all routes for most DI children alive today ever to learn even basic information about their paternal genetic and social heritage. Record keeping on donated gametes varies greatly across Canada. The Commission's research showed that two (2 of 33) DI programs kept no donor records, seven kept no records on the number of children born, and seven did not count the number of women inseminated (see research volume, *Treatment of Infertility: Current Practices and Psychosocial Implications*). Clinics also kept their records for varying periods — three programs kept them for less than five years, while nine kept them for an indefinite period.[24] Children resulting from DI performed outside the health care system are even less likely to have access to any records.

Poor record keeping has also led to situations where it is impossible to determine how many children have been born from the gametes of one donor. This information is important for many reasons. As mentioned above, during private meetings with DI families, donors, and their partners, the Commission heard concerns that individuals could unknowingly marry or have children with a half-sister or -brother. Although statistically such a situation is highly unlikely, it worries many DI participants — and, indeed, it is possible if a clinic has no policies regarding the number of children born from the sperm of one donor (especially if the clinic was the only one serving a particular area).

> In considering this issue of the right to know where you come from, a parallel is often drawn with the adoption process, where, over the past decade, attempts to find relatives have become much more common.
>
> In Quebec, the issue is still a controversial one. The principle of confidentiality persists, despite the fact that there have been constant changes in it since 1960 ... Following the passage of the legislation enacting the new *Civil Code* and amending family law, under article 632 of the Quebec *Civil Code* it is now possible for children and parents to find each other, as long as consent is free and informed, and unsolicited. [Translation]
>
> *S. LeBris, private citizen, Public Hearings Transcripts, Montreal, Quebec, November 21, 1990.*

Better record keeping would afford DI participants a measure of peace of mind without releasing identifying or named information about donors or DI families. Reassurance that a prospective spouse is not genetically related, or that a limit is placed on the number of children born from the sperm of one donor, would go far to ease the concerns of DI participants. The Commission heard that most Canadians believe these limits are necessary — in submissions and public hearings, all groups discussing this option recommended that the number of children per donor be limited.

> All jurisdictions have some means of providing for the release of non-identifying information about birth parents to adoptive families, in recognition of its importance to the emotional well-being of adoptees.

Mechanisms ensuring that information is available to DI children should be a requisite component of the DI process. Only a comprehensive, uniform record-keeping system can take into account the needs of DI families, donors, and Canadian society. A regulatory system is needed to facilitate the release of non-identifying information to DI recipients and children, as well as to ensure proper record keeping for the other reasons just outlined.

Recommendations

The Commission's examination of assisted insemination significantly changed our view of the practice. Like others, we focussed initially on the more complex assisted conception technologies — until our research showed unequivocally that AI is worthy of the same concern, attention, and public policy investment as other technologies. We believe that others must also re-evaluate AI in light of its familial and legal implications and the potential for harm to women, children, and families if it is not practised appropriately.

As we have shown, sperm donation has lifelong implications with a cascade of social, ethical, and legal consequences. The Commission concludes that current shortcomings in the practice of DI must be corrected. Women without a male partner who is fertile have been led to believe that DI is a safe and effective option for them, when in fact there is a patchwork of standards and unsafe practices in this field; as a result, DI recipients are taking chances with their health and the health of their families, often unknowingly. Insemination is being offered under widely varying clinical conditions, sometimes in a dangerous fashion; technical variations in the procedure are being performed with no evidence of their benefit; record keeping is haphazard; some practitioners are not adhering to the standards physicians have set for themselves as a profession; and access criteria differ from clinic to clinic, possibly resulting in discrimination at some. AI has also become a highly medicalized procedure, in many cases unnecessarily, making it increasingly inaccessible to many women for whom it might otherwise be a reproductive option.

Commissioners believe that donor insemination should be available to women and couples who have considered their options and decided to form a family in this way. Few women or couples are likely to choose this option without having given it a great deal of thought or without having considered what the lifelong implications of their choice will be. It will never be an easy decision or one that is taken lightly, nor is it an option that every involuntarily childless woman or couple will be prepared to choose. For these reasons, we believe that relatively few

> The time has come for Canada to implement a donor insemination system; an integrated, uniform approach to this practice can resolve most of the problems and deficiencies the Commission identified and can regulate and standardize sperm collection, service provision, and record-keeping practices.

women, with or without a male partner, are likely to choose this way of having a child; the availability of donor insemination is therefore unlikely to imply major social change, because it will not change how the vast majority of children are conceived and families are formed. Nevertheless, given the need to protect the health and well-being of those who do choose to form a family in this way, as well as the well-being of the resulting children, we believe that steps are necessary to ensure that it is done in a safe manner, with appropriate record keeping and standards, and that the legal status of the resulting families is clarified and standardized across the country.

The Commission therefore believes the time has come for Canada to implement a donor insemination system; an integrated, uniform approach to this practice can resolve most of the problems and deficiencies the Commission identified and can regulate and standardize sperm collection, service provision, and record-keeping practices. This is not a trivial exercise; some practitioners and others will be inconvenienced and restricted by increased regulation, but Commissioners believe this is the only way to eliminate the unsafe practices, poor record keeping, and arbitrary access criteria that have evolved to date.

This is not a trivial exercise; some practitioners and others will be inconvenienced and restricted by increased regulation, but Commissioners believe this is the only way to eliminate the unsafe practices, poor record keeping, and arbitrary access criteria that have evolved to date.

The Commission proposes a system that builds on existing mechanisms within the health care system, and much of the responsibility for adapting them to serve the needs we identify must necessarily lie with provincial/territorial ministries of health. The ministries also have the funding and organizational resources to ensure that AI is offered to women and couples in a manner comparable to other health services — with no direct charges for the procedure and a fee for donor sperm based on cost recovery only. The system we propose will resolve the problems we identified by ensuring that

- all DI recipients and children are protected as much as is medically feasible from sexually transmitted infectious diseases (including HIV) and genetic diseases that are transmittable by donor sperm;

- only sperm that is collected and stored according to established safety standards is used in insemination procedures;

Figure 19.2. Outline of Proposed AI System in Canada

Licensed Collection Facility or Physician (licence granted by NRTC based on testing/record-keeping criteria) →

- collects sample
- interviews donor
- counsels donor
- screens blood and semen (freezes sample for six months for HIV retesting)

- Sends sample to regional bank with:
  - identifying information (name, address, etc.)
  - general medical, social, genetic information
  - test results
  - signed statement by donor that he has read and understood information brochure and consents to donate
  - standard form completed

Licensed Storage and Distribution Facility →

- freezing/storage facility
- attaches code number to general information/test results
- attaches code to stored sample
- maintains name/code link in a secure, separate, and protected file

- sends coded sample out only after receiving name/information of recipient
- requests information on birth outcome
This data/sperm bank thus contains information linking donor and social parents to be forwarded for ongoing storage to the NRTC.

→

Requester (licensed clinic, licensed practitioner, self-insemination recipient)

- receives sample with
  - code number
  - general medical/social information
- performs insemination or instructs for self-insemination

← to receive sample, requester sends to licensed storage and distribution facility:
  - identifying information on the woman
  - standard form completed
  - signed statement that the sperm is for her use
  - signed statement that she has read and understood information brochure
  - signed statement that she will inform facility of the name and birth date of any child that results from the insemination
  - any request that another sample from the same donor be kept in reserve

National Reproductive Technologies Commission

- receives all data (identifying and non-identifying on donors and recipients) for children born each year for ongoing, secure record maintenance.

- no sperm that does not comply with Canadian standards is imported from international sources;

- all sperm donors understand the long-term implications of the act of donation;

- sperm donors have no rights or obligations with respect to children conceived through insemination with their sperm;

- sperm, as a human reproductive material, does not become the object of commercial transactions;

- only practitioners adhering to uniform standards of safety, effectiveness, and informed consent can offer AI services;

- self-insemination is available as a safe, effective, and low-cost alternative to DI carried out in a medical setting;

- secrecy about DI is discouraged while recognizing that families should be free to make their own choices about issues that affect them;

- complete records are collected, stored, and securely maintained on donors, recipients, and DI children, and the needs of DI families and donors are balanced with regard to access to information about each other;

- information on donors and recipients is accessible to those authorized by a court of law in the case of medical necessity; and

- DI record-keeping practices are uniform across the country.

The scheme is further described in Figure 19.2 and in the licensing requirements set out below.

Licensing Requirements for Sperm Collection, Storage and Distribution, and Use

The Commission recommends that

> 83. **The National Reproductive Technologies Commission establish an Assisted Insemination Sub-Committee with responsibility for setting the standards and guidelines to be adopted as conditions of licence and for monitoring developments in this field.**

> 84. **The collection, storage, distribution, and use of sperm in connection with assisted insemination be subject to compulsory licensing by the National Reproductive Technologies Commission.**

85. Sperm collection, sperm storage and distribution, and the provision of assisted insemination services constitute three distinct licensing categories, as described below. Upon meeting the necessary conditions of licence, a single facility may be considered eligible for all three types of licence.

and that

86. Collecting, storing and distributing, or using sperm in providing assisted insemination services without a licence issued by the National Reproductive Technologies Commission, or without complying with the National Commission's licensing requirements, as outlined below, constitute an offence subject to prosecution.

Sperm Collection Facilities

The Commission recommends that

87. The compulsory licensing requirements for sperm collection apply to any physician, centre, or other facility or individual collecting sperm to be used to inseminate a woman other than the social partner of the sperm donor.

and that

88. The Assisted Insemination Sub-Committee of the National Reproductive Technologies Commission develop, with input from relevant bodies, standards and guidelines to be adopted as conditions of licence. The recommendations of the Royal Commission on New Reproductive Technologies should serve as a basis for the guidelines. In particular, the Commission recommends that the following requirements be adopted as conditions of licence for sperm collection:

(a)   Non-identifying information about the donor's medical history, age, and physical and social attributes, including race and ethnicity, should be collected at the time of donation.

(b)   All potential donors should provide a signed, self-administered completed questionnaire providing information about their health and the health of their first-degree relatives (parents, siblings, and offspring), which should be reviewed by a clinical geneticist. Any indication of serious genetic anomalies or other high-risk factors should disqualify a potential donor from participating in the program.

(c)   Identifying information, including the donor's full name, date and place of birth, and address, should be collected from the donor at the time of donation.

(d)   All identifying donor information should be stored securely, so that it remains strictly confidential. When a sperm sample and information related to that sample are forwarded to a licensed sperm storage and distribution facility, no named information should be retained by the collection facility.

(e)   Standard forms and procedures for collecting, recording, and encoding identifying and non-identifying information, and for storing identifying information in strictly confidential and highly secure conditions, should be developed by the Assisted Insemination Sub-Committee of the National Reproductive Technologies Commission.

(f)   Potential donors, who should be of the legal age of consent, should be required to read and discuss information outlining the risks, responsibilities, and implications of sperm donation, including the fact that they will be tested for HIV and other infectious diseases, and should sign a consent form indicating they have done so. Standard information and counselling materials should be developed by the Assisted Insemination Sub-Committee of the National Reproductive Technologies Commission, with a view to ensuring that they are comprehensive, easily understood, and non-directive.

(g) The necessary steps for screening donors and for testing sperm for infectious diseases that could potentially affect the health of the woman using the sperm or her child should be specified by the Assisted Insemination Sub-Committee of the National Reproductive Technologies Commission, and should be strictly followed. Non-compliance with such standards should be punishable by loss of licence.

(h) In setting standards for testing, the Assisted Insemination Sub-Committee should consider inclusion of testing for gonorrhoea, hepatitis A and B, human immunodeficiency virus (HIV) 1 and 2, syphilis, chlamydia, cytomegalovirus, herpes, trichomoniasis, ejaculate C and S, chromosomal analysis, human papillomavirus, and tuberculosis.

(i) Testing for HIV 1 and 2 should include a sperm quarantine period of at least six months before the initial sample is used and further quarantine periods and retesting of the donor at appropriate intervals during any continuing period of donation.

(j) Only sperm from donors with negative results for the diseases tested for should be considered suitable for insemination.

(k) Donors should be compensated only for their inconvenience and for the direct costs of donation. Payment for sperm should not be substantial enough to constitute an incentive to donate.

(l)   Sperm suitable for insemination should be forwarded only to licensed sperm storage and distribution facilities, as described below.

(m)   Sperm forwarded to licensed sperm storage and distribution facilities should be accompanied by the following information:
   (i)   identifying donor information;
   (ii)   the signed donor consent form showing that the donor has read and understood the information and counselling materials;
   (iii)   non-identifying donor information; and
   (iv)   all donor and sperm screening and medical test results, including date of donation.

(n)   Once all sperm from a donor is forwarded to a licensed sperm storage and distribution facility, no identifying information in relation to that donor should be retained in the sperm collection facility.

(o)   Sperm collection facilities should not operate on a for-profit basis. Charges for sperm should cover the costs of collection, testing, record keeping, and related administrative expenses, but should not include a profit.

The Commission further recommends that

89.   Sperm collection facilities report to the National Reproductive Technologies Commission on their activities in a standard form, at least annually.

90.   Sperm collection facilities be required to apply to the National Reproductive Technologies Commission for licence renewal every five years.

and that

91. **Sperm collection licences be revocable by the National Reproductive Technologies Commission at any time for breach of the conditions of licence.**

Sperm Storage and Distribution Facilities

The Commission recommends that

92. **The compulsory licensing requirement for sperm storage and distribution apply to any physician, centre, or other facility providing sperm to be used to inseminate any woman other than the social partner of the sperm donor.**

and that

93. **A licence is also required to treat sperm for the social partner if it is treated with the aim of separating X- and Y-bearing sperm.**

The Commission recommends that

94. **The Assisted Insemination Sub-Committee of the National Commission develop standards and guidelines to be adopted as conditions of licence. The recommendations of the Royal Commission on New Reproductive Technologies should serve as a basis for the guidelines.**
     In particular, the Commission recommends that the following requirements be adopted as conditions of licence:
     (a) All sperm stored or distributed by a sperm storage and distribution facility must be obtained from a licensed sperm collection facility. A licensed sperm storage and distribution facility should also be eligible for a sperm collection licence if it meets the conditions of licence outlined above.

(b) Only sperm accompanied by the following information should be accepted for freezing, storage, and distribution:

    (i) identifying donor information as specified above;

    (ii) the signed donor consent form;

    (iii) non-identifying donor information; and

    (iv) all required donor and sperm screening and medical test results.

(c) Immediately upon receipt, a donor identification code number should be attributed to the sperm sample. All test results, data sheets with non-identifying information, and sperm samples should be identified only by the donor identification code number, and the information linking the name to the code number stored separately and under secure conditions specified by the National Reproductive Technologies Commission.

(d) Sperm suitable for insemination should be cryopreserved in accordance with standards established by the National Reproductive Technologies Commission.

(e) Applications for sperm should be accepted only from an individual or facility licensed to provide assisted insemination services, as described below, or from an individual woman seeking sperm for self-insemination.

(f) Sperm should be provided to individual women for self-insemination without discrimination on the basis of factors such as sexual orientation, marital status, or economic status.

(g) Applications for sperm should be accepted only if accompanied by the following information:

    (i) identifying information, including the name, birth name (if different), date and place of birth, and address of the woman seeking to be inseminated (the recipient);

    (ii) data on the medical history of the recipient;

(iii) in the case of a woman seeking sperm for self-insemination, a signed statement that the sperm is for her own use, that she has received, read, and understood information materials outlining the risks, responsibilities, and implications of donor insemination, and that she consents knowingly to using the sperm;

(iv) a signed undertaking by the recipient, or by the licensed assisted insemination service, that the sperm storage and distribution facility will be informed within 21 days (in accordance with provincial birth registry requirements) of any live birth resulting from the insemination, and be provided with the name, sex, place and date of birth of the child, and information about any significant congenital anomalies or health problems.

(h) Sperm samples distributed to qualified applicants should be accompanied by the following information:

(i) the donor identification code number;

(ii) non-identifying donor information;

(iii) all donor and sperm screening and medical test results (identified only by the donor identification code number);

(iv) the form to be completed and returned to the sperm storage and distribution facility in the event of a live birth, recording:

- the date of birth;
- the sex of the child(ren) born;
- the full name(s) of the child(ren) born;
- any other information that the National Reproductive Technologies Commission deems necessary for adequate record keeping, such as information about any congenital anomalies or significant health problems in the newborn child;

       (v)   informational materials for the recipient explaining the legal status of the donor, the recipient, and her partner, if applicable, and outlining benefits to the child and family of registering the birth of the child(ren) with the National Reproductive Technologies Commission; and

      (vi) in the case of sperm intended for self-insemination by the recipient, directions for thawing the sperm and for self-inseminating.

(i)   Information relating to the donor, the recipient, and the child(ren) should be linked by the licensed storage facility, under secure conditions, pursuant to guidelines established by the National Reproductive Technologies Commission, so as to ensure

      (i)   no more than 10 live births per donor;

      (ii)   the donor or the child(ren) can be contacted in the event of serious medical need (e.g., discovery of a serious genetic disease in either the child or donor that would have implications for the other);

      (iii) access at any time by recipients and the children to non-identifying information about the donor upon providing the identification code number of the donor; and

      (iv) access by qualified researchers to non-identifying data for research purposes.

(j)   Records, including identifying information about the donor, the donor's identification code number, the name of the recipient, and information about the child(ren) born as a result of insemination, should be forwarded to the National Reproductive Technologies Commission annually, for storage by the National Commission for a minimum of 100 years.

(k) All identifying donor information should be stored securely, pursuant to guidelines established by the Assisted Insemination Sub-Committee of the National Reproductive Technologies Commission, so that it remains strictly confidential. Once all sperm samples from a donor have been distributed, no identifying information relating to that donor should be retained by the sperm storage and distribution facility.

(l) Identifying donor information should be released by the National Reproductive Technologies Commission only in the event of serious medical need as determined by a court of law.

(m) Sperm samples should be stored and shipped in accordance with guidelines established by the National Reproductive Technologies Commission.

(n) Sperm storage and distribution facilities should not be permitted to operate on a for-profit basis. Charges for sperm should cover the costs of storage, testing, record keeping, distribution, and related administrative expenses, but should not include a profit.

In addition to the specific conditions of licence outlined above, the Commission recommends that

95. Sperm storage and distribution facilities follow the record keeping, data collection, and data reporting requirements established by the National Reproductive Technologies Commission.

96. Sperm storage and distribution facilities report to the National Reproductive Technologies Commission on their activities in a standard form, at least annually.

97. **Sperm storage and distribution facilities be required to apply to the National Reproductive Technologies Commission for licence renewal every five years.**

and that

98. **Sperm storage and distribution licences be revocable by the National Reproductive Technologies Commission at any time for breach of the conditions of licence.**

Assisted Insemination Services

Access to donor sperm for use in insemination, whether by a clinic or a solo practitioner for use in assisted insemination or by an individual woman for self-insemination, would be contingent upon the provision of identifying information on the recipient as outlined above.

The Commission recommends that

99. **The National Reproductive Technologies Commission develop, with input from relevant bodies, standards and guidelines to be adopted as conditions of licence. The recommendations of the Royal Commission on New Reproductive Technologies should serve as a basis for the guidelines. In particular, the Commission recommends the following requirements:**
    (a) **Only frozen sperm from a licensed sperm storage and distribution facility, obtained upon completion of a form providing the required information on the recipient, should be used. The use of imported sperm is not permissible.**
    (b) **For female participants in assisted insemination programs, invasive exploratory or diagnostic techniques or adjuncts such as hormones should not be used unless there is a reasonable indication of a female fertility problem.**
    (c) **A licence is required to perform insemination at any site other than the vagina even if the recipient is the social partner.**

(d) Criteria for determining access to assisted insemination services should not discriminate on the basis of social factors such as sexual orientation, marital status, or economic status.

(e) Standard information, counselling, and consent forms should be developed by the Assisted Insemination Sub-Committee of the National Commission and should be completed and signed by all recipients before any treatment. Such forms should include

   (i) information on both the physical and psychological effects of assisted insemination and its lifelong implications;

   (ii) information about alternatives to assisted insemination;

   (iii) information about specialized psychosocial counselling services that are available on request to support decision making;

   (iv) a standard section, requiring signature of the recipient, indicating that she has read and understood the above information and that she undertakes to provide the requisite information if she has a pregnancy and birth as a result of the insemination; and

   (v) a standard section where the signature of the partner, if he consents, is provided.

(f) At the time of insemination, the recipient should be provided with the following additional information and materials:

   (i) the donor identification code number;

   (ii) non-identifying donor information (identified only by the donor information code number); and

   (iii) a list of the donor and sperm screening and medical test results.

(g) **Within 21 days of a live birth, the requisite information about the child(ren) born as a result of the insemination should be provided by the recipient to the assisted insemination service, for forwarding to the storage and distribution facility that supplied the sperm.**

(h) **The form to be completed by the recipient and returned to the sperm storage and distribution facility in the event of a live birth should include:**

   (i) **the date and place of birth;**

   (ii) **the sex of the child(ren) born;**

   (iii) **the full name(s) of the child(ren) born;**

   (iv) **details of any significant congenital anomalies or health problems; and**

   (v) **any other information the National Reproductive Technologies Commission deems necessary for adequate record keeping.**

The Commission recommends that

100. **Licensed facilities provide sperm that has been treated with the aim of separating X- and Y-bearing sperm only to individuals who have a clear medical indication for this procedure (for example, X-linked disease). For individuals who do qualify for receipt of sperm treated in this way, there should be**

   (i) **disclosure of objective information to clients about the lack of reliability of any technique used;**

   (ii) **existence of a system of record keeping with respect to the sex of the child that results; and**

   (iii) **submission of an annual report to the National Reproductive Technologies Commission with these data.**

101. **Assisted insemination services report to the National Reproductive Technologies Commission on their activities in a standard form, at least annually.**

102. Assisted insemination services be required to apply to the National Reproductive Technologies Commission for licence renewal every five years.

and that

103. Assisted insemination licences be revocable by the National Reproductive Technologies Commission at any time for breach of the conditions of licence.

The Role of the Assisted Insemination Sub-Committee

We have referred to the Assisted Insemination Sub-Committee in our licensing recommendations for sperm collection, storage, distribution, and the provision of assisted insemination services. However, it is worth providing a brief review of the Sub-Committee's functions, in light of the central role it will play in regulating practices in this area, thereby ensuring a safer and more effective AI system in Canada.

The Assisted Insemination Sub-Committee would be established and chaired by the National Reproductive Technologies Commission. It would be one of six permanent Sub-Committees, along with those dealing with infertility prevention; assisted conception services; prenatal diagnosis; the provision of fetal tissue; and embryo research. Like National Commission members themselves, we recommend that at least half the members of the Assisted Insemination Sub-Committee be women, and that all members be chosen with a view to ensuring that they have a background and demonstrated experience in dealing with a multidisciplinary approach to issues, as well as an ability to work together to find solutions and recommend policies to address the issues raised by assisted insemination and other methods of assisted conception in a way that meets the concerns of Canadian society as a whole.

The Assisted Insemination Sub-Committee would have several functions. It could decide to establish ad hoc working groups to deal with one or more of these functions, if appropriate:

- Setting and revising, from time to time, the licensing requirements for sperm collection; sperm storage and distribution; and the provision of assisted insemination services (including donor and recipient consent requirements; record-keeping procedures; data collection and reporting requirements; etc.) to be applied through the National Reproductive Technologies Commission licensing process. The latest guidelines of the American Fertility Society could be helpful in this regard.

- Developing standard information materials, counselling materials, and consent forms to be used in the provision of AI services.

- Establishing policies and standards for screening donors and testing sperm, and establishing standards for the cryopreservation and safe storage of sperm.

- Developing standards and guidelines for the collection, recording, encoding, and secure storage of identifying and non-identifying donor information, recipient information, and information relating to AI births.

- Overseeing the National Reproductive Technologies Commission's national data base of donors, recipients, and AI births; and establishing appropriate procedures for making identifying information available, under court order, in the case of medical necessity.

- Analyzing the country-wide information that is gathered about technologies and practices, which can be used as a basis for the Assisted Insemination Sub-Committee's guideline- and standard-setting activities, as well as by the provinces in their planning and resource allocation decisions.

- Consulting with the provinces, directly or through the Conference of Deputy Ministers of Health, on matters relating to AI funding and services, where this is useful or needed.

- Discussing and setting policy on new issues as they arise, engaging in direct consultation with the public as needed, and ensuring appropriate levels of regulation on a continuing basis.

- Promoting public awareness and debate regarding assisted insemination in Canada, in part through the publication of relevant data and information in the National Reproductive Technologies Commission's annual report.

The Assisted Insemination Sub-Committee's monitoring, information-gathering, and reporting activities will help to ensure that the Canadian public is better informed about the AI system in Canada. Public accountability in this area will also be enhanced by the composition of the Assisted Insemination Sub-Committee, which should include both National Commission and outside membership, so as to include a broad representation of perspectives and interests. We recommend that the Sub-Committee include membership from relevant professional associations, federal and provincial/territorial health ministries, individuals representing the concerns of donors, recipients, and children born through the use of AI, as well as other interested and affected segments of the public, including, in particular, women. We are of the view that the Sub-Committee's continuing regulatory oversight over sperm collection, sperm storage and distribution, and the provision of assisted insemination services will establish important safeguards in this area, and ensure safe, more effective, and more equitable delivery of AI services in Canada.

Conclusion

The Commission's recommendations in this chapter address the need for action in two broad areas: mandatory licensing of assisted insemination services to ensure that they are provided safely, uniformly, and equitably; and family law reform to clarify and standardize in all provinces the parentage of children born as a result of donor insemination and to protect the integrity of families formed in this way.

Establishing the licensing system we propose will overcome the significant shortcomings the Commission's review revealed in the current provision of assisted insemination services in Canada.   By making standards for safe collection, storage, and use of sperm part of the conditions of licensing for facilities that wish to provide AI services, the health and safety of women and their partners and children will be safeguarded. Women and couples who wish to self-inseminate will also have a source of safe sperm. In addition, people will get the information and counselling they need to make informed decisions about whether they want to have children in this way. Licensing and regulation by the National Reproductive Technologies Commission will also ensure that record-keeping practices are improved and standardized across the country, so that DI children and families have access to the information they need to protect and promote their physical health and emotional well-being.

Assisted insemination has the potential to be a safe, inexpensive, and relatively low-tech reproductive option for Canadian women and couples whose circumstances and values make this an acceptable choice for them in forming a family. The integrated national approach we propose, together with the family law reform we recommend, will help to ensure that this potential is realized.

Appendix 1: International Approaches to DI

The United Kingdom, the United States, and Australia have not implemented an actual DI system; instead, they have dealt with the various issues surrounding DI as separate concerns. Britain's *Human Fertilisation and Embryology Act* (1990) set up a central registry regarding gamete donation, and AI itself is offered both privately and within the public health system.   The act also states that donor information, including donor identities, must be kept on record, and children have access to non-identifying information when they reach the age of majority, although parents are not required to inform children that they originated from DI. The *Family Law Reform Act* (1987) severs the parental rights and responsibilities of the sperm donor and legitimizes the paternity of the male partner of a DI recipient.

In the United States, where DI is offered as a commercial service, regulation falls to the individual states. Most states have addressed the issue of the filiation of the child, but not whether a child should have access to donor information. Fourteen states require that the donor's identity be kept (though under seal unless specified by court order in the case of grave medical importance) but otherwise do not establish a right of children to either identifying or non-identifying information.

South and Western Australia have focussed on the release of donor information. Each has passed legislation requiring that records of donors and recipients be kept; Western Australia allows the release of non-identifying information to the child and to his or her social parents. Both jurisdictions allow the release of identifying information with the consent of the donor.

Other jurisdictions have dealt with DI in a more systematic way. Sweden, for example, has passed a far-reaching *Act on Insemination* (1985), which addresses each stage of DI within a state-controlled framework. All donor sperm collection and cryopreservation is done by public hospitals; donors are given a "gift" of approximately $38.00 Canadian; all inseminations take place in public hospitals under the supervision of a physician qualified in gynaecology and obstetrics and with licensed counselling facilities; and specific practice regulations and guidelines for screening donors, freezing sperm and retesting for HIV, and the insemination procedure itself are adhered to.

The legislation limits DI to married or cohabiting heterosexual couples. The Swedish system does not compel DI parents to tell their children how they were conceived but allows the DI child to have access to the identifying information about the donor upon reaching the age of majority (although DI parents do not have access to this information). If upon reaching the age of majority a DI child requests a meeting with his or her genetic father, the donor is obliged to do so. The donor gives his consent to this meeting at the time of donation. Under the Swedish system, information about the donor and his identity is kept on file for 70 years.

France has regulated the practice of DI within a national framework since the early 1970s. The Centre d'étude et de conservation des oeufs et du sperme humains licenses sperm clinics according to rigorous practice (married donors with children) and record-keeping criteria, and France's state-run health insurance covers all AI costs. A controversial bill (adopted in 1992 in first reading but not passed) places further restrictions on DI — the practice will continue to be limited to heterosexual couples in which the man is sterile or carries a genetic disease. The bill also clarifies the legal status of DI families and reinforces donor anonymity; a married man who has consented to his partner's insemination cannot renounce paternity, a sperm donor cannot demand paternity rights, and the donor's identity is completely protected. The potential French legislation does not allow designated gamete donation.

General Sources

Achilles, R. "Donor Insemination: An Overview." In Research Volumes of the Royal Commission on New Reproductive Technologies, 1993.

Achilles, R. "Self-Insemination in Canada." In Research Volumes of the Royal Commission on New Reproductive Technologies, 1993.

Achilles, R. "The Social Meanings of Donor Insemination." In Research Volumes of the Royal Commission on New Reproductive Technologies, 1993.

American Fertility Society. *Guideline for Practice: Intrauterine Insemination.* Birmingham: AFS, 1991.

Baylis, F. "Assisted Reproductive Technologies: Informed Choice." In Research Volumes of the Royal Commission on New Reproductive Technologies, 1993.

Collins, J., E. Burrows, and A. Willan. "Infertile Couples and Their Treatment in Canadian Academic Infertility Clinics." In Research Volumes of the Royal Commission on New Reproductive Technologies, 1993.

Deber, R.B., with H. Bouchard and A. Pendleton. "Implementing Shared Patient Decision Making: A Review of the Literature." In Research Volumes of the Royal Commission on New Reproductive Technologies, 1993.

Decima Research. "Social Values and Attitudes of Canadians Toward New Reproductive Technologies." In Research Volumes of the Royal Commission on New Reproductive Technologies, 1993.

Decima Research. "Social Values and Attitudes of Canadians Toward New Reproductive Technologies: Focus Group Findings." In Research Volumes of the Royal Commission on New Reproductive Technologies, 1993.

Hughes, E.G., D.M. Fedorkow, and J.A. Collins. "Meta-Analysis of Controlled Trials in Infertility." In Research Volumes of the Royal Commission on New Reproductive Technologies, 1993.

Mullens, A. *Missed Conceptions: Overcoming Infertility.* Toronto: McGraw-Hill Ryerson, 1990.

SPR Associates Inc. "An Evaluation of Canadian Fertility Clinics: The Patient's Perspective." In Research Volumes of the Royal Commission on New Reproductive Technologies, 1993.

Vandekerckhove, P., et al. "Treatment of Male Infertility: Is It Effective? A Review and Meta-Analyses of Published Randomized Controlled Trials." In Research Volumes of the Royal Commission on New Reproductive Technologies, 1993.

World Health Organization Scientific Group. *Recent Advances in Medically Assisted Conception.* Geneva: World Health Organization, 1992.

Specific References

1. Fresh sperm can live up to three days in the optimum conditions present in a woman's vagina — body temperature, structural factors, and cervical and vaginal mucus combine to create the perfect environment to preserve sperm. Outside this environment, two hours is considered the outer limit of sperm life (Noble, E. *Having Your Baby by Donor Insemination: A Complete Resource Guide.* Boston: Houghton Mifflin, 1987).

2. Ontario Ministry of Health, Ad Hoc Group. *Recommended Guidelines for Therapeutic Donor Insemination Services in Ontario.* Toronto: Ministry of Health, 1987; Canadian Fertility and Andrology Society. *Guidelines for Therapeutic Donor Insemination.* Montreal: CFAS, 1988.

3. Human immunodeficiency virus, the virus thought to lead to acquired immunodeficiency syndrome (AIDS).

4. Royal College of Obstetricians and Gynaecologists, Fertility Committee. *Infertility: Guidelines for Practice.* London: RCOG Press, 1992, p. 18.

5. Adapted from Harkness, C. *The Infertility Book: A Comprehensive Medical and Emotional Guide.* San Francisco: Volcano Press Inc., 1986, pp. 189-90. Sperm is evaluated for several qualities; it may be abnormal in more than one of these. Although 100 million sperm per millilitre of ejaculate is the average count in normal men, the sperm count is considered normal if it is between 20 and 100 million per millilitre.

Factor	Evaluation criteria	Results
Sperm count	Sperm is placed, one layer thick, on a counting grid under a microscope. One area of the grid is counted and the number multiplied by 1 million. There is a 10% margin of error.	A count below 20 million is reported as "low sperm count."
Motility	Two to three hours after ejaculation, the percentage of moving sperm in high-power microscopic fields is estimated, and the degree of forward progression is rated 1-4, from none to excellent.	Grades 1 and 2 are reported as "poor motility," grades 3 and 4 as "good motility."
Morphology	100 sperm cells are examined for shape and maturity, and categorized as 1) normal (mature with oval shape), 2) amorphous (immature shape or size), 3) tapered, 4) double-headed, 5) micro (too small), or 6) macro (too big).	If fewer than 60 percent fall into category 1, abnormal morphology is reported.

Viscosity	The liquidity of sperm 20-30 minutes after ejaculation is measured by pouring it drop by drop.	If semen is gelled, poor viscosity is reported.
Volume	Measuring the amount of semen that is ejaculated — 2-5 cubic centimetres (cc) is considered normal.	Less than 2 cc is reported low volume, over 5 cc is reported excessive volume.

6. Ibid., p. 192.

7. MacIntyre, S., and A. Sooman. "Non-Paternity and Prenatal Genetic Screening." *Lancet* 338 (October 5, 1991): 869-71. Non-paternity rates on the general genetic literature are quoted as being "in the range of 10%," but variables that may affect paternity rate are sample ascertainment, birth order, age, cultural and ethnic group, reason for testing, and laboratory technique. Overall, it appears that general population studies in the United Kingdom, France, and the United States are in the range of 1 to 5 percent.

8. United States. Congress. Office of Technology Assessment. *Artificial Insemination Practice in the United States: Summary of a 1987 Survey.* Washington: Office of Technology Assessment, 1988.

9. Wikler, D., and N. Wikler. "Issues and Responses: Artificial Insemination." In Research Volumes of the Royal Commission on New Reproductive Technologies, 1993.

10. Stephens, T., and J. McLean. "Survey of Canadian Fertility Programs." In Research Volumes of the Royal Commission on New Reproductive Technologies, 1993.

11. Ibid.

12. Canada. Statistics Canada. *Demographic and Income Statistics for Postal Areas, Canada.* Cat. No. 17-202. Ottawa: Minister of Supply and Services Canada, 1990.

13. Golombok, S., and J. Rust. "The Warnock Report and Single Women: What About the Children?" *Journal of Medical Ethics* 12 (1986): 182-86.

14. Those who chose known donors wanted the child to have the ability to meet his or her biological father later in life, and wanted to know the donor so that they would be aware of any medical complications that might arise in the future. Some lesbians are using sperm donated by a male relative of their female partner, in order to make a genetic link to the two families.

15. The Commission's readability analysis of education and consent materials used a scale to determine how many years of education were needed to fully comprehend what was written.

16. Canadian Fertility and Andrology Society, *Guidelines for Therapeutic Donor Insemination*, p. 6: "d. In addition to adequate physician, nursing and laboratory staff, the following expertise is also needed: ... i. A clinical geneticist ... ii. A clinical psychologist to provide counselling of recipients at all stages of work-up and treatment."

17. Daly, K.J., and M.P. Sobol. "Adoption as an Alternative for Infertile Couples: Prospects and Trends." In Research Volumes of the Royal Commission on New Reproductive Technologies, 1993, p. 15.

18. Views expressed by the Toronto Branch of the Canadian Adoption Reunion Register, at the Commission's Public Hearings, Toronto, Ontario, November 20, 1990.

19. The Yukon *Children's Act* states that the legal father of a child born through assisted conception is the husband/cohabiting partner of the mother if he has given his consent in advance of the insemination, and that the sperm donor has no parental rights. This means if the mother does not have a partner, the child has no legal father.

Newfoundland law specifies that where the man is married to or cohabiting with a woman at the time she is inseminated and he consents to the insemination, he, and not the donor, is considered the legal father. Even without consent, the man will be considered the father if he has demonstrated his intention to treat the child as his, unless he can prove that he did not know about the DI conception.

The revised Quebec *Civil Code* (in force January 1, 1994) specifies that the use of third-party genetic material does not constitute a filial bond between the third party and the child born of that procreation. The 1981 Code already specified that a child born as a result of DI is presumed to be the legitimate child of the mother and her spouse, if the husband gave his consent to the insemination. According to the revised Code, the husband can challenge the presumption of paternity if he did not consent and did not act as a parent to the child. The Code does not recognize common-law unions; therefore, despite a common-law partner's consent to DI, the Code is of no application and therefore the partner could bring an action to disavow paternity. In other words, a common-law spouse may be presumed to be the father, but, unlike a married spouse, he can attempt to refute the presumption. The revised Code does provide for an action in responsibility against such a common-law partner.

20. Sloss, E., and R. Mykitiuk. "The Challenge of the New Reproductive Technologies to Family Law." In Research Volumes of the Royal Commission on New Reproductive Technologies, 1993. All Canadian jurisdictions, with the exception of Nova Scotia, have legislation that deals with a "rebuttable presumption of paternity" with respect to children born into a stable heterosexual relationship. Legal presumptions are assumptions arising from a given set of facts that require the production of evidence to overcome the assumption. One such assumption is that a husband is the legal father of a child born within a marriage. However, that assumption is at most a starting point and it can be "rebutted," or refuted by evidence that he is not the biological father (such as a blood test). Any "interested person" can bring forth that evidence. In light of the prospect that a person could refute an assumption of paternity, it is therefore theoretically possible that a donor could produce evidence of his biological link to the child so that a "court would likely entertain his action in paternity as against the presumed father of the child." In the situation where a donor seeks custody/access to "his" child, he must refute the presumption *and* persuade the court it would be in the child's best interests that he be granted custody/access. In those jurisdictions with DI-specific consent legislation, the person giving consent to the insemination is legally presumed to

be the father of the child. The difference here is that this presumption is *irrebuttable*, meaning that it is irrefutable, and that person's legal status as father cannot be challenged by anyone. More specifically, in the Yukon, Newfoundland, and Quebec, a sperm donor would not be able to claim any parental rights.

21. Ibid. However, some courts in the United States have decided that in such a circumstance the man could not challenge his paternity. If he renounced paternity later than birth, that is, he acted as a father to the child while knowing he was not genetically linked, he may not be able to absolve himself of responsibility to contribute to the support of the child. In addition, some jurisdictions have legislation defining "parent" as including "a person who has demonstrated a settled intention to treat the child as his or her own even where there is no biological connection." This is an extended definition of the term "parent," and again was for the purpose of support.

22. For some purposes, it is legally possible that a child could have two "parents" of the same sex where support or custody/access legislation provides for extended definitions of the words "parent" and "child." In such a circumstance, should the non-genetically linked woman fall within an extended definition of "parent," she would not be a legal stranger.

23. Sloss and Mykitiuk, "The Challenge of the New Reproductive Technologies to Family Law," refers to one case that seems to support the claim that discrimination in Canadian courts against lesbian families works against the best interests of the child. Although the issue was *child support* not *custody*, the British Columbia case of *Anderson v. Luoma* (1986) is illustrative of where a court has adopted a "conventional, heterosexual conception of the family." Briefly, the genetic/gestational mother applied for child support from her lesbian partner. The women had cohabited for 10 years, and during that time the respondent had supported the plaintiff and the two DI children. The court refused to order support, holding that the relevant legislation "does not purport to affect the legal responsibilities which homosexuals may have to each other to children born to one of them as a result of artificial insemination." The court stated further that the act applies to the "spousal and parental relations of men and women in their role of husband, wife and parent." This limitation of the child's support to their legal mother deprives the child of the opportunity for two lines of support.

24. Stephens and McLean, "Survey of Canadian Fertility Programs," Table 35.

Infertility Treatments: *In Vitro* Fertilization

♦

In vitro fertilization — literally, fertilization in glass — is, perhaps, the best known of all infertility treatments. It captivates the imagination, as it is a dramatic use of advanced technology by skilled practitioners and technicians to treat difficult cases of infertility after other approaches have failed; and, when it is successful, it results in the "miracle babies" so familiar in media images and stories. Among the various treatments for infertility, *in vitro* fertilization has received the most attention, both from researchers and from those critical of infertility treatments in general. More focus is given to IVF than to either fertility drugs or assisted insemination. This is despite the fact that both of these are much more commonly used treatments for infertility and result in the birth of many more children than IVF — from which, in 1991, fewer than 400 infants were born. The most advanced technology, excellent diagnosticians, and skilled practitioners have been devoted to treating the most difficult cases of infertility, the people for whom IVF may be their last chance of conceiving.

For their part, some critics contend that this technology is unproven and dangerous, and that its provision runs counter to women's best interests. They maintain that practitioners and scientists are seeking medical breakthroughs at the expense of women and ignoring the adverse consequences of IVF use, such as multiple pregnancy with its attendant emotional and financial costs, and the short- and long-term health risks of the fertility drugs used to stimulate the production of eggs for IVF. Others are critical of how IVF is offered, saying that IVF is inaccessible to any but urban heterosexual couples with high incomes.

For many people working in the field of new reproductive technologies and for many people observing and commenting on the field, what happens with IVF helps set the context for viewing other infertility treatments. Thus, the Commission was very aware that the implications of its study of and recommendations on IVF would have an impact beyond this treatment itself.

IVF was developed originally to treat fallopian tube blockage resulting from disease. Over the past 15 years, however, it has come to be used and applied in a wider and wider variety of indications. Our research showed that, in the mid- to late 1980s, IVF was being used for indications ranging from unexplained infertility (the "diagnosis" when no apparent fertility problem can be found in either the male or the female partner), ovulation defects, and endometriosis, in addition to tubal blockage (see research volume, *Treatment of Infertility: Current Practices and Psychosocial Implications*). Our survey of fertility programs found that IVF is also used as a diagnostic test of male infertility after assisted insemination has been unsuccessful, to ensure there is no chance the male partner's sperm can fertilize the egg, before the couple stops treatment or turns to donor insemination.

In addition, the technology has been applied in situations not directly related to infertility treatment as commonly understood. For instance, IVF of eggs donated by younger women and then transferred into women past the age of menopause has been used. The technology has also been applied in so-called gestational preconception arrangements (which are discussed in Chapter 23). In this latter use, a zygote* created *in vitro* from the eggs and sperm of a contracting couple is implanted in a woman who gestates and gives birth to a child to surrender to the contracting couple. All these wider applications of the use of IVF raise ethical issues that society has yet to deal with; many of them are alluded to in the section discussing the social context of IVF.

Following a brief explanation of the origins and development of IVF and how the IVF procedure works, the first part of this chapter describes the Commission's work in determining the effectiveness of IVF for various indications and in examining the risks associated with its use. The second half of this chapter examines issues surrounding how IVF is currently being offered in Canada — who is providing it, who has access to it, what kinds of practices are followed in clinics, the counselling and information couples receive, and how success rates are defined and records kept.

To appreciate the Commission's recommendations in this chapter, it is important to understand our two basic findings related to the use of IVF as an infertility treatment:

- First, despite the proliferation of its use for other diagnoses, we found that IVF has been demonstrated to be effective only for the indication it was originally developed to treat — fallopian tube blockage.

- Second, we found marked variations in how treatment facilities are delivering IVF services, and that these variations are not serving the best interests of patients.

---

* See Chapter 22, "Embryo Research," for a discussion of the use of the terms "zygote" and "embryo."

Commissioners believe that the current way IVF is being offered is unacceptable; it is unethical and unsafe to permit IVF to be used as a treatment for indications for which it has not been found effective. Allowing to persist the wide differences in how services are offered gives rise to risk, uncertainty, misinformation,

The current way IVF is being offered is unacceptable; it is unethical and unsafe to permit IVF to be used as a treatment for indications for which it has not been found effective. Allowing to persist the wide differences in how services are offered gives rise to risk, uncertainty, misinformation, and unfairness.

and unfairness. The proliferation of indications for IVF, without demonstration of effectiveness for many of these indications, means that many Canadians, including responsible physicians, share the Commission's concern about the situation.

Such a situation is not unique to IVF, however. Studies of how health care technologies have developed and been disseminated have noted that new technologies that show some promise of effectiveness often become widely disseminated before being rigorously evaluated. Often it is only after a technology has been diffused — if then — that it is evaluated and that some measure of consistency is developed for determining what should be provided and how. Ideally, only those aspects of treatment shown to be effective continue. Unfortunately, once a technology has been widely diffused, it can be very difficult for practitioners to act on findings suggesting the treatment is not of benefit.

Some uses of IVF are unethical when viewed through the prism of our ethical principles, and our approach is to prohibit these (such as IVF in support of preconception arrangements or for post-menopausal women). With regard to the use of IVF to treat infertility, the Commission believes that the time has come to consolidate what we know about IVF and to use that as the basis for shaping the future direction of IVF practice in Canada. In our view, medical procedures should move from the realm of research to that of treatment only if they can be demonstrated to be effective and beneficial and if information on their risks and effects is available. A predominant theme of our entire discussion of IVF is that there is a pressing need for long-term, well-designed research to find out when and for what indications IVF is effective, and what the long-term health effects of its use are, for women and for the children they may have as a result of the procedure. Further, ensuring that IVF services are delivered in a manner that respects the autonomy of patients, enhances their ability to make informed choices, and provides clear information and appropriate support is a necessary component of an ethical approach to infertility treatment. This chapter provides details of the Commission's recommendations on how controls can be put in place to ensure that IVF is used in an ethically acceptable, effective, and safe way.

In reaching our conclusions and recommendations, we based our approach on the precepts of evidence-based medicine set out in Part One of this report, as well as on our ethic of care. We believe that IVF use

> We believe that IVF use presents an ideal opportunity to implement a model system of evidence-based medicine.

presents an ideal opportunity to implement a model system of evidence-based medicine. The practitioner community is relatively small and concentrated, and our publicly funded single-payer health care system provides the means to exercise the control necessary to ensure that services are offered only in ethically acceptable ways. To allow the current situation to continue would be costly for Canadian society — not only in terms of dollars, but also in terms of the potential for harm to individuals and to collective values and goals. Boundaries must be established and, within those boundaries, a regulatory system put in place to guide practice, with compulsory licensing and standards established and enforced by the National Reproductive Technologies Commission. The Commission therefore recommends that

> **104. The provision of assisted conception services in Canada be subject to compulsory licensing by the National Reproductive Technologies Commission.**

and that

> **105. The National Reproductive Technologies Commission establish an Assisted Conception Sub-Committee, with responsibility for setting the standards and guidelines to be adopted as conditions of licence and for monitoring developments in this field.**

We recommend strongly that clinics and the professions begin right away to take the necessary steps to stop inappropriate treatments, pending the establishment of the National Reproductive Technologies Commission and the Assisted Conception Sub-Committee. We recognize that our recommendations will limit the provision of IVF services in Canada, possibly for some time to come. From 1987 to 1991, just under 45 percent of the IVF services provided were for indications other than tubal blockage. Limits on unproven services may cause concern for some people who are infertile, but, as the Commission was told repeatedly, they want safe, effective treatments. Our proposals provide the only means to ensure this goal can be reached. We do not want to reduce the number of successful IVF treatments; rather, we want to prevent unethical uses of technology and to limit the resources devoted to ineffective treatment. It is misleading to patients and costly to the health care system to offer unproven treatments, except in the context of research studies designed to assess their safety and effectiveness, in which participants are fully informed about its experimental nature before consenting to treatment and have the other protections inherent in medical research involving human subjects.

We are not opposed to the further development and application of IVF for diagnoses other than tubal blockage provided those applications are effective and safe. In the section on priorities for IVF research, we have recommended a system that will allow IVF to be used for other diagnoses within the framework of research trials to evaluate whether its use in these situations is both effective and safe. Proven treatments would continue to be offered. Indeed, in light of the importance of children in the lives of individuals, couples, and society generally, Commissioners believe that if ethical, safe, and effective medical procedures are available to assist people to have children, a caring society should provide them through the health care system. Our discussion of how IVF should fit into the health care system follows the section on research priorities. The Commission is recommending that proven treatments be covered by provincial health insurance plans.

> We do not want to reduce the number of successful IVF treatments; rather, we want to prevent unethical uses of technology and to limit the resources devoted to ineffective treatment ... Proven treatments would continue to be offered.

We conclude the chapter with our recommendations for a regulatory system to ensure that IVF technology is used only in an ethical and accountable way. How we reached our conclusions and recommendations is the subject of the remainder of this chapter, beginning with the social context for our inquiry into how IVF is practised in Canada today.

The Views of Canadians

IVF was among the most widely debated technologies in the Commission's mandate and a strong focus of attention in our national surveys, our survey of IVF patients, public hearings, private sessions, roundtables, and letters and submissions. These information-gathering activities produced a large body of material about the views and attitudes of Canadians toward IVF and the issues it raises. Those who took the time and made the effort to present their views helped create a national dialogue on IVF and gave Commissioners a rich and multifaceted basis from which to consider the issues. This multidimensional perspective was necessary, because no single vantage point can provide a comprehensive picture of the personal, medical, social, ethical, economic, and legal dimensions of the issues surrounding the use of IVF.

Any attempt to summarize or categorize the spectrum of views about IVF cannot do justice to all perspectives. It is possible, however, to group the main issues raised into several broad categories. Many of the points made by Canadians with respect to IVF echo the broader discussion of the social context of infertility treatments set out at the beginning of this section.

The Proliferation of IVF

The proliferation of IVF from its original use for blocked fallopian tubes to unproven, and potentially unethical application is of concern to many groups and individuals, some of whom already had reservations about the use of medical technology and the medicalization of women's reproductive health. Many people were concerned that the expanded uses of IVF amount to experimentation on women's bodies without their informed consent.

On the other hand, a national survey of values and attitudes carried out by the Commission found that three-quarters of respondents would be very or somewhat likely to use IVF if they themselves were unable to conceive (see research volume, *Social Values and Attitudes Surrounding New Reproductive Technologies*).

> "Some clinics which offer the procedure *in vitro* fertilization have never succeeded in producing a live birth, yet they claim success rates of up to 25 per cent, basing their statistics on the number of pregnancies achieved rather than the number of births."
>
> *Cited by L. Jones, quoting from CBC Radio "Ideas" 1986 program entitled "Drawing the Line: Reproductive Technologies." Dalkon Shield Survivors Group, Public Hearings Transcripts, Vancouver, British Columbia, November 27, 1990.*

How IVF Services Are Provided

Many people raised concerns about whether consent to IVF treatment is truly informed, whether sufficient information is provided to patients, whether there is enough appropriate counselling, whether women's autonomy is respected, and whether services are provided in accordance with Canadians' values and priorities.

The Commission heard from patients and practitioners alike that information and counselling are vital for patients to make informed choices about their care. Many patients would like information about all the options open to them — not just treatment, but also adoption or coming to terms with not having children.

Risks Associated with IVF

We heard concerns that very little is known about the long-term health outcomes of IVF, both for the women who undergo treatment and for their children. Risks can accrue from the use of fertility drugs (these are outlined in the chapter on fertility drugs), from the surgical and other procedures associated with egg retrieval and transfer of zygotes to the uterus, and from the pregnancy and birth outcomes of treatment.

Any discussion of concerns regarding risk must be understood in the context that no medical treatment is absolutely "safe": patients and practitioners must always weigh the risks against the probable benefits and determine whether the level of risk is acceptable, given the anticipated benefits. We heard that in addition to accurate information about IVF effectiveness, patients, practitioners, and policy makers need accurate information about the risks of IVF as a basis for individual and public policy decisions. Many of the witnesses appearing before the Commission expressed concerns about the safety of the procedures and said that the drugs used in IVF have not been adequately tested or evaluated for their immediate effects on women or their longer-term implications for women or for the children that result from IVF. Intervenors also pointed to the risks involved in the multiple pregnancies often associated with IVF, and many were concerned that the short- and long-term health implications for women and children have not been tracked to date.

> IVF should be classed as experimental [funded through research budgets] and subjected to the high standards of informed choice and consent outlined in the Nuremberg code and the Helsinki Declaration.
>
> *Brief to the Commission from the Canadian Advisory Council on the Status of Women, March 28, 1991.*

> *In vitro* fertilization usually results in the death of a high percentage of embryos; and in many procedures, the deliberate destruction of embryos that are believed to be less healthy ...
>
> We are strongly opposed to the destruction of "unwanted" embryos *in utero* in cases where multiple implantations have resulted from IVF. Therefore, we recommend that IVF programs should be discontinued, except in cases where the woman's own ovum and her husband's sperm are used in the IVF process and where there is no intentional discarding or destruction of embryos.
>
> *H. Hilsden, Pentecostal Assemblies of Canada, Public Hearings Transcripts, Toronto, Ontario, November 20, 1990.*

How IVF Is Paid For

The issue of public funding for IVF has been more controversial than that of funding for other infertility treatments, because it is very expensive, and because of questions about its effectiveness and safety. Even if these were known, however, many people opposed its public funding on the grounds that the health care system cannot afford the "luxury" of expensive, high-technology treatments for infertility, or because they felt it would divert attention and resources from other reproductive services or health priorities, including infertility prevention and basic prenatal care.

To those affected by it, however, infertility is not a trivial concern but a condition with potentially deep and lasting consequences for their well-being throughout their adult lives. We heard testimony that safe and effective procedures that could help those who are infertile should be included in the health care system, on the grounds that infertility is just as important in the lives of those affected as are many other conditions now treated in the health care system.

In an effort to answer the question of how infertility treatment is viewed compared to other medical treatments, data from the Oregon Health Services Commission are often quoted.

Faced with large numbers of the state's population without any medical insurance, Oregon decided to extend public coverage for low-income individuals more widely, so that all citizens without private insurance would be covered. Given the fixed amount of funding they had available, this could be done only by limiting the number of services that would be covered. The state therefore drafted legislation that ranked a large number of health care services, with the highest ranked services being covered and the lowest ranked services being excluded from Medicaid coverage. The list included the use of IVF to treat infertility.

The value attached to each procedure was determined using research into effectiveness, a formula considering cost and benefit, public hearings, and survey data. Ranked first were acute fatal conditions for which

> IVF programs have a responsibility to make sure the participants are left intact by the process, and that goes for anyone involved in the situation of infertility. These are real people with very real life situations you are dealing with.
>
> *N. Newman, IVF Program, University of British Columbia, Public Hearings Transcripts, Vancouver, British Columbia, November 27, 1990.*

> If the [health care] system is going to collapse, it is not going to collapse because IVF has been added as one of the services to which citizens of Canada have access.
>
> *J. Cameron, private citizen, Public Hearings Transcripts, Toronto, Ontario, October 29, 1990.*

treatment provides full recovery, followed by maternity care, acute fatal conditions for which treatment prevents death but without full recovery, and preventive care for children. Ranked as being of low priority were infertility services. IVF in particular ranked 696th out of a total of 709 medical services. This finding is used frequently to suggest, therefore, that IVF should not be funded in our tax-supported system.

Precisely because this ranking is so often quoted, it is important to recognize that it is likely to be misleading, because of the methodology used. Respondents were asked to rank treatments for diseases that all of us are at risk of contracting. As long as the possibility exists that treatment may be needed, great importance is attached to its availability. While it was possible for any person responding to become ill with most of the conditions listed — a heart attack, or diabetes, or kidney disease, or a stroke — it was fairly obvious to respondents when they were not going to need IVF. If they already had children, it was unlikely that they would see the need for IVF services applying to themselves. The only way to get a true estimation of the relative value of infertility treatment would be to ask people who have not yet had children about the relative importance of this treatment. Only then would their responses be comparable to asking them about other treatments they may need. They are only "at risk" of needing this particular service if they do not have children.

The telephone survey that was carried out as part of the Oregon priority-setting exercise surveyed 1 000 households. Of these, 405 households had members under the age of 18, and 135 households had more than two members 18 years of age and over, most of whom were probably adult children still living at home. It is also likely that some of the other households with only two members 18 years of age and over were, in fact, a single parent and an adult child. One hundred and ninety-nine people, or about 20 percent, lived alone, in a household of one. This obviously could be young people who have not yet attempted to have children, but it could also include the elderly, divorced, or widowed, many of whom have had children or are past the age where it is a possibility.

What all these numbers, taken together, indicate is that the majority of respondents to the survey already had children. Thus, although they were a representative sample of Oregonians, they were not a representative sample of people who are as likely to require infertility treatment as treatment for some other condition. They were asked to place a value on treatment for disorders they are at risk for, in comparison to a treatment they knew they were not likely to need. This means the ranking of infertility treatment was not done on a comparable basis.

We heard various views from Canadians on how IVF should be funded. A Commission survey found that about one-quarter of those interviewed thought that people seeking treatment should pay the entire cost; just over half the respondents said that the cost of infertility treatment should be shared by the province and the individuals seeking treatment; and 10 percent said public health insurance should cover the entire procedure.

Access to IVF*

In contrast to access to donor insemination, access to IVF by single women or lesbians is not a major issue. This is because these women want access to safe sperm, but not usually to IVF, as their problem is not infertility, but the lack of a male partner. We heard concerns, however, that implicit or explicit program criteria could be used by clinics in a discriminatory way with respect to other groups — for example, women with disabilities.

> Most IVF patients talk of the inconvenience of daily trips to the clinic and the hours off work. Most northern patients must book a vacation to get enough time for a treatment cycle.
>
> J. Smart, private citizen, Public Hearings Transcripts, Ottawa, Ontario, September 19, 1990.

Because of the highly technical nature of IVF, which makes it necessary to provide the procedure in specialized clinics, we heard that access is a critical issue for those who live outside southern Ontario (where most IVF clinics are concentrated) and the few other major urban centres.

We also heard that those with low incomes have problems with access to IVF. Ontario is the only province that provides health insurance coverage for IVF. As well as the procedure itself, there are drug costs and travel and accommodation costs that may put it out of reach for many.

Decision Making About IVF

Individuals can make decisions about whether to undergo IVF only within the parameters of the decisions that society has already made about whether the treatment should be available, to whom, and under what conditions. Canadians told the Commission that they want more opportunities to influence decisions about the use of technologies and the allocation of public resources to them; they do not want to leave decisions about technologies like IVF solely in the hands of practitioners and researchers. Although we heard the view that society should look to the medical profession as both the repository of knowledge about reproductive technologies and the best source of decisions regarding their use, more often we heard the view that practitioners and researchers should not be

---

* See Annex for dissenting opinion.

the ones making moral and ethical judgements for the rest of society.

The Commission developed its social and ethical perspective on the provision of IVF in light of this social context. Taken in concert with current knowledge about effectiveness and risk, this enabled the Commission to recommend a public policy framework within which IVF could be offered to Canadians who are infertile in a safe and ethical manner — that is, in a way that protects and promotes the well-being of women, couples, and children and respects principles of equality, appropriate use of resources, non-commercialization of reproduction, and accountability. The remainder of this chapter is devoted to the conclusions emerging from the Commissioners' review of the evidence on IVF technology and its use in Canada today and to our recommendations to address the concerns brought before us.

> Right now, there is [an] arbitrary screening process. For example, in *in vitro* fertilization, the screening process is determined by the medical people in control of the clinic. And, therefore, they have set up what criteria they choose in order for people to access that technology ... Right now, you have to be a married couple. You have to have financial means to gain access to the clinic ... not all society can afford $5 000 or $10 000 per attempt at *in vitro* fertilization; not all society live in Calgary and can, therefore, gain immediate access to the technology; and not all society who want children are married, heterosexual couples.
>
> *P. Corbett, Social Issues Committee, YWCA, Calgary, Public Hearings Transcripts, Calgary, Alberta, September 14, 1990.*

Origins and Development

If a woman's fallopian tubes are blocked, the egg cannot travel from the ovary, be fertilized in the tube, and continue on to implant in the uterus (see Chapter 7). IVF technology was developed originally to give women who had blocked fallopian tubes a chance at becoming pregnant by circumventing the tubal problem. Zygotes created outside the body, using the woman's eggs and her partner's sperm, are transferred to her uterus.

As described in greater detail in the Commission's research volumes,* the first steps in the development of human IVF (though this was not the immediate goal of the research) occurred in the United States in the 1930s and 1940s, using eggs from ovaries removed at hysterectomy. In February 1944, biologist Miriam Menken, who worked as an assistant to Harvard

---

* See, in particular, *Treatment of Infertility: Assisted Reproductive Technologies.*

gynaecologist and researcher John Rock, isolated a viable egg, mixed it with sperm collected from medical students, and observed by microscope the first human *in vitro* fertilization.

During the 1960s, the development of laparoscopy enabled researchers to see the uterus and fallopian tubes and allowed them to retrieve eggs directly from the ovaries. Ovulation induction drugs, which became generally available in 1967, were used soon after that to increase the number of eggs produced during a menstrual cycle. In the early 1970s the first successful retrieval, culture, and fertilization of human eggs was achieved, and researchers began their attempts to transfer the resulting zygotes to a woman's uterus, where it was hoped they would implant and develop.

During this period, researchers in Britain, Australia, and the United States were developing similar techniques and alternately reported procedural breakthroughs. Although much of the early work was pioneered in the United States, public concern about the ethical and social implications served to limit private and public funding for such research, and U.S. research progressed less quickly than that going on in Britain and Australia.

By the mid-1970s it was clear that although ovulation induction drugs permitted the retrieval of many eggs during a cycle, these hormones also made the lining of the uterus less suitable for zygote implantation. In 1977, British researchers Robert Edwards and Patrick Steptoe collected one naturally produced egg from Lesley Brown, fertilized it with her husband's sperm, and transferred it to her uterus. In July 1978, Louise Brown, the first IVF child, was born in England.

Over the next months and years, IVF technology was incorporated in medical practice throughout the Western world. Australian researchers and clinicians developed more effective egg retrieval methods and adjusted fertility drug doses and combinations to increase the number of eggs produced without sacrificing too much in uterine receptivity. They also initiated the practice of egg donation, where one woman's egg was retrieved, fertilized *in vitro*, and transferred to another woman's uterus. Canada, too, joined the countries involved in this field. In 1982, an Ontario woman gave birth to the first Canadian children born as a result of IVF, although the twin boys were conceived in England. The first IVF children conceived in Canada (also twin boys) were born in Vancouver in 1983. The mid-1980s also saw the first public funding of IVF in Canada, by Ontario's medicare program.

Another significant event of the 1980s was the development in Australia of zygote freezing (cryopreservation) and thawing techniques. Although successful cryopreservation of animal zygotes had been possible since 1972, the first pregnancy from a frozen then thawed human zygote was not achieved until 10 years later, and it was not until 1984 that the first live birth from a frozen zygote occurred.

IVF Procedures

Ovulation induction: Fertility drugs are usually prescribed to stimulate the production of several eggs in one menstrual cycle. Egg growth inside the ovary is monitored through blood or urine tests or ultrasound, and retrieval is timed just before ovulation occurs. Another drug may be given to lessen the chances of spontaneous ovulation before retrieval. Drug levels are monitored, and the woman is watched for signs of ovarian hyperstimulation syndrome. About 15 percent of IVF cycles are cancelled because eggs do not develop adequately, or because the woman ovulates before the retrieval.

Egg retrieval: When the eggs are ripe, but before they are released by the ovary, they are retrieved. The woman is given a light anaesthetic, and the physician uses an ultrasound probe to guide a needle to the location in her vagina closest to the ovary. The needle is passed through the vaginal wall to aspirate the fluid from each follicle (the ovary structures in which the eggs mature). The fluid is examined under a microscope to determine whether any mature eggs were retrieved. Any found are transferred to a prewarmed culture medium. (Immature eggs are transferred to an incubator to see whether they will mature further.) Eggs are found in about 80 percent of retrieval procedures.

Once the eggs have been removed from the woman's body, the following choices are available:

Disposal or research: If the egg is immature, abnormal, or surplus, it may be disposed of or used in research (for example, research into egg freezing).

Manipulation of gametes: Sperm and eggs can be treated to improve the chances of fertilization. The experimental techniques for eggs include *zona cutting* — the cells surrounding the egg are removed by passing it back and forth through a narrow pipette to shear off the adhering cells; then the egg is punctured with a needle to make a hole in the zona pellucida, the "shell" of the egg, so that sperm can penetrate more easily; *zona drilling* — surrounding cells are removed as with zona cutting, followed by an application of an acid solution to create a "drill hole" in the zona pellucida; *partial zona drilling* — after the cells are removed, instruments are used to create a series of gaps in the zona pellucida; and *microinjection* — sperm cells are injected directly into the egg.

Gamete intrafallopian transfer (GIFT): If the woman has a functioning fallopian tube, the egg may be transferred back into her body before being fertilized. In GIFT, the egg is transferred to the fallopian tube, and sperm is also put there in the hope that fertilization will occur in the tube.

Direct oocyte sperm transfer (DOST): A variation of GIFT in which eggs are collected from the ovary and placed immediately in the uterus. Sperm is then added, and, if fertilization occurs, this is in the uterus instead of in the fallopian tube.

(continued in next box)

IVF Procedures *(continued)*

Donation: Eggs can be donated to a recipient, to be fertilized with the sperm of the recipient's partner, with the intention of implanting the embryo in the recipient's uterus for gestation.

Egg fertilization and embryo culture: A semen specimen is collected from the woman's partner (or donor sperm is thawed), and the sample is concentrated by sperm wash. Four to 12 hours after the egg retrieval, a drop of sperm is added to medium with the eggs, which are returned to the incubator. Within 20 hours of insemination, each egg is examined to determine whether fertilization has occurred. With normal sperm, an estimated 70 to 80 percent of the eggs will be fertilized. On the third day, each zygote is assessed and the following choices are available as well as embryo transfer to the uterus:

Cryopreservation: Zygotes can be frozen in liquid nitrogen for later use.

Disposal or research: If a zygote does not develop properly, is abnormal in appearance, or is surplus, it can be disposed of or used in research. From various studies, an estimated 20 to 50 percent of IVF zygotes have chromosomal abnormalities. They may also have abnormalities in shape. Those with identifiable abnormalities are rejected for transfer.

Preimplantation diagnosis: Zygotes can be analyzed to identify single-gene or chromosomal conditions. Preimplantation diagnosis is still at an experimental stage, it is invasive and expensive, and it reduces their survival rate (see Chapter 27).

Donation: Zygotes can be donated to another woman or couple who are infertile.

Embryo transfer: When the zygote reaches the two- to eight-cell stage, it can be transferred to the uterus using a fine catheter inserted through the cervix, or to the fallopian tube using laparoscopy (a more invasive option requiring general anaesthesia). About 20 percent of embryo transfers result in implantation measurable by elevated hormone levels in the woman's blood, called a "chemical pregnancy." The live birth rate per zygote transferred, however, is about 17.5 percent.*

Zygote intrafallopian transfer (ZIFT): This procedure was developed to try to improve implantation rates by transferring zygotes to the fallopian tube earlier in their development. Only two Canadian programs offer ZIFT.

Implantation and beyond: Ideally, implantation takes place and the pregnancy proceeds to birth normally.

---

*   Society for Assisted Reproductive Technology, The American Fertility Society. "Assisted Reproductive Technology in the United States and Canada: 1991 Results from the Society for Assisted Reproductive Technology Generated from the American Fertility Society Registry." *Fertility and Sterility* 59 (5)(May 1993): 956-62.

From the mid-1980s on, IVF practice expanded quickly throughout Europe, Australia, and North America. Because of the technical demands of the procedures, infertility clinics were developed where expertise and equipment could be centralized. In Britain and the United States, these clinics emerged as private, often free-standing, commercial enterprises; in other European countries, as in Canada, IVF programs were most often added to the existing services of teaching hospitals.

As IVF developed in the laboratory and in medical practice, many women's groups, as well as organizations representing the medical, legal, religious, and other communities, began to examine the ethical, social, and legal issues surrounding IVF. An extensive literature on the implications of IVF for Western cultures and social systems has emerged, identifying a range of issues that using the technology raises.

IVF Procedures

As noted earlier in this chapter, IVF has been used in an expanding range of situations as its practice has evolved. Regardless of why it is being used, IVF practice in Canada consists generally of the same basic stages, with some variation in the details of procedures from program to program. Each stage leads to several possible results and options. The stages and options are described in the accompanying boxes and flow chart (Figure 20.1); readers interested in a more detailed examination should consult the research volumes. Numbers cited in these boxes are general statistics based on international evaluations of IVF; they do not take into account variations in success rates for each infertility diagnosis or for different patient groups (see section on The Effectiveness of IVF).

Practitioners offering IVF usually see the most complex and difficult infertility cases — patients are often those for whom other treatments have failed and who may see IVF as their last chance for pregnancy. Many cases of infertility are "cured" before a couple reaches an IVF program — the woman might become pregnant without treatment or following fertility drug treatments prescribed by her general practitioner or gynaecologist; pregnancy might follow tubal surgery or less invasive techniques such as assisted insemination; or the couple might decide to adopt or to accept not having children.

The Effectiveness of IVF

One of the major areas of our investigations involved assessing the available data from the world literature of all published clinical studies about the effectiveness of IVF for specific diagnoses or indications.

Figure 20.1.   One IVF Cycle

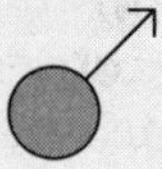

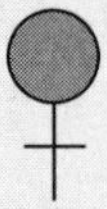

Ovulation induction: Fertility
drugs prescribed and egg growth
monitored.

Semen analysis: A semen
sample collected through
masturbation is analysed for
viability of the sperm.

CYCLE CANCELLED: In
15% of cycles, eggs do not
develop properly and are
lost to ovulation.

Egg retrieval: Just before ovulation
the eggs are retrieved using a needle
guided by ultasound. Depending on
the drug regime used, the number
can range from 5 to 10 or more eggs.

Sperm wash: The sperm are
concentrated and impurities in
the semen are removed.

Immature eggs are transferred to
a culture medium to mature.

Egg fertilization: Four to 12 hours after the egg retrieval, 50 000 to 500 000 sperm are
added, and eggs are returned to an incubator. Within 20 hours of insemination, each egg is
examined to determine if fertilization has occurred.

CYCLE CANCELLED: In
13% of cases, a viable zygote
does not result.

Embryo transfer: In about three days, when the zygotes have reached the two- to eight-cell stage,
they are evaluated for viability. A number of them are transferred to the uterus using a fine catheter
inserted through the cervix (or to the fallopian tubes using laparoscopy for GIFT).

CYCLE CANCELLED: About 80% of
transfers do not result in implantation.

Implantation: If the zygote implants successfully in the wall of the uterus, a gestational sac can be
detected by ultrasound and elevated hormone levels will be present in the woman's blood, indicating
pregnancy.

CYCLE CANCELLED: About 20% of
clinical pregnancies are lost to miscarriage,
and 5% are ectopic and must be terminated.

Pregnancy: Pregnancy proceeds normally. More than one embryo may implant successfully and
multiple pregnancy is common. About 30% of IVF deliveries are multiple (in Canada, 39% of those
born are from a multiple pregnancy).

LIVE BIRTH: For every 100 cycles initiated in 1991, 13 resulted in a live birth.

Source: Statistical estimate based on data from the Society for Assisted Reproductive
Technology/American Fertility Society central registry, 1991, summarizing statistics collected from 215
Canadian and U.S. IVF programs.

Until now, an overall assessment of this information in a way that is readily available and useful in guiding policy has not been carried out. The Commission set out to remedy that gap. Our findings about the effectiveness of IVF are described later in this section — but in essence IVF has been found effective only for fallopian tube blockage; for other indications, there is a need for additional and more rigorous research. This finding is central to our conclusions about the direction public policy should take and is a driving force behind our recommendations.

We conducted our assessment by evaluating the results of all published trials of IVF that met certain criteria through a technique known as meta-analysis. This was supplemented by the findings of the Canadian Infertility Therapy Evaluation Study, the

> **Meta-analysis:** Pooling the results from studies with similar methodologies when each study on its own may not include sufficiently large sample sizes to provide reliable results.

largest study ever conducted on infertility treatments in Canada. We used this information to assess the effectiveness of IVF for blockage of the fallopian tubes, ovulation disorders, endometriosis, male infertility, and unexplained infertility. We outline the results of our meta-analysis later in this section.

We should begin, however, by noting the difficulty of statistical analysis in this area and hence the difficulty of assessing the effectiveness of infertility treatment on the basis of trials that meet our usual criteria for reliability. These problems are inherent in the chance nature of infertility and the characteristics of people seeking infertility treatment. As a result, the design and execution of appropriate randomized control trials are very difficult, involving such methodological problems as finding people who are willing to be part of the control ("no treatment") group.

Answering the question "does the treatment work?" is seldom straight-forward. For example, even couples who are fertile have a 4 percent chance of not conceiving in their first year of trying. It is therefore often difficult to tell whether an outcome (a pregnancy or birth) was the result of treatment or the result of the chance nature of fertility at work. If everyone in the treatment group were sterile, that is, unable to have a pregnancy without treatment, then any birth that occurred would obviously have been the result of receiving treatment. But the reality is that

> One of the major concerns regarding *in vitro* fertilization worldwide, as well as in this country, is the perceived absence of quality assurance and ethical guidelines for the practice of IVF.
>
> *S. Brown, Reproductive Endocrinology and Infertility Committee, Society of Obstetricians and Gynaecologists of Canada, Public Hearings Transcripts, London, Ontario, November 1, 1990.*

those having infertility treatment include a mix of people who are sterile and people with low fertility. To complicate matters even further, the proportion of these two groups will vary according to the diagnostic category.

This means that the number of births following treatment is not a direct measure of the effectiveness of treatment, because the likelihood of birth among the same or similar patients who have not had treatment must also be known — hence the need for a control group, which can be very difficult to assemble. Sometimes couples are willing to be their own control — accepting random assignment to a "waiting" group or postponing the beginning of treatment. But some couples are understandably unwilling to do this. Multicentre trials are therefore needed in order to generate large enough numbers to permit statistically significant and reliable conclusions to be drawn.

> The number of births following treatment is not a direct measure of the effectiveness of treatment, because the likelihood of birth among the same or similar patients who have not had treatment must also be known.

Despite these methodological difficulties, good information about the effectiveness of IVF is needed for decision making at both the societal and the individual level, and until the Commission investigated this area comprehensively, the existing information had simply not been collated and analyzed in one overall assessment, making rational decisions difficult or impossible.

At a societal level, policy makers and others making resource allocation decisions need good information about the effectiveness of medical procedures, the population to be served, and the cost and resource implications compared with the potential health benefits. Information about these elements helps to determine whether IVF should be offered and, if so, under what circumstances.

At the individual level, practitioners and couples have to take what is known about the broad effectiveness of IVF and apply it to the couple's specific circumstances to determine whether IVF is an appropriate treatment for them. To establish an accurate assessment of whether IVF is likely to work in their case, and whether the chance of a live birth is worth the risk of treatment, information about four elements is essential. These are

- *the natural force of pregnancy* — the couple's chance of conceiving naturally, given their age, diagnosis, and other relevant factors;

- *the effectiveness of treatment* — the couple's chance of conceiving with IVF, given their age, diagnosis, and other relevant factors;

- *the known risks of treatment* — including the short-term health implications and the possible long-term effects of treatment; and

- *the relative effectiveness, risk, and cost of alternative treatments or strategies.*

In the absence of information about each of these elements, practitioners and patients are unable to weigh the options, and patients cannot make informed choices.

Commissioners decided that if the evidence showed that IVF did not pass assessment after evaluating these four elements for a given diagnosis, we would recommend that it not be offered as a treatment for that diagnosis, regardless of the demand. If IVF showed promise with respect to a given category of diagnosis, but the evidence was not sufficient to demonstrate that it was more effective than receiving no treatment, we would recommend that it be considered a priority for research. If the evidence derived from well-designed research studies showed that it was effective for a particular category of diagnosis, we would recommend that it be considered for funding as a medical service. However, the ethical, social, and legal implications would also have to be weighed in reaching an appropriate policy decision in this regard.

When assessing the effectiveness of IVF in achieving a live birth, it is important to keep in mind that natural conception rates in couples from the general population are also far from 100 percent. The average monthly chance of conception leading to a live birth is about 20 to 25 percent. There is a range in couples' ability to conceive, so that the peak conception rate is 33 percent in the first month of trying; then it falls quickly, settling to about 5 percent each month. Fertilization may occur more frequently than this, but about half of all fertilized eggs never result in a live birth (see Chapter 7).

The Natural Force of Pregnancy

Although some couples have virtually no chance of conceiving without treatment, some infertility conditions have a known rate of "spontaneous remission" — that is, the woman becomes pregnant without intervention. The Commission's research found that time elapsed between diagnosis and treatment can affect this natural force of pregnancy. A meta-analysis of randomized control trials found that if a couple's infertility could be traced to partial fallopian tube blockage, mild endometriosis, male-factor infertility (low sperm count), unexplained infertility, or tubal blockage that had been treated with surgery, their chances of conceiving naturally during the first three years after diagnosis were almost as high as if they underwent IVF. After three years' duration of infertility, however,

> I think it's unfair for society to expect medicine to offer a better outcome than what nature has to offer, and what I will try to show you is that *in vitro* fertilization offers, in fact, with the current technology, approximately what a couple would have if their fallopian tubes were normal.
>
> *P. Claman, GOAL Program, Ottawa Civic Hospital, Public Hearings Transcripts, Ottawa, Ontario, September 19, 1990.*

their chances of conceiving naturally declined markedly. This seems to indicate that IVF may not be called for in these categories until a couple's chances of conceiving naturally have been virtually eliminated — that is, after three years of infertility.

Another factor affecting the natural force of pregnancy is whether a couple has primary or secondary infertility. Couples with secondary infertility (that is, they have previously had a child together or one member of the couple has had a child with another partner) may be slightly more likely than those with primary infertility to become pregnant without intervention.

The Age of the Female Partner

A significant factor determining the chances of pregnancy without intervention is the age of the female partner. We have already seen that increasing age is associated with declining fertility in women (see Chapter 12). For couples whose fertility is already declining because of age, a three-year wait to let nature take its course may not be acceptable — if an older couple does wait and remains infertile, there is good evidence that treatment will be less effective.

Every stage in the IVF process has been shown to be less effective when the source of the egg is an older woman. A study of *in vitro* fertilization in the Netherlands, for example, showed that effectiveness dropped by one-third for women aged 35 to 40 and by two-thirds for women over the age of 40.[1] Thus, the age of the female partner is a very important aspect to be taken into account in decisions about whether it is appropriate to offer IVF to a particular couple.

Behavioural and Environmental Factors

Although there has been little research examining the relationship between behavioural or environmental factors and the results of IVF, we would expect that factors that have been shown to reduce male or female fertility would also reduce the likelihood of a couple conceiving and giving birth to a healthy child following IVF. These factors include smoking, substance abuse, weight and eating disorders, excessive exercise, and stress, as well as exposure to harmful agents in the workplace or the environment. Preliminary research in several countries indicates, for example, that infertile women who smoke are less likely to have a live birth following IVF. Infertility specialists told the Commission that good practice would involve providing counselling or referring couples for counselling when such behavioural or environmental factors are present in one partner or both.

Effectiveness by Infertility Diagnosis

A couple's diagnosis is the most important element influencing the outcome of IVF, so it is disturbing that it is often neglected in analyses of the effectiveness of IVF. Because IVF may be effective for one category of diagnosis but not for another, Commissioners considered it essential to determine the effectiveness of IVF for each category of diagnosis (or "indication") currently used to justify IVF.

The Commission examined the existing evidence about IVF and associated techniques, by indication, to see whether they met either of the criteria below. We structured our investigation according to the five diagnostic categories usually used — fallopian tube problems, ovulatory problems, endometriosis, seminal defects, and unexplained infertility. These five categories account for a very large percentage of the infertility for which couples seek treatment at Canadian IVF clinics. For example, data collected from 10 Canadian IVF clinics[2] on 3 107 egg retrieval cycles indicate that

- 1 600 (51 percent) were performed on women with tubal problems only (complete or partial blockage or tubal adhesions);

- 369 (12 percent) were performed on women with other female infertility factors only (endometriosis, ovulatory problems);

- 227 (7 percent) were performed on women whose male partner had an infertility problem only;

- 464 (15 percent) were performed on women with multiple causes of infertility, whether in one member of the couple or both; and

- 446 (14 percent) were performed on women in couples with unexplained infertility.

We decided that IVF should satisfy one of two criteria before we would categorize it as effective or, in other words, as a treatment that is of benefit for a specific indication:

1.   IVF would have to be shown to be effective for a specific indication (for example, blocked fallopian tubes, unexplained infertility) through appropriately designed randomized clinical trials that allowed meta-analysis of combined studies with a total of at least 200 couples in both the control group and the treatment group; or

2.   if a specific mechanism is known to be causing the infertility, IVF would have to be shown to correct it in a way that is biologically convincing.

We decided that if either of these two criteria is not met, then the treatment was not of proven value and should no longer be offered, except in the context of controlled clinical trials.

Our information about the effectiveness of specific infertility treatments was drawn both from the Canadian Infertility Therapy Evaluation Study and from extensive reviews and analysis of existing randomized control trials conducted in Canada and elsewhere. Researchers for the Commission identified a total of 501 randomized trials in infertility treatment in the literature (41 different journals) over a 24-year period (1966-1990). We found relatively few were of sufficient quality to allow meta-analysis — for example, the method of randomization was unstated or pseudo-randomized in 200 of the 501 "randomized" trials. In fact, relatively few studies done to date have been well designed and carried out, or produced data that allow reliable conclusions to be drawn and comparisons to be made with other studies, although this is changing, with three times as many published clinical trials for infertility treatment in 1990 as in 1986. Nevertheless, we found that most of the studies conducted do not permit reliable conclusions because of methodological weaknesses or lack of a control group. Small sample sizes, even when study results are aggregated to do meta-analysis, also limit the conclusions that can be drawn.

Because the goal of couples seeking IVF is to have a child, we defined IVF as effective if couples who underwent the procedure had a greater likelihood of having a live birth than those in a similar group of couples who were infertile who did not undergo the procedure. This was not always possible to determine, however, because many studies reported on pregnancy rates, not live births. Notwithstanding the shortage of good data, our conclusions were influenced by five major studies providing evidence relevant to IVF in particular.[3] Based on the evidence we collated and analyzed for each of the five diagnostic categories, we assigned IVF and associated technologies to one of the following groups: (1) proven effective; (2) proven ineffective; or (3) not enough evidence to categorize the treatment as either effective or ineffective (see Table 20.1).

Table 20.1. Effectiveness of IVF for Various Infertility Diagnoses

Indication	Effective*	Ineffective	Not enough evidence to categorize as effective or ineffective
1. Ovulatory defects			
oligomenorrhea and irregular cycles			IVF/GIFT/ZIFT
2. Tubal defects			
bilateral (complete) tubal obstruction	IVF		GIFT/ZIFT/DOST
partial (incomplete) tubal obstruction			IVF/GIFT/ZIFT/DOST
tubal adhesions			IVF/GIFT/ZIFT/DOST
3. Endometriosis			
minimal and mild endometriosis			IVF/GIFT/ZIFT/DOST
moderate and severe endometriosis	IVF (if tubes are blocked)		IVF/GIFT/ZIFT/DOST
4. Seminal defects			
azoospermia (absence of sperm in semen)		IVF	IVF with egg manipulation
oligospermia			IVF/GIFT/ZIFT/DOST IVF with micromanipulation
5. Unexplained infertility			IVF/GIFT/ZIFT/DOST

* See explanation in text.

As shown in this table and described in greater detail in the accompanying research volumes, our review of the available evidence permitted two main conclusions about the effectiveness of IVF: First, IVF is effective only in cases of complete fallopian tube blockage resulting from tubal disease or defect, severe endometriosis, or previous surgical sterilization. IVF has not been proven effective for any of the other diagnoses it is currently being used for. Second, only IVF itself has been shown to be effective for blocked tubes — variations such as GIFT and ZIFT have not been shown to be of benefit.

Our data collation and analysis showed clearly that in 1990, more than a decade after IVF was first offered, IVF procedures for most infertility diagnoses fall into the category of not enough evidence — there simply is not enough reliable evidence to categorize them as effective or ineffective; we do not know if the treatment is more likely to result in a live birth than no treatment. This is not the same as saying that IVF does not work; rather, additional and better data are

> There is simply not enough evidence to determine whether IVF or its variants are effective or ineffective when diagnoses other than fallopian tube blockage are present, such as ovulatory defects, partial tubal blockage, tubal adhesions, seminal defects, or unexplained infertility.

required before firm conclusions can be drawn about the appropriateness of IVF as a treatment for most types of infertility.

Our review of the evidence showed that IVF is effective when a woman has blocked fallopian tubes as a result of a disease, such as endometriosis, or surgical sterilization. By "effective" we do not mean that IVF will necessarily result in a live birth in every given case; however, when the results of treating many women with this diagnosis are taken together, IVF has been shown to be more effective (that is, more likely to result in a live birth) than receiving no treatment.

In Britain, data were collected for the period 1984-1989 on the outcomes of 5 055 IVF cycles in 2 735 women. The data were broken down by indication and showed that 15 percent of women undergoing IVF for tubal blockage conceived, and 10 percent had a live birth.[4] In comparison, the natural pregnancy rate for couples who are fertile is 20 to 25 percent per cycle. However, it must be remembered that couples who are fertile who are trying to become pregnant will have coitus more than once in the month, while a woman undergoing IVF has only one chance to become pregnant each month. In addition, a woman with blocked fallopian tubes has an extremely low chance of conceiving without treatment, since sperm cannot reach the egg, so the comparison with that baseline shows clearly that IVF does make a difference.

Although based on small sample sizes, Canadian data confirm that IVF is more effective than no treatment for women who have complete tubal obstruction. Forty-eight such women who underwent IVF in Canadian infertility programs were 11 times more likely to have a live birth than 66 women who were untreated, and these results were statistically significant.[5]

While we cannot regard these results as conclusive, because of the small size of the groups in the study, they are biologically plausible. In women who have two completely blocked fallopian tubes, fertilization of an egg cannot take place. Since IVF bypasses the fallopian tubes by allowing fertilization to take place outside of the woman's body, we would expect that the procedure would result in a higher proportion of live births than no treatment. In other words, IVF satisfies our criteria for classification as an effective treatment for this indication because it corrects a specific mechanism known to cause infertility.

When other diagnoses are present, such as ovulatory defects, partial tubal blockage, tubal adhesions, seminal defects, or unexplained infertility, there is simply not enough evidence to determine whether IVF or its variants are effective or ineffective. That is, studies have not been done or, if they have been done, they contain methodological weaknesses that make them an inadequate basis on which to make judgements about effectiveness or ineffectiveness. Moreover, for diagnoses other than complete tubal blockage, IVF does not overcome a specific mechanism that makes conception impossible. For example, with partial tubal obstruction there is still some possibility that sperm may fertilize the egg, and that the fertilized egg may travel to the uterus.

In effect, a substantial proportion of women undergoing IVF at fertility programs across the country are doing so when there is no evidence that, given their diagnosis or that of their partner, IVF will help them conceive. In other words, unproven and quite possibly ineffective procedures are being offered as medical treatment, and women are undertaking the risks of these procedures without knowing whether they are more likely to have a child than if they received no treatment. Moreover, treatment is being offered and these risks undertaken without any comprehensive and consistent collection and analysis of information on outcomes, so that these uncertainties could be reduced.

> A substantial proportion of women undergoing IVF at fertility programs across the country are doing so when there is no evidence that, given their diagnosis or that of their partner, IVF will help them conceive. In other words, unproven and quite possibly ineffective procedures are being offered as medical treatment, and women are undertaking the risks of these procedures without knowing whether they are more likely to have a child than if they received no treatment.

In summary, Commissioners conclude that Canadians are justified in their concerns about the effectiveness of IVF as a treatment for many categories of infertility. The Commission believes this situation cannot be allowed to continue, and we make detailed recommendations to remedy it at the end of this section. We recognize, however, that it will take some time to put the proposed system in place and to establish the National Reproductive Technologies Commission; in our view, action should not wait until this has occurred. We therefore urge practitioners, professional bodies, and provincial/territorial governments to act now to ensure that unproven uses of IVF are discontinued as treatments and offered only in the context of research trials.

Our recommendation is that IVF be provided as treatment only for bilateral tubal blockage. Its use for any other indication should be considered research. We recognize, in making these recommendations, that we are proposing to subject IVF to a degree of rigour not generally required in other areas of medicine. As we have stated, however, we believe that infertility treatments in general, and IVF in particular, provide models for evidence-based medicine and that in this approach lies the future of ethical, responsible, and accountable health care management.

Relative Cost-Effectiveness

In addition to assessing effectiveness from the perspective of patients — that is, whether IVF increases their chances of having a child — the Commission looked at the issue of effectiveness from the perspective of health policy makers (see research volume, *New Reproductive Technologies and the Health Care System: The Case for Evidence-Based Medicine*). Effective use of limited resources is becoming increasingly necessary, and policy makers have to take into account not only whether a treatment works, but whether its provision through the health care system constitutes an appropriate use of resources.

> There isn't all that much health money to go around these days, and right now in the province of Ontario, at least to date, I understand there's been about seven million spent on funding IVF clinics ... if you shut down the clinics, then the money can be used for something I think that is much more worthwhile.
>
> K. Kozolanka, private citizen, Public Hearings Transcripts, Ottawa, Ontario, September 19, 1990.

The Commission analyzed the cost-effectiveness of IVF as it is currently offered at a large Canadian IVF program affiliated with a teaching hospital. Researchers compared live birth rates and costs incurred by 205 couples undergoing IVF (the IVF group) and 194 couples who were either undergoing other infertility treatments, such as fertility drug therapy or assisted insemination, or receiving no treatment (the standard therapy group). The patients in the study, like those enrolled in IVF programs around the country at the time of the study, had varying durations of infertility and a variety of diagnoses. The two groups of couples under observation in the study were of comparable age and were similar in their range of diagnoses and duration of infertility. In the standard therapy group, IVF was not offered for at least six months, and both groups were followed for up to three years.

The results of the study were of significance, despite the relatively small size of the study sample. At first glance the treatment group had a higher rate of pregnancy and live birth, but, after adjusting for the difference in observation time, there was no difference in the rate of successful confinements (that is, pregnancies leading to at least one live birth) per month at risk of pregnancy.

The difference in costs, however, was great. The researchers compared the costs to the patient/couple (both direct and indirect) and to the insurer (since the program was in Ontario, physician and clinic costs were covered by provincial health insurance). This is the perspective most widely advocated for economic evaluations. The types of costs analyzed were direct medical costs, such as diagnostic, physician, and clinic costs; direct patient costs, such as drugs and travel; and the costs of associated medical treatment, such as the treatment of spontaneous abortions, ectopic pregnancies, excessive bleeding, or other complications. Costs associated with premature and multiple births (which are more common following IVF — see section on Risks of IVF) and chronic care for long-term disabilities were not factored in.

Table 20.2. Average Costs (in Canadian Dollars) per Patient (Six Months' Observation) — 1990

	Cost to patient		Cost to insurer		Cost to society*	
Cost category	IVF treatment	No IVF treatment	IVF treatment	No IVF treatment	IVF treatment	No IVF treatment
Direct medical	n.a.	n.a.	3 827.44	1 345.40	3 827.44	1 345.40
Direct patient	1 214.37	81.88	n.a.	n.a.	1 214.37	81.88
Associated medical	n.a.	n.a.	63.91	0.00	63.91	0.00
Indirect	360.68	101.26	n.a.	n.a.	360.68	101.26
Total	1 575.05	183.14	3 891.35	1 345.45	5 466.40	1 528.55

* Total of cost to patient and cost to insurer.

Source: Goeree, R., et al. "Cost-Effectiveness of an *In Vitro* Fertilization Program and the Costs of Associated Hospitalizations and Other Infertility Treatments." In Research Volumes of the Royal Commission on New Reproductive Technologies, 1993.

Although the overall live birth rate was not significantly better, as Table 20.2 indicates, for the current mix of patients receiving IVF, this treatment was considerably more expensive than alternative treatments or no treatment (the control group). The researchers concluded, based on costs over six months' observation, that IVF is not cost-effective when used to treat the wide variety of diagnoses for which it is

For many couples, waiting longer before beginning treatment could be as effective as the treatment itself.

now used. If IVF had been provided only for bilateral tubal blockage, costs would have been different; this study does not provide data on that point. The study shows that, overall, both the natural force of pregnancy and alternatives such as fertility drug treatment and assisted insemination are less expensive than IVF, yet equally effective for the current mix of patients. The Commission therefore concludes that many of the people currently participating in IVF programs should be considering other approaches to dealing with their infertility. For many couples, waiting longer before beginning treatment could be as effective as the treatment itself. Furthermore, factors such as the duration of infertility, the infertility diagnosis, and the chances of success of the particular couple, given their diagnosis and the woman's age, should be weighed carefully before IVF treatment (or referral to a well-designed controlled trial) is considered a reasonable approach to dealing with their infertility.

Cost-Effectiveness of IVF Compared to Tubal Surgery

The data gathered by the Commission show clearly that IVF as it is now being used is not cost-effective; this is not surprising, given that patients in IVF programs have a range of diagnoses, ages, and other characteristics, while IVF has been proven effective only in the case of complete tubal blockage. We also considered it useful to compare the cost of IVF with the traditional treatment for this condition, tubal surgery, to determine whether IVF is more or less cost-effective (see research volume, *New Reproductive Technologies and the Health Care System: The Case for Evidence-Based Medicine*).

Surgery is usually the first line of treatment for women with blocked fallopian tubes and is an insured service under provincial medicare plans. Because surgery is covered by provincial health insurance and IVF is not (except in Ontario), women with tubal defects are usually advised to "try" surgery first. Although surgery can repair damaged tubes in 80 percent of cases, this does not necessarily restore the functioning that will permit fertility — only 20 to 25 percent of women eventually become pregnant after surgery. This is in line with the pregnancy rate per cycle of IVF (18 percent). However, women who undergo more than one cycle of IVF have a higher probability of having a live birth than women who undergo tubal surgery. A Norwegian study found that 72 percent of women who had a complete IVF treatment (three to five cycles of IVF, unless a live birth was achieved after fewer treatments) had a live birth, compared to 24 percent of women who had tubal surgery.[6]

When the risks of IVF and tubal surgery are compared, women who have surgery have a much higher level of physical pain and longer recovery time. They also have a higher rate of ectopic pregnancy (23 percent) than women undergoing IVF, although the rate associated with IVF is still 2 percent (likely because of the presence of tubal damage in many women undergoing IVF). However, spontaneous abortion rates are higher in IVF patients (28 percent) than in post-surgical pregnancies (15 percent).[7] We would also expect IVF to be associated with a higher incidence of multiple births than tubal surgery.

Tubal surgery is associated with a lower cost than IVF. Hospital costs for surgery and the patient's stay have been estimated at $4 200 per patient; in addition, the surgeon's fee is in the range of $324 to $500, for a total of approximately $4 500 to $4 700. Accurate comparisons for IVF are almost impossible because of the different factors involved (such as type of drugs used), but a rough estimate is that one cycle of IVF costs between $5 400 and $7 500 per patient.

However, comparing the costs of each procedure does not tell us which is more cost-effective. To calculate this, we must consider the cost to achieve a live birth. A recent Dutch survey compared IVF and tubal surgery for tubal blockage and found that their treatment costs, per ongoing pregnancy achieved, were very similar.[8] The Norwegian study discussed earlier found that the costs per live birth were higher for tubal surgery ($17 000) than after IVF treatment ($12 000).[9] In other words, IVF appears to be at least as cost-effective as, if not more cost-effective than, tubal surgery.

Depending on their condition and prognosis, then, some women may be better off with IVF, others with tubal surgery; given that tubal surgery is an insured medical service, there are no cost-effectiveness arguments for not insuring IVF as well.

Given that both IVF and tubal surgery increase the likelihood of having a liveborn child in cases where the diagnosis is complete tubal blockage, it would be desirable to ensure that the choice between them is based on medical factors, not financial considerations related to insurance coverage. The choice of treatment for this diagnosis should be based on the prognosis for the individual. Our data show that the cost of a treatment has a strong influence on people's treatment choices when the options offer roughly comparable results but at widely differing costs. After analyzing the data on tubal surgery and comparing the results with data on IVF for tubal blockage, the Commission concluded that IVF may in fact be an appropriate first treatment in some cases where the diagnosis is complete tubal blockage. Although IVF is not a cost-effective procedure when, as at present, it is offered for a wide range of diagnoses, IVF is as cost-effective as the alternative, tubal surgery, in cases of tubal blockage and is a useful treatment for that diagnosis. However, its inclusion under public health insurance plans must take other factors into consideration (see section on Health Insurance Coverage).

Another reason for blocked tubes is tubal ligation (tying of the fallopian tubes), the most widely used form of female contraception in Canada — 66 percent of women undergo this procedure at some point during their reproductive lives. Some eventually regret their decision, especially if they have a new partner, and they may attempt to have the sterilization reversed through microsurgery. Live birth rates after tubal surgery to reverse sterilization (60 percent) are higher than after surgery for tubal blockage resulting from disease, and the surgery is less complex. However, if the sterilization reversal is unsuccessful, IVF may be the next treatment sought. The Commission found that between 5 and 15 percent of patients

> Although IVF is not a cost-effective procedure when, as at present, it is offered for a wide range of diagnoses, IVF is as cost-effective as the alternative, tubal surgery, in cases of tubal blockage and is a useful treatment for that diagnosis.

requesting IVF at Canadian infertility clinics in 1991 had had tubal ligation.

The Commission believes that surgical sterilization should be considered permanent, and those considering it should be counselled appropriately. Appropriate counselling and sufficient time to reflect on the implications of surgical sterilization will help to minimize the number of men and women who later regret their decision and attempt to regain their fertility. It would be unrealistic to assume, however, that all such decisions will not be regretted; even with proper counselling and consideration of the implications of sterilization, a small number of people will still wish to reverse their decision, as their life situations may change markedly. Commissioners believe that this option should be available to them.

In light of all these considerations, as well as our findings reported in the next section with regard to risk, the Commission recommends that

> **106. IVF be offered as treatment only to women with a diagnosis of complete fallopian tube blockage resulting from disease, defect, or surgical sterilization. Prior tubal surgery should not be a prerequisite for IVF; the choice of procedure should be based on medical prognosis for that woman.**

and that

> **107. Variations of IVF, and IVF for diagnoses other than fallopian tube blockage, be offered only in the context of research, and that the Assisted Conception Sub-Committee of the National Reproductive Technologies Commission facilitate multicentre collaborative trials in this regard.**

Later in this chapter we return to the issue of the nature and scope of research required on variations of IVF and IVF for diagnoses other than blocked fallopian tubes before they could be considered for inclusion in the health care system.

Risks of IVF

The second factor the Commission assessed in examining whether and under what conditions IVF should be provided were the risks involved. As noted earlier, no medical procedure can ever be entirely risk-free. There is, however, a need to reduce the risk to the minimum acceptable level while maintaining effectiveness. The risks outlined in this section are the known effects of IVF, which include multiple pregnancies and the risks of the drugs and procedures surrounding IVF.

Multiple Pregnancies

Among the most serious risks of IVF are those associated with multiple pregnancy, a risk that is also associated with the use of the ovulation drugs, which are often used in conjunction with IVF (see Chapter 18). The usual practice in IVF is to transfer more than one zygote to the woman's uterus, as this increases the likelihood that at least one will implant; there have been reports of as many as seven zygotes being transferred at the same time, and often more than one implants and develops. Using American Fertility Society registry figures, which included both Canadian and U.S. data, the result of the practice is that about 30 percent of IVF deliveries, 24 percent of GIFT deliveries, and 23 percent of ZIFT deliveries are multiple, compared to a rate in the general population of about 1 percent. In fact, this way of counting understates the problem, as one confinement may give rise to several infants. For example, in Canada for 1991, although 23 percent of live birth confinements after IVF were multiple, one liveborn IVF child in three was part of a multiple

> In addition to these risks, there are the effects associated with hormonal stimulation, which cannot be guaranteed to be innocuous in the long term. Hormonal stimulation, resulting in multiple pregnancies that lead to complications for the child, is controversial. This practice produces headaches, fatigue, and insomnia, among other things, and is associated with the formation of ovarian cysts.
>
> Also, little is said about the disappointment of women for whom assisted reproduction has raised hope and led to feelings of failure and guilt after each unsuccessful try. [Translation]
>
> *Brief to the Commission from Ordre des infirmières et infirmiers du Québec, April 1991.*

birth (81 of 213 infants born after IVF or 38 percent). This is the more relevant statistic, because it is these individuals and their families who must deal with the consequences of multiple births.

Most of the multiple births reported in our survey of fertility programs were twins, with one set of triplets and one set of quadruplets. In a sample of this size (171 deliveries), however, no higher-order births would normally be expected — a set of triplets is expected to occur less than once in 10 000 deliveries, and a set of quadruplets less than once in a million deliveries.

Multiple pregnancies pose serious health risks for both women and their children. For women, multiple pregnancy increases the risk of anaemia, miscarriage, toxaemia, high blood pressure, kidney trouble, difficult delivery, and post-birth haemorrhage. In Canada, a woman carrying three or more fetuses usually spends the last 4 to 12 weeks of the pregnancy in hospital, and most undergo a Caesarian delivery with its attendant risks. Just as important, multiple pregnancies present risks for fetuses: miscarriage, accidents during delivery, and premature births are much more common in multiple pregnancies. Prematurity brings with it another risk — low birth weight. The incidence of low birth weight in the Canadian population is between 6 and 8 percent,[10] but studies have found that 12 percent of IVF singletons, 55 percent of IVF twins, and 94 percent of IVF triplet or higher-order births result in low birth weight (less than 2 500 grams). Moreover, one-third of triplets and higher-order births result in very low birth weight (less than 1 500 grams).[11]

The consequences of low birth weight can be serious and long-lasting: breathing problems are common in low birth weight infants, who are also more likely to have cerebral palsy, poor eyesight, short attention span, and poor learning skills as they grow up. Hyperactivity, reading difficulties, and poor coordination and motor skills in childhood are also more common. A three-year Canadian study of children with very low birth weights born between 1984 and 1986 found that 20 percent suffered some form of serious disability.[12] More recently, U.S. studies have shown that 25 percent[13] of very low birth weight children have serious disabilities, while an additional half have other problems, such as those requiring special education services.[14,15] In other words, a substantial proportion of very low

> Our triplets are IVF children. This was really the last thing we tried in an eight-year process of infertility treatments, infertility work-ups. And right from the first time I took Clomid®, I was informed that there was a chance of multiple births. And I interpreted that as twins. It didn't occur to me that people have triplets or quads or quints, it doesn't happen to anyone you know until you've had them yourself and then you do meet others.
>
> *S. Picard, Parents of Multiple Births Association of Canada, Public Hearings Transcripts, London, Ontario, November 2, 1990.*

birth weight children will need continuing attention or care in varying degrees for a good part of their lives.

In addition to posing risks to the physical health of women and children, then, the consequences of multiple births can also strain the psychological and social health of the family after birth and place additional demands on the health, education, and social services systems. Parents of multiple-birth children cope with demands on their time, energy, and finances that are much greater than those of other parents. Although there are few Canadian studies of multiple-birth families, parents of "multiples" told the Commission that they had paid a price in raising their children. Despite the joy most parents derive from having children, these parents also felt overwhelmed by the demands on them. Families often need the support of paid and volunteer caregivers after the children leave hospital. In addition to pressures on the family, multiple births also involve added costs for health and social services systems. Provincial health insurance, for example, pays for the woman's longer hospital stay before and after birth, for Caesarian delivery, and for extended neonatal intensive care for the children.

Recognizing the risks involved in multiple pregnancies and the fact that if too many embryos implant they are all likely to die, some IVF clinics (5 of the 16 surveyed by the Commission) offer a procedure known as selective reduction in the situation of multiple pregnancy; some embryos are aborted to give the others a chance to survive. As well as

> People seeking reproductive medical services need to be informed before making reproductive decisions ... There are long-term social consequences ... Recently the POMBA [Parents of Multiple Births Association] prepared a first-year cost comparison between a three-person family with one infant and families with triplets, quadruplets, and quintuplets. Our cost comparison showed that the first year... start-up costs of having triplets are $8 000 higher, quadruplets is $11 000 higher, and quintuplets is $16 000 higher than giving birth to a single baby. This cost comparison does not allow for transportation needs like the purchase of a van to properly facilitate four infant car seats safely within the law, the housing needs — our family ... had to move to a larger home — or paying for the cost of part-time paid assistance ... Because of [the] extraordinary time commitment involved in caring for three or more babies at once, our families also found it necessary for at least one of the parents to relinquish the security of a second income yet assume these extraordinary costs. All these unique additional stresses put the family at risk.
>
> *D. Launslager, Parents of Multiple Births Association of Canada, Public Hearings Transcripts, London, Ontario, November 2, 1990.*

ethical dilemmas, the procedure has risks, including loss of all the developing fetuses.

To avoid the physical and psychological risks of multiple pregnancy and selective reduction, Canadian associations of practitioners working in this field have recommended limits on the number of zygotes transferred, but they have not specified a standard. Most but not all IVF practitioners are now limiting the number of zygotes they transfer. Furthermore, the World Health Organization analysis of international data found that the live birth rate after IVF declines if more than three zygotes are transferred, and the guidelines of the European Society of Human Reproduction limit the number of embryos transferred to three.

After considering the health risks to women, fetuses, and children, the emotional and financial costs, and the dubious benefits of transferring larger numbers of embryos, the Commission recommends that

> **108. No more than three zygotes be transferred during IVF procedures, and then only after counselling of the couple to ensure that they understand the possibility and implications of having triplets. Patients should give their consent in writing if more than one zygote is to be transferred and should be assured that no more than three will be transferred.**

Drug Risks

Most patients at Canadian IVF clinics undergo "stimulated" cycles; that is, ovulation induction drugs are used to stimulate the woman's ovaries to produce more than one egg. This increases the chances of at least one viable embryo being created *in vitro* and means that some can be frozen for use in a future cycle, thus avoiding the need for additional egg retrieval at that time while still giving another chance at pregnancy. We discussed what is known about the risks of fertility drug use in Chapter 18. As we noted in that chapter, although ovulation induction drugs increase the number of eggs produced, their use can also make the uterus less hospitable to implantation; as a result, even if more zygotes can be created *in vitro*, fewer may survive transfer in a stimulated cycle.[16]

One Canadian clinic is currently conducting a trial to determine the effectiveness of "natural cycle" IVF without drugs; the one egg produced naturally during an unmedicated cycle is retrieved for fertilization. Although the drug risks are avoided and the uterus is more hospitable to implantation, only one egg is available for fertilization; thus, there is less of a chance of obtaining a viable zygote for transfer. U.S. statistics indicate that success rates for natural cycle IVF are increasing, but they are still less than half that of stimulated cycles.[17]

There is evidence, however, that the beneficial aspects of stimulated and unstimulated cycles can be combined to improve success rates and reduce risks. The ovaries are stimulated to produce multiple eggs, which are retrieved and fertilized and the zygotes cryopreserved until the woman's hormone levels have returned to normal. Then she has the opportunity to have one or two zygotes transferred, during several natural cycles if necessary, with only the one invasive egg retrieval procedure needed. Some believe that this is the only ethical way to perform IVF; drug risks are reduced, the chances of implantation are maximized, and only the most viable zygotes may be transferred. It is with this background that some physicians have expressed the view that cryopreservation of zygotes should be made mandatory in all IVF programs.

The question of whether frozen zygotes are as viable as fresh remains unanswered, but recent U.S. data show that the number of live births after fresh and frozen zygote transfer are similar.[18] Moreover, as cryo-preservation techniques are refined, rates of successful transfer are increasing.[19] There appears to be no increase in spontaneous abortion or birth anomalies compared to pregnancies established with fresh zygotes, although more evidence is still required to confirm this.

The Commission believes that the benefits offered by cryopreserving zygotes for later implantation in an unstimulated cycle outweigh the risks. Cryopreservation reduces the use of ovulation induction drugs, gives more transfer opportunities during several cycles, and thus increases the likelihood of implantation. It also reduces the risks of multiple births resulting from the transfer of larger numbers of zygotes. The Commission therefore recommends that

> **109. The Assisted Conception Sub-Committee of the National Reproductive Technologies Commission monitor developments and make recommendations regarding cryopreservation and natural cycle IVF as knowledge and practice evolve.**

Procedural Risks

All invasive procedures carry some risk of infection, bleeding, damage to internal tissues, and pain; IVF is no exception. In addition, the rate of extra-uterine pregnancies (ectopic or "tubal" pregnancies) — although quite low at a few percent — is still at least 25 times more common in IVF patients than in the general population. This may be because of the characteristics of IVF patients, however, rather than being a result of IVF

procedures. Many IVF patients
have tubal problems, are older,
and have had trouble conceiving,
so that the rate of ectopic pregnancy would be expected to be
higher even if IVF had not been
used. The Commission believes
that data on the incidence of
these various outcomes following
IVF use — both ovulation induction and the procedure itself —
should be collected by all facilities offering IVF. Having this
information available will facilitate more informed decision
making by patients, practitioners, regulators, and policy makers.

> In the *in vitro* clinic where I am a
> consultant, only one couple of the 185
> I have seen decided against IVF when
> informed of the profound physical,
> emotional, and financial costs which
> are part and parcel of the treatment.
> For me this underscores the emotional
> intensity of the infertility experience.
>
> *P. Gervaize, private citizen, Public*
> *Hearings Transcripts, Ottawa, Ontario,*
> *September 18, 1990.*

Psychosocial Effects of Treatment

Being treated for infertility is stressful and difficult for couples.
Sociological studies carried out for the Commission showed high stress
levels in couples involved in IVF treatment. How much of this stress is
attributable to the treatment process and how much results from their
infertility are hard to disentangle. An examination of 686 couples
undergoing IVF found that patients ranked higher than the general
population on a list of 29 symptoms of psychological distress. Although IVF
treatment places couples under greater than normal pressure in a very
personal part of their lives, the study also found that the vast majority of
couples were well adjusted in terms of marital happiness (see research
volume, *Treatment of Infertility: Current Practices and Psychosocial
Implications*). This supports the findings of other studies showing that
infertility does not have a significant effect on the quality of marital life, but
rather has indirect negative effects by lowering individuals' self-esteem and
sense of control over their lives. The stress of repeated failures of treatment
is particularly difficult for couples to deal with.

Social support, or the lack of it, plays an important role in reducing or
adding to the stress felt by couples in treatment. Couples reported three
common stress-causing situations: friends or family members asking each
month whether the woman was pregnant yet; hints that the couple needed
only to "relax" to get pregnant; and suggestions of folk cures to increase the
couple's fertility. Women were more likely than their partners to discuss
their infertility with others, but most women and men reported that they
were not interested in taking part in support groups.

Since the female partners in couples undergoing IVF experience the
most painful and invasive aspects of diagnostic and treatment procedures,
not surprisingly women undergoing IVF report more stress than men do.

Women also said they feared being dropped from the program if their bodies did not seem to be responding normally to treatment, and this created stress as well. The male partners tended to report more negative consequences on privacy and feelings of control.

Not all the psychosocial implications of IVF treatment are negative. The majority of IVF patients surveyed reported positive effects on their relationship with their partner and on their feelings about themselves. Even if treatment proved unsuccessful, they felt they had done everything they could to overcome their infertility.

Long-Term Outcomes

One of the repeated messages we heard from Canadians was the need for information about longer-term risks and outcomes following IVF. As with most new medical treatments, the lack of follow-up data on IVF makes it difficult to determine whether there are any long-term adverse effects on women or children. Although some infertility practitioners have made great efforts, at present no organization or agency in Canada gathers information on the outcomes after IVF or tracks its effects over time. As described in our research volumes, record-keeping practices vary markedly among clinics and practitioners, with some clinics not even having data on whether a given IVF procedure resulted in a live birth.

One of the questions that must be asked about IVF is whether it poses any risk to the children born through its use. The many studies to date show no increased risk of congenital anomalies in IVF infants. One Australian study revealed a higher incidence of neural tube defects, but this result has not been confirmed by other studies, including a large recent case-control study by the National Institute of Child Health and Human Development.[20] We have

> There should be some way of monitoring the future health of couples using the NRTs and the offspring born to them so that problems that occur can be tied back to those technologies and appropriate action taken.
>
> *D. Allen, private citizen, Public Hearings Transcripts, Toronto, Ontario, October 29, 1990.*

already alluded to the high incidence of low birth weight infants following IVF, and perinatal death is three to four times higher for IVF births than for other births.[21] Because the technology is relatively new, however, long-term tracking of large numbers of IVF children has not yet been possible — the oldest child born as a result of the procedure is now 15.

It is essential that data on IVF — on treatment cycles, immediate outcomes, and long-term outcomes — be collected in a systematic and consistent manner. Data are needed to evaluate whether there are longer-term implications for women and what the actual outcomes are with respect to the health of IVF children as they grow up. To assess these outcomes in the least intrusive manner would require linkage of coded IVF patient data bases with coded data on the same individuals from health-related and other data bases to draw conclusions about long-term outcomes for both women and their children (see section on Measuring Health Outcomes).

> The federal and provincial governments should provide the funds and resources to develop a "new reproductive technologies" data base.
>
> *Brief to the Commission from the Manitoba Association of Registered Nurses, January 7, 1991.*

In summary, the Commission's review of the effectiveness and risks of *in vitro* fertilization showed that IVF is effective for one diagnostic category only — complete fallopian tube blockage — and that the risks of the technology, though real, are manageable from the perspective of service providers through the establishment of guidelines for practice and the careful monitoring of individual patients as treatment proceeds. From the perspective of individuals seeking treatment, however, each patient must make a fully informed decision about whether the identified level of risk is acceptable to her. It is therefore essential that anyone contemplating treatment be fully informed of what is known and what is not known about risks. These issues are discussed later in this chapter (see section on Patient Information, Consent, and Counselling).

Issues in Current IVF Practice in Canada

Based on our analysis of the effectiveness and risks of IVF, the Commission has recommended that it be offered only for bilateral fallopian tube blockage. In keeping with our ethic of care, however, we are also concerned with the conditions under which treatment is offered.

The Commission investigated current practices in Canadian infertility programs through two surveys — one of the programs themselves, the other of patients who participated in those programs. As will become clear in the next few pages, our review of the way IVF is offered in Canada today shows that there is little consistency or uniformity in the IVF treatment community. Although professional organizations have set guidelines, and some physicians in the field have worked hard to try to ensure high standards and comprehensive reporting of data, it is clear that the current situation results in little standardization of practices, little accountability, and unacceptable record-keeping practices. Compliance with recommended standards is patchy, information is not collected in a format that allows comparison or aggregation of clinic data, and definitions of success vary widely, resulting in confusion for prospective patients and great difficulty in assessing outcomes. The Commission believes that this patchwork of practices and standards is detrimental to women and couples, prevents needed analysis of the results of IVF research and treatment, and makes meaningful comparison between clinics impossible.

It was this situation, as well as the potential for harm to Canadians if it is not rectified, that led Commissioners to recommend a system of mandatory licensing for clinics offering IVF and other assisted conception services, as well as an Assisted Conception Sub-Committee within the National Reproductive Technologies Commission to establish standards and guidelines to be adopted as conditions of licence and monitor developments in the field of IVF treatment and practices.

As a condition of licensing, centres would have to comply with guidelines to be established by the Assisted Conception Sub-Committee of the National Reproductive Technologies Commission. As outlined below, these would include such aspects as standards of practice, record-keeping procedures, and participation in national information gathering, the qualifications of practitioners employed by assisted conception programs, and standards for information provided to patients and informed consent procedures.

Licensing will achieve our goals of ensuring that the non-medical implications of IVF are considered, that country-wide standards for practices and procedures are set and complied with, and that appropriate record keeping occurs. The requirement of standardized record keeping will allow ongoing evaluation of outcomes so that results can be fed back into practice and used to inform prospective patients. The collection and publication of data in the National Commission's annual report will provide evidence that guidelines are being complied with. Licensing will also provide the opportunity for wider perspectives to be brought to bear in formulating guidelines. As in other areas, National Commission hearings of applications for assisted conception licences should be open to the public, with the opportunity for parties with relevant information to participate.

We base this recommendation for compulsory licensing of assisted conception facilities on our extensive review of current clinic practices, the conclusions of which are described below. The studies conducted for the Commission in the course of this review, which are available in the accompanying research volumes, suggested several areas Commissioners needed to address in our recommendations if treatment is to be provided in an ethical and beneficial way.

Although professional organizations have set guidelines, and some physicians in the field have worked hard to try to ensure high standards and comprehensive reporting of data, it is clear that the current situation results in little standardization of practices, little accountability, and unacceptable record-keeping practices.

Although for clarity we address these areas separately, they are not in reality separable — without good record keeping on clearly defined outcomes, effectiveness cannot be known and risks cannot be assessed. This means appropriate information cannot be given to patients and cannot be used to shape good practice, which requires

- adherence to practice standards;

- clear definitions of how success rates are calculated and used;

- appropriate record keeping on patients, procedures, and the results of treatment — at present data on clinic practices are not recorded in a standard manner, so it is impossible to know the number of people treated, the number of pregnancies, the number of confinements, or the number of live births. These data are needed not only for public policy but also to permit evaluation, development, and refinement of clinical standards;

- information about risks — we have some information about procedural and short-term risks but less information about long-term risks, and at present most clinics are not structuring their operations to provide the information that will enable these data to be gathered and analyzed;

- appropriate information provision, counselling, and consent procedures in clinics — at present some practices may be hindering people's ability to make informed choices about their options with respect to treatment and other strategies; and

- equitable access to treatment.

We consider each of these areas in turn.

Clinic Practices

The Commission's survey found many differences in the practices, standards, and protocols followed by IVF programs. Although the Canadian Fertility and Andrology Society has established guidelines for practice, there is no national body to require adherence to such standards or monitor the provision of services. In addition, IVF programs change over time, as the director and staff at each clinic make independent

> Some flexibility and variation in practice may be needed to take individual situations into account, but what emerges clearly from our study is a picture of large differences in practice and procedures across the country.
>
> *T. Stephens and J. McLean, "Survey of Canadian Fertility Programs," in Research Volumes of the Commission, 1993.*

decisions about policy, protocols, procedures, and services offered as part of their program.

For example, half the programs surveyed did not limit the number of times IVF could be attempted, but 7 of the 16 limited patients to fewer than five cycles. Whether a "rest" between cycles (to allow the woman's body to return to normal before another IVF attempt) was required also differed from program to program, with three programs requiring patients to wait more than three months between IVF attempts, six clinics requiring a three-month wait, six programs requiring two months, and one clinic specifying one month.

One clinic reported that it offered patients "natural cycle" transfer, cryopreserving all zygotes for three months to allow the woman's body to return to normal after ovulation induction, then transferring them to her uterus during an unstimulated cycle. One other clinic offered natural cycle IVF with fresh zygotes; only the one naturally produced egg is fertilized and transferred.

We also found variations in clinic practices with respect to whether they used donated gametes (sperm and eggs) and whether they offered cryopreservation of zygotes (and thus whether they could offer natural cycle IVF) (Table 20.3). In the five clinics offering cryopreservation, time limits on zygote storage ranged from four months to 10 years, and one clinic's policy was to store them until the woman who was the source of the eggs used to create the zygotes had turned 60.

Table 20.3. Services Offered at 16 IVF Programs, 1991	
IVF-ET	15
GIFT	6
ZIFT	2
IVF with donor sperm	13
IVF with donor egg/embryo	8
IVF surrogacy	1
Selective reduction	5
Embryo cryopreservation	5
Embryo genetic diagnosis	2

Source: Stephens, T., and J. McLean. "Survey of Canadian Fertility Programs," Table 1. In Research Volumes of the Royal Commission on New Reproductive Technologies, 1993.

"Success" Rates

Given that we found insufficient evidence to conclude whether IVF is effective for most indications, concerns about how "success" rates are calculated and used by IVF clinics come into sharper focus.   Many Canadians appearing before the Commission questioned the accuracy and reliability of the success rates quoted by IVF clinics, expressed concern that the methods used to calculate success rates were misleading to prospective participants in IVF programs, and asked the Commission to determine why different IVF clinics and practitioners quote such widely varying rates for the effectiveness of their procedures.

Measuring and Reporting "Success" Rates

"Success" in IVF treatment is defined differently by patients, by clinics, and by practitioners, which creates confusion for patients and policy makers alike.   As a result, prospective patients cannot assess their likelihood of having a child through the use of IVF. Without clearly defined and universally used definitions of success, it is impossible to know what is being compared — is it successful fertilization, a clinical pregnancy, or a live birth — and meaningful evaluation is impossible. People are misled about their probability of having a child when "success" rates are quoted with no frame of reference. Couples considering IVF should have access to objective information about the record of a clinic in treating conditions comparable to their own, as well as overall effectiveness rates at various clinics for the treatment they are contemplating, given their diagnosis.

In response to concerns raised about this situation in the United States, the U.S. Congress, which had heard testimony from the Federal Trade Commission that the success rates claimed by IVF clinics (up to 80 percent success in some cases) routinely misled couples who are infertile and considering IVF, passed a law in 1992.   The legislation, which will come into effect in 1994, will initiate an accreditation program to ensure uniformity in the definition of success and in the measurement of success rates.   Accreditation of the approximately 200 private IVF clinics in the United States will be accorded only to programs that define their success rates in a standardized and clear way, based on the total number of patients treated, categorized by the age of the women treated and by the infertility diagnosis. The legislation will also ensure that clinics report the number of births following IVF (live births per cycle initiated; and live births per egg retrieval procedure). As we have seen, unless these definitions are clear, such statistics can be misleading because of the frequency of multiple births following IVF.

Consumer protection is not the only aspect to be considered, however. Records on outcomes and complications are also needed to guide practice and for research and policy making, to allow analysis that gives rise to better decisions about whether a procedure should be offered as treatment, whether it should be abandoned, whether it should be considered experimental, and whether it should be an insured medical service.

Record-Keeping Practices

The Commission investigated the record-keeping practices of Canadian clinics. The "success" rates at a particular clinic may be much higher or lower than the average for all clinics solely because of differences in the characteristics of its patient group. Probably for similar reasons there are great differences in the success rates quoted between countries — even if the procedures used are identical.[22] Thus, simply knowing a clinic's overall success rate is not sufficient to judge its record.

> The accuracy and completeness of record-keeping, and the categories by which statistics are collected, leave much to be desired in many programs. This makes it difficult to judge the outcomes and quality of service being delivered. The varied and often unclear ways in which success rates are defined by different clinics make it hard for potential patients to assess programs, and mean that consent may not be fully informed.
>
> *T. Stephens and J. McLean, "Survey of Canadian Fertility Programs," in Research Volumes of the Commission, 1993.*

We found that, in Canada, clinics record data on patients and procedures, define success, and calculate success rates differently from one to another, making it impossible to compare or analyze the effectiveness of IVF on a national or international basis. Half the IVF programs surveyed by the Commission defined success as achieving pregnancy (8 of 16), but four different definitions of pregnancy were used (results from a blood test; evidence of conception from ultrasound scanning; a urine test; or a tissue test). Other clinics defined success as live birth (6 of 16), egg retrieval and fertilization (1 of 16), or embryo transfer (1 of 16). The clinics also conveyed information to patients about their chances of success in different ways; 6 of the 16 clinics gave a percent chance of pregnancy based on a certain number of cycles or embryos transferred. Some clinics (4 of 16) gave patients a percentage without specifying a number of cycles or embryos transferred. Others told patients their chances of a live birth per cycle, per egg retrieved, or per embryo transferred. These differing methods of calculation led to "success rates" ranging from 10 percent at some clinics to 26 percent at others, but in no way are these rates comparable to each other.

To complicate the picture still further, we found clinics use different definitions of "cycle," making it impossible to determine how many treatment cycles were actually initiated for every live birth that occurred. Some clinics (6 of 16) defined "cycle" as ovulation induction, some (2 of 16) defined it as egg retrieval and fertilization, while others (5 of 16) defined a cycle as having occurred only if the embryo transfer stage was reached. Most clinics also did not keep records on the outcomes of treatment by specific diagnostic indications (such as tubal blockage, unexplained infertility, etc.). Current methods of calculating success rates are outlined in Table 20.4.

Table 20.4. Different Success Rate Definitions in Current Use in Canada

Number of clinical pregnancies per	patient entering program
	patient receiving treatment
	treatment cycle initiated
	egg retrieved
	embryo transferred
Number of confinements (e.g., triplets counted as 1) per	patient entering program
	patient receiving treatment
	treatment cycle initiated
	egg retrieved
	embryo transferred
Number of children born (e.g., triplets counted as 3) per	patient entering program
	patient receiving treatment
	egg retrieved
	embryo transferred

The Commission's survey of 750 past and current IVF patients across Canada confirmed the findings of the clinic survey. Most patients (80 percent) were given a percent chance of pregnancy, not of live birth. A few (8 percent) said they were not told their chances of pregnancy. Some said they were given a percentage, but they "were not sure how it applied," while others were told simply that there was a "high success rate." Although most were told their chances of pregnancy were less than 25 percent, 62 percent of patients said they were confident or very confident that their treatment would result in the birth of a child.

Commissioners understand the need for clinics to record results at various endpoints — this enables practitioners to understand where in the process problems and obstacles are occurring and allows them to adjust their practices accordingly. However, the current variations in the way clinics record their results and calculate the rate of various outcomes preclude any substantive analysis of effectiveness and have led to a situation where policy and treatment decisions must be based on limited and deficient data.

Patients should not be put in the position of having to make a decision about participating in IVF treatment based on false assumptions about their chances of having a child. For couples who are infertile, the birth of a child is the measure of success; it is therefore misleading to present success rates based on the number of clinical pregnancies, as half the Canadian IVF clinics do, because only 70 percent of clinical pregnancies end in live births. It is also misleading to base success rates on the total number of children born, because multiple births inflate that rate. Similarly, it is inappropriate to give prospective patients figures based on the number of eggs retrieved or zygotes transferred, as fewer than half the patients treated actually reach the embryo transfer stage. It is also important to give patients a context for the rates quoted, as some clinics will not have treated enough patients with a particular diagnosis to make meaningful predictions for a given couple. Thus, it is also important for patients to have access to national data about the results of treatment with IVF (or a related technology) for their diagnostic category.

Patients are most interested in the likelihood of the birth of a healthy child, but for some this is not the only measure of success; for some women, simply achieving pregnancy represents an affirmation of their capacity to do so. Whatever their personal definition of success, patients need clearly explained and standard measures of the likelihood that treatment will result in particular outcomes — especially live birth. This measure must be the same from clinic to clinic. Thus, the Commission concurs with the World Health Organiza-

> Patients' expectations of having a baby were generally substantially higher than the estimates provided to them by the clinics. This finding, as well as the fact that patients want to know their probability of success, points to the need for more explicit, formal systems for informing patients.
>
> *SPR Associates Inc., "An Evaluation of Canadian Fertility Clinics: The Patient's Perspective," in Research Volumes of the Commission, 1993.*

tion recommendation that the most appropriate rates to use from patients' perspective are the number of live births and the number of pregnancies per 100 treatment cycles initiated at a clinic.[23] Because most clinics do not treat enough patients with similar diagnoses and of similar ages to produce reliable figures, ideally patients should also be given national statistics on the number of live births per 100 treatment cycles initiated in couples with a similar diagnosis and age of the female partner. Such statistics should be included in the National Commission's annual report. The Commission therefore recommends that

> **110. As a condition of licence, all IVF programs collect, maintain, and report to the National Reproductive Technologies Commission annual statistics on pregnancies per 100 treatment cycles initiated and live births per 100 treatment cycles initiated at that clinic.**

> **111. All IVF programs assemble and submit annual statistics on live births per cycle initiated by the age and diagnostic indication of each woman treated with IVF. These statistics should be published and distributed to contributing clinics in an accessible form for use in patient information materials.**

and that

> **112. The success rate used by all clinics in patient information materials relate only to the chances of live birth per treatment cycle initiated.**

Physicians are interested in rates of particular outcomes at various stages of a treatment, to help clarify what is working and at what stage. Knowing where problems occur in the treatment process enables problems to be addressed and improvements to be made. Thus, physicians need outcome data on a range of factors: whether elevated hormone levels are present; whether ovulation has occurred; whether egg extraction has been successful; whether eggs have been fertilized; whether zygotes have been transferred and have implanted successfully; whether biochemical pregnancy occurs; and whether clinical pregnancy results. Information on whether pregnancies are carried to term, whether they are multiple, and whether live birth results is also essential, as is information about the health of the resulting children. Outcome rates for these events can be calculated using different denominators — for example, the relevant outcome per number of stimulation cycles, per number of treatments attempted, or per 100 *in vitro* fertilization cycles attempted or completed — but these rates will be for specialized use by those working in this field.

Funders and policy makers have still different needs with respect to data collection. They are interested, for example, in the costs to the health care and social service systems of particular treatments. This may include costs associated with the treatment itself, such as drugs, hospital days, and physician fees for specific services. It may also include costs associated with treatment complications, such as spontaneous losses, pre-term delivery, low birth weight, multiple births, and the continuing costs associated with chronic illness or disability. This information helps to form an assessment of the opportunity costs of allocating public resources to a treatment and its effects, relative to directing them to other public sector purposes. This assessment is part of the process taxpayers expect policy makers and funders to complete if they are to be accountable for their responsible use of public resources.

The Commission concludes that it is essential for all IVF programs to collect data that allow rates for various outcomes to be calculated in a standard and comparable way. The International Working Group for Registers on Assisted Reproduction has developed a comprehensive and useful model to collect information and has been perfecting this model since 1987. Some Canadian practitioners have made strenuous and commendable attempts to develop a Canadian registry using this model, but participation by most of the treatment community has been haphazard, with only 2 of 16 clinics submitting data in 1991. The organization created in 1991 to collect the data, the Canadian Voluntary Registry Association, could not secure adequate funding and has since dissolved.

> Some Canadian practitioners have made strenuous and commendable attempts to develop a Canadian registry using this model, but participation by most of the treatment community has been haphazard, with only 2 of 16 clinics submitting data in 1991.

Commissioners believe that the model proposed by the International Working Group is a good basis on which to begin collecting the relevant data for analysis and output in various forms to meet the needs of patients, practitioners, researchers, and policy makers. This model could serve as a basis on which to begin consistent country-wide record keeping on IVF practice in Canada. The Commission therefore recommends that

> **113. All facilities offering IVF be required, as a condition of licence, to provide information in standard form to the Assisted Conception Sub-Committee of the National Reproductive Technologies Commission, which will maintain a data base building on the model of the International Working Group for Registers on Assisted Reproduction.**

Measuring Health Outcomes

We have already alluded to the need to fill the many gaps in our knowledge about the outcomes of IVF and of the use of drugs to stimulate ovulation. As IVF and other reproductive technologies could potentially affect the next generation, it is essential that their effects be monitored and evaluated taking this into account. Monitoring encompasses the reporting of data, the tracking of selected outcomes or indicators over time, and the independent audit of these data. This process provides feedback information useful in setting licensing conditions and regulating the provision of services and in the development of practice guidelines.

The need for information about whether IVF has long-term health consequences is not being met by current systems and mechanisms. It would be possible, however, to assess health outcomes in those affected or potentially affected by fertility treatment (patients and their children) by linking their records to other population-based data banks on health outcomes, such as hospitalization data and vital statistics data. As the information needs in this area are similar for all infertility treatments, the Commission's proposals on how best to obtain information on long-term outcomes are dealt with elsewhere in the report (see Chapter 18).

Clinic Staff

In teaching hospitals, the IVF program usually falls under the responsibility of the department of obstetrics and gynaecology. Most IVF programs employ a director, a nurse/coordinator, administrative staff, and treatment teams of physicians, technicians, and other personnel. If laboratory services are offered on-site, then a laboratory manager and technicians are also part of the program staff. Some clinics also employ the services of a social worker or counsellor.

The Commission was told that IVF patients are usually assigned to an attending physician upon acceptance into the program, and he or she makes the final decisions with the couple about the couple's treatment. Attending physicians usually have a treatment team, consisting of an assistant physician, an administrator, and a nurse/clinician. In most cases it is the nurse/clinician who supervises women during ovulation induction, while the physicians (usually gynaecologists) perform egg retrieval and embryo transfer.

We believe that any assisted conception program should include, as a minimum, personnel with the following expertise:

- An individual with training and experience in reproductive endocrinology, particularly in the use of ovulation-inducing agents and the hormonal control of the menstrual cycle. An individual who has a certificate of competence in reproductive endocrinology and infertility from the Royal College of Physicians and Surgeons, or the equivalent, would fulfil this requirement.

- An individual with expertise in laparoscopic techniques and in ultrasound-guided egg retrieval techniques.

- A director of the embryology laboratory with personal experience in the organization and maintenance of a basic or clinical embryology laboratory as well as in tissue culture techniques.

- An ultrasonographer (or obstetrician/gynaecologist with specialized training and experience in gynaecologic sonography) who provides the monitoring of follicular development and supervises ultrasound-directed egg retrieval.

- A designated overall program director. If the overall program director is not a licensed physician, then there must be a designated medical director who is responsible for the clinical aspects of the treatment program.

- Nursing and support staff sufficient to perform the counselling and record-keeping functions necessary for licensing.

A single individual could fulfil the requirement for expertise in one area or more. It is also important that the clinic have available referral to social services to assist in counselling if such trained individuals are not on clinic staff.

The Commission believes that this list, adapted from the guidelines of the American Fertility Society, offers a reasonable basis on which to develop guidelines for Canadian clinics. The Commission therefore recommends that

> **114. The Assisted Conception Sub-Committee of the National Reproductive Technologies Commission establish, as a condition of licence, the requisite staff qualifications and expertise for facilities offering IVF and related services.**

Patient Information, Consent, and Counselling

Information provision, consent to treatment, and counselling procedures that enable patients to make informed choices about their care are important components of IVF services. The ideal situation for patients is to be given full information about their treatment options in the context of other options — such as adoption or coming to terms with not having children. Counselling and social support are also needed to evaluate and weigh the options fully and make choices about treatment in light of what is important to them personally. Informed choice is best assured when decisions about treatment are shared between patients and physicians.

Individual decisions about IVF are complex. Some aspects involve the assessment of technical information as the basis for an appropriate decision, while other aspects contributing to the decision must be based on women's and couples' values, goals, and priorities. Technical information may also be inconclusive, lacking, or unhelpful in reaching some decisions, which are neither straightforward nor solely health care decisions. While patients themselves are in the best position to evaluate their own needs, beliefs, and resources in relation to the expected results of treatment, the practitioner has greater knowledge and experience with the technical aspects of treatment and its results. Both types of knowledge — the patient's and the practitioner's — need to be brought to bear in a partnership to allow the patient to make choices about treatment.

Studies have concluded that facilitating women's and couples' capacity to assume a more active role in their care improves the results of treatment.[24] This may be related to patients' increased sense of control and the fact that they are more likely to comply with any requirements of treatment if they have had an active role in decisions surrounding it. More active patient participation in treatment and more effective communication between patient and doctor may also enable practitioners to monitor the effects of treatment more accurately and hence to make adjustments as appropriate to improve the results of treatment. A lack of information or choice may have a detrimental effect, by increasing the patient's anxiety about treatment and its results.

To assess the quality of information and informed consent protocols now in use in Canadian infertility programs, the Commission analyzed patient information materials provided by 16 IVF programs. Researchers evaluated the readability of English-language materials and judged the reading level required to understand them. We found that, overall, IVF patients receive more information and better counselling than patients receiving assisted insemination or other treatments. In addition, informed consent procedures in IVF programs are generally more detailed and documented than those in other types of infertility treatment. We also found, however, that there was no uniformity in programs' information and procedures and that many did not measure up to the standard of informed choice for patients.

Patient Information Materials

The Commission heard repeatedly, from individuals and groups with varying views of IVF, about the need for high-quality, readable, and readily understandable information for people considering or undergoing the procedure. Lack of information was seen as seriously hindering people's ability to make informed choices. Providing such information enables patients to participate more fully in their treatment. It does not, however, remove the onus from practitioners. The burden of providing quality care rests with health care professionals. It is their responsibility to ensure that medical treatments are provided in a safe and ethical manner. Good information is a vital component of this. The Commission considers it unethical not to explain procedures and to ensure that patients understand the implications of procedures that may not have occurred to them.

Women undergoing IVF told the Commission that four areas of information were most important to them: their personal chances of having a child as a result of treatment (85 percent of those surveyed); the long-term effects of treatment (82 percent); the emotional demands of treatment (81 percent); and short-term effects of treatment (80 percent). Fewer than half the patients surveyed were satisfied with the information they received in these areas.

The information patients need to make informed decisions about their care includes the nature and objectives of the procedure and alternatives to it; the nature and probability of the known and possible consequences of the procedure; and the costs of the procedure. They also need to know that only qualified personnel will be offering the service. (The licensing system we propose will ensure that.)

Very few programs addressed all these aspects. Most of the information materials mentioned adoption as an alternative to IVF but did not give sources of information about it,[25] and one program did not inform patients about the costs they would incur as part of the IVF program.

The Commission also found that patient information materials were not written in readily understandable language. Although the nature of the subject matter is technical, and this makes it challenging to present in an easily understandable way, the materials could be made more readable with help of those expert in communicating technical information to a non-technical audience. For example, essential technical vocabulary could be identified and defined, and efforts could be made to identify patients' information needs and design the contents of the material accordingly. Researchers have found, for example, that

> The use of a clinical, technical style in conveying medical information is not unusual ... It reflects the kind of technical, scientific writing with which most health ... professionals are comfortable and familiar. It uses the passive voice, deals with facts rather than feelings, and is concerned primarily with transmitting information rather than experience.
>
> *J. Wood Catano, "An Assessment of the Readability of Patient Education Materials Used by Genetic Screening Clinics," in Research Volumes of the Commission, 1993.*

people have more difficulty absorbing information when they are in anxiety-producing or stressful situations. It would be appropriate, therefore, if IVF programs could get expert assistance in writing the material to be given to patients to ensure that they are completely informed in a sensitive and compassionate way.

One of the characteristics affecting patients' understanding of the information materials was the general style of the writing. Our analysis showed that most information about IVF was written in a very clinical and directive style, inadvertently conveying the message that patients could not hope to understand this complicated treatment, but should in any case comply with the directions of clinic staff. Our analysis concluded that a more informal and less directive style would be easier for most patients to understand and would reflect a commitment by clinics to promoting patients' informed choice.

Although every question patients might have cannot be anticipated and answered in written materials, written information should answer the basic questions about treatment. Gaps in existing research, evaluation, and record keeping may make it impossible to provide full information in all areas, but where information needs cannot be met, materials written for patients should state explicitly that reliable data are not available. Therefore, the Commission recommends that

> **115. The Assisted Conception Sub-Committee of the National Reproductive Technologies Commission, in consultation with relevant professional and lay groups, develop standard information materials explaining IVF procedures; and that these materials be analyzed for readability, content, and non-directiveness and distributed routinely to all patients accepted into IVF programs as a basis for discussion between patients, practitioners, and counsellors. Patients should be given time to discuss and fully comprehend information materials before any treatment is initiated.**

Consent Procedures

It is standard medical practice and a legal requirement to obtain consent to treatment from patients, indicating that they are fully informed about, and agree to, the treatment course outlined by the attending physician. We found no standard procedure at Canada's IVF programs for obtaining informed consent; policies vary widely from clinic to clinic. Some have detailed written consent forms for each stage or procedure in the IVF process; at the other extreme, one clinic gained written consent for only one procedure (egg retrieval), considering all others routine medical care for which consent is implied by consent to egg retrieval.

Consent procedures should entail the following elements or criteria:

- the patient must be legally competent to consent to treatment;
- the patient must possess the mental capacity to authorize care;
- the patient must receive proper disclosure of information from the caregiver;
- the authorization should be specific to the procedure to be performed;
- the patient should have an opportunity to ask questions and to receive understandable answers;
- the authorization obtained should be free of undue influence and coercion; and
- the authorization obtained should be free of misrepresentation of material information.

**Types of Consent Forms Completed by
IVF Patients***

▲ Authorization for surgery (standard consent form)
▲ Consent to drug therapy
▲ Consent for results of treatment to be used in a study/trial of treatment
▲ Consent to IVF (verifies that alternatives have been considered and patient is free to withdraw from treatment at any time)
▲ Consent to egg retrieval
▲ Consent to cryopreservation and disposition of embryos (outlines clinic's protocols with respect to embryos)
▲ Authorization for embryo transfer
▲ Authorization for release of information (for research)

---

* Not all forms are completed by all patients; consent procedures and forms vary from clinic to clinic.

Although the Commission's survey of IVF patients showed that they were more likely to experience a rigorous consent procedure than were patients undergoing other types of treatment, the consent forms they were given were difficult to read and understand. The forms used by four programs (4 of 16) were rated as requiring at least one graduate degree to understand, while six others were rated as requiring at least two years of post-secondary education. It was also disturbing that many of the forms required patients to consent to procedures that were not explained in the information materials provided. In addition, few patients were told that consent could be withdrawn at any time, nor were they given copies of the signed consent forms. Therefore, the Commission recommends that

> **116. The Assisted Conception Sub-Committee of the National Reproductive Technologies Commission develop standard patient consent materials to be distributed routinely to all patients accepted into IVF programs as a basis for discussion between patients, practitioners, and counsellors.**

> **117. Patients should be given time to discuss and fully comprehend the meaning and implications of consent to treatment before any treatment is initiated. They should be given copies of all consent forms they sign and should be informed of their right to withdraw consent at any stage of treatment without jeopardizing future care or treatment.**

and that

> **118. Adherence to these standards should be a condition of licence for facilities offering IVF.**

Counselling

Counselling is a central issue in the provision of infertility treatment. Although two-thirds of IVF programs have a counselling specialist on staff, such as a psychologist or social worker, the patients we surveyed found this aspect of their experience at the clinics the least satisfying. They told the Commission that they would have liked more counselling, especially during and after treatment.

Most of the information gathered by the Commission indicates that the majority of IVF clinics use the terms "counsel" and "educate" interchangeably. In some clinics, the role of "counsellor" was filled by in-house doctors, nurses, and administrators. It was not clear whether any of these staff members had specialized training in infertility or medical counselling.

Some of the clinics indicated that they would refer couples to outside counselling if it was requested, if staff members observed "inappropriate" behaviour during treatment, or if a history of physical or sexual abuse was suspected. Other clinics organized self-help groups for patients and encouraged patients to contact local or national infertility support groups.

Most programs offered professional counselling only when the patient requested it specifically, but one clinic reported that 94 percent of IVF patients took advantage of professional counselling when it was offered. The Commission's survey of patients indicated a similar desire for counselling; patients told the Commission they wanted more time to discuss their treatment with physicians or professional counsellors. In particular, post-treatment counselling was identified as important; 80 to 91 percent of those who did not receive post-treatment counselling would have wanted it. Many patients would have liked more counselling both during and after treatment; only 35 percent were satisfied with the counselling they received, and only 31 percent were satisfied with the counselling offered to their partners.

As we have recommended elsewhere, supportive counselling should be available on referral from infertility clinics if a social worker/counsellor is not attached to the clinic. The Commission therefore recommends that

> **119. Counselling be an integral part of assisted conception services and be offered either on-site or by referral to appropriate professionals.**

and that

> **120. Standard written materials to be used in counselling be developed and made available by the Assisted Conception Sub-Committee. These materials should include information about alternatives to medical treatment, such as adoption and living without children; avoiding exposure to risk factors that could affect the results of treatment (for example, smoking); some exploration of questions related to values and goals that patients may wish to factor into decisions; and the physical and psychological effects of treatment.**

Access to Treatment

Two factors that could constitute barriers to IVF for some people are the cost of treatment and the location of IVF programs. Our recommendations with respect to the inclusion of IVF in provincial health care systems for diagnoses for which it has been demonstrated effective will go some way toward addressing the financial barriers to access. Even when a service is insured, however, other costs are involved, such as unpaid time away from work, travel, and accommodation costs, the costs of related services or treatments (particularly drugs), and so on. Canada is a large country; it is not appropriate that highly specialized services such as IVF be provided in every area, and, consequently, a service may not be available close to a prospective user. Some provinces are taking measures to assist in this regard when people live in remote communities. As Canadians pointed out in our public hearings, however, cost and distance are not the only barriers.

Two other types of potential barriers to access to new reproductive technologies emerged in our hearings and research. The first were criteria used by the clinics themselves to refuse treatment. We found that possible and probable reasons for refusing IVF treatment varied from clinic to clinic. Some of these criteria may be appropriate, given that age, diagnostic category, duration of infertility, and other characteristics may affect the results of treatment. However, other reasons given by clinics for refusing treatment bear no relation to the likelihood of having a child (see Table 20.5).

Table 20.5. Possible or Probable Reasons Clinics Would Refuse Patients for IVF Treatment, 1991

	Teaching hospital (11)	Private and other (5)
Doubtful parenting ability	8	3
Psychological immaturity	5	3
Unmarried (with partner)	0	0
Unmarried (no partner)	7	3
Lesbian	7	2
Below average intelligence	2	1
Physically disabled	3	2
Other living children	2	1
Low income	1	0
Province of residence	1	1
Country of residence	1	1
Other	2	1
Not stated	1	0

Source: Stephens, T., and J. McLean. "Survey of Canadian Fertility Programs," Table 16. In Research Volumes of the Royal Commission on New Reproductive Technologies, 1993.

In the Commission's estimation, policies and guidelines should not be arbitrary, they should be applied to everyone equally, and they should not be misused in a discriminatory way to deny services. Lack of a partner, sexual orientation, or disability should not be reasons in and of themselves to deny access, yet, as Table 20.5 shows, they clearly are in some clinics.

If a woman is diagnosed as having bilateral tubal blockage, we have recommended that she have access to IVF to treat it. As with any other medical service provided through the publicly funded health care system, this would be available whether she is married or single, heterosexual or homosexual. However, as the diagnosis of tubal blockage is usually made following a failure to conceive by natural means, it is likely that very few women not in heterosexual relationships would be aware that they have this problem. It is theoretically possible that a woman would find out, for instance, following failure to conceive using donor insemination, and in such a case there are no grounds for denying a single woman or a lesbian access to IVF using donor sperm as a medical treatment available to any woman with this diagnosis.

The second category of potential obstacles consists of factors in the health care delivery system that make gaining access to infertility services more difficult. For example, Canadians whose first language is neither English nor French may be reluctant to approach an infertility treatment program, or less likely to be able to make fully informed decisions if they do, if services are not designed with the pluralistic nature of Canadian society in mind. Similarly, level of education influences income, awareness, empowerment, and other attitudes and characteristics. These character-istics are significant factors in allowing people to negotiate the complex and unclear route to new reproductive technology services and therefore in gaining access to them.

Workplace policies can also influence access to services depending on whether paid sick leave or vacation leave is available and whether sick leave can be used when undergoing infertility treatment; the degree of flexibility in work schedules and the amount of time off that can be taken, when it can be taken, and how much notice is required; and the existence or nature of employer-sponsored supplementary health insurance (to cover services and drugs not included under public health insurance).

Admission policies are set by IVF clinic directors and treatment teams, and individual cases are usually decided upon by the attending physician and the rest of the treatment team. Our review of current practices showed that admission policies set by clinics do present barriers to treatment and that they vary from clinic to clinic. We found that speed of access to IVF also varies widely across Canada; private clinics and four of the five non-teaching hospitals had no waiting list at all. Patients at most (16 of 20) teaching hospitals, however, could expect to wait at least a week for an initial appointment, and five hospitals reported waiting lists of 30 weeks or more for treatment. Close to half the programs (7 of 16) told the

Commission, however, that they turned away fewer than 5 percent of applicants in 1991. Only one clinic reported that more than 10 percent of applicants were turned away. Most programs told applicants who were refused treatment about other clinics — referral to U.S. clinics was almost as common as referral to other Canadian programs. Six clinics said they did not refer to other programs.

Clinics told us that they accepted patients who had been infertile for varying lengths of time. Couples with a clear diagnosis of the cause of their infertility were accepted right away, but for couples with no clear diagnosis (about 20 percent of IVF patients have "unexplained" infertility), some clinics would allow admission after one year of infertility, while others accepted patients only after three years of infertility. Although most programs considered previous fertility treatment (fertility drug treatment or assisted insemination using the partner's sperm) before deciding to admit a patient to the IVF program, there were few fixed criteria in this regard. If there was no clear diagnosis — and if drugs or insemination with the partner's sperm had not worked — some clinics offered IVF as a method that might enable the couple to have a child related to them both.

Many groups and individuals told the Commission that upper middle class, well-educated, married couples are more likely than other people to use IVF treatment. The Commission's survey of patients based on voluntary return of questionnaires confirmed this. Of the 750 IVF patients surveyed by the Commission, 66 percent were employed full-time, 41 percent had professional occupations (compared with 31 percent of the general population), and 80 percent had annual family incomes over $50 000 (compared to 33.3 percent of the general population).

The Commission believes that no medical treatment offered through the publicly funded health care system should be limited to a select group of people. Although physicians may encounter instances where non-medical factors mean it is appropriate to refuse access, these instances should be rare, and the use of discriminatory criteria such as marital status, income, or sexual orientation in and of themselves to deny access violates fundamental constitutional and human rights guarantees. If the situation is one into which any child born would clearly be harmed, then a physician may in conscience refuse to provide access, but decisions about who is "worthy" of treatment should not be made in an ad hoc way using such discriminatory criteria by practitioners. The Commission therefore recommends that

> **121. Access to IVF treatment be determined on the basis of legitimate medical criteria, without discrimination on the basis of factors such as marital status, sexual orientation, or economic status.**

Referring Physicians

The physicians practising in the community — family or general practitioners and obstetricians/gynaecologists — are relevant to our consideration of the issues surrounding IVF for two reasons. First, these are the physicians usually consulted first by couples having difficulty conceiving. The doctor may offer to prescribe fertility drugs or to refer the couple to an infertility specialist or facility. We dealt with the issue of fertility drugs in an earlier chapter (see Chapter 18).   Here we are concerned with referral practices.

Our survey showed that twice as many patients reach a fertility clinic on referral from a gynaecologist as from a general practitioner (see Table 20.6). Patients are likely to have seen several different physicians before entry into an IVF program; sometimes they are referred from one professional to another over a period of years before they receive a firm diagnosis.   In the Commission's survey of patients, 86 percent had attempted previous fertility treatments before being admitted to an IVF program.

Table 20.6. Source of Referral to Clinic* (Sample Size 750 IVF Patients)	
Family physician/general practitioner	25%
Gynaecologist	52%
Self-referred	19%
Spouse/partner	7%
Friends	8%
Other family member	4%
Other specialist	2%
Other fertility clinic	4%
Other	1%

* Multiple responses were possible.

Source: SPR Associates Inc. "An Evaluation of Canadian Fertility Clinics: The Patient's Perspective," Figure 3.3. In Research Volumes of the Royal Commission on New Reproductive Technologies, 1993.

Shuttling patients needlessly from professional to professional is stressful and wastes valuable time and resources. It is doubly important, then, that gynaecologists and family practitioners have adequate information about the management of infertility, how to evaluate fertility effectively through history, examination, and infertility investigation, and how to assess whether referral to a fertility program is indicated.   The

Commission endorses the model for general practitioners proposed by the British Royal College of Obstetricians and Gynaecologists, which outlines the steps in evaluating fertility and the circumstances under which a referral to a fertility specialist is indicated. This useful guide sets out the steps involved in diagnosing infertility, the various risk factors for infertility, and the types of treatments available. It also provides guidance on counselling infertile patients. We find the model to be clear and logical and that it promotes responsible use of resources by discouraging premature or unnecessary referrals while ensuring a rational step-by-step approach to investigating and treating infertility. Such a guide may also be useful to those practising obstetricians and gynaecologists not focussing on infertility. The Commission therefore recommends that

> **122. A practical referral guide for general practitioners, modelled on that of the British Royal College of Obstetricians and Gynaecologists, be developed by the College of Family Physicians of Canada.**

and that

> **123. The guide be distributed widely and that knowledge of its content be examined in qualifying examinations for family practitioners.**

Priorities for IVF Research

Fallopian tube blockage is the only indication for which IVF has been demonstrated effective; the evidence now available is insufficient to permit a determination of effectiveness for all other uses. Any use of IVF to treat other diagnoses must, therefore, be done only in the context of research, so that these uses can be evaluated further in well-designed research studies before being considered for inclusion in the health care system as medical treatment.

Several factors differentiate clinical trials from standard medical services. In particular, clinical trials require prior ethical review, a more rigorous consent procedure for patients, and funding from research agencies, as opposed to health care budgets. Commissioners believe that any clinical trials done with the participation of licensed clinics should be funded at arm's length from organizations with a vested interest in the results (for example, pharmaceutical companies).

The Medical Research Council already has guidelines for research involving human subjects, which include, among other aspects, full disclosure of the nature of the research and counselling about the known and potential risks of the experimental treatment, leading to informed consent on the part of participants. The clinical trials necessary to assess the effectiveness of IVF treatment for diagnoses other than tubal blockage should comply with these guidelines.

As IVF and related technologies have developed, they have sometimes been referred to as "innovative therapy." In the Commission's view, this is misleading to prospective patients. A procedure is not "therapy" unless it has been shown to be of demonstrable benefit; experimental treatments should not move from the realm of research to the realm of therapy unless and until effectiveness and risks have been identified. Providing treatment under the guise of "innovative therapy" thus has two undesirable consequences, both arising from the fact that it involves the provision of experimental treatment outside the context of research, with its concomitant standards and protections for research subjects.

First, "innovative therapy" may expose women to risk without their full awareness that the treatment is not of proven benefit and may have unknown risks. Second, "innovative therapy," provided in an ad hoc way by individual practitioners working independently, will never generate the answers patients, practitioners, and policy makers need about the effectiveness and risks of treatment; thus, it creates a situation where women are being exposed to risk, sometimes unknowingly, without the data being gathered that could, when aggregated with data on others, provide the knowledge on which to base evaluation or further refinement of the technology. In the Commission's view, therefore, if IVF and related technologies are to be provided ethically and beneficially, this must be either as treatment or as research, depending on the current state of the evidence. The rubric "innovative therapy" must not be allowed to obscure this fundamental means of protecting the health and well-being of women and children.

> The Commission sees the development of multicentre randomized control trials as one essential approach to clarify the effectiveness of IVF for diagnostic categories other than tubal blockage, and to ensure progress in the field while minimizing unnecessary exposure to risk. These trials will help to ensure that couples with negligible chances of success do not waste precious time, energy, and resources on IVF or incur the risks without a probability of benefit.

As to the form this research should take, the Commission sees the development of multicentre randomized control trials as one essential approach to clarify the effectiveness of IVF for diagnostic categories other than tubal blockage, and to ensure progress in the field while minimizing unnecessary exposure to risk. These trials will help to ensure that couples with negligible chances of success do not waste precious time, energy, and resources on IVF or incur the risks without a probability of benefit.

One priority for research is whether IVF and GIFT are effective treatments for couples with unexplained infertility of more than three years' duration. Preliminary results indicate this may be the case. Although the conventional wisdom among practitioners currently favours GIFT, there is in fact no concrete evidence demonstrating that it is more effective than IVF — or, indeed, than no treatment at all — in increasing the likelihood of pregnancy in cases of unexplained infertility. Therefore, the Commission recommends that

> **124. IVF and GIFT be evaluated for the treatment of three-year unexplained infertility in the context of a randomized control trial organized by licensed IVF clinics, facilitated by the Assisted Conception Sub-Committee of the National Reproductive Technologies Commission and funded by provincial/territorial ministries of health.**

Although gamete intrafallopian transfer is contra-indicated in cases of tubal disease because of poor tubal function and the risk of ectopic pregnancy, after reviewing the evidence the Commission believes that a priority for research should be to determine the effectiveness of GIFT and the related technologies ZIFT and DOST for unexplained infertility. Preliminary results indicate they may be promising, and the Commission therefore recommends that

> **125. Randomized control trials be organized by licensed IVF clinics, facilitated by the Assisted Conception Sub-Committee of the National Reproductive Technologies Commission and funded by provincial/territorial ministries of health, to investigate the effectiveness of gamete intrafallopian transfer and zygote intrafallopian transfer as treatments for unexplained infertility.**

Using the criteria outlined earlier, there is not enough evidence to conclude whether IVF is effective or ineffective as a treatment for minimal, moderate, or severe endometriosis, unless the disease has resulted in blockage of the fallopian tubes. More data are needed before IVF can be assessed as a treatment for infertility associated with endometriosis. Therefore, the Commission recommends that

> **126. IVF for the treatment of minimal, moderate, and severe endometriosis that has not resulted in fallopian tube blockage be evaluated in a randomized control trial organized by licensed IVF clinics, facilitated by the Assisted Conception Sub-Committee of the National Reproductive Technologies Commission and funded by provincial/territorial ministries of health.**

There is no evidence that IVF is an effective treatment for ovulation disorders, and it is not biologically plausible that IVF would overcome a problem with ovulation — rather, appropriate diagnosis of hormonal problems and relevant fertility drug treatment make sense. IVF for infertility resulting solely from ovulation disorders is not a treatment that has been shown to be effective, it is not promising for the reasons just discussed, and it should not therefore be a priority for research.

We found that there is insufficient evidence to categorize IVF as either an effective or an ineffective treatment for cases in which the male partner has oligospermia (low sperm count). Further, it is not biologically plausible that IVF would overcome male-factor infertility, as the sperm must have the capacity to fertilize, whether *in vitro* or *in vivo*. Given as well the paucity of data demonstrating benefit, the Commission concludes that *in vitro* fertilization should not be offered as a treatment in cases of oligospermia. This conclusion is beginning to be recognized in practice — at least one major Canadian centre does not offer IVF if the male partner has a sperm count under 5 million, because the probability of fertilization is too low. We consider the procedure to have relatively little promise in such cases. It is not a treatment, and it should not be a priority for research.

Micromanipulation of the egg is currently being explored as a means of increasing the effectiveness of IVF in cases of oligospermia; micromanipulation (of necessity, in combination with *in vitro* fertilization) is of unproven benefit in such cases. Its risks are unknown, as relatively few live births have been documented to date. Although we recognize the possibilities offered by micromanipulation, the techniques may pose risks. It is possible, for example, that micromanipulation may allow sperm with deficiencies to fertilize an egg or may cause subtle damage to the egg, with long-term consequences for any resulting child. Nevertheless, given the potential of micromanipulation to be an effective treatment in cases of oligospermia, the Commission recommends that

> **127. Research and evaluation of micromanipulation of eggs be conducted under strict research protocols. Outcome studies on primates should be available before such research studies are considered in human beings. Any such studies should be conducted only at a licensed IVF facility and should be reviewed and approved by local research ethics boards, and by the Embryo Research and Assisted Conception Sub-Committees of the National Commission working in concert.**

Health Insurance Coverage

We have recommended that IVF be offered as treatment only in cases of tubal blockage; for other diagnoses it should be offered only in the context of research because it is not a treatment of proven benefit. It is possible, however, that IVF will be demonstrated effective through multicentre clinical trials, at acceptable levels of risk for indications other than tubal blockage; thus, the issue of whether IVF should be an insured service for a greater range of indications will arise again. When we considered the arguments for and against public health insurance coverage of IVF, two major considerations emerged: the arbitrary nature of existing criteria for public health insurance coverage, and the implications of a two-tier private/public health care system.

Criteria for Coverage

The Commission examined a range of medical procedures to determine whether there are common criteria determining which are insured and which are not. We found many unexplained discrepancies: some elective services are insured, while others are not. Some very high risk treatments are covered, while others are labelled "experimental" and are not covered. Some insured services have very low rates of effectiveness — many much lower than IVF — and many were insured without any evidence that they were effective at all. Our most disturbing finding about public health insurance coverage, however, is that once a treatment becomes an insured service, it is extremely difficult to remove it from the list of insured services

— even when the evidence shows subsequently that it is ineffective, excessively expensive relative to its effectiveness, or dangerous.

Health economists often evaluate medical services by examining their cost per quality-adjusted life year (QALY): that is, the cost of the service is divided by the number of years the procedure adds to the patient's life, adjusted to take into account whether the patient was pain-free and mobile during those years. Such measures provide a basis for evaluating emerging technologies relative to traditional treatments (although they may not be suitable for evaluating IVF). Some procedures have a very high cost per QALY but are nevertheless used extensively and frequently.

Given the current cost pressures on the health care system, and given its capacity to expand indefinitely in response to the availability of new treatments if rational limits are not set, our findings with respect to IVF indicate that the provinces would benefit from a re-evaluation of their current criteria for extending health insurance coverage generally. Technology assessment and cost-benefit analyses have proven very effective in determining the relative value of medical procedures and would constitute valuable input to future decisions about which services should be insured. Commissioners therefore believe, and we have recommended with respect to research on IVF, that provinces fund studies to generate data on which to base such decisions and ensure that they will be in the best interests of Canadians.

Dangers of a Two-Tier System

To help guide the policy makers who will make decisions about extending public health insurance coverage to IVF for tubal blockage and funding clinical trials of IVF for other diagnoses, it is instructive to examine the alternatives to public funding. Many of those who believe that we cannot afford to provide infertility treatment within the health care system have suggested that private clinics could step in to provide such treatments. This is the situation that has developed in the United States and some other countries, where IVF is provided primarily by this method. Even in Canada there are now four private IVF clinics in existence.

> The Commission has serious ethical and public policy objections to the establishment of a parallel system for providing IVF or, indeed, other medical procedures.

The Commission has serious ethical and public policy objections to the establishment of a parallel system for providing IVF or, indeed, other medical procedures. First, there can be no such thing as a purely private system. As we discussed in Chapter 4, the publicly funded system unavoidably ends up bearing financial costs generated by the private system, with no means of recovering those costs from the private system.

This means that the existence of a parallel private system leaves the public system without control over its costs. The nature and number of privately provided services are determined solely by the private providers, but they have unavoidable consequences for the publicly funded system, which has no way of controlling them in light of its own priorities or spending constraints. This is precisely what is happening with private IVF provision in Britain; it has the potential to happen in Canada as well if policy makers are not vigilant.

IVF service delivery in Ontario is in some ways an instructive case of how private health care affects the public system. Patients at private IVF clinics in Ontario pay physicians directly for certain services, but physicians also bill the provincial health care plan for a wide range of related laboratory and diagnostic services. These costs include much of the fertility investigation and follow-up to IVF, such as blood tests, ultrasound, and laparoscopies. The line between investigating infertility and treating it is vague and is left to the physician to determine. In addition, the public system bears the cost of treating adverse health affects resulting from IVF — the extra pregnancy monitoring and delivery care needed for the more frequent premature and multiple births and the subsequent cost of neonatal care. These costs, while significant, are short-term costs. There are also longer-term costs that arise from private provision of IVF. For instance, chronic disease or disability in low birth weight children resulting from IVF pregnancies also generates ongoing costs to the public purse. The key point, however, is that the public system is obliged to cover these costs without having any control over the number or nature of the procedures that generated them in the first place.

In summary, a great deal of the cost of IVF is already being funded by provincial health plans, whether the procedure itself is performed in a public or a private setting. The "private" clinics are never truly outside the public system and can operate only because part of their cost of doing business is subsidized by these additional payments from the public system. Moreover, the training of personnel for these clinics (physicians, nurses) is heavily subsidized by society.

If the amount charged to patients at private infertility clinics reflected all costs actually involved in the provision of treatment (including training of personnel; laboratory tests and other diagnostic procedures; and the additional costs of health care arising from complications, multiple births, and other consequences of the provision of treatment), the cost would be so prohibitive as to discourage clinics from opening. Fees would have to be set so high that very few prospective patients would be able to afford them.

The existence of private IVF clinics also gives rise to other concerns. The three private clinics in Ontario — Toronto Fertility Sterility Institute, C.A.R.E. Centre (Mississauga and its affiliated referral centre in southern Ontario), and IVF Canada (Scarborough) — are owned and operated by physicians. Studies have shown repeatedly that physician ownership of medical facilities providing services increases the use of services when the physician is in a position to recommend to patients that they need these services. This increases the cost of care substantially, while the quality of care has been observed to stay the same or decline. Although no studies have examined IVF clinics specifically, evidence from several other fields of medicine indicates that physician ownership of health care facilities has generally negative consequences.

If the amount charged to patients at private infertility clinics reflected all costs actually involved in the provision of treatment (including training of personnel; laboratory tests and other diagnostic procedures; and the additional costs of health care arising from complications, multiple births, and other consequences of the provision of treatment), the cost would be so prohibitive as to discourage clinics from opening.

Some of the private clinics also provide commercial laboratory services to their patients. This situation raises a conflict of interest, as well as concerns about quality control, because some such facilities do not have to be licensed. Ontario regulations, for example, do not require physicians doing simple testing procedures in their offices or testing for the sole purpose of diagnosing and treating their own patients to undergo the rigorous licensing and monitoring requirements for free-standing laboratories.

Perhaps most important, however, from the Commission's perspective is the fact that private ownership of clinics places assisted reproduction technologies in the realm of

Private ownership of clinics places assisted reproduction technologies in the realm of consumer-driven markets.

consumer-driven markets. In the Commission's view, this is inappropriate, primarily because it is at odds with the principle of non-commercialization of reproduction, one of our guiding principles. Commercialization also leads to inequality because only those who can afford it have access. Access to safe and effective procedures should not be determined by ability to pay; having children is too important in people's lives to allow such a situation to persist.

If a technique is of benefit, it should be available to Canadians on an equitable basis; if it is unproven, then it is in the realm of research and should not be provided as a service, but only in the context of research, with the protections of more stringent standards and informed consent inherent in research. Moreover, if treatment is being provided in the context of research, patients should certainly not be charged for it. Adopting our recommendations in this regard should protect Canadians from the potential dangers of research involving treatment of unknown benefit by ensuring that it is conducted only in the context of well-run trials that have been subject to prior scrutiny by research ethics boards — trials that will generate information of use in evaluation while minimizing risk.

In summary, the Commission sees a two-tier or mixed private/public medical care system as both inappropriate and unacceptable to the vast majority of Canadians. As we have discussed, IVF has been shown to be an effective medical treatment for one type of infertility; as such it should be offered within the public health care system, where priorities can be set, equitable access can be maintained, and standards can be promulgated and monitored. The Commission therefore recommends that

> **128. IVF for bilateral fallopian tube blockage be an insured service under provincial medicare programs within the regulatory framework recommended by the Royal Commission on New Reproductive Technologies.**

and that

> **129. The province of Ontario discontinue coverage of IVF for indications other than bilateral fallopian tube blockage and that the resources now devoted to those services be reallocated to fund clinical trials of unproven but promising techniques.**

Recommendations

The Commission has concluded that *in vitro* fertilization should be offered as treatment only for indications for which it has been proven effective. To date, this includes only one category of infertility disorders — those involving complete blockage of the fallopian tubes. We have recommended clinical trials and evaluation of other uses of IVF, or variations of IVF technology, before they can be considered for introduction as services. We have identified those we consider to be of highest priority for such trials.

We have shown the need for rigorous and thorough data collection on outcomes to enable development and refinement of clinical standards in response to findings. We have also shown that no mechanism exists to collect these data on a continuing basis, despite the dedicated efforts of some physicians and organizations such as the Canadian Fertility and Andrology Society and the Society of Obstetricians and Gynaecologists of Canada. The guidelines for practice they have developed are simply not being adhered to in some cases, nor are clear and standard definitions being used to record and collect data, thus making it very difficult to compare or aggregate data from different clinics. Our investigation also revealed wide variations in standards and practices; voluntary self-regulation has not led to consistency of standards and practice in the treatment community, but rather to practice ranging from excellent to completely unacceptable.

We have also shown the need for ongoing evaluation of the results of IVF treatment across the country. The great inadequacy of current record keeping makes it necessary to require that all clinics and practitioners conform to specified guidelines and standards as a condition of obtaining and maintaining a licence to offer IVF services. In our view, the experience with IVF in Canada to date demonstrates that a voluntary system is not adequate to protect the well-being of Canadians; instead, the standards developed and established by practitioners must become part of the licensing conditions under which IVF practice will be permitted.

Finally, we found that the criteria used to limit access to IVF treatment differ from clinic to clinic and that those who are admitted to IVF programs are not always given the information and support they need to make informed choices about their treatment. To provide a good standard of care for IVF patients, clinics require not only highly trained medical and technical personnel, but also access to a range of other specialized personnel, including individuals with psychosocial counselling expertise. Our data show wide variations in the quantity and quality of information, counselling, and consent procedures, with the result that patients' needs may go unmet.

We have examined the resource implications of offering IVF as an insured medical treatment and judge that in cases of diagnosed bilateral fallopian tube blockage, coverage of IVF as a medical service under provincial health insurance plans is justified. Other uses of IVF should be evaluated for effectiveness before being considered for public health insurance coverage. We also believe that IVF should not be offered except through the public health care system. To permit the development of a parallel private system would put serious burdens on the public system, as well as violating principles of equality and non-commercialization of reproduction.

We recognize that some of our recommendations set a more rigorous standard for IVF than exists in many other areas of medical practice. This is clearly necessary, however, given the nature and goals of infertility treatments, the fact that they are intended to influence human reproduction, their many social implications, the vulnerability of participants, and the need to consider the potential effects on children and on future generations — all these factors justify rigorous standards of practice and care. At the same time, the standards we recommend are entirely achievable. This approach could also be applied to other areas of health care, particularly in emerging areas of medical technology but also in long-established areas of practice. Indeed, in our view, assuring the health and safety of Canadians and the integrity of the health care system requires such an approach.

Licensing Requirements for Assisted Conception Services*

The Commission recommends that

> **130. The compulsory licensing requirements for assisted conception services apply to any physician, centre, or other individual or facility providing any of the following services or any other service related to assisted conception:**
> * ***in vitro* fertilization (IVF);**
> * **embryo transfer (either to the woman who was the source of the egg giving rise to the embryo or to another woman);**
> * **gamete intrafallopian transfer (GIFT);**
> * **zygote intrafallopian transfer (ZIFT);**
> * **preimplantation diagnosis;**
> * **insemination at sites other than the vagina; and**
> * **direct egg/sperm transfer (DOST).**

> **131. Providing assisted conception and related services without a licence issued by the National Reproductive Technologies Commission, or without complying with the National Commission's licensing requirements, constitute an offence subject to prosecution.**

---

* The following section contains only those recommendations related to the proposed licensing scheme. Recommendations not related to licensing appear only in the body of the text, while some licensing recommendations appear both in the text and in the following listing. The goal was to enable the reader to see the licensing regime in its entirety and also to have recommendations follow on from their rationale in the text where necessary.

132. The Assisted Conception Sub-Committee of the National Reproductive Technologies Commission develop standards and guidelines to be adopted as conditions of licence, with input from relevant professional bodies and individuals and groups representing patients and other key sectors of the community. The recommendations of the Royal Commission on New Reproductive Technologies should serve as a basis for these guidelines.

133. Only drugs and procedures of proven effectiveness for the infertility condition in question should be offered as treatment. Procedures whose effectiveness has not yet been clearly established should be offered only in the context of clinical trials.

134. Guidelines for determining which drugs and procedures are of sufficiently proven effectiveness to be offered as treatment (by indication), and which interventions require further research, should be established by the Assisted Conception Sub-Committee of the National Reproductive Technologies Commission, in consultation with relevant professional bodies and other interested groups.

135. In particular, the following treatments shown as being of unproven effectiveness should not be offered except in the context of research, unless or until their effectiveness is established:
    - IVF (for any indication other than complete tubal obstruction);
    - GIFT;
    - ZIFT; and
    - DOST.

and that

136. Drugs and procedures now in use that are of unproven benefit should be offered only in the context of multicentre clinical trials. The Assisted Conception Sub-Committee should facilitate participation by licensed centres in such trials, which should have prior research ethics board approval. Funding from provincial/territorial ministries of health would be desirable for those trials designated as of highest priority. Projects involving the micromanipulation of eggs should also have express approval of the Assisted Conception Sub-Committee in concert with the Embryo Research Sub-Committee of the National Commission.

Conditions of Licence Applicable to Assisted Conception Services

The Commission recommends that

137. Assisted conception services should not be offered without assessment of the male as well as the female partner to determine the probable cause of infertility.

138. IVF should be offered only after less intrusive and costly options have been discussed and considered.

139. Sperm for use in assisted conception services (with the exception of the partner's) must be obtained from a licensed facility, as outlined in our recommendations on assisted insemination.

140. IVF should be offered as treatment only in cases of diagnosed bilateral fallopian tube blockage, and tubal surgery should not be a precondition for IVF in such cases.

141. IVF treatment should not be offered to women who have experienced menopause at the usual age.

142. Treatment should be offered only after counselling regarding behaviours or personal habits that could render successful treatment less likely.

143. A maximum of three zygotes should be transferred to a woman's uterus in any IVF attempt, in order to minimize the risk of multiple pregnancies.

144. Any proposal to use preimplantation diagnosis on zygotes should be approved by the Assisted Conception Sub-Committee in consultation with the Prenatal Diagnosis and Genetics Sub-Committee, and no proposal should be approved for preimplantation diagnosis to determine the sex of the embryo for non-medical reasons.

Impermissible Barriers to Treatment

145. Access to IVF treatment should be determined on the basis of legitimate medical criteria, without discrimination on the basis of factors such as marital status, sexual orientation, or economic status.

Patient Information, Consent, and Counselling

146. Standard information materials and consent forms should be developed by the Assisted Conception Sub-Committee in consultation with professional, patient, and other interested groups and distributed by licensed centres to all persons contemplating or receiving assisted conception services.

147. Information materials should include clear information on the nature of the proposed treatment and its alternatives; the nature and probability of known and possible consequences of the procedure; and the costs of treatment.

148. Consent forms should identify fully the specific procedures and treatments being consented to, including egg retrieval and fertilization, zygote cryopreservation, embryo transfer, zygote donation to another recipient, donation for research, or disposal.

149. Patients should be given time to discuss and fully comprehend consent forms, which should be signed by the patient before any treatment is initiated.

150. Patients should also be informed of their right to withdraw consent at any stage of treatment, without affecting their access to future care or treatment in any way.

151. **Counselling should be an integral part of assisted conception services and should be offered either on-site or by referral to appropriate professionals. Standard counselling materials should be developed by the Assisted Conception Sub-Committee and should include information about alternatives to medical treatment such as adoption and living without children; avoidance of exposure to risk factors that could affect the results of treatment (for example, smoking); some exploration of questions related to values and goals that patients may wish to take into account when making their decisions; and the physical and psychological effects of treatment. Specific additional counselling materials for donors and recipients of eggs and zygotes should also be offered.**

Calculation of Clinic Success Rates

The Commission recommends that

152. **Clear definitions for rates of pregnancy and live birth rates per treatment cycle initiated, by categories of indication, should be specified by the Assisted Conception Sub-Committee as the basis upon which licensed facilities would submit data annually.**

153. **All information provided to prospective patients about clinic rates for live birth or pregnancy per treatment cycle initiated should be based on clear and standard definitions established by the Assisted Conception Sub-Committee.**

Non-Commercialization of Assisted Conception Services

The Commission recommends that

> 154. Assisted conception services should not operate on a for-profit basis.

Reporting and Record Keeping

The Commission recommends that

> 155. Licensed assisted conception services should report to the National Reproductive Technologies Commission on their activities in a standard form, annually and in the event of any change (such as the departure or replacement of qualified personnel) substantially affecting the conditions of licence.

and that

> 156. In particular, the following be reported annually to the National Commission:
> - data to allow rates per treatment cycle initiated and by diagnostic category to be established for the following outcomes: biochemical pregnancy, clinical pregnancy, live birth (number of confinements as well as number of individuals born), stillbirth, and ectopic pregnancy. Information on pre-term birth, birth weight, and congenital anomalies should also be submitted;
> - written diagnostic criteria should be developed by the Assisted Conception Sub-Committee and be used by clinics to allocate patients to diagnostic categories for purposes of data reporting;
> - frequency of pregnancies in patients on the waiting list; and
> - social and geographic categories of data.

157. **Confidential records should be kept on individual cases, including patient history, examination, investigation, procedures, operations, and treatments.**

Licence Renewal and Revocation of Licences

The Commission recommends that

158. **Licensed assisted conception facilities be required to apply to the National Commission for licence renewal every five years. At the outset, the Commission should grant licences of varying duration, so that applications for five-year licence renewals would be staggered over several years.**

and that

159. **Assisted conception licences be revocable by the National Commission at any time for breach of conditions of licence.**

The Role of the Assisted Conception Sub-Committee

The Assisted Conception Sub-Committee would be established and chaired by the National Reproductive Technologies Commission. As discussed in Chapter 5, it would be one of six permanent sub-committees, along with those dealing with infertility prevention; assisted insemination services; prenatal diagnosis; embryo research; and the provision of fetal tissue for research and other designated uses. Like the other sub-committees, the Assisted Conception Sub-Committee should include both National Commission members and non-members, and, like the National Reproductive Technologies Commission itself, at least half the members of the sub-committee should be women. All sub-committee members should be chosen with a view to ensuring that they have a background and demonstrated experience in taking a multidisciplinary approach to issues, as well as an ability to work together to find solutions and recommend policies to address the issues surrounding assisted conception in a way that meets the concerns of Canadian society as a whole.

The Assisted Conception Sub-Committee would have several functions. It could decide to establish ad hoc working groups to deal with one or more of these functions, if appropriate:

- Setting and revising, from time to time, the licensing requirements for individuals and centres providing assisted conception services (including staff qualifications and expertise; guidelines for recognized and experimental procedures; protocols for prescribing drugs to patients undergoing fertility treatments; record keeping and reporting requirements; etc.), to be applied through the National Reproductive Technologies Commission hearing process. As noted earlier, relevant professional associations, patient, and other interested groups would have input into this process.

- Developing standard information materials, counselling materials, and patient consent forms to be used in the provision of assisted conception services.

- Monitoring the assessment and introduction of new assisted conception technologies; advising on which clinical trials are most urgent; and facilitating and funding, or coordinating provincial/territorial funding, for such trials.

- Developing guidelines and standardized definitions for the collection and reporting of data on the results of treatment.

- Gathering relevant country-wide data and information about facilities, technologies, and practices, consistent with the registry model proposed by the International Working Group for Registers on Assisted Reproduction. This information will serve as a basis for the Sub-Committee's guideline- and standard-setting activities. It will allow evaluation of long-term health outcomes for women using assisted conception and related drugs and services, and for children born as a result of such technologies. It will also be of use to the provinces in their planning and resource allocation decisions, and to medical and other researchers undertaking primary and academic research in this field.

- Consulting with the provinces and territories, directly or through the Conference of Deputy Minsters of Health, on matters relating to technology assessment and the funding or provision of assisted conception services, where this is useful or necessary.

- Discussing and setting policy on new issues and dilemmas as they arise, including training and education issues, ethical and legal concerns, and international issues; monitoring practices in referral to IVF and ensuring appropriate levels of regulation on an ongoing basis.

- Providing advice, in the revised federal drug approval system, on issues relating to fertility drugs, and monitoring marketing and other activities in this sector.

- Working with the Assisted Insemination and Prenatal Diagnosis Sub-Committees on issues related to sex-selective assisted insemination and prenatal diagnosis, preimplantation diagnosis on zygotes, the implantation of zygotes subject to manipulation, and eggs subject to micromanipulation.

- Promoting public awareness and debate regarding IVF and related technologies and services in Canada, in part through the publication of the National Commission's annual report.

- Establishing protocols for screening egg donors and testing eggs for sexually transmitted diseases and other infections; developing standards and guidelines for the collection, recording, encoding, and secure storage of identifying and non-identifying egg donor information, recipient information, and information relating to children born through the use of donated eggs. (These functions are discussed in the next chapter, "Handling of Eggs and Embryos.")

- Overseeing the National Commission's information registry system relating to egg donors, recipients, and births; and establishing appropriate procedures for making such information available, pursuant to court order, in the case of emergency. (These functions are discussed in Chapter 21.)

Increasing the level of informed public debate about assisted conception technologies and services is a particularly important part of the role we foresee for the Assisted Conception Sub-Committee. Public input into the monitoring and control of assisted conception services will be promoted by the Sub-Committee's information gathering, reporting, and public consultation functions. Public accountability will also be enhanced by the composition we have recommended for the Sub-Committee, which should include members both from the National Commission and from outside the National Commission, ensuring broad representation of the various interests involved. In particular, we recommend that the Assisted Conception Sub-Committee have a multidisciplinary make-up, including membership from relevant professional bodies, federal and provincial/territorial health ministries, and individuals representing the concerns of patients and other key segments of the community, particularly women.

We are of the view that the Assisted Conception Sub-Committee's activities in regulating and monitoring technologies and practices, in gathering and disseminating much-needed information, and in bringing together the various interests involved will help to ensure that assisted conception services are delivered in a safe, ethical, and effective way, consistent with the expectations of those directly affected and of Canadian society at large.

Conclusion

The breadth and detail of the Commission's recommendations demonstrate the seriousness with which we view how IVF is being provided in Canada today. We believe that there is a place in our health care system for effective, safe infertility treatments, but that IVF as it is now being offered does not meet those criteria. We also believe that IVF has been overemphasized in terms of the resources and public policy attention devoted to it relative to other infertility treatments, such as drug therapy and assisted insemination. For example, currently at least twice as many children are born each year in Canada after assisted insemination than after IVF.

In some areas, such as the cessation of unsafe or ineffective treatments, we have called for immediate action. Our long-term goal, however, is the creation of a system in which individuals who are infertile can be helped, where possible, to conceive, with a treatment that promises the greatest chances of success based on their diagnosis and other characteristics; in which practitioners are free to practise within well-defined parameters; and in which scientists and researchers can carry out approved research to expand the boundaries of infertility treatment without harm to women. We believe that our recommendations will lead to the creation of that system; we look to governments and practitioners to implement them.

General Sources

Abbey, A., L.J. Halman, and F.M. Andrews. "Life Quality, Psychosocial Factors, and Infertility: Selected Results from a Five-Year Study of 275 Couples." In Research Volumes of the Royal Commission on New Reproductive Technologies, 1993.

Angus Reid Group Inc. "Reproductive Technologies — Qualitative Research: Summary of Observations." In Research Volumes of the Royal Commission on New Reproductive Technologies, 1993.

Canadian Press. "In Vitro Fertilization: Medical Bills Huge for Multiple Births." *The London Free Press*, June 15, 1992.

Caplan, A.L. "Arguing with Success: Is In Vitro Fertilization Research or Therapy?" In *Beyond Baby M: Ethical Issues in New Reproductive Techniques*, ed. D.M. Bartels et al. Clifton: Humana Press, 1989.

Decima Research. "Social Values and Attitudes of Canadians Toward New Reproductive Technologies." In Research Volumes of the Royal Commission on New Reproductive Technologies, 1993.

Decima Research. "Social Values and Attitudes of Canadians Toward New Reproductive Technologies: Focus Group Findings." In Research Volumes of the Royal Commission on New Reproductive Technologies, 1993.

de Groh, M. "Reproductive Technologies, Adoption, and Issues on the Cost of Health Care: Summary of Canada Health Monitor Results." In Research Volumes of the Royal Commission on New Reproductive Technologies, 1993.

Feeny, D. "New Health Care Technologies: Their Effect on Health and the Cost of Health Care." In *Health Care Technology: Effectiveness, Efficiency, and Public Policy*, ed. D. Feeny, G. Guyatt, and P. Tugwell. Montreal: The Institute for Research on Public Policy, 1986.

Goeree, R., et al. "Cost-Effectiveness of an *In Vitro* Fertilization Program and the Costs of Associated Hospitalizations and Other Infertility Treatments." In Research Volumes of the Royal Commission on New Reproductive Technologies, 1993.

Hughes, E.G. "Cigarette Smoking — Does It Reduce Fecundity?" *Journal of the Society of Obstetricians and Gynaecologists of Canada* 14 (November 1992): 27-37.

Hughes, E.G., D.M. Fedorkow, and J.A. Collins. "Meta-Analysis of Controlled Trials in Infertility." In Research Volumes of the Royal Commission on New Reproductive Technologies, 1993.

Hull, M.G.R. "Indications for Assisted Conception." *British Medical Bulletin* 46 (1990): 580-95.

Millar, W.J., S. Wadhera, and C. Nimrod. "Multiple Births: Trends and Patterns in Canada, 1974-1990." *Health Reports* 4 (3)(1992): 223-50.

Mitchell, J.M., and J.H. Sunshine. "Consequences of Physicians' Ownership of Health Care Facilities — Joint Ventures in Radiation Therapy." *New England Journal of Medicine* 327 (November 19, 1992): 1497-1501.

Muir, E. "Review of the Literature on the Psychosocial Implications of Infertility Treatment on Women and Men." In Research Volumes of the Royal Commission on New Reproductive Technologies, 1993.

Mullen, M.A. "Medically Assisted Reproductive Technologies: A Review." In Research Volumes of the Royal Commission on New Reproductive Technologies, 1993.

Mullens, A. *Missed Conceptions: Overcoming Infertility*. Toronto: McGraw-Hill Ryerson, 1990.

Ontario. Panel on Health Goals for Ontario. *Health for All Ontario*. Toronto: The Panel, 1987.

Oregon State Legislature. Oregon Health Services Commission. *Prioritization of Health Services: A Report to the Governor and Legislature*. Oregon: State Legislature, 1991.

Rachlis, M.M. "The Canadian Health Care System." In Research Volumes of the Royal Commission on New Reproductive Technologies, 1993.

Rowlands, J., N. Saby, and J. Smith. "Commercial Involvement in New Reproductive Technologies: An Overview." In Research Volumes of the Royal Commission on New Reproductive Technologies, 1993.

Royal College of Obstetricians and Gynaecologists. *Infertility: Guidelines for Practice*. London: RCOG Press, 1992.

Society for Assisted Reproductive Technology, The American Fertility Society. "Assisted Reproductive Technology in the United States and Canada: 1991 Results from the Society for Assisted Reproductive Technology Generated from the American Fertility Society Registry." *Fertility and Sterility* 59 (5)(May 1993): 956-62.

SPR Associates Inc. "An Evaluation of Canadian Fertility Clinics: The Patient's Perspective." In Research Volumes of the Royal Commission on New Reproductive Technologies, 1993.

Stephens, T., and J. McLean. "Survey of Canadian Fertility Programs." In Research Volumes of the Royal Commission on New Reproductive Technologies, 1993.

Trounson, A.O. "Cryopreservation." *British Medical Bulletin* 46 (1990): 695-708.

United States. Congress. Senate Committee on Labor and Human Resources. *Senate Report No. 102-152, to accompany Bill H.R. 4773, Fertility Clinic Success Rate and Certification Act of 1992*. Washington: U.S. Government Printing Office, 1992.

Vandekerckhove, P., et al. "Infertility Treatment: From Cookery to Science: The Epidemiology of Randomized Controlled Trials." In Research Volumes of the Royal Commission on New Reproductive Technologies, 1993.

World Health Organization. Regional Office of Europe. *Summary Report: Consultation on the Place of In Vitro Fertilization in Infertility Care*. Copenhagen, June 18-22, 1990. Geneva: World Health Organization, 1990.

Wright, J. "The Psychosocial Impact of New Reproductive Technology." In Research Volumes of the Royal Commission on New Reproductive Technologies, 1993.

Specific References

1. Haan, G. "Effects and Costs of In-Vitro Fertilization: Again, Let's Be Honest." *International Journal of Technology Assessment in Health Care* 7 (4)(1991), p. 587.

2. Data on IVF cycles presented at the September 1993 IVF World Congress in Kyoto, Japan, by Arthur Leader, Chief, Division of Reproductive Endocrinology and Infertility, Ottawa Civic Hospital, Ottawa, Ontario.

3. These five studies are the following: Tan, S.L., et al. "Cumulative Conception and Livebirth Rates After In-Vitro Fertilisation." *Lancet* 339 (June 6, 1992): 1390-94; Collins, J., E. Burrows, and A. Willan. "Infertile Couples and Their Treatment in Canadian Academic Infertility Clinics." In Research Volumes of the

Royal Commission on New Reproductive Technologies, 1993; Holst, N., et al. "Handling of Tubal Infertility After Introduction of In Vitro Fertilization: Changes and Consequences." *Fertility and Sterility* 55 (1)(January 1991): 140-43; Marana, R., and J. Quagliarello. "Distal Tubal Occlusion: Microsurgery Versus In Vitro Fertilization — A Review." *International Journal of Fertility* 33 (2)(1988): 107-15; and Hughes, E.G., D.M. Fedorkow, and J.A. Collins. "Meta-Analysis of Controlled Trials in Infertility." In Research Volumes of the Royal Commission on New Reproductive Technologies, 1993.

4. Tan et al., "Cumulative Conception and Livebirth Rates After In-Vitro Fertilisation."

5. Collins et al., "Infertile Couples and Their Treatment in Canadian Academic Infertility Clinics."

6. Holst et al., "Handling of Tubal Infertility After Introduction of In Vitro Fertilization."

7. Marana and Quagliarello, "Distal Tubal Occlusion: Microsurgery Versus In Vitro Fertilization — A Review."

8. Haan, "Effects and Costs of In-Vitro Fertilization: Again, Let's Be Honest," 582-93.

9. Holst et al., "Handling of Tubal Infertility after Introduction of In Vitro Fertilization."

10. Millar, W.J. "Trends in Low Birthweight Canada 1971 to 1989." *Health Reports* 3 (4)(1991): 311-17.

11. Mickleburgh, R. "Rising Rate of Multiple Births Creates Burden for Taxpayers." *The Globe and Mail*, January 6, 1993, A6.

12. Lyons, J. "Tiny Tots: Prognosis Healthier as HSC Study Focuses on Underweight Babies." *Winnipeg Free Press*, August 17, 1992, C17.

13. Escobar, G.J., B. Littenberg, and D.B. Petitti. "Outcome Among Surviving Very Low Birthweight Infants: A Meta-Analysis." *Archives of Disease in Childhood* 66 (1991): 204-11.

14. Halsey, C.L., M.F. Collin, and C.L. Anderson. "Extremely Low Birth Weight Children and Their Peers: A Comparison of Preschool Performance." *Pediatrics* 91 (4)(April 1993): 807-11.

15. Eilers, B.L., et al. "Classroom Performance and Social Factors of Children with Birth Weights of 1250 Grams or Less: Follow-Up at 5 to 8 Years of Age." *Pediatrics* 77 (1986): 203-208.

16. Porter, J.B., P.J. Manberg, and S.C. Hartz. "Statistics and Results of Assisted Reproductive Technologies." *Assisted Reproduction Reviews* 1 (1)(1991): 28-37.

17. Ibid.

18. McGuire, R. "Big Surprise; Frozen Embryos Make Better Babies." *The Medical Post*, December 1, 1992, p. 24.

19. There remains some question about the viability of cryopreserved embryos. Australian data indicate that the rate of clinical pregnancies is significantly improved when frozen and thawed embryos are implanted during natural cycles

(cited in Mullen, M.A. "The Use of Human Embryos and Fetal Tissues: A Research Architecture." In Research Volumes of the Royal Commission on New Reproductive Technologies, 1993). Past studies have indicated that frozen embryos are only half as viable as fresh. A study published in the *New England Journal of Medicine* concluded that freezing embryos significantly reduces their capacity for implantation (Levran, D., et al. "Pregnancy Potential of Human Oocytes — The Effect of Cryopreservation." *New England Journal of Medicine* 323 (17)(October 25, 1990): 1153-56); and one researcher concluded that embryo freezing is much more difficult and time consuming and much less successful than might have been anticipated (Ashwood-Smith, M.J. "The Cryopreservation of Human Embryos." *Human Reproduction* 1 (5)(1986), p. 330).

20. Lancaster, P.A.L. "Congenital Malformations After In-Vitro Fertilisation." *Lancet* (December 12, 1987): 1392; Mills, J.I., et al. "Risk of Neural Tube Defects in Relation to Maternal Fertility and Fertility Drug Use." *Lancet* (July 14, 1990): 103-104.

21. Stephenson, P.A., and P.G. Svensson. "In Vitro Fertilisation and Infertility Care: A Primer for Health Planners." *International Journal of Health Sciences* 2 (3)(1991): 119-23.

22. American figures for 1989 show that 15.6 percent of embryo transfers resulted in the birth of a healthy baby. In Australia and New Zealand, where statistics are compiled in more detail and IVF is generally agreed to be more advanced, the clinical pregnancy rate per treatment cycle initiated was 13.4 percent, and the live birth rate per treatment cycle initiated was 9.4 percent.

23. World Health Organization. Scientific Group. *Recent Advances in Medically Assisted Conception.* Geneva: WHO, 1992, p. 53.

24. Deber, R.B., with H. Bouchard and A. Pendleton. "Implementing Shared Patient Decision Making: A Review of the Literature." In Research Volumes of the Royal Commission on New Reproductive Technologies, 1993.

25. One clinic stood out in the depth and accessibility of the information provided about other options. In addition to listing the options, their risks, and their benefits, the information materials from this clinic also instructed patients on how to arrange public, private, and international adoptions.

Handling of Eggs and Embryos

◆

As we saw in the previous chapter, the process of *in vitro* fertilization involves removing eggs from a woman's body, fertilizing them in the laboratory, and returning the resulting embryos* to her body where, it is hoped, they will implant and a pregnancy will result. If many eggs are retrieved, or if more viable zygotes are created than can be transferred safely, the situation of "excess" or "surplus" eggs or zygotes arises. The possible uses of these eggs and zygotes raise social, ethical, and legal dilemmas that have not been adequately considered by society to date.

These possible uses of surplus eggs and zygotes include donating them to another couple who is infertile, donating them for use in research, or allowing the clinic to dispose of them. We look at the issue of embryo research in the next chapter. Our focus in this chapter, therefore, is egg and embryo donation.

While recognizing that egg and embryo donation can be beneficial for some individuals and couples who are infertile, Canadians expressed concern about aspects of these practices, such as whether the donors fully understand the implications of donation, and whether appropriate counselling and consent procedures are available.

---

* There is a problem with terminology, as the term "embryo" is used in different ways. In the language of biologists, before implantation the fertilized egg is termed a "zygote" rather than an "embryo." The term "embryo" refers to the developing entity after implantation in the uterus until about eight weeks after fertilization. At the beginning of the ninth week after fertilization, it is referred to as a "fetus," the term used until time of birth. The terms embryo donation, embryo transfer, and embryo research are therefore inaccurate, since these all occur with zygotes, not embryos. Nevertheless, because the terms are still commonly used in the public debate, we continue to refer to embryo research, embryo donation, and embryo transfer. For accuracy, however, we also refer to the developing entity during the first 14 days as a zygote, so that it is clear that we mean the stage of development before implantation and not later.

We also look at the issues raised by the potential to cryopreserve surplus zygotes. If a couple undergoing IVF has more eggs fertilized than they need for their current cycle, they may be able to have these surplus zygotes frozen for use in a later cycle. These cryopreservation techniques have created ethical and legal dilemmas of their own. For example, if the couple later decides they do not wish to have their frozen zygotes transferred, do they want to make them available for donation? If the couple's relationship ends, what is the status of the frozen zygotes? If the male partner dies, is it ethical to transfer a zygote later, with the resulting child to be raised by the woman? If it is the woman who dies, could the surviving male partner use the zygotes with a subsequent partner and raise the resulting child?

These concerns are discussed in the next section, where we examine what we learned about the views and attitudes of Canadians toward egg and embryo donation, and toward zygote freezing.

The Views of Canadians

The Commission heard a great deal about egg and embryo donation during its public consultation activities. Many people recognized the potential benefits of donation but were concerned about the circumstances under which donations are made and the implications of donation for the people concerned.

The Commission heard from both practitioners and individuals who are infertile, who believe that egg or embryo donation offers opportunities to help another woman or couple who is infertile in cases where a donation would be their only chance of becoming pregnant. In some cases, for example, the woman may not produce any eggs herself; in other cases, she may be at risk of passing on a genetic disease to her children. For instance, women with Turner syndrome are born with ovaries containing eggs, but the eggs degenerate before the women reach reproductive age, rendering them infertile.

> *In vitro* fertilization, egg donation and embryo transplants are now [currently] the only forms in which Turner's syndrome women can conceive ... Not everyone with Turner's syndrome would want to go this route of egg donation and bearing children ... But there are lots of women with Turner's syndrome who have been unable to adopt because of the long waiting lists and the other various reasons that they feel that this is an option that they don't want to have the door closed on them.
>
> *D. Galszechy and S. Rowden, The Turner's Syndrome Society, Public Hearings Transcripts, Toronto, Ontario, November 19, 1990.*

Canadians were concerned that women might be pressured into donating eggs. For instance, some intervenors thought that women might agree to donate eggs in the belief that access to infertility treatment would be restricted if they did not agree. The Commission heard strong representations about the need to ensure that women's autonomy is respected and that the choice to donate eggs or zygotes is made independent of treatment decisions or other factors, and with appropriate counselling and consent procedures.

The Commission also heard that a woman should not undergo the risks and discomforts of invasive procedures such as ovulation induction and egg retrieval solely for the purpose of donating the resulting eggs to someone else.

> The women who are the candidates [to receive] egg donations are women who have gone through premature ovarian failure or whose ovaries have been removed, who have no possible source of eggs on their own, or women who have genetic indications, who do not wish to pass on a serious or potentially lethal genetic disorder.
>
> *M. Fluker, private citizen, Public Hearings Transcripts, Vancouver, British Columbia, November 26, 1990.*

There were questions about whether donation should be anonymous, or whether women should be permitted to designate a recipient for their eggs or zygotes. Some clinics currently permit designated donation. One Canadian clinic said that it would prefer anonymous donation, but that it did not have the organization in place to facilitate this. Many concerns were raised about the future relationship between the child, the birth mother, and the donor in circumstances where the donor's identity was known to the recipient.

Still other issues were raised by the question of who receives donated eggs or zygotes. Canadians seemed to believe that donation is justified to help women who are infertile because of ovarian damage resulting from disease or medical treatment, or women at risk of passing on a genetic disease to their children. However, they had many difficulties with the question of whether post-menopausal women should be recipients of donated eggs. Many people were concerned about women becoming parents at a later stage of life and the implications of this for the children. Others pointed out, however, that there are no barriers to

> We support the use of egg donation in circumstances where a woman is not able to produce her own eggs.
>
> *R. Reid, Society of Obstetricians and Gynaecologists of Canada and Canadian Fertility and Andrology Society, Public Hearings Transcripts, Montreal, Quebec, November 22, 1990.*

men becoming parents at any age, and that this was not necessarily considered a detriment to the child.

There was also opposition to the practice of a woman contracting with a couple to gestate a zygote created from their egg and sperm and to surrender the resulting child to them at birth. This use of technology is discussed in Chapter 23, "Preconception Arrangements."

Like donor insemination, egg and embryo donation raise legal and social issues for families and for the children who are born. Socially, the family must deal with the fact that the child is not genetically related to at least one of his or her parents. And just as family law has not caught up to the implications of donor insemination, it is not structured adequately to deal with the issues raised by egg and embryo donation — for example, the possibility that a zygote could be gestated and a child born several years after his or her genetic parents are dead. Many people pointed to the need for appropriate record keeping to enable children to find out about their genetic origins.

> Each fertilized egg must be given its due respect and protection whether in the laboratory or in the body of its mother. Eggs which are not utilized for introduction to the maternal uterus must continue to be protected. They must not be discarded as mere tissue but preserved for embryo adoption at some time in the future when they can be introduced into the uterus of some other infertile mother.
>
> *J. Bromley, Fort Smith Pro-Life Group, Public Hearings Transcripts, Yellowknife, Northwest Territories, September 12, 1990.*

The Commission heard opinions on whether those donating eggs or zygotes should be paid for their donation. Sperm donors are usually compensated for their donation, to cover the time and inconvenience involved. The risk, time, and inconvenience are far greater in the case of egg or embryo donation if it is done specifically for this reason (and not in the context of a woman's own infertility or other treatment). If this is to be allowed and compensation is to be provided, many Canadians wondered how decisions about it would be made and identified many dangers of commercializing this area.

> The treatment of embryos, like all other human genetic materials, semen and ova, must be similar to the treatment of blood by the Canadian Red Cross. The donation of an embryo must be considered as a gift.
>
> *C. St. Peter, Canadian Research Institute for the Advancement of Women, Public Hearings Transcripts, Ottawa, Ontario, September 20, 1990.*

Other jurisdictions have also grappled with the question of when, if ever, people should be able to donate eggs and zygotes and who should receive them. The international consensus appears to be that donation is permissible, as long as appropriate counselling and consent procedures are in place.[1]

There is also widespread international acceptance of zygote freezing. Storing frozen zygotes may be of considerable benefit to the couple whose gametes were used to create them. As we explained in the previous chapter, if the transfer of zygotes in the first IVF cycle is not successful, the woman does not have to undergo egg retrieval a second time if zygotes created after the first retrieval are frozen for future use. Similarly, a couple wishing to have a second child through IVF may also avoid the need for additional egg retrieval.

However, the ability to freeze zygotes means that they can be maintained for a considerable period of time outside the human body. The Commission heard that there is a pressing need to decide who has the legal authority to make decisions about the disposition of the zygotes, including how long they should be stored and whether, if they were not used by the couple, they could be donated to another couple, disposed of, or donated for research purposes.

We discuss these issues and concerns, beginning with egg donation, then turning to embryo donation and zygote freezing.

> In those cases where a couple have jointly decided to bear responsibility for children potentially conceived through IVF/ET, they should jointly decide, prior to the commencement of their procedure, on what they desire to be done with nonimplanted embryos; their wishes should be specified in writing as part of the consent procedure. Where an individual woman has decided to undergo IVF/ET, the decision should rest with her solely. At the health facility, the individual woman or couple should be given standard consent forms which grant the choice of discarding the embryos, donating them to research, or designating donation to other infertile people. The disposal of eggs or sperm also should be governed by the patients' wishes with the same range of available options.
>
> *Brief to the Commission from the Canadian Advisory Council on the Status of Women, March 1991.*

Egg Donation

Egg donation became possible only when IVF procedures became available. The Commission heard about four categories of egg donors: women who donate their "excess" eggs after undergoing egg retrieval for their own IVF treatment; women paid specifically to undergo procedures to donate their eggs; women about to undergo surgery on the uterus and/or ovaries who agree to egg recovery for donation at the same time; and volunteers willing to undergo the procedure specifically to donate to individuals or couples who are infertile, often a relative. The processes of ovulation stimulation and egg retrieval are the same for the latter three categories of egg donors as they are for women undergoing IVF. Some have speculated that another source of eggs may be possible in the future: maturing the eggs of female fetuses to a point where they can be fertilized and used for donation.

U.S. studies of IVF using donated eggs have shown a higher overall success rate than IVF using the eggs and sperm of a couple who is infertile;[2] this is probably because the egg donors tended to be younger than most IVF patients, with the result that their eggs are more likely to be viable. As with IVF pregnancies generally, however, record keeping by Canadian clinics has left us with no way to know reliably how many children have been born in this country through egg donation. U.S. estimates for 1990 indicate that at least 547 zygotes created with donated eggs were transferred to recipients at 67 clinics in that country, although no rates of live birth were available.[3]

Egg donation raises significant ethical and legal questions. How these issues are perceived depends in part on the motivations of participants. For example, when the egg "donor" intends to raise the resulting child gestated by another woman, we refer to the situation as a preconception arrangement. When the recipient intends to raise the child, however, we refer to egg donation or embryo donation. Thus, it is clear that the intentions of participants influence the way we view the process and its participants, and hence how we assess the legal and social implications.

> If more ova are removed than can be reimplanted from a woman who is herself undergoing IVF, she should retain the right to decide whether the surplus are to be donated.
>
> *D. Day, Nova Scotia Advisory Council on the Status of Women, Public Hearings Transcripts, Halifax, Nova Scotia, October 17, 1990.*

We examine the social, ethical, and legal questions raised by egg donation, beginning with the most well-known form — anonymous egg donation from a woman undergoing IVF to another couple who is infertile. We then consider other forms of egg donation, payment for egg donation, and legal issues.

Anonymous Egg Donation by Women Undergoing IVF*

Donors

It is essential to ensure respect for the autonomy of women donating "spare" eggs after undergoing egg retrieval as part of their IVF treatment. We have noted the concerns we heard that women could be subject to undue pressure to donate eggs, believing that they might be rejected from the program or that their future care could be jeopardized if they did not agree to donate. This situation could arise, given the call for donated eggs; Commission research found that 8 of the 15 IVF clinics participating in our survey offer IVF with donor eggs, and there are waiting lists of up to 120 prospective recipients (see research volume, *Treatment of Infertility: Current Practices and Psychosocial Implications*). Since one woman can produce many more eggs in a stimulated cycle than she can have transferred, the possibility exists that clinic staff could pressure women to donate eggs not needed for their own IVF treatment for use by other couples.[4]

As we have shown, counselling protocols for IVF patients are inadequate at some clinics and, as discussed in relation to assisted insemination using donor sperm, gamete donation can have psychological repercussions for the donor, the child who results, and their families. This situation could also lead to women donating eggs without being fully informed and considering all the implications of this act.

A third dilemma for a woman considering egg donation while undergoing fertility treatment is the possibility that her donated egg may fertilize, implant, and gestate successfully in the recipient woman, while her own treatment could prove unsuccessful. Even if she is unaware of the fate of her donated eggs, the possibility could cause psychological distress for the donor if she remains childless.

Finally, we must take into account that any eggs deemed "surplus" during an IVF cycle may not be of the highest quality; presumably, the practitioner would reserve for the donor those eggs considered most viable for fertilization and transfer. In addition, as cryopreservation becomes more reliable and available (or, indeed, if cryopreservation of eggs becomes available), many women may choose to have their eggs fertilized and the resulting zygotes cryopreserved for their own use in future cycles instead of donating them.

Recipients

Couples who receive anonymously donated eggs face many of the same concerns as couples undergoing donor insemination: many of the psychosocial issues discussed with regard to DI also apply to the children

---

* See Annex for dissenting opinion.

and families that result from egg donation. These issues include secrecy about the child's origins, access to information about the donor, how records are compiled and stored, and what the best interests of the child are.

As discussed with respect to donor insemination (see Chapter 19), the Commission believes the best interests of the family and the child are served if non-identifying information about the gamete donor is available to the parents and child at any time and if identifying information on children and donors is preserved for 100 years, so it is available if ordered by a court in cases of medical necessity. As outlined in Chapter 19, we believe donors should not have access to identifying information about their genetic offspring.

The Commission does not consider, however, that sperm donation and egg donation are completely parallel situations. In egg donation, both parents have a physical link to the child — the male partner is genetically linked, and the woman is the gestational mother. This is not the case with donor insemination. Cultural attitudes and other pressures are also different for women and men with respect to their genetic links to their children. The Commission therefore believes that distinct programs of prior counselling, consent, and post-treatment counselling and support are necessary for couples involved in egg donation.

For some infertility-related conditions, a donated egg may be a woman's only chance of achieving pregnancy. Women with premature ovarian failure, ovarian failure after radio- or chemotherapy, or a genetic disease they could pass on to their children could therefore be candidates to receive donated eggs.[5] This may be ethically justified if done within accepted protocols and with fully informed consent. We are more troubled, however, by the prospect that the technique could be used not to help overcome infertility at a time of life when the ability to become pregnant is normal, but to expand the human reproductive lifespan. Studies have shown that, with hormone treatment, post-menopausal women can successfully gestate a fetus from a donated egg or embryo and carry it to term.[6]

> We are more troubled, however, by the prospect that the technique could be used not to help overcome infertility at a time of life when the ability to become pregnant is normal, but to expand the human reproductive lifespan.

Egg donation to post-menopausal women raises concerns about whether older women are physically and psychologically prepared for the demands of pregnancy and parenthood, as well as concerns about the best interests of the resulting child. The Commission's objections to this practice rest not on these types of considerations, but rather on a more fundamental principle regarding the appropriate circumstances in which finite societal resources should be used to provide medical services. We find the use of donated eggs for post-menopausal women inappropriate — it is invasive, expensive, and an inappropriate use of resources. Moreover, because it is normal for women to be infertile at this age, there is no medical justification for the practice.

Finally, where zygote cryopreservation is not available, recipients of donated eggs would have to be informed of the potential for the transmission of HIV through donated eggs and be fully informed of the nature and extent of this risk before deciding about whether to proceed with treatment using donated eggs. Because egg cryopreservation and thawing have not been successful to date, is not possible to establish an egg quarantine period, with testing of the donor six months after the donation, before the donated eggs are used in treatment. The Commission's conclusion with respect to the use of fresh eggs differs from that on fresh sperm because egg cryopreservation is not available at this time and zygote cryopreservation is available only in some clinics. This means the only option for some women who want donated eggs will be the use of fresh eggs. (They will be unable to have the donated eggs fertilized with their own partners' sperm and frozen for six months if zygote freezing is not available.) We do have concerns about the potential for transmitting HIV through donated eggs, but we believe that steps can be taken to minimize this risk, for example by ensuring that thorough medical and social histories are obtained from donors. We have also emphasized the importance of fully informing the recipient about this risk. As zygote cryopreservation becomes available at all facilities offering IVF, however, we believe that the use of fresh donated eggs should be phased out. In any event, donated eggs will likely be difficult to obtain, because most women undergoing IVF will want to have their "surplus" eggs fertilized by their partners' sperm and the resulting zygotes cryopreserved for their own use in future cycles.

In summary, the Commission recommends that

> **160. Egg donation by women undergoing IVF be permitted only if**
>
> **(a)   the woman has read, understood, and discussed her consent to donate and has been informed that a decision not to donate eggs will in no way jeopardize or affect her current or future care; and**
>
> **(b)   the woman has had appropriate counselling to assist her in understanding the implications of egg donation and has given her informed consent to it.**

161. The Assisted Conception Sub-Committee of the National Reproductive Technologies Commission, with input from experts, develop protocols for evaluating egg donors, with the donor being tested for sexually transmitted diseases potentially transmissible to the recipient or the child; with zygotes created using donated eggs being cryopreserved for six months where possible and the donor retested for HIV; and with the donor providing identifying and non-identifying information for purposes of inclusion in a national data base for gamete donations.

162. Women who have experienced menopause at the usual age should not be candidates to receive donated eggs.

163. Record-keeping protocols should be developed and followed for egg donors; non-identifying information about the egg donor would be maintained and be available to the parents and child(ren) of families that result from the donation, and regulations about access to identifying information would be comparable to those governing families created through donor insemination.

and that

164. The Assisted Conception Sub-Committee, with input from relevant experts, develop interim protocols for counselling and obtaining the informed consent of prospective recipients of fresh donated eggs, in particular regarding the risk of transmission of HIV given the impracticability of an egg quarantine period and the fact that zygote freezing is not available in

some clinics. These interim protocols should be used until zygote cryopreservation becomes available as a safer option.

Egg Donation Before Surgical Sterilization

British and U.S. practitioners have obtained eggs for donation from women about to undergo surgical sterilization.[7] From the practitioner's perspective, women undergoing surgical sterilization are good candidates for egg donation. The women have usually proven their fertility, there is no risk of jeopardizing their health by ovulation induction or egg retrieval, and they have presumably completed their families.[8] Eggs from this source would be a safer option for couples who need egg donation because, unlike IVF patients, the donors would not want the eggs for their own future treatment. The donated eggs could therefore be fertilized with the recipient's partner's sperm and the resulting zygotes frozen and quarantined for six months until the egg donor was retested for HIV.

Commissioners have concerns about this practice. Although women undergoing surgical sterilization may be less psychologically vulnerable than women undergoing fertility treatment, Commissioners would not want to see them feel pressured in any way to donate eggs. If a woman is to be asked to consider this, it is essential she too have appropriate counselling to enable her to make an informed choice about egg donation. The Commission therefore recommends that

> **165. Egg donation by a woman undergoing a surgical sterilization be subject to the same protocols regarding informed consent, donor testing, and record keeping as those for women donating eggs in the context of IVF procedures.**

"Altruistic" Egg Donation

Some women have been willing to undergo ovulation induction and egg retrieval in order to donate the eggs retrieved for use in an unknown recipient. Mount Sinai Hospital in New York has reported that some women are motivated to participate in their donor program because they have a friend or relative who is infertile.[9] Our survey of Canadian clinics revealed that although women who need ova sometimes find their own donors (for example, a friend or a relative), there is no evidence that women are being recruited by the clinics as donors.

The Commission does not believe that it is ethical to permit such an invasive surgical procedure, with its attendant risks, on an otherwise healthy woman for the benefit of someone else, particularly in the absence of information about the long-term effects of these procedures. We therefore conclude that voluntary anonymous egg donation is appropriate only in the context where women would be having the egg retrieval procedure anyway — that is, in IVF programs or during surgical procedures that are to be carried out for reasons unrelated to egg donation. The Commission therefore recommends that

> It is essential to ask, for example with respect to oocyte donation and contract motherhood, what is altruism? What kinds of altruism are good, and what kinds may be problematic for those, primarily women, who are expected to be altruistic? Why should there not be more emphasis on male altruism in reproduction?
>
> *C. Overall, reviewer, research volumes of the Commission, 1992.*

> **166. Eggs for donation be obtained only from women already undergoing surgical procedures or egg retrieval as part of their own treatment. Egg retrieval exclusively for purposes of donation should not be permissible.**

Designated Egg Donation

Designated egg donation refers to the situation where a known donor, often a sister or close friend of the recipient, donates an egg for use in IVF. Seven of the eight Canadian programs offering IVF with donated eggs permit designated donations, and two have reported live births from sister-donated eggs. Some clinics encourage women to find their own donors because of the scarcity of anonymously donated eggs. One hospital-based clinic, however, explicitly forbids designated donations in its program.

There appears to be somewhat greater acceptance of designated egg donation than designated sperm donation.[10] Surveys have shown, for example, that couples are more comfortable with the idea of the sister of a woman who is infertile providing an egg for IVF than with the notion of the brother of a man who is infertile providing sperm for use in donor insemination.[11] The former is usually depicted as a "gift," while donor insemination still carries some of the cultural connotations and psychological implications associated with adultery.

Advocates of designated egg donation cite advantages: there is first-hand knowledge of the donor's physical, psychological, family, and social history; no third party or "broker" has to be involved; and relationships between the parties can be discussed and clearly defined before the donation takes place.[12]

But the practice also raises serious concerns. The potential for coercion of the women involved exists, especially between family members, who may feel it is their "duty" to supply eggs. The potential donor may be subject to overt or covert pressure from the recipient or from other family members. Most important, donation would require her to undergo the risks, discomfort, and inconvenience of medical procedures that will be of no benefit to her and may even cause her harm.[13]

> Oocyte donation programs must also operate using anonymous donors. The use of known donors is still acceptable, however, since obtaining oocytes is more complex than obtaining sperm, and follows an in-depth psychological assessment of the receiver and the donor. [Translation]
>
> *C. Duchesne, Section de reproduction du département d'obstétrique-gynécologie, Hôpital Saint-Luc, Public Hearings Transcripts, Montreal, Quebec, November 21, 1990.*

The most troubling aspect of such arrangements is the potential for harm to the eventual child. Although egg donation is relatively new, and we therefore have little knowledge on which to base an assessment of the likely effects on children, there is reason to believe this could cause considerable difficulties in relationships between the child and its parents, the child and its genetic mother, and the social parents and the egg donor.

The Commission believes that the potential for coercion and exploitation of the donor, as well as the potential adverse effects on the resulting child, are too great to justify designated egg donation. Therefore, the Commission recommends that

> **167. Designated donation of eggs to a named recipient not be permissible.**

Payment for Egg Donation

Although the Commission is not aware of any Canadian cases of payment for egg donation, U.S. clinics regularly advertise for egg donors and pay them a fee. There are also cases where U.S. clinics have offered free medical care to women who want a tubal ligation, provided they agree to undergo ovulation induction and egg retrieval.[14] As we have recommended with respect to sperm donation, payment for human gametes is inappropriate, as it would constitute commercialization of human reproductive material, a situation that the Commission considers ethically unacceptable.

The Commission considers payment for eggs unacceptable on other grounds as well; multiple egg induction and retrieval are accompanied by medical risks, pain, and the possibility of long-term health effects. As already established with respect to organ and tissue donation, it is unethical to allow people to risk their health to sell parts of their bodies. The potential for exploitation is simply too great to justify this practice. Thus, the Commission concludes that payment in connection with egg donation is never acceptable. Only women who would be having invasive procedures anyway (egg retrieval during IVF procedures; surgery for other reasons) would be in a position to consent to donate eggs. The Commission therefore recommends that

168. Payment for egg donation not be permissible.

Potential Use of Eggs from Fetuses

We would object strongly to fertilization of eggs obtained from female fetuses, even if it becomes technically feasible to retrieve and mature them. We find this suggestion deeply offensive to all notions of human dignity and have recommended that it be among the activities prohibited outright in the *Criminal Code* of Canada (see Chapter 5).

Legal Issues

Before the introduction of IVF, legal motherhood was attributed unequivocally to the woman who gave birth to a child. There was no need to determine whether that presumption was grounded in genetics or gestation. Thus, egg donation challenges existing legal principles that define who is a child's mother. When donated eggs are involved, two women are physically involved in the creation of the same child, one as the source of the genetic material and one as the person who gestated the fetus and gave birth to the child. In other words, it would be possible for the egg donor to seek to establish her biological link with the child and to pursue a legal declaration of motherhood, just as it is possible,

> Who has control of the embryo? The researcher who made its creation possible or the donors of the gametes? If it is accepted that the embryo may be owned, who is the owner? At what point does the embryo become a person or a human being? The controversy surrounding "humanization" is far from being resolved. [Translation]
>
> *Brief to the Commission from Ordre des infirmières et infirmiers du Québec, April 1991.*

in the absence of legal rules to the contrary, for a sperm donor to seek a declaration of paternity in cases of assisted insemination.[15]

If egg donation is permitted, the most important step in resolving the legal issues surrounding egg donation is the determination of legal parenthood. In Canada, because there is no legislation dealing specifically with egg donation (although some provinces/territories have taken legislative steps to clarify parenthood in cases of sperm donation), it is difficult to say with certainty who currently would be accorded the status of legal mother. This must be the first legal principle established with regard to egg donation. For example, the provisions of the revised Quebec *Civil Code* state explicitly that "contribution of genetic material to medically assisted procreation does not allow the creation of any bond of filiation between the contributor and the child born of that procreation." The Commission recommends that

> We would object strongly to fertilization of eggs obtained from female fetuses, even if it becomes technically feasible to retrieve and mature them. We find this suggestion deeply offensive to all notions of human dignity and have recommended that it be among the activities prohibited outright in the *Criminal Code* of Canada.

> **169. Provinces and territories that have not already done so amend their family law legislation to clarify legal parenthood in cases of egg donation, with the recipient gestating and giving birth being declared the legal mother of the resulting child.**

In the Commission's view, an egg donor should have no parental rights or responsibilities toward any child born as a result of the donation. The woman who receives donated eggs or zygotes should be deemed to be the mother of any resulting child. The male partner of the recipient, if he has given his consent to the procedure, should be deemed to be the father of the resulting child. In other words, the legal principles that should govern parenthood in cases of egg donation are similar to those that should govern legal parenthood in cases of sperm donation.

Dealing with "Spare" Embryos

IVF patients are usually asked to determine before the eggs are retrieved what they want done with any "spare" zygotes resulting from IVF procedures. If the clinic does not offer cryopreservation, the couple can usually choose to donate the zygotes for use by other couples who are infertile or to donate them for research; or they can ask the clinic to dispose of them. If the facility offers cryopreservation, other decisions have to be made about the disposition of frozen zygotes. If the couple later decides they do not wish to have their frozen zygotes transferred, do they want to make them available for donation? If the couple's relationship ends, what is the status of the frozen zygotes? If the male partner dies, is it ethical to transfer a zygote later, with the resulting child to be raised by the woman? If it is the woman who dies, could the surviving male partner use the zygotes with a subsequent partner and raise the resulting child?

Embryo Cryopreservation

After an egg has been fertilized, the resulting zygote can survive for only a few days at most outside the body, even when kept in the special medium developed for this purpose. The advent of techniques making it possible to freeze and thaw zygotes successfully has extended the period that they can remain *ex utero*, but these techniques have created ethical and legal dilemmas of their own. In particular, whether human embryos are categorized as property, as potential human beings, or otherwise will have an effect on the way rights with respect to their control are formalized. Resolving these issues is of fundamental importance to the creation of a coherent and cohesive approach to the regulation of new reproductive technologies.

Embryo (Zygote) Cryopreservation

The practice of IVF changed dramatically after 1984, when the first child developed from a frozen zygote was born in Australia. Zygote freezing is now a routine component of many assisted conception programs. Before the advent of cryopreservation, IVF clinics had three options for dealing with excess zygotes: implanting them all, running the risk of multiple pregnancy; using the extra ones for research; or disposing of them. The ability to freeze zygotes now means that clinics can transfer fewer embryos in a given cycle and freeze the remainder for the couple's use in later cycles. This avoids the need for another invasive egg retrieval procedure and gives more chances of pregnancy from a single retrieval.

1. The zygote is introduced to increasing concentrations of cryoprotectant agents to dehydrate the zygote and replace the water with agents that do not promote ice formation.
2. The zygote is slowly cooled to sub-zero temperatures.
3. The zygote is then stored in liquid nitrogen.
4. When needed, the zygote is thawed rapidly in a warm bath.
5. The zygote is rehydrated and the cryoprotectant solution removed. It can then be transferred to the uterus.

Legal Control and Informed Consent

The main issue with respect to the legal status of embryos is who may exercise decisional authority and what the scope of that authority is — in other words, who has the authority to decide among legally available alternatives in relation to the zygote, such as transfer, storage, disposal, donation, and research. Questions that must be answered include not only who has authority, but whether that authority can be exercised in advance, when and how that authority can be transferred to others, and how disputes are to be resolved. At present, Canadian law and jurisprudence are largely silent on these issues, and although there have been U.S. court cases, their application to the Canadian situation is uncertain. Because the technologies and the law in this area are so new, the answers to these questions are not clear when the embryo (meaning the zygote) exists outside a woman's body.

It has been suggested that property law may be an appropriate mechanism to achieve the goal of giving the two individuals who were the source of the gametes joint control over what happens to a zygote created from their gametes. Yet, in the Commission's view, reproductive material should never be characterized as property, because terms such as "ownership" and "property" suggest that human zygotes can be treated as objects, which is contrary to principles such as respect for human life and dignity and non-commercialization of reproduction. The Commission therefore believes that the complex issues of control and decisional authority with respect to human zygotes must be addressed in a conceptual framework that makes it clear that they are not "property." (We discuss this in more detail in Chapter 22, "Embryo Research.")

> The complex issues of control and decisional authority with respect to human zygotes must be addressed in a conceptual framework that makes it clear that they are not "property."

The Commission concludes that the two individuals who were the source of the gametes should have joint authority to determine what happens to zygotes created from their gametes and that decisions in this regard should be taken before egg retrieval and fertilization — that is, before the zygotes are created. This means that information, counselling, and consent procedures for those contemplating IVF must take into account the fact that surplus zygotes could result and that decisions about them are necessary before treatment can proceed.

This is also the position of the American Fertility Society, whose ethical statement on IVF holds that only the gamete sources have the right to decide on the disposition of resulting zygotes, and of the Warnock Committee in the United Kingdom, which stated that "the couple who have stored an embryo for their use should be recognized as having rights to the use and disposal of the embryo."

Because Canadian law is so uncertain at this stage, however, clear rules are necessary to establish this principle and to ensure that zygotes do not become the object of disputes. Our proposal would also make it unnecessary for the courts to sort out disagreements with respect to the disposition of embryos, a situation that has the potential to create conflicts of the type the Commission believes should be prevented with respect to human reproductive tissues and capacities. In other words, from the Commission's ethical perspective, these rules are a matter for society, through its legislators, to decide — not for the courts to decide through an adversarial process.

As far as the Commission has been able to determine, IVF clinics in Canada that offer cryopreservation of "spare" zygotes have consent procedures regarding the disposition of these zygotes in the event that the couple decides not to have them transferred or in circumstances (such as the death of the partners) that make this impossible. Some of these consent procedures include a provision directing the clinic what to do with the embryos after a specified period of storage — the choices are donation to others for use in infertility treatment, donation for research, or disposal by the clinic. What is happening to "excess" zygotes in clinics that do not offer cryopreservation varies from clinic to clinic.

We believe that the rules regarding the handling of surplus zygotes must be clarified and standardized. Moreover, patients should not be subject to pressure to consent to any particular use of their zygotes, be it donation or research, and they should be assured that refusal to donate zygotes or to consent to their use in research will not in any way affect their current or future treatment. The Commission therefore recommends that

> **170. Decisions regarding the disposition of zygotes be made by women and couples before any gametes are retrieved or zygotes created, with such decisions being binding on the IVF clinic or facility involved. The Assisted Conception Sub-Committee of the National Reproductive Technologies Commission should develop standardized consent forms listing the decisions required from donors.**

This will, however, be in the context of what is allowable. Given that the outcomes of longer-term storage are unknown, we believe it makes sense to set a limit of five years for the duration of storage. Another issue is whether storage should be permitted after the death of one partner. The wish to transfer a stored zygote after the death of a partner may be understandable. It is relevant, though, that for all other couples pregnancy is not an option when one partner has died.

Enabling the use of stored zygotes to establish a pregnancy after the death of one of the partners would require societal resources to be used for the storage and transfer. It would also require legal reform to ensure clear succession and inheritance rights if the interests of already existing children are not to be harmed; the distribution of estates could be considerably delayed, and administration of an estate difficult. If embryo transfer is allowed after the death of a man, it should also be allowed after the death of a woman, provided a subsequent female partner consented to gestate the zygote. The potential complexities, consequences, and ramifications are unclear. Given this, it seems to Commissioners necessary to have some limits, and the death of either partner is a clear and practical limit. It is moreover a limit that does not deprive people of an option that most people have. If transfer is not allowed, they are simply like all other couples when one dies. This position may seem contradictory when we have recommended allowing single women to have donor insemination; however, we do not know the social and psychological effects on the child of coming from a father known to be dead. The Commission therefore recommends that

> **171. Zygotes not be stored for more than five years from the date they are frozen, or beyond the death of one of the gamete donors.**

Embryo Donation

As now constituted, IVF programs are not set up to deal with the implications of embryo donation. Social and medical data about the egg donor, who would usually be an IVF patient, would have to be collected, as would information about the sperm donor. This information would be necessary if zygote recipients and the resulting child were to have access to information similar to that given to recipients of donated sperm or eggs. Information about the genetic health, physical characteristics, identity, ethnic origin, and other characteristics of potential embryo donors would have to be available. This information is not routinely attached to cryopreserved zygotes, however, and the decision to donate could potentially be made months or years after the zygote was created.

Embryo donation raises concerns about the psychosocial implications for the donor and recipient couples and the best interests of any child who results. In the Commission's view, if donated eggs are available and the recipient's partner's sperm can be used to fertilize them, with freezing of the resulting zygotes to allow for donor testing, this would be the preferred alternative so that both parents raising any child born have biological links — one has gestated the child and one is the genetic parent. In practice, however, we recognize that zygotes, rather than eggs, are more likely to be available for donation. Even so, we believe that it is only under unusual circumstances that embryo donation, rather than egg donation, should be considered the preferred course of action if donated eggs are available. These circumstances would all entail situations where both partners have medical conditions that make pregnancy using their own gametes inadvisable or impossible — for example, if the female partner has ovarian failure or a genetic disease and the male partner has one of the indications for donor insemination.[16]

We believe that embryo donation is permissible, subject to safeguards similar to those discussed earlier in the context of egg donation, such as the prohibition of designated donation and payment for donation, and the requirements for informed consent and proper record keeping.

Recommendations

Egg and Embryo Donation

The Commission recommends that

172. **Designated donation of eggs and zygotes to a named recipient is not permissible.**

173. **Women who have experienced menopause at the usual age should not be candidates to receive donated eggs or zygotes.**

174. **Eggs and zygotes for donation or research should be obtained only from women already undergoing surgical procedures or egg retrieval as part of their own treatment. Egg retrieval solely for purposes of donation is not permissible. Any woman asked to donate (whether in the context of IVF or a surgical procedure) should be subject to protocols regarding counselling, informed consent, donor testing, and record keeping established by the Assisted Conception Sub-Committee of the National Commission.**

175. (a) Full and informed consent to any egg or embryo donation should be obtained under circumstances that make it clear that a decision not to donate will in no way affect the patient's current or future care or access to treatment.

   (b) Counselling and informed consent of potential embryo donors must include the fact that donors will be tested for HIV antibodies at the time of donation and six months later and that their embryos will be quarantined for six months to allow for this testing.

176. (a) In the case of eggs and zygotes for donation, identifying information, including the donor's full name, address, and date and place of birth, should be collected from the donors as soon as they consent to donation under specified conditions (for example, in the event of their deaths). Immediately upon collection of the identifying information, a donor identification code number should be attributed to it.

   (b) Non-identifying information about the donor's medical and genetic history, age, and physical and social attributes, including race and ethnicity, should be collected in a standardized form once consent to donation has been obtained. Non-identifying donor information, all test results, and the donated eggs and zygotes should then be identified only by the donor identification code number. Appropriate record storage procedures should be in place to preserve confidentiality.

(c)   Where a child is born as a result of a donation, identifying information about the donor, the donor's identification code number, the name of the egg or zygote recipient, and information about the child born as a result of the donation should be forwarded to the National Reproductive Technologies Commission, for storage under secure conditions for a minimum period of 100 years.

177. All necessary steps for testing donors of eggs and zygotes for infectious diseases or other conditions that could potentially affect the health of the woman receiving the donated egg, of the zygote, or of the resulting child should be strictly followed.

178. Testing for HIV 1 and 2 should include a zygote quarantine period of at least six months, with re-testing of the donor's blood for antibodies to HIV at the expiry of that period.

and that

179. Egg and embryo donors should not be compensated in any way.

Disposition of Unused Eggs and Zygotes

The Commission recommends that

180. Zygotes should be disposed of in accordance with the wishes of the gamete donor(s), expressed in writing before gamete retrieval. Zygotes should not, however, be stored for more than five years from the date they are frozen. Zygotes stored for a couple's own use should be stored only up to the death of either partner.

> 181. **Surplus eggs should not be fertilized or used without the express permission of the egg and sperm donors.**

and that

> 182. **Adherence to these requirements, set by the Assisted Conception Sub-Committee of the National Reproductive Technologies Commission, with respect to the handling of eggs and embryos would be a condition of licence to offer assisted conception services. Failure to comply would result in loss of licence.**

Conclusion

The Commission considers that donating eggs and zygotes could enable women who are infertile and who would not otherwise be able to conceive to have children. We believe, however, that the interests of the donating woman or couple must be protected, and we have recommended a system of controls to ensure that women's autonomy in deciding whether to donate is protected, and to prevent what we consider to be unethical uses of the act of donation. We also consider that the interests of the children born would mean that appropriate donor testing and record keeping be put in place.

In this chapter we alluded to the fact that frozen zygotes can also be donated for use in research. Chapter 22, "Embryo Research," examines the aims of embryo research, the uses to which it may be put, and the ethical and social issues it raises.

General Sources

Stephens, T., and J. McLean. "Survey of Canadian Fertility Programs." In Research Volumes of the Royal Commission on New Reproductive Technologies, 1993.

Specific References

1. Inquiries in various Australian states, the United Kingdom, and Ontario (the Ontario Law Reform Commission) throughout the 1980s have considered both egg and embryo donation acceptable within guidelines. An inquiry in South Australia found egg donation acceptable, but not embryo donation. The U.S. Department of Health, Education and Welfare found in 1979 against the acceptability of either egg or embryo donation (Walters, L. "Ethics and New Reproductive Technologies: An International Review of Committee Statements." *Hastings Center Report* (June 1987): 3-9). A 1988 working committee on new reproductive technologies in the Quebec Department of Health and Social Services was not able to come to a unanimous conclusion on the freezing of embryos or donation of eggs.

2. Squires, S. "Motherhood: It's Never Too Late." *Washington Post Health*, September 8, 1992.

3. Sauer, M.V., and R.J. Paulson. "Understanding the Current Status of Oocyte Donation in the United States: What's Really Going On Out There?" *Fertility and Sterility* 58 (1)(July 1992), p. 16.

4. *Personal Experiences with New Reproductive Technologies: Report from Private Sessions.* Ottawa: Royal Commission on New Reproductive Technologies, 1992, p. 8.

5. Harvey, J.C. "Ethical Issues and Controversies in Assisted Reproductive Technologies." *Current Opinion in Obstetrics and Gynecology* 4 (1992): 750-55.

6. Grainger, D.A. "Oocyte Donation: 1988-1991." *Assisted Reproduction Reviews* 1 (4)(November 1991): 104-109.

7. Serhal, P. "Oocyte Donation and Surrogacy." *British Medical Bulletin* 46 (3)(1990), p. 797; Gordon, M. "Inconceivable?" *Mirabella* (July 1991), p. 60; Grainger, "Oocyte Donation," p. 105.

8. Great Britain. Interim Licensing Authority for Human In Vitro Fertilisation and Embryology. *Report of the Meeting for Centres and Ethics Committees.* London: Interim Licensing Authority, 1990.

9. Gordon, "Inconceivable?" p. 62.

10. Sauer, M.V., et al. "Survey of Attitudes Regarding the Use of Siblings for Gamete Donation." *Fertility and Sterility* 49 (4)(April 1988): 721-22.

11. Ibid., p. 722.

12. Sauer, M.V., et al. "Oocyte and Pre-Embryo Donation to Women with Ovarian Failure: An Extended Clinical Trial." *Fertility and Sterility* 55 (1)(January 1991), p. 42.

13. American Fertility Society. Ethics Committee. "Ethical Considerations of the New Reproductive Technologies: Donor Eggs in In Vitro Fertilization." *Fertility and Sterility* (Suppl.) 53 (6)(June 1990): 48S-50S.

14. Gordon, "Inconceivable?" p. 60.

15. Except in three jurisdictions where there is consent to DI legislation.

16. American Fertility Society. Ethics Committee. "Ethical Considerations of the New Reproductive Technologies: Pre-Embryos from In Vitro Fertilization." *Fertility and Sterility* (Suppl.) 53 (6)(June 1990), p. 51S.

Embryo Research

♦

Researchers in the United States observed a human egg being fertilized in a glass dish (*in vitro*) for the first time in 1944. By the late 1960s, researchers in Great Britain were able to bring about fertilization of human eggs *in vitro* fairly reliably. This work led to the first live birth of a child having its beginnings outside the human body, which occurred in Britain in 1978. Since then, techniques for fertilizing human eggs have developed rapidly. Among the factors that have contributed to the development of this technique are the use of fertility drugs to stimulate human egg production and improvements in the procedures that enable sperm and egg cells to mature successfully *in vitro*.

One result of these developments is that more embryos* (or, more accurately, zygotes**) are created *in vitro* than are actually needed for assisted conception.[1] The existence of embryos *in vitro* has made it possible, for the first time in history, to conduct research on human zygotes

---

* There is a problem with terminology, as the term "embryo" is used in different ways. In the language of biologists, before implantation the fertilized egg is termed a "zygote" rather than an "embryo." The term "embryo" refers to the developing entity after implantation in the uterus until about eight weeks after fertilization. At the beginning of the ninth week after fertilization, it is referred to as a "fetus," the term used until time of birth. The terms embryo donation, embryo transfer, and embryo research are therefore inaccurate, since these all occur with zygotes, not embryos. Nevertheless, because the terms are still commonly used in the public debate, we continue to refer to embryo research, embryo donation, and embryo transfer. For accuracy, however, we also refer to the developing entity during the first 14 days as a zygote, so that it is clear that we mean the stage of development before implantation and not later.

** See discussion in this chapter (section on The Aims of Embryo Research and the section on The Ethical Uses of Human Zygotes in Research) on the use of the terms "embryo" and "zygote."

at this very early stage of development. Such research is less than 30 years old and was made possible only because the use of *in vitro* fertilization makes zygotes available. Conducted in many countries, including Canada, this research has facilitated advances in infertility treatments, provided insights into the early stages of human development, and increased our understanding of fertility and contraception.

The research also raises questions, however, about the moral and legal status of the embryo (meaning the zygote) and about how society's respect for human life should apply to this situation. What form of respect is owed to the zygote and at what stage of its development? What forms of research, if any, are consistent with respect for human life? What is the legal status of zygotes *ex utero*? Are they property or something else altogether? What legal or other rules should govern who has access to them and how they are treated? Should distinctions be made between *in vitro* and *in utero* zygotes? If a particular status is ascribed to embryos *in vitro*, how would this affect the status of zygotes *in utero*? These are some of the specific questions that have been raised in this area.

In general, concerns have been expressed about the potential impact of embryo research on women and on society. For example, some people are concerned that women may be pressured to donate zygotes not needed for implantation during IVF procedures for research, or to undergo fertility drug treatment to obtain eggs for research into fertilization. Some have also expressed concerns that development of the field could lead to an international trade in human zygotes, or that techniques currently used in animal embryo research, such as cloning and ectogenesis, could be applied to human beings. In addition, there is concern that the long-term social implications of embryo research are unknown; for example, could future applications of knowledge alter our current notions of humanness or parenthood? Can research be regulated in such a way as to prevent such misuse or abuse?

Embryo research in Canada has been conducted to date without a clear legal and public policy context. Research proposals are assessed on their individual merits by research ethics boards in hospitals and universities where research is going on. There is a growing public conviction, however, that consistent policies are needed to guide individual ethics committees. Because human embryo research is a relatively new field in Canada, the Commission had an unusual opportunity to examine relevant ethical and legal questions while the field is still young and to make recommendations that will anticipate rather than react to new developments. Commissioners believe it is important to seize this current opportunity to put in place limits and boundaries and to regulate within those boundaries, ensuring that only ethically acceptable, accountable use of technologies involving human zygotes occurs in Canada. During our consultations with Canadians the Commission heard a range of views about the acceptability and appropriate regulation of embryo research. Although many people expressed hope about the potential benefits of such research, others expressed fears about the potential for harm and concern about the ethical and social implications.

To help assess the arguments presented to us, we commissioned various research studies to obtain as definitive a picture as possible of embryo research as it is practised in Canada and elsewhere. We also reviewed the legislation adopted in other jurisdictions and sought the views of theologians, ethicists, and legal scholars on the moral and legal status of the human embryo. In the remainder of this chapter, we document what we learned in consultations with Canadians across the country and from our inquiry into the current and future uses of human zygotes or embryos in research. We then review some of the laws, regulatory mechanisms, and government policies that have shaped research in this field. With this background, we discuss the ethical, legal, and social implications of embryo research. Our recommendations for policy conclude the chapter.

The Views of Canadians

Commission Survey

In the spring of 1990, the Commission conducted a national survey of Canadians to help us gauge attitudes toward various aspects of new reproductive technologies. We also conducted a later qualitative study involving 10 focus groups across the country in which participants were asked what they knew and thought about the use and disposal of sperm, eggs, and zygotes. The study revealed that participants had no ethical concerns about the freezing or disposal of sperm and unfertilized eggs or their use in research. By contrast, fertilized eggs were seen as having the potential for life or, by some, as being the beginning of life. As such, participants thought that the use of fertilized eggs in research should be restricted more than the use of sperm or unfertilized eggs.

Some participants argued that the techniques used in IVF should be modified to ensure that no surplus zygotes are created; they considered it unethical to produce fertilized eggs that cannot be transferred to a woman's body with the aim of establishing pregnancy. Others thought it was acceptable to produce surplus zygotes under certain conditions. According to the Commission survey, 63 percent of respondents would permit surplus

> If more ova are removed than can be reimplanted from a woman who is herself undergoing IVF, she should retain the right to decide whether the surplus are to be donated (at which time she relinquishes control), frozen, used for regulated research purposes or destroyed.
>
> *D. Day, Nova Scotia Advisory Council on the Status of Women, Public Hearings Transcripts, Halifax, Nova Scotia, October 17, 1990.*

zygotes to be frozen for later transfer to the woman from whom the egg came; 47 percent would allow surplus zygotes to be donated to another woman who is infertile; and 46 percent would permit their use in research in some circumstances. Almost all participants had many questions and concerns and called for some controls or limits in this area.

Submissions to the Commission

The Commission also sought the views of Canadians in public consultations and private meetings from Vancouver to St. John's and received many written submissions from individuals and groups. These consultations revealed that Canadians have a range of views on the question of when a human life begins, a life to which society has legal and moral obligations. Some argued that legal personhood should be recognized at fertilization, and hence that a zygote should not be subjected to research that is not for its own benefit. Other intervenors either argued that the developing human entity develops personhood gradually with gestational development or pointed to legal rulings by Canadian courts that it achieves personhood only at birth. They supported embryo donation and research but felt restrictions should be placed on researchers, such as ethical review of research proposals and prohibition of research beyond a certain point in development (proposing, for example, that research be prohibited beyond 14 to 17 days of development).

We also heard a range of views about the acceptable sources of embryos for use in research. Among those that accept embryo research, some thought research should be permissible only on zygotes not implanted during IVF; others believed zygotes could be created specifically for research, provided there were limitations on that research. Many women's groups disagreed with the creation of zygotes for research, stating that it could lead to the exploitation of women, including pressure to undergo ovulation induction to produce eggs to make zygotes.

Virtually all those who commented on these issues pointed out that traditional mechanisms of peer review and research ethics board review may not provide sufficient safeguards against inappropriate use of embryos in research. Many were of the view that the public, particularly women, should have more opportunity to participate in decisions about the restrictions or requirements that should apply to such research. The Commission heard many suggestions about how the public could participate in such

> We request that the law tolerate no treatment whatsoever of any human embryo as an experimental subject in the practice of either *in vitro* fertilization or *in vivo* fertilization. [Translation]
>
> *Brief to the Commission from l'Association féminine d'éducation et d'action sociale, November 1990.*

decisions, ranging from increased public representation on institutional ethics committees, to a multidisciplinary permanent advisory committee at the federal level, to a voluntary or statutory licensing authority with public representation.

We also heard a range of views on the desirability of legislation as a means of regulating research in this field. Many doctors and researchers, as well as the Medical Research Council of Canada, argued that a voluntary system — under which research is monitored through federal granting agencies, provincial licensing bodies, research ethics boards, and peer review — provides effective protection while allowing the freedom needed to

> [In] experimentation and research, parents or researchers may not freely dispose of the physical integrity or life of the unborn child. Accordingly, corpses of human embryos and fetuses must be respected.
>
> *J. Penna, Roman Catholic Diocese of Saskatoon, Public Hearings Transcripts, Saskatoon, Saskatchewan, October 25, 1990.*

promote progress in knowledge and therapy. These intervenors argued that legislative controls might impede progress in research and therapy. Representatives of legal and human rights groups expressed concern about the absence of legal direction on issues such as "ownership" of zygotes, the storage and disposal of zygotes, and the interests and responsibilities of donors and physicians with respect to embryos.

There was widespread agreement among all intervenors that any commerce or trafficking in human gametes or embryos should be prohibited, and that certain forms of research, such as the division of human zygotes ("cloning"), the formation of animal/human hybrids, and the gestation of human zygotes in the uterus of another species, were totally unacceptable.

These public consultations gave us a broad picture of the views and concerns of Canadians about embryo research. To evaluate these concerns, in the next few sections we discuss our findings from a series of studies examining the aims of embryo research, its future directions, its current practice in Canada, the source of embryos for research, and current regulations in Canada and abroad.

The Aims of Embryo Research

Nearly all documented human embryo research to date has taken place well before 14 days after fertilization (the stage by which a zygote created in a woman's body [*in vivo*] implants in the uterus) (see Figure 22.1). In fact, technical limitations make it difficult to keep a fertilized egg alive and developing *in vitro* normally after six days.

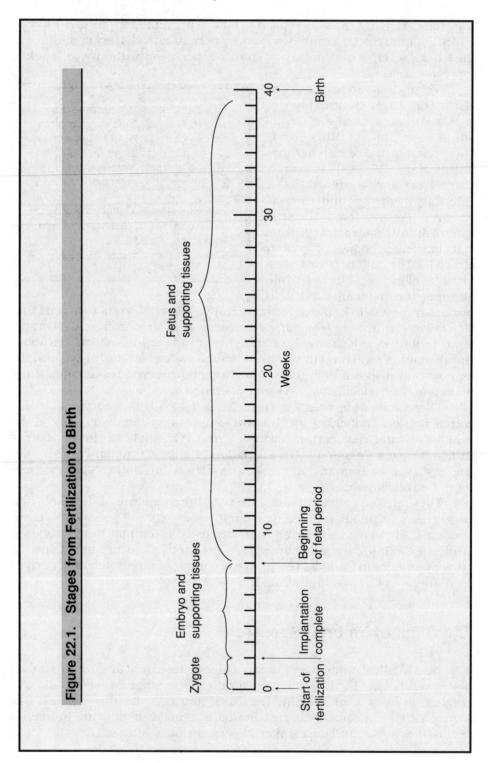

Figure 22.1.   Stages from Fertilization to Birth

As we have outlined, there is a problem of terminology. Embryo research, embryo donation, and embryo transfer are not accurate terms, since these in fact occur at the zygote stage. The term "pre-embryo" has also been used to refer to the zygote. This is a more accurate term in some respects because, as discussed in Chapter 7 "The Biology of Human Reproduction," there are important changes in identity between the zygote and the post-implantation embryo (for example, 99 percent of the fertilized egg develops into supporting tissues, while 1 percent develops into the embryo proper). The term "pre-embryo" has been a source of controversy, however, as some people believe that it diminishes the humanity of the developing entity. To avoid this possible bias, we have chosen the more neutral term "zygote."

Evaluating whether research on zygotes is acceptable requires an understanding of the goals of this research. What sort of knowledge are researchers seeking to discover, and how will this knowledge contribute to human health? In this section, we outline the major types of embryo research and their objectives. Currently, biomedical research involving human zygotes is undertaken for one or more of the following reasons:

- to improve existing infertility treatments and develop new technologies for assisted conception;

- to learn more about human infertility (including implantation failure and ectopic pregnancy) and develop better ways to diagnose it;

- to detect and prevent genetic and chromosomal anomalies in human beings;

- to investigate new methods of contraception; and

- to advance knowledge about human development and its disorders.

We look at each of these in turn. Before examining them, however, it is worth noting that the question of what constitutes "research" is not straightforward. In the field of embryo research, it is difficult to distinguish between basic and applied research, between clinical investigation and new therapy. For example, research into new methods of fertilizing eggs *in vitro* or freezing zygotes has often gone hand in hand with clinical practice. It may be very difficult, therefore, to say whether the use of a new procedure for zygote freezing constitutes research or treatment improvements. Classifying embryo research according to whether it is clinical, pre-clinical, or basic is therefore next to impossible and not very meaningful. The Commission documented dozens of approaches to this problem. Although each system of classification has its own internal logic, they are often inconsistent with each other, and each suffers from the difficulties just outlined.

Although many commentators and international reports emphasize a distinction between therapeutic and non-therapeutic embryo research, for the reasons discussed below we found this an inappropriate distinction and not useful for purposes of discussing the acceptability of research or what the public policy response should be. "Therapeutic" embryo research has been defined as research performed on a zygote to improve its chances of successful implantation and healthy development. Non-therapeutic research, on the other hand, is not intended to promote the developmental chances of a particular zygote; zygotes that have been the subject of non-therapeutic research are disposed of rather than implanted. As we have seen, some participants in the Commission's public hearings argued that therapeutic embryo research should be allowed, while non-therapeutic research should be prohibited.

The therapeutic/non-therapeutic distinction is common in other areas of biomedical research. In our view, however, this distinction cannot provide a basis for regulating research on human embryos. Research involving a zygote could have diagnostic or curative potential for that zygote only if it was subsequently transferred to a woman's uterus with the aim of establishing a pregnancy. However, transferring a zygote after it has been subjected to research poses unknown dangers for both the woman and the eventual fetus. This procedure should be allowed, therefore, only if there is evidence of its safety. The only way to establish such evidence would be through non-therapeutic research on zygotes, that is, observing *in vitro* the development of zygotes that have undergone a particular technique, to see whether they develop normally.

In other words, the only way to develop therapeutic embryo research is to allow for some non-therapeutic embryo research. Thus, the regulatory options are either to allow some forms of non-therapeutic research or to preclude research using zygotes altogether. Allowing therapeutic research while at the same time prohibiting non-therapeutic research would not be workable, nor would it be ethical, because of the risks it would create for women and children. In distinguishing between various types of embryo research, therefore, we found it more useful to classify by area of study than to talk about basic and applied research or therapeutic and non-therapeutic research.

Treating Infertility

The most common area of research using human zygotes is aimed at improving the success of IVF as a clinical treatment for infertility or testing new procedures for the treatment of infertility. Although the fertilization rate of human eggs exposed to sperm *in vitro* is between 70 and 80 percent, many fertilized eggs never develop to the stage at which they can be transferred to the uterus. In addition, there is significant attrition after transfer, with many zygotes not implanting, so that the average rate of live births per zygote transferred is only about 17.5 percent. Also, as is discussed in Chapter 20, most IVF practitioners transfer three or even four zygotes during each treatment cycle, with the goal of improving the chances of a live birth; this is a significant factor in the increased rate of multiple pregnancies and premature births associated with IVF.

Improving the rate of live births would help reduce the need to transfer several zygotes. Research projects in various countries have therefore sought to improve the chances that transfer of a zygote will lead to a live birth. Among these projects are studies seeking to

- improve zygote freezing, storage, and thawing techniques;

- diagnose which gametes will fertilize successfully and which zygotes will result in live births;

- discover the optimal conditions for maturation and survival of gametes and zygotes *in vitro*; and

- assess the optimal stage of growth at which to transfer a fertilized egg and where in the woman's reproductive tract to place it (the uterus or the fallopian tube, for example).

Studies in zygote freezing include the comparison of various substances (cryoprotectants) and freezing techniques, with the aim of improving upon the current 50 to 70 percent rate for zygotes that survive freezing and thawing. Researchers are also studying how to freeze and thaw unfertilized eggs. If successful, this research would dramatically reduce the need to create and freeze surplus zygotes. The only way to test the safety of this technique, however, is to conduct research involving zygotes produced using frozen eggs that have been donated for research purposes. Eggs frozen in different ways are thawed and fertilized, and the chromosomes and rates of cleavage of the resulting zygotes are studied to see whether they develop normally.

One example of diagnostic research is the development of chemical gradients to select the healthiest sperm for insemination *in vitro* — but fertilization is the only way to test which gradient works best. Another example is the study of the metabolism of the zygote as a predictor of future viability.

An example of research into the optimal conditions for the survival and maturation of zygotes involves fertilizing donated eggs *in vitro* to study whether the use of different fertility drugs to induce ovulation has an effect on the likelihood of fertilization. In a British study, women having tubal ligations volunteered to undergo ovulation induction before the sterilization procedure. Their eggs were retrieved during the procedure and were fertilized *in vitro* to permit study of the effects of various fertility drugs on the resulting zygotes.[2] Again, fertilizing eggs may be the only way that research projects studying fertilization can be carried out.

Researchers are also testing new procedures to treat certain previously untreatable forms of infertility. Techniques are being developed, for example, to treat male infertility in which otherwise apparently normal sperm are unable to penetrate an egg's outer membrane. Several techniques have been investigated, including both chemical and mechanical drilling through the egg's outer coat or shell (the zona pellucida) to ease the entry of sperm. Microinjection of a single sperm cell into the cytoplasm of the egg has also been attempted. Zona drilling has also been used to rupture the shell in the hope that it will improve the chance of implantation. Live births resulting from the use of each of these methods have been reported. Although these techniques may ultimately be used in treatment, their safety must first be assessed through embryo research on zygotes that are not subsequently transferred to a woman's uterus. Only if zygotes resulting from these experimental fertilization techniques are observed and assessed *in vitro* can it be known whether they develop normally, at least initially. A further phase of clinical research to assess any longer-term effects of these manipulations on the health of the potential individual born will also be needed before it can be viewed as "treatment."

Understanding Infertility

There is great interest in understanding the subtle mechanisms of human reproduction — for its own sake, but also to permit the development of better approaches to infertility and healthy reproduction.

In vitro study of human zygotes has shown that they manufacture and release numerous biochemical compounds. Very little is known about these growth factors released by the zygote and how they affect development and interaction with the woman's body. It is known that the zygote binds substances from its environment as it travels along the fallopian tube toward the uterus, but why it does so is not clear. Identification and functional analysis of these growth factors and chemical messengers may provide clues to understanding "unexplained" infertility. They may also help to define what is necessary for normal growth, both in laboratory culture and in the woman's uterus. Preliminary research has begun to reveal the metabolic behaviour of human zygotes; tests are being developed to show what type of and how much nutrient a zygote takes up from the medium in which it is being cultured.

Another area of human embryo research centres on the mechanisms and conditions necessary for successful implantation of the zygote in the wall of the uterus. This research may help explain why implantation fails, leading to relatively high rates of early loss or miscarriage. Understanding implantation may also help to explain ectopic pregnancies where no obvious tubal or structural defects exist. Ectopic pregnancy affects thousands of Canadian women each year, is a serious risk to their life and health, and remains an important clinical problem, in terms of both treating this medical emergency and the future fertility of a woman who experiences such a pregnancy (see Chapter 10, "Sexually Transmitted Diseases and Infertility").

Inherited Disorders

A new step in embryo research is the very recent development of "preimplantation diagnosis" techniques — that is, techniques for diagnosing the presence or absence of genetic disease in the human zygote. This experimental technique has been offered to women and couples at high risk of passing on a genetic disease, such as cystic fibrosis. Researchers at University Hospital in London, Ontario, are now evaluating the clinical feasibility of this procedure for women who are known carriers of a sex-linked genetic disease. This technique constitutes research at the current state of knowledge.

We discuss preimplantation diagnosis of genetic disease in future chapters; however, it is important to note its relationship to embryo research. For example, preimplantation diagnosis requires washing the zygote to remove surrounding cells, removing the zona pellucida, then gently lifting away one cell and analyzing its DNA to detect the particular gene. This "biopsy" technique was developed through research on zygotes, and any future clinical application of this procedure will depend on continued research into such biopsy techniques.

Regulating Fertility

Research on zygotes may be relevant to understanding new contraceptive methods. For example, the contraceptive RU-486, developed in the 1980s, works by countering the effects of the hormone progestin, which promotes the maturation of eggs. A potential risk of using RU-486 is that eggs might still mature and fertilize, despite the effects of RU-486, but develop abnormally. A study to assess the chances of this occurring involved recovering unfertilized eggs from women who volunteered to take RU-486 prior to undergoing laparoscopic sterilization and studying their maturation, fertilization, and cleavage *in vitro*.[3] The study showed that RU-486 did not affect fertilization and cleavage of zygotes, but further research is needed to evaluate whether RU-486 has any effect on developing embryos later.

Other research of relevance to the regulation of fertility involves studies on antigens and other proteins in the zygote as part of the search for contraceptives that work by provoking an immune response. This research may also throw light on the problem of recurrent spontaneous abortion.

Studying Human Development and Its Disorders

Scientists are investigating the mechanisms by which the cells of the early zygote — which have the capacity to give rise to any type of body tissue — differentiate into cells that are "committed" to be one type of tissue or another. Why do some cells give rise to the embryo itself and others give rise to the placenta? Why do some cells then give rise to liver cells and others to brain cells? Elucidating these mechanisms is of great interest to basic biologists and scientists involved in human reproduction and may have relevance to our understanding of cell growth, differentiation, and cancer. Research to date has shown that certain observable shape differences in the zygote are correlated with later impaired development; chromosomal abnormalities have also been correlated with abnormal development of various kinds, but much more research will be required before these mechanisms are understood completely or even partially.

Future Directions in Embryo Research

The areas of embryo and gamete research discussed in the previous sections are expected to remain the focus of research internationally for many years to come, but it is likely that new areas of study, such as the effects of people's age on the viability of their gametes, identification of hitherto undiscovered mechanisms that cause infertility, and the roles of viruses and chemical substances in causing congenital anomalies, may also be explored. Many aspects of this research could have important preventive and clinical applications. In addition, the study of stem cells derived from zygotes and cultured *in vitro* could yield information about cell division and its control, which could help researchers understand the proliferation of cancer cells.

Technology Transfer Between Animals and Humans

In discussing future directions in embryo research, it is important to distinguish human embryo research from animal embryo research. It is also relevant to consider the relationship between animal research and use of the technologies in human beings.

There are two issues with regard to technologies transferred from animals to human beings. In the first category of technologies are those that would be unethical in and of themselves if applied to human beings (such as ectogenesis, parthenogenesis, and inter-species crosses). Areas of current research with animal embryos include "cloning" by nuclear substitution, modification of the embryo's genetic make-up, partheno-genesis (creation of a zygote from the female gamete alone), fusion of female gametes, ectogenesis (development of a fetus to viability outside the uterus), and transfer of the zygote to another species for gestation. Transfer of these technologies for use with human embryos would be unacceptable. Use of human zygotes in this way would contravene the Commission's stated ethical principles and be contrary to the values of Canadians; indeed, such uses have been condemned by the various bodies that have issued recommendations on research involving human embryos. We recommend prohibition of these.

In the second category are technologies that are not unethical in and of themselves, but whose use would be unethical if they were used in human beings for the same purposes as they are used in animals (for example, IVF done with the goal of producing many "high-quality" zygotes from one animal, to be gestated by less commercially valuable animals; or alteration of the genetic make-up of zygotes in order to produce a commercially valuable strain of animals). This category of technologies and techniques could be transferred ethically only if their goals were not transferred with them. It is in fact desirable to transfer knowledge gained through animal research to human beings, provided this knowledge and the technologies that result from it are applied in ethically acceptable and beneficial ways for women and for society.

In short, there has been, and will likely continue to be, a great deal of technology transfer between human medical research and veterinary research related to assisted reproduction. But it is important to remember that the aims of using reproductive technology in animals are very different from its goals when undertaken in human beings. In farm animals, the objective is not to circumvent infertility but to produce as many offspring as possible from a valuable selected animal or group of animals, with the goal of benefiting producers and consumers. IVF is used in cattle, for example, to obtain as many offspring as possible from commercially valuable genetic parents, using ordinary animals for many gestations. IVF zygotes are being used, for example, to establish entire populations of European cattle breeds in developing countries, by transfer to indigenous breeds for gestation. In our meeting with a large commercial breeding laboratory, Commissioners learned that frozen cattle zygotes are shipped around the world for this purpose. IVF in cattle is also used to produce large numbers of early cleavage-stage zygotes, which are used in studies of early development.

> It is in fact desirable to transfer knowledge gained through animal research to human beings, provided this knowledge and the technologies that result from it are applied in ethically acceptable and beneficial ways for women and for society ... If borrowing knowledge from animal studies contributes to ethically acceptable goals in human medicine, then it is appropriate and indeed desirable to use this knowledge.

In human beings, by contrast, the ultimate goal is to maximize the probability of obtaining a viable and healthy pregnancy from use of a given technology. Although the conditions for which IVF is used in human beings have broadened, all are still concerned with remedying infertility, with the ultimate aim being to allow a woman to have a healthy child.

The goals of IVF in human beings and domestic animals, therefore, are very different. What IVF-related research efforts involving human and animal embryos have in common is the goal of perfecting the various tools and strategies that make IVF and manipulation of the embryo possible in each species. In the view of the Commission, if borrowing knowledge from animal studies contributes to ethically acceptable goals in human medicine, then it is appropriate and indeed desirable to use this knowledge. Improvements in human IVF should not be refused simply because they originated in animal breeding. IVF has enabled people to circumvent infertility and to have a child. By itself, and as a medical intervention, this does not commodify or exploit women or reproduction.

But it is essential that the values underlying the use of these technologies in animals not be transferred along with the technologies. If a given line of animal embryo research has no beneficial or morally acceptable human application, the use of human zygotes for similar research should be prohibited. Given that there are vulnerable interests to be protected, and consistent with our guiding principles, we make recommendations later in this chapter that would ensure that only ethically acceptable use of these technologies is allowed.

> It is essential that the values underlying the use of these technologies in animals not be transferred along with the technologies. If a given line of animal embryo research has no beneficial or morally acceptable human application, the use of human zygotes for similar research should be prohibited.

As discussed in Chapter 24, situations involving commercial interests in health care require that vulnerable individual or societal interests be protected by public policy or regulation. In agribusiness, the owner of the animal and the provider of reproductive technology services have commercial interests and goals; the animal itself has no recognized goals. The wider society has a general concern for animal welfare (so there are some regulations in place) and an interest in cheaper and better food products. In the human situation, however, there is no "owner" — the woman or couple have their own interests and goals but are not necessarily in a position to advance or defend themselves. Interposed here as well is the physician, who has a professional obligation to serve the interests and goals of the patient, but the interests of the patient may still be vulnerable interests in the face of commercial interests promoting technology. This means additional safeguards may be needed; adoption of our recommendations would put these in place. Our recommendations throughout this chapter would protect vulnerable interests by preventing inappropriate transfer of commercial technologies or goals from animal to human embryo research. Further detailed discussion of particular technologies being used in animals (such as zygote splitting, cloning by nuclear substitution, sex-selective zygote implantation, transgenic animals, ectogenesis) and our assessment of whether transfer is appropriate are provided in Chapter 25. Accurate information on these techniques must be available for Canadians, as there is much misinformation in the public domain. An important aspect of the public policy response to embryo research is accountability, which requires that information be available to Canadians on what is being done in embryo research. Our recommendations include measures to bring this about — most importantly, the requirement that any facility conducting research on human zygotes/embryos be licensed and comply with conditions of licence.

Current Uses of Zygotes in Research in Canada

Although the future use of human zygotes in research is speculative, we wanted to determine how they are being used today in Canada. Early in our mandate, however, the Commission discovered there was no comprehensive information on how zygotes — or human reproductive tissues generally — are being used in research in Canada. We therefore undertook primary research to obtain these data. We sought to track the use of reproductive tissues — including gametes, embryos, fetal tissue, and placentas — to see how health care facilities, medical laboratories, and medical disposal firms are handling these tissues. In this section we discuss the use of gametes and zygotes; our findings regarding the use of fetal tissue and placentas are described in Chapter 31.

Handling and Use of Eggs and Embryos*

Because of the clinical circumstances in which human eggs are recovered and fertilized, and because of the specialized technologies required to sustain them outside the body, the facilities from which eggs and embryos can be obtained are limited. In Canada, fertilized and unfertilized eggs can be generated only in hospitals performing obstetric and gynaecological surgery and in clinics specializing in treating infertility. We decided to survey every health care facility in Canada that offers obstetric and gynaecological services, including those with fertility clinics attached to them.

Canada's hospitals and health care facilities offering obstetric and gynaecological services were surveyed between November 1991 and February 1992. Among the 642 facilities on which the survey results were based, 8 handled eggs and 8 handled embryos (for example, retained them for a patient's future fertility treatment or other treatment) (see research volume, *Treatment of Infertility: Current Practices and Psychosocial*

---

* The developing human entity is usually available only at the zygote stage. We use the term "embryo" in this section because it was the term used in the questionnaire of our research.

Implications). One facility reported retaining eggs for research purposes, and one reported retaining embryos for research purposes. None of the facilities reported providing either eggs or embryos to outside institutions, researchers, or agencies.

The questionnaire used in this survey did not ask about the movement of eggs or embryos *within* the facility. The location to which they would be sent most commonly within a facility, however, is the pathology laboratory. (All spontaneously aborted tissue, tissue from induced abortions, and tissue from surgical procedures are routinely examined in the pathology laboratory). The research team expressed concern that those designated to complete the questionnaire may not always have been the most knowledgeable about the distribution of reproductive materials by or within the facility.

Given this, and in an attempt to develop a clear picture of the use of human reproductive tissue in Canada, the Commission decided to conduct a follow-up survey with a sample of Canadian medical laboratories. Questionnaires were sent to 60 medical laboratories (primarily regional facilities affiliated with larger hospitals and universities), of which 48 (80 percent) responded. Of the 48 laboratories that responded, 2 reported handling eggs for purposes of pathology analysis, and 19 reported handling embryos (such as early pregnancy losses) for pathological examination. This shows there is some "internal" movement of eggs and embryos within hospitals and their associated clinics and laboratories, largely for pathological examination. However, these tissues are used for research purposes only very rarely — only one laboratory used embryos in research; none used eggs.

As a final check on the possible distribution of eggs and embryos, the Commission also conducted a survey of 23 medical waste firms (which included regional offices of larger national firms), of which 16 (70 percent) replied. None of the medical waste firms reported any handling of eggs or embryos, but much of what is disposed of through these waste firms is delivered to them in sealed containers, so that they may be unaware of the precise nature of the tissues handled.

The original survey of health care facilities as well as the follow-up survey of medical laboratories confirmed that there is relatively little human embryo research being conducted in Canada. Results from both these surveys identified one health care facility engaged in research on eggs, one facility engaged in research using embryos, and one medical laboratory involved in embryo research. Within these facilities, several distinct research projects have been undertaken. Research on embryos included studies of the development of cell motility, the process of division of embryonic cells *in vitro*, and the preimplantation diagnosis trial at University Hospital in London, discussed above. Research on eggs included a project analyzing unfertilized eggs for errors in chromosome number and structure; the frequency of chromosomal abnormality is then analyzed statistically for correlation with such factors as the woman's age, the use of various fertility drugs, and heavy cigarette smoking. Another group is doing research on egg freezing.

It is evident that the data we were able to gather from these surveys are limited and inaccurate in various ways. For example, one of the more interesting results of the survey of health care facilities was that many hospital administrators seemed unaware of what their own institutions were doing with eggs or embryos. Moreover, respondents to both surveys may have interpreted questions differently. The survey asked about the use of eggs and embryos in "research," "treatment," and "pathology." But as we have seen throughout this report, these terms can be defined in various ways — new treatments and pathology analyses may be defined in certain contexts as "research" by some people but not others. Such data limitations are unavoidable in surveying areas that have never been surveyed before. We believe it is important to develop clear information on these questions, however, and our recommendations will help generate a better data base regarding the handling and disposition of eggs and zygotes in Canada.

Research by Pharmaceutical Manufacturers and Biotechnology Companies

There has been a persistent rumour, particularly in Europe, that human embryos are used by the pharmaceutical and cosmetics industries. Although investigations suggest that these rumours are unfounded,[4] we felt it was important to determine whether private sector companies in Canada are using eggs or embryos. The Commission surveyed all 67 member companies of the Pharmaceutical Manufacturers Association of Canada. Of these, 55 companies (82 percent) provided written responses. None reported any use of human eggs or embryos. One company is using human sperm. This research project ($100 000 annual expenditure) is being conducted in collaboration with a non-profit body outside Canada. It involves the use of sperm in research into a contraceptive method using the immune system.

The Commission also surveyed 26 biotechnology companies identified as potential users of human reproductive tissues. Of the 20 respondents (77 percent), none reported any research involving eggs or embryos. These findings lead us to conclude that little or no embryo research is being done by industry in Canada. This is consistent with the findings of a recent international study of embryo research. Partly in response to the rumours regarding the use of human zygotes in industry, the Council of Europe commissioned a survey of the commercial and industrial uses of human reproductive tissues. The study revealed extensive medical research involving zygotes, concentrated in England, France, the United States, and Australia, but there was no evidence of the use of embryos for commercial or industrial purposes.[5]

This could change. Industry respondents to the Commission's survey speculated that research involving human gametes or zygotes could be undertaken by the pharmaceutical industry in the next five years; research would likely focus on fertility controls for both men and women and more effective infertility treatments. It is important, therefore, to establish safeguards to ensure that research on zygotes in the private sector is regulated and that zygotes are not commercialized. Our recommendations later in this chapter are intended to address these issues.

Sources of Zygotes Used in Research

In Vitro Creation of Zygotes

The two potential sources of human zygotes for use in research are donations from women or couples being treated at fertility clinics and zygotes created specifically for research purposes. As we have noted, because the number of eggs that will fertilize *in vitro* is unpredictable, often all the eggs retrieved are exposed to sperm to help ensure that enough zygotes will be available for transfer to the uterus. As a result, more eggs are usually fertilized than can be transferred safely during that cycle. The extra zygotes may be cryopreserved for use in a future cycle if the current cycle is unsuccessful or if the couple plans to have more than one IVF child. If some zygotes turn out not to be needed, however, a couple may decide to donate them for research. Sometimes the zygotes intended for future use may be rejected for cryopreservation because of damage or an obvious anomaly, such as fertilization by more than one sperm; or cryopreservation may not be available. In these cases, too, the couple may decide to donate the zygotes for research.

The second potential source of zygotes is eggs fertilized expressly for the purpose of using the resulting zygote in research. This requires that donated gametes be available and that donors consent to this use of their gametes. This source of zygotes is less common, since women undergoing infertility treatment generally prefer to use their scarce eggs for their own treatment. However, women whose ovaries are being removed for medical reasons may be willing to donate any eggs that become available as a result of surgery.

Uterine Flushing

Zygotes can be "flushed" from a woman's uterus if less than seven days have elapsed since intercourse. This technique was first developed to recover zygotes from commercially valuable breeding livestock, with those recovered being transferred to less valuable stock for gestation. Only a limited number of uterine flushings have been performed in human beings — because of differences in uterine structure and the time between fertilization and implantation, the procedure is much more dangerous and less successful in human beings. The procedure can result in ectopic pregnancy if the zygote is flushed into a fallopian tube, for example, instead of out of the body; or the zygote may implant in the uterus, leading to a normal (but unintended) pregnancy. Because of these risks to the woman, guidelines developed by the Canadian Fertility and Andrology Society and the Society of Obstetricians and Gynaecologists of Canada recommend against the use of uterine flushing to retrieve eggs and zygotes.

Potential Availability of Zygotes

Since the vast majority of eggs fertilized *in vitro* are intended for use in establishing a pregnancy, there is a relative scarcity of zygotes for research. If zygote freezing becomes a routine adjunct of IVF programs, the availability of viable zygotes for research is likely to decline further. On the other hand, as increasingly accurate, non-invasive viability tests for zygotes are developed, the availability of non-viable zygotes (that is, those unlikely to survive transfer and develop to term) for research may increase.

Some have raised the concern that the demand for zygotes for research purposes may affect women's clinical care, that women will be pressured to donate surplus IVF zygotes for research, or that women will be pressured to undergo unnecessary ovulation induction to produce eggs that can be fertilized for use in research. We have no evidence that this is occurring, but it is nevertheless important to have clear and appropriate safeguards in place to ensure that any demand for zygotes does not affect clinical care. Our recommendations later in this chapter address this need.

Alternatives to Research on Human Zygotes

Animal models have provided the starting point for most of the research areas described here. There is ample evidence, however, of the limitations of generalizing results from animal models to human beings. For example, it is now possible to freeze, thaw, fertilize, and transfer mouse eggs, and the resulting offspring are normal. Investigations into freezing human eggs have been far less successful, owing to subtle but critical structural differences between the eggs of the two species. Although animal models can provide insights for application to preliminary basic human embryo research, animal research alone is not enough; human embryo research is also needed to safeguard the health and well-being of women and the resulting children. Similarly, the use of human cell lines can provide important insights into certain questions, but it cannot eliminate the need for human embryo research.

Regulation of Embryo Research in Canada

On the basis of the evidence we assembled regarding the aims of embryo research, we believe that it can provide important health benefits. We are also aware, however, that allowing embryo research raises difficult ethical and legal questions and concerns. We need to determine whether it is possible to answer these concerns and acquire the benefits of embryo research in an ethically acceptable manner. In approaching this question, we looked first at the current state of laws and professional guidelines related to embryo research in Canada.

Legislation

No legislation directly regulates embryo research in Canada. Several federal and provincial inquiries have made recommendations in the area of embryo research (discussed below), but none has led to legislation.[6] In the absence of specific legislation, a variety of existing federal and provincial laws might apply. For example, provincial human tissue gift acts require the informed consent of tissue and organ donors to the use of tissue for research in certain contexts (for example, the transplantation of tissue from one person to another, or the post-mortem donation of tissue for transplantation, medical education, and research). These acts also preclude the buying and selling of human tissue. However, it is not clear that these laws apply to gametes or zygotes, which are often excluded, implicitly or explicitly, from legal definitions of "human tissue."

Hence, the legal requirements regarding the handling of zygotes are far from clear. In fact, the legal status of zygotes *ex utero* is itself unclear. As discussed in greater depth in Chapter 30, under Canadian law the embryo and the fetus are not legal persons before live birth. In law, what is not considered a "person" is often classified as "property," and recent court cases in the United States have characterized

> Commissioners believe that it would be highly undesirable for zygotes or embryos to be characterized as property, with all the social and legal implications such a classification implies. Rather, we think that legal rules relating to the zygote and embryo should be designed to ensure that they are treated with respect as a form of potential human life.

zygotes *ex utero* as the "property" of the gamete donors, at least for certain purposes.[7] Some IVF clinics in Canada have adopted this characterization in their consent forms, which state that couples enrolled in their programs are considered joint owners of the zygotes created from their gametes.

However, the legal classification of zygotes and embryos has not yet been addressed explicitly by the courts in Canada.

Commissioners believe that it would be highly undesirable for zygotes or embryos to be characterized as property, with all the social and legal implications such a classification implies. Rather, we think that legal rules relating to the zygote and embryo should be designed to ensure that they are treated with respect as a form of potential human life.

An analysis prepared for the Commission suggested that a property model may be appropriate, since the core of property law is the idea of an exclusive right of control (see research volume, *Overview of Legal Issues in New Reproductive Technologies*). Characterizing embryos as property would vest exclusive control of gametes, and joint control over zygotes *ex utero*, in the gamete donors. This would protect donors' autonomy and privacy interests by requiring that they give their consent to any use of their gametes or zygotes for research (or indeed any other purpose). However, using a property law model for reproductive materials would have very significant drawbacks. A pure property law regime would give the "owners" of zygotes not only a right of control, but also all the other standard incidents of property ownership.   For example, owners of property are generally allowed to give property away or sell it, bequeath it to inheritors, destroy it or experiment on it, store it, and share in the profits of research on it.

> None of the reports reviewed by the Canadian Bar Association recommended a prohibition on experimentation. The general approach, typified by the recent report of the Law Reform Commission of Canada, is in favour of allowing experimentation on gametes and embryos, subject to certain restrictions. The advantages of increased knowledge, benefits to childless couples and therapeutic development outweigh concerns related to genetic manipulation and duplication of the species within the controlled experimental environment. The Canadian Bar Association is of the opinion that experimentation upon gametes and embryos is both appropriate and desirable.
>
> *Brief to the Commission from the Canadian Bar Association, November 1990.*

These implications of a pure property law regime for embryos are clearly unacceptable. As discussed later in this chapter, there is clear international consensus that the buying and selling of zygotes are inconsistent with respect for human life, as are certain kinds of research involving zygotes. Moreover, the buying and selling of zygotes could promote the exploitation of women, the commodification of women and children, and the alienation of women from their bodies.

Some people suggest that zygotes could be seen as a unique kind of property in which the right to exclusive control applied, while the other standard incidents of ownership, such as the right to sell one's property, would be restricted. These other incidents of ownership could be restricted either by explicit legislation or by allowing the courts gradually to develop a common law conception of the rights of ownership with regard to *ex utero* zygotes. This is, in effect, what is occurring in the United States, as the courts adapt property law to fit the distinctive situation of *ex utero* zygotes. However, as the U.S. experience shows, relying on the courts to develop a new definition of property rights with respect to *ex utero* zygotes is unpredictable and leads to a lack of uniformity, as judges in different states develop the common law in different directions. Moreover, courts are limited to the specifics of the case before them, whereas legislators can take into account a wider range of circumstances and interests.

We believe, therefore, that explicit legislation is needed to address the issue of control over zygotes *ex utero*, but we do not see property law as an appropriate model for thinking about who should have what kinds of decision-making powers with respect to them. We can address those issues directly, by asking why we think certain people should have particular powers of decision, and by seeing how this would affect the relationships of concern to us. Talking about "property" is not helpful here, because it gives rise to inappropriate assumptions about the interests and rights at stake.

The Law Reform Commission of Canada also argued that leaving these issues to be resolved on the basis of property law principles would be unethical. It recommended that Canadian lawmakers should

> develop special legal rules that will protect embryos but also permit the ethical debate to continue. Such rules could be developed on the basis of the written, signed consent of the producers [the gamete providers] given before the embryos are conceived ... [who should be] allowed to change their decision regarding the ultimate fate of the embryos before the embryos are used for the purpose for which they were intended.[8]

The Commission concludes that legal rules should be developed that adequately protect the interests of those whose gametes are used to create the zygote, including their right to understand fully and consent to the retrieval and subsequent use of their gametes and resulting zygotes. Our recommendations later in this chapter are intended to address these requirements.

Professional Guidelines

In the absence of legislation, the only existing Canadian policy related to embryo research is the voluntary guidelines of the Medical Research Council. In its 1987 report on *Guidelines on Research Involving Human Subjects*, the MRC endorsed "non-therapeutic" embryo research, for up to 14 to 17 days following fertilization, if approved by a local research ethics board. It recommended that zygotes not be created solely for research purposes and that embryo research be undertaken only to improve knowledge and treatment of infertility.[9] Compliance with these guidelines is a requirement only when the research in question is funded by the MRC, but the guidelines have also been adopted widely by research institutions, universities, hospitals, and other granting agencies in Canada.

Although the MRC guidelines have served Canada well to date, we believe that additional measures are needed. For example, they do not provide much guidance about how informed consent should be sought for embryo research, or about appropriate standards for handling and storing human zygotes. Moreover, research ethics boards are likely to differ in the way they approach decisions regarding embryo research, giving rise to potential inconsistencies. As well, local research ethics boards may lack the expertise to evaluate certain kinds of research proposals and may be unduly vulnerable to pressure from advocacy groups. Furthermore, there is no mechanism for centralized record keeping regarding embryo research, so the public can know what is occurring in this field, and the MRC guidelines do not apply to research not funded by universities or government bodies.

Some of the limitations with respect to research ethics boards are being addressed. For example, the Royal College of Physicians and Surgeons recently established the National Council on Bioethics in Human Research (NCBHR), funded by the MRC, to assist in the implementation of MRC guidelines. It is intended, in part, to function as the voluntary and unofficial standard-setter for university research ethics boards.[10] However, the efficacy of this mechanism is not yet clear. Although the NCBHR has lay input, it is still established and funded by the medical research community, and it is not yet known whether this mechanism will be seen by the public as capable of resolving conflicts of interests in the public interest, or as assuring adequate public input. Moreover, these guidelines and review mechanisms do not apply to research done in settings where there is no research ethics board — for example, in industry.

> The same ethical guidelines that apply to medical experimentation on humans and the use of human tissues for experimentation, transplantation or other therapies should apply to the embryo and foetal tissues. Thus the only embryo experimentation and research that is ethically defensible is that which will potentially benefit the embryo itself.
>
> *J. Bromley, Fort Smith Pro-Life Group, Public Hearings Transcripts, Yellowknife, Northwest Territories, September 12, 1990.*

For these and other reasons, we believe that embryo research should be evaluated in a national context, as well as at the local level. Most federal and provincial inquiries in Canada that have addressed embryo research have emphasized the need for standardized and centralized monitoring of it. Some recent reports have endorsed a system of national standards and national approval of embryo research and/or national accreditation or licensing for facilities where such research occurs.[11] This is also true of the 1990 report of the two major associations of professionals involved in embryo research (the Canadian Fertility and Andrology Society and the Society of Obstetricians and Gynaecologists of Canada).[12]

Regulation of Embryo Research Internationally

The Commission also reviewed current public policies on embryo research in other countries; for a detailed discussion, see Appendix 1. Our review revealed a range of responses to this issue: some countries allow non-therapeutic research for up to 7 or 14 days (provided the zygote is not subsequently transferred for implantation), while others ban it; some countries restrict research to surplus zygotes, while others allow the creation of zygotes for research purposes.

In other areas, however, there is consensus. For example, it is widely agreed that certain forms of embryo research are inherently impermissible (for example, cloning; formation of cross-species hybrids). Moreover, it is widely accepted that if embryo research is to occur, it must be subject to limitations such as the following:

- the research project must be approved by an ethics committee;
- the informed consent of the embryo or gamete donors must be obtained before donation;
- zygotes that have been the subject of research cannot be transferred to a woman's uterus;
- research on human zygotes is permissible only if the information sought cannot be obtained in any other way (for example, research using animal embryos or cell lines);
- zygotes must not be bought or sold; and
- the aim of embryo research should not be commercial profit.

Moreover, as in the Canadian inquiries, there seems to be a trend internationally toward some form of national monitoring of embryo research, through legislation, licensing, or accreditation. We have examined these international models carefully in considering our recommendations.

Issues and Recommendations

The Commission's guiding principles, elaborated below as they pertain to embryo research, helped to shape the Commission's recommendations about the kinds of embryo research that should be permitted in Canada, the limitations that should be imposed on embryo research, and how these activities should be regulated.

As discussed earlier in this chapter, the use of zygotes in medical research has the potential to provide important medical knowledge and to improve the quality of health care for Canadians. To the extent that such research can help alleviate harms and the effects of disease, then it promotes ethically valid goals. Zygotes are not, however, simply "things" to be used however we like. They are connected to the human community in many ways. Human zygotes come from a human source — indeed, from particular human beings; they share certain basic biological qualities with human beings; and they may have the potential to become fully developed human beings. To treat a zygote as merely a thing would be to deny the reality of these connections.

In deliberating about zygote and embryo research and in applying our guiding principles, we took these considerations into account. We sought to allow for the attainment of the benefits of increased medical knowledge, while ensuring that these benefits are obtained only in a way that respects the connections between zygotes and the human community and that avoids undermining our sense of respect for the dignity of human life.

We have divided our recommendations into six areas: the ethical uses of zygotes in research; obtaining zygotes and informed consent; the use of zygotes following research; the funding of embryo research; commercialization; and accountability.

The Ethical Uses of Human Zygotes in Research*

At the heart of the debate on the ethics of research involving human zygotes are fundamental questions about when a developing entity acquires a distinctive moral status and how we ought to treat it as a result. According to the chairperson of the Warnock Commission, this is the most important issue raised by the reproductive technologies.[13] We agree that it is a vital issue, partly because of its relationship to other issues that are equally fundamental to our mandate, such as the rights and status of women, the interests of families, and the collective interests of society at large.

Canadians have differing views on the moral status of the zygote and embryo. Although there is strong agreement on a commitment to the principle of respect for human life, Canadians differ about what form that respect should take and what level of protection is owed to human life at its different stages of development. There is also a wide range of answers to these questions in the history of moral philosophy.

Some people argue that human life acquires full moral status at the moment of fertilization. Others argue that moral status changes and

---

* See Annex for dissenting opinion.

increases as a fertilized egg achieves the various stages of development from zygote to embryo to fetus and, eventually, to a child. Various stages of development have been proposed as marking a crucial change in moral status, including sperm penetration of the egg, syngamy, implantation, development of the primitive streak, development of sentience, quickening, viability, and birth. Each of these various "marker events" has been said to be relevant in assessing the moral status of the zygote, embryo, fetus, or child.

Commissioners recognize that no amount of deliberation on our part will definitively answer the question of the moral status of the embryo. Philosophers and theologians have grappled with the issue for centuries, as have scientists, legal scholars, and politicians in our own time. As noted by one researcher who prepared a paper on this issue for the Commission,

> Definitions of "person" or "human being" ... are imbued with subjective considerations ... that in turn are informed by differing cultural standards, parental teachings, and religious pronouncements, regarding the morality of certain practices ... Consequently, arguments, evidence, and other forms of justification may be advanced in support of a particular understanding of the concept of personhood or humanhood, but the evaluation itself can neither be proven nor disproven.[14]

Although there is no way to "prove" any particular view on this question, we believe it is important to state clearly our position on the ethics of embryo research and to explain our reasons for rejecting alternative views.

We believe that the moral status of the embryo before day 14 after fertilization does not preclude research under certain defined conditions. We judge that given clear and stringent protections and regulation, it is ethically permissible to conduct research on human zygotes up to this stage, and that such research is in fact an essential part of ensuring the quality of health care and thus the safety and well-being of patients. We recommend the 14-day limit on research for several reasons: it recognizes the developmental stage at which the primitive streak appears, establishing the start of one or more distinct entities; it is also the point at which the zygote has normally completed its implantation in the uterine wall; and it is the most widely accepted international standard for embryo research.

We are aware that many Canadians will disagree with this conclusion. Many intervenors in our public hearings told us that embryos should be treated with respect because they are living entities with the potential to develop into full members of the human community; hence, they should be accorded the same legal protection against potentially harmful research as children or adults. We considered this argument very carefully and respect the depth of conviction of those who advance it. We share the concern that zygotes be treated with due respect. It is clear that the zygote is human, in the sense of having the genetic, biochemical, and cellular composition of the species *Homo sapiens*. Similarly, there is no doubt that the zygote is alive, although it is not viable outside a woman's reproductive tract for more than a few days. Zygotes are further connected to humanity because they may have the potential to become human beings. (A zygote does not necessarily have the potential to become a human being, as a significant percentage have a genetic make-up that means they could never develop to that stage, as discussed in Chapter 7.) These criteria alone confer a degree of moral status on the fertilized egg, even at its earliest stages of development. As a living entity that may have the potential to become a human being, a measure of respect and protection should be extended to it.

However, as noted in Chapter 30, Canadian law does not recognize embryos or fetuses as "persons." Embryos may have the potential to become persons, and we agree that this is grounds for treating the embryo with respect. But the idea of potentiality is complex, as is the relationship between potentiality and moral status. Potentiality has been used to justify different, even contradictory, policies on embryo research. It is appealed to not only by advisory bodies or policies banning embryo experimentation after fertilization or syngamy,[15] but also by those that allow experimentation for 7 or 14 days.[16] This suggests that the idea of potentiality is not simple or straightforward. In the debate over embryo research, it has been interpreted in at least two very different ways.

First, those who defend the 14-day limit argue that potentiality is not an all-or-nothing matter. They adopt the principle of graduation, according to which the zygote/embryo/fetus deserves more respect as it develops, up until viability or birth, at which point it becomes a full member of the moral community. In this view, various forms of research are acceptable at early stages, since the zygote is a potential human being only in a very remote sense. As development progresses, however, this potential comes closer to being realizable, and at some point non-therapeutic research would violate the respect owed a potential human being. Fourteen days is often chosen as the dividing line, since this marks the development of the primitive streak, which fixes the individual identity of the embryo and forms the basis for its nervous system.

We are sympathetic to this line of argument, but we do not agree that the 14-day limit on research should be understood exclusively in terms of the development of potentiality. In natural conception, a zygote starts the process of implantation in the woman's uterus at about 7 days after fertilization; *if implantation does not occur around that time*, the possibility of successful implantation and development *in utero* soon disappears. Zygotes *in vitro* actually *lose* their potential to become human beings after 14 days. Focussing exclusively on potentiality, therefore, would suggest that there is no moral objection to research involving zygotes *in vitro* after day 14. If we consider it permissible to do research on zygotes only when they have little or no potential to become persons, then, it can be argued, this tells us that research on zygotes should occur only *after*, not before, 14 days.

The 14-day limit does not rely, therefore, solely on a measurement of potentiality. A 14-day-old embryo *ex utero* deserves moral respect not for what it *can* become, but rather for what it *has already* become. After 14 days zygotes are closer to humanness, not in the sense that they have greater potential to become a human being, but in the sense that they have already developed two key components of a fully formed human being — a fixed individual identity and the precursor of a nervous system. (Researchers have not to date been able to keep human zygotes developing normally *in vitro* beyond 7 days, so there is no realistic possibility, for the foreseeable future, of experimenting on zygotes that have reached the stage of individuation.)

Those who argue for a complete ban on any embryo research not intended to benefit the particular zygote offer a different interpretation of the zygote's potential. In this view, the potential of the zygote is clear from fertilization, and the process of development is continuous. There is no marker event that is so significant that it justifies distinguishing the level of respect owed a zygote at different stages of development. As the Australian Senate Select Committee stated, from conception the zygote "may be properly described as genetically new human life organised as a distinct entity oriented towards further development," and so "the stance and behaviour proper to adopt towards it would include not frustrating a process which commands respect because its thrust is towards the further development of a biologically individuated member of the human species."[17]

We do not accept this view. Again, one difficulty is that the sense in which a zygote is a potential person is very remote. At day 4 a zygote may have the potential to become a person, but it is not *likely* that this will in fact occur, even in the most propitious circumstances. The probability of a zygote developing to birth depends on many factors, but generally half of all eggs fertilized *in vivo* do not result in a live birth (see Chapter 7). The likelihood is far smaller in the case of *in vitro* fertilization, as only about 17.5 percent of transferred zygotes result in a live birth.

People's intuitive commitment to respect for potentiality is unlikely to hold in circumstances where the likelihood of realizing that potential is so remote. As the British Royal College of Obstetricians and Gynaecologists observed, large numbers of fertilized eggs are aborted spontaneously, and "it is morally unconvincing to claim absolute inviolability for an organism with which nature itself is so prodigal."[18]

A second difficulty lies in determining the point at which the "new life" first exists. People who see fertilization as a critical landmark for assigning full moral status must decide at what point in the process of fertilization this "personhood" occurs. Is it the entry of the sperm? pronuclei formation? syngamy? or the "turning on" of the genes?

Historically, the passage of the sperm through the egg cell wall was often identified as the point at which a new life came into existence. However, recent advances in embryology have established that it takes about 24 hours after fertilization for the nuclei of the egg and sperm to break down and for the chromosomes of the egg and sperm to come together on a common spindle. When this process is complete, "syngamy" is said to have occurred. Hence, many proponents of this argument now identify syngamy as the point at which development begins, on the grounds that this is when genetic identity is established.[19]

However, as discussed in Chapter 7, individual embryonic development cannot be said to have begun until the appearance of the primitive streak, after the fourteenth day following fertilization. Before this stage of gestation, the developmental singleness of the zygote has not yet been established. Occasionally two or even three primitive streaks may form within a single embryonic plate. Conversely, but more rarely, what initially appears to be twins may combine into a single embryo. Furthermore, some fertilized eggs have a genetic constitution that means they will develop into tumours or into empty sacs, so no embryo develops at all. (This is termed "blighted ovum" and is a very frequent finding in early spontaneous abortions.) Hence, it is only with the development of the primitive streak that individuation occurs. It is therefore inaccurate to identify syngamy as the moment at which a specific individual human being comes into existence, since the process of establishing this identity continues after syngamy.

In addition, the subtle changes gametes undergo before and during fertilization and syngamy are steps in a developmental process that begins before fertilization. Moreover, the entire process of development from unfertilized gamete through fertilization to syngamy is both continuous and highly regulated by the reproductive cells involved. Thus, the process by which human life develops its potentiality begins before fertilization.

In summary, the complexity of these processes and of the notion of potentiality means that the moral status of the zygote or embryo cannot be seen simply as a function of its potentiality. We believe that they deserve respect because of their connections to the human community; potentiality is one form of connection, but not the only one and not necessarily the most important one. Zygotes are connected to the human community by their past and their present, not only by their potential future. As we have seen, these forms of connection may run in opposite directions. Zygotes at a later stage of development may be closer to the human community than earlier zygotes in terms of their present characteristics, but farther away in terms of their future potential. In this case, the future of the zygote (its potential) is less important, morally speaking, than its present stage of development.

The 14-day limit, we believe, respects all these forms of connection. It also recognizes the legitimate value of medical knowledge and the need to find a morally acceptable compromise in a pluralistic society in which there are various views about the relative importance of different stages of embryo development. People disagree about issues such as the role of potentiality, the importance of individuation, or the value of medical knowledge, and the 14-day limit is a prudent and legitimate compromise among these differing views and interests.

Indeed, many recent reports that adopt the 14-day limit place less emphasis on the idea of potentiality and more emphasis on the idea that this limit is simply a reasonable compromise among varied interests and perspectives. For example, the British Columbia Branch of the Canadian Bar Association argues that "Although arbitrary, the limit is at a natural point of evolution when the embryo would implant in the womb and satisfactorily balances the concerns against genetic engineering and in favour of beneficial experimentation."[20] The Medical Research Council points out that the recommended limit of about 14 days may accord with a "pragmatic sense of ethical acceptability."[21] Moreover, the 14-day limit has now become the international consensus. As the Law Reform Commission of Canada notes, "given the current state of knowledge, it is appropriate to agree to a standard that enjoys broad international support, if only to ensure that research done in Canada will be as respected as that done in the rest of the world."[22] Similar statements about the importance of international consensus on the 14-day standard can be found in the reports of the Canadian Bar Association, the Conseil d'État in France, various Australian state committees, the American Fertility Society, and many others.

> Zygotes are connected to the human community by their past and their present, not only by their potential future ... The 14-day limit, we believe, respects all these forms of connection.

Some people consider this limit arbitrary, and indeed it is — just as many other rules or limits adopted by society are necessarily arbitrary — the speed limit, for example, or the amount of time allowed to appeal a court decision. The decision to establish a limit of 14 days does not rest on any precise assessment of a specific single criterion, such as potentiality, to determine the degree of moral status. However, the fact that so many recent reports have endorsed the 14-day limit suggests that it has found widespread acceptance, based on its complex balancing of interests and views. We believe that in a pluralistic society, this approach is reasonable, and indeed is the only realistic basis for resolving certain ethical issues. In light of these considerations, the Commission recommends that

> ## 183. Approved research on human zygotes/embryos be restricted to the first 14 days of development.

Although research on zygotes in the first 14 days is ethically permissible, any such research must always respect the zygote's connections to the human community. Commissioners believe that certain kinds of research, such as cloning and formation of cross-species hybrids, deny these connections and so violate basic norms of respect for human life and dignity. These are unacceptable and should be prohibited. We found widespread agreement on this among Canadians.

As noted earlier and discussed in detail in Chapter 25, forms of zygote manipulation that would be unethical in human beings are being researched in the context of animal embryo studies. These include "cloning" by nuclear substitution, parthenogenesis (creation of a zygote from the female gamete

> Certain kinds of research, such as cloning and formation of cross-species hybrids ... violate basic norms of respect for human life and dignity. These are unacceptable and should be prohibited. We found widespread agreement on this among Canadians.

alone), fusion of female gametes, ectogenesis (development of a fetus to viability outside the uterus in an "artificial womb"), and transfer of zygotes to another species for gestation. These manipulations may serve valuable scientific and commercial purposes. However, transfer of these technologies to human zygotes would contravene the Commission's ethical principles, would be contrary to the values of Canadians, and has been condemned by the various bodies that have issued recommendations on research involving human zygotes.

The idea that human zygotes could be incubated and develop to term in an artificial womb is seen as reprehensible by most Canadians. Even in the unlikely event this were possible, its pursuit would dehumanize motherhood; some have even suggested it could lead to "baby farms." Equally forceful objections apply to the idea of transferring human zygotes to the uterus of another species, cross-species fertilization, or cloning by nuclear substitution, all of which would deny the zygote's connections to the human community. The Commission therefore recommends that

> **184. Human zygote/embryo research related to ectogenesis, cloning, animal/human hybrids, and the transfer of zygotes to another species be prohibited, under threat of criminal sanction.**

Commissioners also believe that no research involving the genetic alteration of human zygotes or embryos should be permitted or funded in Canada. Genetic alteration need not be a violation of the zygote's moral status, if it is done to treat a genetic disease diagnosed through preimplantation diagnosis. However, we believe that the risks of such a procedure far outweigh its potential benefits, and that there are safer and more appropriate ways for couples to manage the risk of passing on a genetic disorder. (We discuss our views on this matter in Chapter 29.) The Commission recommends that

> ## 185. Research involving genetic alteration of human zygotes or embryos not be permissible.

Finally, we considered the question of whether zygotes should be created for research purposes. On the one hand, we believe that this would create the danger of promoting instrumentalization of zygotes, thereby potentially undermining commitment to respect for human life and dignity. On the other hand, it is not clear whether we can distinguish effectively between zygotes that become available because they are "surplus" to the needs of couples undergoing IVF treatment and zygotes created specifically for research. Some commentators argue that the distinction is unworkable, since doctors can stimulate the maturation of more eggs than are needed for purposes of IVF by using fertility drugs. According to a submission to the Australian Senate Select Committee, "any intelligent administrator of any IVF program can, by minor changes in his ordinary clinical way of going about things, change the number of embryos that are fertilized. So in practice there would be no purpose at all in enshrining in legislation a difference between surplus and specially created embryos."[23]

Moreover, some important forms of embryo research can be done only if unfertilized eggs are donated specifically for research. For example, studies on new fertilization techniques — such as changes in the fluid in which unfertilized eggs are kept before being mixed with sperm — would be impossible if research was permitted only on surplus zygotes, because some aspects of fertilization can be understood only by carrying out fertilization.

In the light of these considerations, Commissioners conclude that it is acceptable for zygotes to be created for research purposes, provided that appropriate research safeguards are in place. The conditions to be met include the following:

- informed consent of the gamete donors must be obtained before donation;

- a zygote that has been the subject of research not intended to benefit that zygote is not to be transferred to a woman's body;

- research is permissible only if the knowledge sought cannot be obtained through studies on animal embryos or cell lines;

- the research must be done in a facility licensed for such research;

- the aim of the research is to benefit human health, not to seek commercial profit; and

- no egg retrieval procedures are undertaken specifically to obtain eggs for this purpose; only eggs retrieved during procedures already being performed for the health of the woman can be used.

These conditions are discussed in greater detail below.

Obtaining Zygotes and Informed Consent

Although most of the public debate about embryo research has centred on the moral status of the embryo, other important ethical issues have been raised as well. These include respect for the autonomy of the donors whose gametes are used to create the zygote. We are particularly concerned about the possibility that the pursuit of embryo research could put pressure on women and couples enrolled in IVF programs to donate eggs or zygotes for research.

The principle of autonomy says that every individual has a right to control his or her own body, subject to the limits imposed by law. In the context of embryo research, this principle would give gamete donors a right to prohibit any use of zygotes created from their eggs or sperm, since they have a unique moral interest in the use of their genetic material. They are also entitled to full disclosure of the risks and

> The question of what you do with an embryo clearly is not the doctor's decision. I think it has to be the decision of the patient.
>
> D. Cumming, Department of Obstetrics and Gynaecology, Faculty of Medicine, University of Alberta, Public Hearings Transcripts, Edmonton, Alberta, September 13, 1990.

benefits of potential uses of their gametes. Thus, the informed consent of gamete or zygote donors must be required for all decisions about the storage and disposition of zygotes. Their consent will necessarily be circumscribed by legislation and regulations pertaining to embryo research. For example, donors could not consent to donate gametes or zygotes for research that is illegal. The Commission recommends that

> **186. Clinics and researchers be permitted to use human zygotes for research only with the fully informed consent of the persons who have donated the gametes used to create the zygote.**

Donors' consent should be provided in writing, and consent must be as informed as possible. The Commission recognizes that it may not always be possible to predict all possible research uses in advance. Nevertheless, all information available about the particular research use must be disclosed to donors.

There is increasing recognition that discussions of embryo research cannot take place in abstraction from the health and well-being of the women who produce the eggs. Doing research on zygotes could put women enrolled in IVF programs under pressure to consent to donate unused eggs or zygotes. This pressure could be particularly acute if the creation of zygotes for research purposes were prohibited. Women or couples could feel compelled to donate zygotes so as not to be seen as uncooperative or because they believe that to refuse could cost them their place in the IVF program. Such situations, if they arose, would clearly contradict principles of autonomy and medical ethics.

In addition, the ethic of care tells us that a woman should not undergo the risks of invasive procedures unless they offer the possibility of benefit to her. This is why surgical procedures intended only to retrieve eggs for research should not be permitted. A fully informed woman having surgery for other reasons and who agrees to donate eggs would not be subject to any additional risk from egg retrieval; we therefore consider this ethically permissible. However, procedures specifically to retrieve eggs for research from women not already undergoing surgery for other reasons would not be ethically acceptable. The Commission recommends that

> **187. A woman's or couple's consent to donate zygotes generated but not used during infertility treatment for research never be a condition, explicit or implicit, of fertility treatment. Potential donors must be informed that refusal to consent does not jeopardize or affect their continuing treatment in any way.**

and that

> **188. Zygotes be created for research purposes only if gametes for this purpose are available without conducting any additional invasive procedures.**

Some commentators suggest that the only way to ensure that women in IVF programs are not pressured to donate unused eggs or zygotes is by banning embryo research altogether. We do not accept this view. On the contrary, we believe that prohibiting research on zygotes could create a situation where women are subject to new IVF techniques whose safety has not been adequately tested.

For example, legislation in the Australian state of Victoria does not permit testing of the chromosomes of zygotes produced using new techniques such as micro-insemination and egg freezing. If these zygotes were subsequently implanted in women, the outcome for the developing fetus and the woman carrying it would be unknown. Preventing non-therapeutic research on embryos would therefore mean that women were subject to additional risks from new procedures.[24] As the MRC observes, "It may be viewed as unethical not to conduct supportive research designed to assess and improve the safety and efficacy of such procedures as *in vitro* fertilization and embryo freezing. Without such research, therapeutic advances become limited and haphazard."[25] The Commission concurs, and we believe that women's health and autonomy are best protected by carefully circumscribing and regulating, rather than prohibiting, embryo research.

Use of Zygotes Following Research

If eggs are being fertilized and the resulting zygotes frozen or biopsied in experimental ways as part of research to improve IVF techniques or preimplantation diagnosis techniques, it is impossible at the outset to know whether or how this would affect the normal process of zygote development. If such a zygote were transferred to a woman's uterus and a pregnancy established, the resulting child could be born with anomalies or impaired functioning.

At some point in the development of knowledge, however, it will be necessary to conduct clinical trials of new fertilization, freezing, or preimplantation diagnosis techniques. The children born as a result would be vulnerable to unknown risks. To minimize these risks, we believe that any research that involves transferring zygotes that have been manipulated must be preceded by research on animal zygotes and embryos, as well as on human zygotes that are not subsequently transferred in the uterus, to establish that the procedure is feasible and of acceptable risk.   There should be full disclosure to the adults participating in the research, and any such proposal would have to be approved by the National Reproductive Technologies Commission. The Commission recommends that

> **189. Human zygotes that have been subjected to manipulations of any kind for research purposes not be transferred to a woman's body. If knowledge reaches the point where manipulations are likely to increase the woman's chances of conceiving or be of a therapeutic nature, application to conduct a clinical trial in a licensed facility should be made to the National Reproductive Technologies Commission.**

and that

> **190. No transfer of zygotes that have been the subject of research be undertaken without the approval of the National Reproductive Technologies Commission.**

Funding Embryo Research

The focus of most international debate has been on concerns about embryo research. It is equally important to understand, however, why this research is needed in the first place. All else being equal, there are valid reasons to fund research related to areas in which treatment is being provided. If IVF is being offered as treatment, it is desirable to engage in research to help ensure its safety and efficacy. However, we cannot research all conditions and treatments, so choices have to be made about where to allocate resources. These decisions have to be made in light of the priority assigned to other calls on limited research funds — for example, prevention and health promotion research.

Is embryo research an important health priority? What benefits are expected from embryo research? Where do these benefits fit within our larger health care priorities? This is a matter of some debate. Some argue that to ban such experimentation would go against the interests of humanity. Others argue, however, that almost all the information currently acquired through embryo research could be acquired in other ways.

We believe that, depending on its aim, embryo research can provide important benefits not available through other research means.[26] We concur with the position embodied in the MRC guidelines, which state that the purpose of proposed embryo research is "a critical element" in deciding whether such research is acceptable.[27]

Policies in some countries require that embryo research be directed only to improving infertility treatment; others have a broader definition of allowable research. As noted earlier, improving infertility treatment is likely to remain the most common aim of embryo research. However, we believe that embryo research may also prove useful in studying contraception and fertility; it could also promote women's health by improving knowledge about the causes of ectopic pregnancy and other threats to women's reproductive health and about how to reduce the incidence of spontaneous abortion. Since we recommend below that all facilities involved in human embryo research be licensed by the NRTC, which would monitor research projects done anywhere in the country, we do not believe it is necessary to specify further restrictions in law on the aims of research.

> Public funding of embryo research is appropriate, provided the research is duly approved by institutional ethics boards using a clear framework developed by the NRTC and conducted in a licensed facility.

We believe that public funding of embryo research is appropriate, provided the research is duly approved by institutional ethics boards using a clear framework developed by the NRTC and conducted in a licensed facility. In this area, as in any other decision about public funding, granting agencies should be guided by the principle of the appropriate use of resources. Hence, they should ensure that the research will benefit our understanding and treatment of human health and should weigh these benefits against the benefits of alternative uses of the funds. However, since we propose that the conditions for receiving a licence to conduct human embryo research include that the research must benefit human health and that the information sought cannot be obtained in other ways, we see no reason why support for embryo research in licensed facilities should not qualify as an appropriate use of public funds.

Indeed, public funding can help ensure that public priorities are respected in this area of research. According to the U.S. Office of Technology Assessment, the former ban on federal funding of embryo research in the United States meant that questions fundamental to an understanding of human reproduction remained largely uninvestigated by U.S. researchers; research into the efficacy and risks associated with infertility treatments such as IVF and GIFT also remained largely uninvestigated. For these reasons, the Commission recommends that

> **191. Research projects involving the use of human zygotes and carried out in licensed facilities be eligible for public funding.**

Commercialization

As we have emphasized throughout this report, it is inappropriate for decisions involving human reproduction to be motivated by the prospect of financial gain. Thus, the buying and selling of gametes and zygotes would be unacceptable, and we recommend their prohibition. This prohibition is essential, not only as a matter of respect for human dignity, but also to protect anyone who might be pressured or induced to sell gametes or zygotes. However, fees to recover the cost of related services, such as freezing, storage, testing, handling, and transport, may be acceptable. The Commission recommends that

> **192. The sale of human eggs, sperm, or zygotes be prohibited, under threat of criminal sanction.**

In addition to prohibiting the buying and selling of zygotes, we also wish to make it clear that human zygotes, embryos, and fetuses are inappropriate subject matter for intellectual property protection. Inherent in the moral point of view and respect for human life is abhorrence of any recognition of property interests of one human being in another; as entities that may have the potential for human life, zygotes should not be patentable.

Prohibiting the patenting of human zygotes or embryos does not necessarily preclude the patenting of innovative products derived from embryo research. For example, embryo research may lead to the discovery or development of cell lines with important diagnostic or therapeutic uses, and if patent protection were available, private companies might provide funds for this research that would not be available from public funding sources. Allowing patenting in this context raises important issues that require further consideration and study leading to policy decisions. We discuss these issues, and the principles that should underlie patent policy, in Chapter 24.

Accountability

Society has a right and a responsibility to ensure that embryo and zygote research is circumscribed by appropriate ethical boundaries. At present, however, there are no specific federal or provincial/territorial laws governing embryo research in Canada. Proposals for embryo research are reviewed by local ethics review boards, but these differ in composition, expertise, and approach, and their deliberations and decisions are not always made public. Moreover, if embryo research were to occur in the private sector, it might escape ethical review entirely.

Commissioners believe that the implications of embryo research are so profound that they warrant a shift from the current system of medical and scientific self-regulation toward a more active regulatory system in the context of policy making with greater public participation. The principle of accountability suggests that the public has a right to know what is going on in this area and to be assured that research complies with social and ethical as well as medical and scientific standards.

We believe that a more open and participatory system would not only promote more informed public debate, but would also provide the greatest protection against misuse. One essential ingredient of such a system is the availability of clear and accurate information — information that should be provided on a regular basis by a body without a particular vested interest. The debate about embryo research is not only about whether such research is acceptable in principle, but also about whether it can be regulated appropriately in practice. Many Canadians share the concern of the Working Party on Human Fertilisation and Embryology of the Church of England, which questioned whether "society possesses the maturity as well as the means for restricting research work within acceptable bounds."[28] We believe that society does have the wisdom and the will to establish and enforce these limits. We therefore need to put in place the means to do so — an open and participatory system of national regulation and monitoring to prevent abuse and to provide public

> The implications of embryo research are so profound that they warrant a shift from the current system of medical and scientific self-regulation toward a more active regulatory system in the context of policy making with greater public participation. The principle of accountability suggests that the public has a right to know what is going on in this area and to be assured that research complies with social and ethical as well as medical and scientific standards.

assurances that misuse or abuse is not occurring. The Commission therefore recommends that

> **193. All research using human zygotes be subject to compulsory licensing by the National Reproductive Technologies Commission.**

Such licensing would not replace institutional ethics committees in universities and hospitals. Rather, it would serve as an additional and nationally consistent check on the acceptability of research using human zygotes before its commencement. It would also ensure that private sector researchers are subject to the same oversight as those in the public or quasi-public sector. Licensing by the NRTC would also afford a greater degree of public accountability than professional self-regulation, reassuring Canadians that embryo research in this country is not violating widely held social values and norms.

Facilities that applied and met the NRTC's licensing conditions would receive a licence to conduct research using human zygotes for a period of five years. Once the clinic was licensed, it would then seek approval for individual projects from a local institutional ethics review board, which would use guidelines drawn up by the NRTC to assess such proposals. We do not consider it necessary to require researchers to obtain a separate licence for each research project.

We believe that this combination of national licensing of facilities and local approval of projects in the context of clear NRTC guidelines would provide the most appropriate blend of safeguards and flexibility for human embryo research in Canada. Since one of the conditions of licensing, discussed below, would be that the research facility provide an annual report to the NRTC on its research projects, it would be possible for the NRTC to ensure that local ethics review boards across the country are applying the basic principles and guidelines consistently in their assessments of individual projects. Publication of such information in the NRTC's annual report would allow for public education and feedback on the issues surrounding embryo research and its evolution in practice.

Commissioners believe, however, that the extra risks to women and children involved in any research that involves transfer of a zygote that has been subject to manipulation warrant an extra level of approval. The Commission therefore recommends that

> **194. Any research project involving the transfer of a zygote that has been subject to experimental manipulation receive approval from both a local research ethics board and the National Reproductive Technologies Commission.**

In summary, Commissioners conclude that the area of embryo research has far-reaching implications for all of society and therefore warrants a comprehensive response. We recommend that the federal government use its legislative powers to establish boundaries around this area of research and to set limits on what is acceptable and then, within those limits, to put in place regulation ensuring appropriate and accountable use. Both Commissioners and the Canadian public are concerned that measures be put in place that ensure any embryo research that is carried out is conducted in the best interests of women, children, and society. The details of the licensing regime we recommend in this regard are set out below.

Licensing Requirements for Research Using Human Zygotes

The Commission recommends that

195. Licensing requirements for zygote/embryo research apply to any physician, centre, or other individual or facility using human zygotes in research. Both experimental and "innovative" therapies for human zygotes should fall under the rubric of research. Any individual or institution engaged in such manipulation would therefore be subject to licensing.

196. Engaging in research using human zygotes without a licence issued by the National Reproductive Technologies Commission, or without complying with the National Commission's licensing requirements, as outlined below, constitutes an offence subject to prosecution.

and that

> **197. The National Reproductive Technologies Commission establish a permanent Embryo Research Sub-Committee,* with responsibility for developing standards and guidelines to be adopted as conditions of licence and for overseeing the implementation of the National Commission's licensing program.**

The Commission recommends that

> **198. The following requirements be adopted as conditions of licence for zygote/embryo research:**
>
> **(a)   All approved research must be restricted to the first 14 days of development of the human zygote.**
>
> **(b)   The use of surplus human zygotes for research purposes is permissible, provided the prior informed consent of the donors has been obtained. Consent to the use of surplus zygotes for research must not, however, operate as a condition of participation in an assisted conception program.**
>
> **(c)   The creation of human zygotes specifically for research purposes is permissible. The use of invasive procedures specifically to retrieve eggs for purposes of creating zygotes for research is, however, prohibited; only eggs retrieved during procedures already being performed can be used.**
>
> **(d)   Standard gamete donor information materials and consent forms should be developed by the Embryo Research Sub-Committee of the National Reproductive Technologies Commission.**

---

* This is termed the Embryo Research Sub-Committee, as this is how such research has been referred to in the public debate. As we have noted, the research is actually done at the zygote stage. However, the term Embryo Research Sub-Committee should be read to refer to both zygote and embryo research.

(e) Proper documentation showing the source of gametes, and signed donor consent forms, must accompany all gametes used to create zygotes for research. This documentation must be retained in the documentation relating to the research project and kept in a secure manner to protect confidentiality and the privacy of donors.

(f) Human zygotes that have been subject to manipulation of any kind for research purposes cannot be transferred to a woman's body without the specific approval of the National Reproductive Technologies Commission, and then only in the context of a clinical trial. Such approval should be contingent on the ability to demonstrate that the manipulations in question are likely to increase the woman's chances of conceiving or be of a therapeutic nature. The Embryo Research Sub-Committee would act in concert with the Assisted Conception and Prenatal Diagnosis Sub-Committees in reviewing any such application.

(g) All research on human zygotes must be undertaken only for purposes of promoting understanding and treatment of human health. No such research may be undertaken for commercial gain.

(h) The objectives of research on human zygotes should be achievable only through the use of human zygotes.

(i) Research involving genetic alteration of human zygotes is not permissible.

(j) Any research project involving the use of human zygotes undertaken by a licensed researcher or facility must be approved by a local institutional research ethics board. Guidelines for approving such research projects should be developed by the Embryo Research Sub-Committee. The onus would be on researchers to demonstrate that the proposed research complied with the guidelines.

(k)   Individuals or facilities engaging in human embryo research report to the National Reproductive Technologies Commission on their activities in a standard form annually, and that a summary of such projects be included in the National Commission's annual report. The data required annually should include, for example, a summary of each research protocol, documentation of research ethics board approval, the number of zygotes involved, the facility or source from which they were obtained, and funding source(s) for the research.

(l)   Individuals or facilities engaging in human embryo research be required to apply to the National Reproductive Technologies Commission for licence renewal every five years.

(m)   Human embryo research licences be revocable by the National Reproductive Technologies Commission at any time for breach of the conditions of licence.

The Role of the Embryo Research Sub-Committee

It is useful to reiterate the Embryo Research Sub-Committee's other functions, given its crucial role in ensuring adequate and accountable oversight of this increasingly important area of research. Given that the field will continue to evolve, as well as its implications for society, the Embryo Research Sub-Committee will have a crucial role in maintaining vigilance and promoting public dialogue about the directions such research should be allowed to take and how collective values and goals should be embodied in decisions about it.

The Embryo Research Sub-Committee would be established and chaired by the NRTC. It would be one of six permanent Sub-Committees, along with those dealing with infertility prevention; assisted conception services; assisted insemination services; prenatal diagnosis; and the provision of fetal tissue for research and other designated purposes. Like National Commission members themselves, we recommend that at least half the Sub-Committee members be women, and that all members be chosen with a view to ensuring that they have a background and demonstrated experience in dealing with a multidisciplinary approach to issues, as well as an ability to work together to find solutions and recommend policies to address the difficult issues raised by research on human zygotes in a way that meets the concerns of Canadian society as a whole.

As well as setting and revising the licensing requirements for human embryo research to be applied through the NRTC licence hearing process, the Sub-Committee would also

- develop standard information materials and standard requirements for donor consent forms to be used in all research projects;

- establish guidelines to be applied by institutional research ethics boards in reviewing and approving embryo research projects;

- analyze the data and information provided about projects and practices to help in the Sub-Committee's guideline- and standard-setting activities;

- discuss and develop policy on new issues and problems as they arise, monitor new research techniques, and ensure appropriate levels of regulation on an ongoing basis;

- work together with members of the Assisted Conception and Prenatal Diagnosis Sub-Committees in approving clinical trials involving the transfer of human zygotes that have been subject to manipulation; and

- promote public awareness and debate regarding human embryo research in Canada, through the publication of the NRTC's annual report, the circulation of draft discussion or policy papers for comment, or direct consultation with the public, as required.

In addition to enhancing public awareness and debate by providing more and better information about research using human zygotes currently under way in Canada, public accountability in this area would be promoted by the composition of the Embryo Research Sub-Committee. This should include both NRTC and outside membership, with a multidisciplinary make-up, including membership from the relevant medical and research communities as well as from groups familiar with the reproductive health concerns of women and other key segments of the public. Such broad representation will, we believe, enhance public confidence that any research undertaken on human zygotes in Canada reflects widely shared social concerns and values.

Conclusion

In summary, the Commission concludes that the use of human zygotes in research can be considered acceptable when that research is directed to promoting understanding of human health and disease and developing treatment. However, any use of human zygotes must be within the strict guidelines we have outlined — which include clear limits on the way zygotes or eggs are acquired (informed consent, no invasive procedures specifically to retrieve eggs for research) and handled, as well as limits on the purposes for which research is conducted. Moreover, there must be a national system of licensing for this research, to ensure its compliance with ethical, legal, and scientific standards. Certain kinds of research would be expressly prohibited, and research would be permissible only up to 14 days after fertilization.

A consistent theme throughout our report has been the ethical imperative of providing treatment only if risks and effectiveness are known or in the context of research to obtain this knowledge. We have determined that *in vitro* fertilization should be offered as treatment for women with fallopian tube blockage, and that IVF for other diagnoses be considered a research priority. Commissioners consider that offering this treatment without also allowing research aimed at improving its safety and effectiveness would be unethical. In other words, prohibiting research on human zygotes would create a situation where the health of women and their children was put at risk, because it would close off an avenue to knowledge that could contribute to the development and evaluation of safer, more effective ways of performing IVF. We therefore believe that research involving human zygotes not only is acceptable but is an important component of the ethical provision of IVF and related techniques of assisted conception. It is for these reasons that we have determined that such research should be permitted within the framework of licensing, ethical review, public accountability, and other safeguards we recommend.

Appendix 1: Current Public Policies on Embryo Research in Eight Countries

Great Britain

Embryo research in Britain is now governed by the *Human Fertilisation and Embryology Act*, which was introduced in 1989 and passed in 1990. Under the act, all embryo research must be approved by the new Human Fertilisation and Embryology Authority. This body has the authority to issue three types of licences, one of which is a research licence to permit the creation of zygotes and their use for approved research projects, as well as such use of surplus zygotes. These licences must be renewed each year. Research is permitted only up to 14 days after fertilization, and a zygote that has been the subject of research cannot be transferred to a woman's uterus. The informed consent of the zygote donors is required, and certain kinds of research are expressly prohibited, including trans-species fertilization.

This system of statutory licensing replaces the Voluntary Licensing Authority (VLA) (which changed its name in 1989 to the Interim Licensing Authority), an interim body established by the medical profession in the wake of the Warnock Committee's report (1984).

Australia

Because medical research falls under state jurisdiction in Australia, most public policy regarding embryo research exists at the state level. Three of the six Australian states have recently enacted legislation covering embryo research.

The state of Victoria passed the *Infertility (Medical Procedures) Act* in 1984. It permits research on surplus zygotes with the informed consent of the zygote donors if properly approved by a state licensing body, but it prohibits the creation of zygote for research purposes. Regulations under the act set limits on the permissible aims of research. Uncertainty about the definition of an embryo led to a legislative amendment in 1987, which specifies that a fertilized egg becomes an embryo only at the point of syngamy (that is, the actual coming together of chromosomes of sperm and egg), which occurs 22 to 24 hours after the sperm has penetrated the egg. This means that researchers can fertilize eggs solely for the purpose of research, if the research is performed before syngamy.

The other two states to pass legislation covering embryo research are Western Australia (*Human Reproductive Technology Act, 1991*) and South Australia (*Reproductive Technology Act, 1988*). Both effectively prohibit embryo research not intended to benefit the particular zygote that is the subject of the research.

The other three states do not yet have legislation. However, they did establish inquiries that covered embryo research. The New South Wales report endorsed embryo research for up to 14 days, as well as the creation of zygotes for research purposes; the Tasmania report rejected all embryo research; the Queensland report left the issue undecided. There is no indication that legislation is imminent in any of these states.

Given the wide range of state responses to this issue, there has been considerable pressure for the federal government to legislate in the area. Several federal reports have recommended that restrictions on embryo research be applied uniformly across the country through a system of national licensing of IVF and related research. However, no system for statutory national regulation has yet been implemented. In 1985, a private member's bill was introduced in the federal Senate to prohibit embryo research under the *Criminal Code*, but it did not receive legislative approval.

The only existing federal policy is the voluntary guidelines of the National Health and Medical Research Council (NHMRC), developed in

1982. According to these guidelines, embryo research is permissible for up to 14 days if approved by a local institutional ethics review board, and zygotes can be created solely for the purpose of such research. These guidelines are binding only on researchers who receive funding from the NHMRC. However, the NHMRC guidelines have been adopted by the medical profession itself. In the absence of a national system of statutory licensing, the Fertility Society of Australia set up its own system of voluntary licensing. Adherence to the NHMRC guidelines is required to receive a licence from the Reproductive Technology Accreditation Committee. However, this too is a voluntary system; there are no professional or legal sanctions against researchers who do not seek a licence.

United States

No federal regulation or legislation in the United States directly concerns embryo research, other than a de facto moratorium on the public funding of such research. Although several federal reports have endorsed the ethical permissibility of embryo research, and the legitimacy of its public funding, the institutional mechanisms required for processing funding requests do not exist. This may change under the new Clinton administration, which lifted a similar ban on public funding of fetal tissue transplantation research.

There is some regulation by both state governments and the medical profession. The Ethics Committee of the American Fertility Society recommended in 1990 that research on human zygotes, for up to 14 days, be considered ethically acceptable, with the consent of the donor and if reviewed by a properly constituted institutional review board. Creating zygotes for research purposes is also allowed, under certain circumstances. These guidelines are purely voluntary.

Several states have enacted legislation that deals with embryo research and research involving the use of fetal tissue. Most are concerned with research on aborted fetuses, and their relevance to research on zygotes *in vitro* is unclear. The state of Louisiana passed legislation specifically to prohibit the creation of zygotes for research purposes, but this was struck down as unconstitutional by a federal court, partly on the grounds that the legislation was too vague (for example, the term "experimental" was not defined).[29] Other states prohibit the donation of fetuses or zygotes for research.

Germany

In 1986, a draft law to regulate embryo research was introduced in the German legislature. In October 1990, after several years of debate, the *Embryo Protection Act* was passed; it came into force in January 1991. This act prohibits the creation of zygotes for research purposes and prohibits non-therapeutic experimentation on surplus zygotes. It also prohibits cloning, the creation of chimeras, and preimplantation diagnosis. Zygotes can be created *in vitro* only to bring about a pregnancy in the woman whose egg is used to create the zygote. Once created, zygotes can be frozen and used for future pregnancy attempts by the woman whose egg was used originally to create the zygote.

The act allows an exception to this ban on embryo research for zygotes that are dead or incapable of development. However, if the zygote displays "developability," then research is limited to non-invasive observation that does not affect the possibility of successful implantation. Although the act states that an embryo exists only from the point of syngamy, it extends protection to the fertilized egg before this point. It states that for the first 24 hours after penetration by the sperm, before syngamy, the egg shall be assumed to be capable of development and hence protected from experimentation.

France

The current system of voluntary licensing for reproductive technology centres, established by the French government in April 1988, does not specifically cover embryo experimentation. However, a non-binding moratorium was placed on preimplantation diagnosis by the National Advisory Committee on Ethics for the Life and Health Sciences in 1986 and was reaffirmed in 1990.

Two major government reports have recommended comprehensive legislation, including the regulation of embryo research. In its 1986 report, the Conseil d'État endorsed embryo research for up to 14 days, subject to a system of case-by-case authorization by a national ethics committee. The creation of zygotes for research purposes was deemed impermissible, as were certain forms of research such as ectogenesis, cloning, and parthenogenesis. A 1989 draft bill, known as the *loi Braibant* and based on the Conseil d'État report, was never passed.

Subsequently, the Task Force on Biomedical Ethics and Life Sciences released a report entitled *Aux frontières de la vie*. It recommends the initiation of a legislative debate on whether embryo research should be allowed. If the National Assembly accepts embryo research, the task force recommends that such research then be required to comply with the following conditions: (1) there should be no production of zygotes solely for research purposes; (2) there should be no transfer of a zygote that has been the object of experimentation; and (3) the consent of donors should be required. Similar proposals, though with a seven-day limit on embryo research, were made by the National Advisory Committee on Ethics for the Life and Health Sciences in 1989. In March 1992, the *Projet de Loi #2600*, which deals with the donation and use of human body parts, stipulated that zygotes be donated only for therapeutic reasons. However, further details about what is meant by this are not provided, and in fact this bill, as well as two others submitted to the National Assembly in March 1992, have been put on hold during the recent change of government in France. Another committee has been established to look at the issue, and its report is due by the end of 1993.

Spain

The Spanish Law 35, *Health: Assisted Reproduction Techniques*, was passed in November 1988. It was largely based on the Report of the Special Commission set up by the Spanish legislature to study IVF and assisted insemination. The Spanish law allows research on non-viable surplus zygotes for up to 14 days, and on viable zygotes provided it is "applied research of a diagnostic character or if it has a therapeutic or prophylactic purpose." It is left to scientists to determine non-viability, but generally this would be when the zygote fails to cleave or when there are more than two pronuclei. The creation of zygotes for research purposes is forbidden. Research involving cloning, parthenogenesis, or genetic manipulation is not allowed.

Sweden

The Swedish *In Vitro Fertilization Act*, introduced in January 1989, sets out the conditions under which embryo research may be undertaken. Research is permitted up to 14 days after the fertilization of the egg, but only if the research is related to the improvement of IVF techniques. Couples may consent to the use of unused zygotes for research. Research projects must be approved by an ethics committee.

Norway

The Norwegian Act No. 628, passed in 1987, prohibits embryo research. This law may be amended to allow for research up to seven days after fertilization. When the bill was originally drafted, the minister of health suggested the seven-day limit, but this was not accepted by the legislature. A legislative committee of inquiry is now looking at embryo research issues.

General Sources

Benjamin, M. *Splitting the Difference: Compromise and Integrity in Ethics and Politics.* Lawrence: University of Kansas Press, 1990.

Betteridge, K.J., and D. Rieger. "Embryo Transfer and Related Technologies in Domestic Animals: Their History, Current Status, and Future Direction, with Special Reference to Implications for Human Medicine." In Research Volumes of the Royal Commission on New Reproductive Technologies, 1993.

Boué, A. "Spontaneous Abortions and Cytogenetic Abnormalities." In *Progress in Infertility*, 3d ed., ed. S.J. Behrman, R.W. Kistner, and G.W. Patton. Boston: Little, Brown and Company, 1988.

Edwards, R.G. "The Galton Lecture, 1982: The Current Clinical and Ethical Situation of Human Conception In Vitro." In *Developments in Human Reproduction and Their Eugenic, Ethical Implications*, ed. C.O. Carter. Proceedings of the Nineteenth Annual Symposium of the Eugenics Society. London: Academic Press, 1983.

Handyside, A.H., et al. "Birth of a Normal Girl After In Vitro Fertilization and Preimplantation Diagnostic Testing for Cystic Fibrosis." *New England Journal of Medicine* 327 (September 24, 1992): 905-909.

Litman, M.M., and G.B. Robertson. "Reproductive Technology: Is a Property Law Regime Appropriate?" In Research Volumes of the Royal Commission on New Reproductive Technologies, 1993.

McLaren, A. "Human Embryo Research: Past, Present, and Future." In Research Volumes of the Royal Commission on New Reproductive Technologies, 1993.

Owen, K.D., and Z. Rosenwaks. "Current Status of *In Vitro* Fertilization and the New Reproductive Technologies." *Current Opinion in Obstetrics and Gynecology* 4 (June 1992): 354-58.

Singer, P., et al., eds. *Embryo Experimentation*. Cambridge: Cambridge University Press, 1990.

SPR Associates Inc. "Report on a Survey of Use and Handling of Human Reproductive Tissues in Canadian Health Care Facilities." In Research Volumes of the Royal Commission on New Reproductive Technologies, 1993.

SPR Associates Inc. "Report on a Follow-Up Survey of Use and Handling of Human Reproductive Tissues (Survey of Medical Laboratories and Medical Waste Disposal Firms)." In Research Volumes of the Royal Commission on New Reproductive Technologies, 1993.

Steptoe, P.C., and R.G. Edwards. "Birth After the Reimplantation of a Human Embryo." *Lancet* (August 12, 1978): 366.

Walters, W. "Personhood and the Human Embryo." In *Moral Priorities in Medical Research: The Second Hannah Conference*, ed. J.M. Nicholas. Toronto: The Hannah Institute of the History of Medicine, 1984.

Specific References

1. Whereas researchers in the 1970s might have been able to retrieve and fertilize one egg per cycle, doctors today can retrieve 5, 10, or more eggs per cycle and expect a 70 to 80 percent fertilization rate. As a result, many human zygotes exist for at least a brief period outside the human body (*ex utero*) in Canada. An *ex utero* zygote will die within a day or two if it is not transferred to a woman's body. Only a few embryos can be implanted without risks to the woman and to the children if they survive; this means that unless the remaining zygotes are frozen and stored they will not survive.

It is impossible to calculate the exact number of *ex utero* zygotes, in part because there are no precise data on the average number of eggs retrieved or the average fertilization rate. However, a variety of sources suggest that an average of six eggs is retrieved per cycle and about 70 to 80 percent of these eggs fertilize. This would mean that in Canada in 1991 approximately 13 500 zygotes were created through the retrieval and fertilization of eggs for 3 000 *in vitro* fertilization patients. Of these 13 500 zygotes, just over half were transferred with the aim of establishing a pregnancy. This leaves some 6 000 *ex utero* zygotes that were not transferred, though many of these would not have been viable, would not have shown normal cell division, or would have had anomalies that meant they could not have developed further. Some were also frozen.

2. Templeton, A.A., et al. "Oocyte Recovery and Fertilization Rates in Women at Various Times After the Administration of hCG." *Journal of Reproduction and Fertility* 76 (2)(1986): 771-78. It is important to note that the women involved in this study were also the subjects of research, since the ovulation induction was not done for their personal direct benefit.

3. Messinis, I.E., and A. Templeton. "The Effect of the Antiprogestin Mifepristone (RU 486) on Maturation and In-Vitro Fertilization of Human Oocytes." *British Journal of Obstetrics and Gynaecology* 95 (6)(June 1988): 592-95.

4. Council of Europe. Select Committee of Experts on the Use of Human Embryos and Foetuses. *Report on the Use of Human Foetal, Embryonic and Pre-Embryonic Material for Diagnostic, Therapeutic, Scientific, Industrial and Commercial Purposes.* Strasbourg: Council of Europe, 1990, para. 74-75.

5. Ibid., para. 107.

6. Legislation on embryo research has been considered in Quebec. In 1989, following the report of its Working Committee on New Technologies in Human Reproduction, the Quebec Department of Health and Social Services proposed a supervisory framework for embryo research that would require official approval for current projects and prohibit trade in embryos or the creation of human embryos solely for the purpose of research. Legislation was being considered by the Quebec Justice Department, but as of September 1992 no such legislation had been presented.

7. Most recently, *Davis v. Davis* (1989) WL 14 0495 (Tenn. Circ), also *Davis v. Davis* 15 Fam L. Rep. (BNA) No. 46, at 2097 (Blount Country Cir. Ct. Tenn., Sept. 26, 1989).

8. Law Reform Commission of Canada. *Medically Assisted Procreation.* Working Paper 65. Ottawa: Minister of Supply and Services Canada, 1992, p. 141.

9. Medical Research Council of Canada. *Guidelines on Research Involving Human Subjects.* Ottawa: MRC, 1987.

10. For a discussion of the role of the NCBHR, see Dossetor, J.B., and J.L. Storch. "Roles for Ethics Committees in Relation to Guidelines for New Reproductive Technologies: A Research Position Paper." In Research Volumes of the Royal Commission on New Reproductive Technologies, 1993.

11. The reports of the Law Reform Commission of Canada (*Biomedical Experimentation Involving Human Subjects,* 1989), the Working Committee of the Quebec Department of Health and Social Services (*Rapport du comité du travail sur les nouvelles technologies de reproduction,* 1988), the Bar of Quebec (*Rapport du comité sur les nouvelles technologies de reproduction,* 1988), the Ontario Law Reform Commission (*Report on Human Artificial Reproduction and Related Matters,* 1985), and the Canadian Bar Association, British Columbia Branch (*Reproductive Technologies,* 1989), generally support the substance of the MRC guidelines (that is, the 14-day limit, the need for donor consent and for local research ethics board approval, the unacceptability of transferring zygotes that have been experimented on, and the limitations on certain forms of research — for example, cloning). However, they all recommend more systematic regulation and monitoring of embryo research, to ensure that these guidelines are being respected and applied consistently.

12. Canadian Fertility and Andrology Society and the Society of Obstetricians and Gynaecologists of Canada. Combined Ethics Committee. *Ethical Considerations of the New Reproductive Technologies.* Toronto: Ribosome Communications, 1990, pp. 43-45.

13. Warnock, M. *A Question of Life: The Warnock Report on Human Fertilisation and Embryology.* Oxford: Basil Blackwell, 1985, p. xvi.

14. Baylis, F.E. "The Ethics of Ex-Utero Research on Spare 'IVF' Embryos." Ph.D. dissertation, University of Western Ontario, London, 1989, p. 69.

15. See Australia. Tasmanian Government. *Report of the Committee to Investigate Artificial Conception and Related Matters.* Tasmania: Government Printing Office, 1985.

16. United Kingdom. Committee to Review the Guidance on the Research Uses of Fetuses and Fetal Material. *Report* (The Polkinghorne Report). London: HMSO, 1989.

17. Australia. Senate Select Committee on the Human Embryo Experimentation Bill 1985. *Human Embryo Experimentation in Australia.* Canberra: Australian Government Publishing Service, 1986, para 3.7.

18. Royal College of Obstetricians and Gynaecologists. *Report of the RCOG Ethics Committee on In Vitro Fertilisation and Embryo Replacement or Transfer.* London: RCOG, 1983.

19. Buckle, S. "Arguing from Potential." In *Embryo Experimentation,* ed. P. Singer et al. Cambridge: Cambridge University Press, 1990, p. 95.

20. Canadian Bar Association, British Columbia Branch. *Report of the Special Task Force Committee on Reproductive Technology of the British Columbia Branch, The Canadian Bar Association.* Victoria: The Association, 1989.

21. MRC, *Guidelines on Research Involving Human Subjects.*

22. Law Reform Commission of Canada. *Biomedical Experimentation Involving Human Subjects.* Working Paper 61. Ottawa: Minister of Supply and Services Canada, 1989.

23. Australia, *Human Embryo Experimentation in Australia,* para. 3.31.

24. Gaze, B., and K. Dawson. "Who Is the Subject of the Research?" In *Embryo Experimentation,* ed. P. Singer et al. Cambridge: Cambridge University Press, 1990.

25. MRC, *Guidelines on Research Involving Human Subjects,* p. 34.

26. For accounts of the aims of recent embryo research, and why embryo research is necessary to achieve those aims, see Interim Licensing Authority. *IVF Research in the UK: A Report on Research Licensed by the ILA,* 1989; and Trounson, A. "Why Do Research on Human Pre-Embryos?" In *Embryo Experimentation,* ed. P. Singer et al. Cambridge: Cambridge University Press, 1990.

27. MRC, *Guidelines on Research Involving Human Subjects.*

28. *Personal Origins: The Report of a Working Party on Human Fertilisation and Embryology of the Board for Social Responsibility.* London: CIO Publishing, 1985, p. 137. Similarly, the Family Law Council of Australia suggests that once we allow the creation of embryos for research, we will start down a slippery slope, and that "no end can be set on the dangers" (Australia. *Creating Children: A Uniform Approach to the Law and Practice of Reproductive Technology in Australia.* Canberra: Australian Government Publishing Service, 1985, p. 84).

29. *Margaret S. v. Edwards* 794 F.2d 994 (5th Cir., 1986).